CARDIOVASCULAR ANESTHESIA AND POSTOPERATIVE CARE

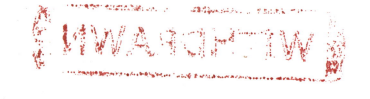

Cardiovascular Anesthesia and Postoperative Care

Edited by

SAIT TARHAN, M.D.
Professor of Anesthesiology
Mayo Medical School
Consultant in Anesthesiology
Mayo Clinic and Mayo Foundation
Rochester, Minnesota

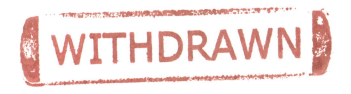

YEAR BOOK MEDICAL PUBLISHERS, INC.
CHICAGO • LONDON

Copyright © 1982 by Mayo Foundation. All rights reserved. No part of this publication may be reproduced, stored in a retrieval system, or transmitted, in any form or by any means, electronic, mechanical, photocopying, recording, or otherwise, without prior written permission from the publisher. Printed in the United States of America.

Reprinted, April 1983
Reprinted, July 1984

Library of Congress Cataloging in Publication Data
Main entry under title:

Cardiovascular anesthesia and postoperative care.

    Includes index.
    1. Anesthesia—Complications and sequelae.
2. Cardiovascular system—Surgery—Complications and sequelae. 3. Postoperative care. I. Tarhan, Sait. [DNLM: 1. Anesthesia. 2. Postoperative care. 3. Cardiovascular system—Surgery. WG 460 T185c]
RD87.3.C37C37   617'.9674101   81-11695
ISBN 0-8151-8702-5   AACR2

This book is dedicated to a friend, DWIGHT C. MCGOON
by
THE CONTRIBUTORS

Contributors

FROUKJE M. BEYNEN, M.D.
Assistant Professor of Anesthesiology
Mayo Medical School
Consultant in Anesthesiology
Mayo Clinic and Mayo Foundation
Rochester, Minnesota

ROY F. CUCCHIARA, M.D.
Associate Professor of Anesthesiology
Mayo Medical School
Consultant in Anesthesiology
Mayo Clinic and Mayo Foundation
Rochester, Minnesota

RONALD J. FAUST, M.D.
Assistant Professor of Anesthesiology
Mayo Medical School
Consultant in Anesthesiology
Mayo Clinic and Mayo Foundation
Rochester, Minnesota

GLENN A. FROMME, M.D.
Instructor in Anesthesiology
Mayo Medical School
Consultant in Anesthesiology
Mayo Clinic and Mayo Foundation
Rochester, Minnesota

ANDREW J. KULESZA, M.D.
Associate Professor of Anesthesiology
Department of Anesthesiology
State University of New York
Upstate Medical Center
Syracuse, New York
(Former Resident in Anesthesiology, Mayo Medical School)

PAUL F. LEONARD, M.D.
Associate Professor of Anesthesiology
Mayo Medical School
Consultant in Anesthesiology
Mayo Clinic and Mayo Foundation
Rochester, Minnesota

H. MICHAEL MARSH, M.B., B.S.
Associate Professor of Anesthesiology
Mayo Medical School
Consultant in Anesthesiology and Respiratory
    Intensive Care
Mayo Clinic and Mayo Foundation
Rochester, Minnesota

JOSEPH M. MESSICK, Jr., M.D.
Associate Professor of Anesthesiology
Mayo Medical School
Consultant in Anesthesiology
Mayo Clinic and Mayo Foundation
Rochester, Minnesota

W. EUGENE MILLER, M.D.
Associate Professor of Radiology
Mayo Medical School
Consultant in Diagnostic Radiology
Mayo Clinic and Mayo Foundation
Rochester, Minnesota

CARL R. NOBACK, M.D.
Assistant Professor of Anesthesiology
Emory University School of Medicine
Department of Anesthesiology
Emory University Clinic
Atlanta, Georgia.
(Former Instructor in Anesthesiology, Mayo Medical School)

HUGO S. RAIMUNDO, M.D.
Assistant Professor of Anesthesiology
Mayo Medical School
Consultant in Anesthesiology
Mayo Clinic and Mayo Foundation
Rochester, Minnesota

DUANE K. RORIE, M.D.
Associate Professor of Anatomy and
    Anesthesiology
Mayo Medical School
Consultant in Anesthesiology
Mayo Clinic and Mayo Foundation
Rochester, Minnesota

JOHN CHRISTOPHER SILL, M.B., B.S.
Assistant Professor of Anesthesiology
Mayo Medical School
Consultant in Anesthesiology
Mayo Clinic and Mayo Foundation
Rochester, Minnesota

PETER A. SOUTHORN, M.B., B.S.
Assistant Professor of Anesthesiology
Mayo Medical School
Consultant in Anesthesiology and Respiratory
    Intensive Care
Mayo Clinic and Mayo Foundation
Rochester, Minnesota

ANTHONY W. STANSON, M.D.
Assistant Professor of Radiology
Mayo Medical School
Consultant in Diagnostic Radiology
Mayo Clinic and Mayo Foundation
Rochester, Minnesota

SAIT TARHAN, M.D.
Professor of Anesthesiology
Mayo Medical School
Consultant in Anesthesiology
Mayo Clinic and Mayo Foundation
Rochester, Minnesota

ROGER D. WHITE, M.D.
Associate Professor of Anesthesiology
Mayo Medical School
Consultant in Anesthesiology
Mayo Clinic and Mayo Foundation
Rochester, Minnesota

DAVID M. WILSON, M.D.
Associate Professor of Medicine
Mayo Medical School
Consultant in Internal Medicine
Division of Nephrology
Mayo Clinic and Mayo Foundation
Rochester, Minnesota

Contents

Foreword	xv
Preface	xvii

1 / Preoperative Assessment of the Patient. *Sait Tarhan, Joseph M. Messick, Jr., and Ronald J. Faust* 1
    Preoperative Evaluation 1
    Pulmonary Dysfunction 3
    Hypertension 4
    Electrolyte Disturbances 5
    Drugs Taken Before Surgery 10
    Bleeding Disorders 11
    Cardiovascular Surgery and Hematologic Disorders 13
    Diabetes 13
    Cigarette Smoking 15
    Reoperations 15

2 / Radiology. *Anthony W. Stanson and W. Eugene Miller* 19
    The Preoperative Chest Roentgenogram 19
    Angiography 25

3 / Preoperative Medication. *Sait Tarhan and Froukje M. Beynen* . . . 35
    Premedicant Drugs 35
    Premedication of Patients with Coronary Artery Disease . . . 39
    Premedication of Children 39

4 / Anesthetic Agents and Anesthesia for Cardiac Surgery.
    Carl R. Noback and Hugo S. Raimundo 41
    Cardiovascular Effects of Anesthetic Drugs and Neuromuscular
        Blocking Agents 41
    Induction of Anesthesia 48

5 / Monitoring During Cardiovascular Surgery. *Duane K. Rorie* 55
    Arterial Pressure 55
    Electrocardiogram 59
    Central Venous Pressure 59
    Left Atrial Pressure 66

    Cardiac Output 68
    Temperature 70
    Arterial Blood Gases, pH, and Serum Potassium 71
    Urinary Output 71

6 / Anesthesia for Surgical Repair of Congenital Heart Defects
    in Children. *Froukje M. Beynen and Sait Tarhan* 73
    Classification of Congenital Heart Defects 73
    Preoperative Evaluation and Premedication 74
    Induction of Anesthesia 78
    Anesthesia for Closed-Heart Surgery 85
    Anesthesia for Open-Heart Surgery 104

7 / Valvular Heart Disease, Cardiovascular Performance,
    and Anesthesia. *John Christopher Sill and*
    Roger D. White 181
    Valve Replacement 181
    Determinants of Cardiac Performance 183
    Circulatory Compensation for Valvular Lesions 190
    Mitral Valve Disease 191
    Aortic Valve Disease 200
    Tricuspid Valve Disease 209
    Anesthesia 210

8 / Coronary Circulation and Anesthesia for Coronary
    Artery Bypass Graft Surgery. *Sait Tarhan and*
    Hugo S. Raimundo 227
    Coronary Circulation 227
    Anesthesia for Coronary Artery Bypass Graft Surgery 231

9 / Oxygenators and Hemodilution in Cardiopulmonary Bypass.
    Andrew J. Kulesza and Roger D. White 245
    Oxygenators 245
    Comparisons Among Oxygenators 247
    Complications 250
    Hemodilution 250

10 / Anesthesia for Closed Cardiac Operations in Adults.
    Hugo S. Raimundo and Sait Tarhan 257
    Closed Mitral Commissurotomy 257
    Pericarditis 259
    Adult Coarctation 260
    Reoperation in the Early Postoperative Period ("Reopening") 261

Contents

11 / **Anesthesia for Abdominal Aortic Aneurysm.**
    Sait Tarhan and Hugo S. Raimundo 265
    Preoperative Assessment 265
    Preoperative Preparation 266
    Anesthesia 267
    Cross-Clamping of Aorta 267
    Symptomatic and Ruptured Abdominal Aneurysm 268
    Surgical Control of the Bleeding Aorta 269
    Blood Transfusions 270
    Cardiac Arrest 270
    Acute Aortovenous Fistula Due to Rupture of
        Abdominal Aortic Aneurysm 270
    Postoperative Care 272

12 / **Anesthesia for Thoracic Aneurysm.** *Sait Tarhan and*
    Hugo S. Raimundo 275
    Pathogenesis of Thoracic Aneurysms 275
    Surgical Classification of Dissecting Aneurysm 275
    Clinical Features 276
    Prognosis 276
    Anesthesia for Ascending Aortic Aneurysms 277
    Resection and Prosthetic Replacement of Aneurysms
        of the Aortic Arch 277
    Dissecting Aneurysms 280
    Traumatic Ruptured Thoracic Aorta 285

13 / **Anesthesia for Carotid Artery Surgery.** *Roy F. Cucchiara*
    and Joseph M. Messick, Jr. 289
    Surgical Considerations 290
    Anesthetic Considerations 291
    "Critical" Human Cerebral Blood Flow 296
    Anesthetic Technique 297
    Recommendations 299

14 / **Myocardial Preservation.** *Glenn A. Fromme and*
    Roger D. White 303
    Myocardial Changes Occurring With Ischemia 303
    Interventions Affecting Myocardial Preservation 304
    Efforts at Protecting the Heart During Cardiac Surgery . . . 306
    Infusion of Cardioplegic Solution (Technical Aspects) 311

15 / **Protection of the Brain from Ischemic and Embolic**
    Phenomena. *Roy F. Cucchiara, Carl R. Noback,*
    and Ronald J. Faust 315

  Cerebral Ischemia 315
  Neurologic Sequelae of Cardiopulmonary Bypass 317
  Embolic Phenomena During Cardiopulmonary Bypass 317

16 / Renal Function and Cardiovascular Anesthesia.
  Joseph M. Messick, Jr., David M. Wilson,
  and Roy F. Cucchiara 325
  Renal Function 325
  Renin-Angiotensin-Aldosterone System 327
  Antidiuretic Hormone 328
  Diuretics 329
  Acute Renal Failure 330
  Renal Dysfunction Associated with Cardiac Surgery 335
  Free-Water Clearance 336

17 / Mechanisms, Diagnosis, and Treatment of Cardiac Arrhythmias.
  Roger D. White 341
  Normal Mechanisms of Impulse Formation and Conduction 341
  Abnormal Mechanisms 342
  Diagnosis and Treatment 346

18 / Support of the Circulation During and After Cardiac
  Operation. *Glenn A. Fromme and Roger D. White* 357
  Terminology 357
  Primary Determinants of Cardiac Performance 358
  Physiologic Changes With Decrease in Cardiac Output 359
  Intraoperative Hypotension 360
  Agents Used to Treat Intraoperative Hypotension 361
  Emergence From Bypass 364
  Inotropic Support During Emergence From Bypass 365
  Mechanical Support: Intra-aortic Balloon Pump 368
  Postoperative Low Cardiac Output 368
  Conclusions 373

19 / Intra-aortic Balloon Counterpulsation. *Sait Tarhan and*
  Ronald J. Faust 377
  Cardiogenic Shock 377
  Postcardiotomy Cardiogenic Shock 379
  Technique and Equipment 380
  Balloon Management 382
  Complications of Intra-aortic Balloon Counterpulsation 385

20 / Blood and Cardiovascular Anesthesia. *Ronald J. Faust,*
  Roy F. Cucchiara, and Joseph M. Messick, Jr. 387
    Hematology of the Red Blood Cell 387
    Immunohematology 387
    Hemolytic Transfusion Reactions 391
    Other Types of Transfusion Reactions 396
    Autologous Transfusion 398
    Blood Components 398
    Hemostasis and Coagulation 404
    Controlling the Coagulation System 406

21 / Cardiac Pacemakers and Anesthesia. *Paul F. Leonard* 413
    Indications for Electronic Pacing 413
    Unipolar Versus Bipolar Leads 413
    Pacemaker Placement and Reliability 414
    Types of Pacemakers 414
    Electromagnetic Interference 417
    Anesthesia for the Pacemaker Patient 418

22 / Anesthesia for Cardiovascular Diagnostic Procedures.
    Carl R. Noback, Hugo S. Raimundo, and Sait Tarhan 421
    The Steady State and the Role of the Anesthetist 421
    Anesthesia for Cardiac Catheterization 422
    Anesthesia for Angiocardiography 429
    Anesthesia for Arteriography 430
    Anesthesia for Related Procedures 431
    Conclusion 431

23 / Postoperative Management of the Cardiac Surgical
    Patient: General Introduction. *H. Michael Marsh*
    and Peter A. Southorn 435
    Postoperative Cardiac Care Unit 435
    Staffing 436
    Transfer From Operating Room to Postoperative
      Cardiac Unit 436
    Initial Assessment 437

24 / Postoperative Management of the Cardiac Surgical
    Patient: Respiratory Care. *H. Michael Marsh*
    and Peter A. Southorn 439
    Pathophysiology of Problems Encountered 439
    Conduct of Prolonged Mechanical Ventilation in
      the Adult 458
    Conduct of Prolonged Mechanical Ventilation in
      Infants 464

25 / Postoperative Management of the Cardiac Surgical
    Patient: Cardiovascular Care. *Peter A. Southorn
    and H. Michael Marsh* 475
    General Principles 475
    Monitoring 478
    Low Cardiac Output—Pathophysiology 480
    Systemic Hypertension 488
    Arrhythmias 489
    Special Considerations in Care of Infants and
        Small Children 490

Index 499

Foreword

It is an immense privilege for me, as a surgeon, to make these few introductory comments to this impressive text prepared by my respected colleagues in anesthesiology. There are few partnerships so intensely interdependent, so intimately intertwined, and so personally poignant as that which exists between a cardiovascular anesthesiologist and a cardiac surgeon. Especially is this true if these professionals have been blessed by a long and respectful relationship. As they wrestle with the mutually relevant case-by-case decisions that attend the daily drama of the operating room, instinctive interactions and intercommunications develop almost as though through a single brain. Such is one of the greatest rewards of their distinctive careers, and perhaps one of the greatest benefits they could confer on their patients.

Similar also is the relationship between the disciplines themselves—cardiac anesthesiology and cardiac surgery. This may undoubtedly be true of other branches of surgery, too, but a subtle difference seems to exist. The elegantly manipulable variables of the cardiovascular system, and the sense of immediacy fostered by the moment-by-moment dependence of the patient's life and health on the proper control of the circulation, all serve to excite and illuminate the interdependence of these disciplines.

Immense progress has been made during the past few decades in the management of the cardiac surgical patient. Many texts have dealt with the surgical arm of this subject, but a place remains for a thoroughly comprehensive compilation of the theory and the techniques of cardiovascular anesthesiology. What is particularly advantageous in such an endeavor is the ideal blending of that which is theoretical and that which through experience has proved to be practical.

Aristotle struggled 24 centuries ago with the proper blending of experience and theory with respect to teaching (Book I of *Metaphysics*). He said, "With a view to action, experience seems in no respect inferior to [theory], and men of experience succeed even better than those who have theory without experience . . . [yet men with theory] can teach, and men of mere experience cannot."

This book on cardiovascular anesthesiology exposes the incompleteness of Aristotle's apparent assumption that theory and experience are isolated qualities, interdependent but not cohabitable in the same person. Each of the contributors to this text is involved in the busy day-by-day application to clinical practice of the theory and art that his or her writings encompass. The various chapters comprehensively organize the many facets of knowledge and experience pertaining to the field of cardiac anesthesiology. The authors of these chapters, each having a special area of expertise, are orchestrated into a single team of specialists from one institution whose concepts and methods are constantly being stressed by the demands of clinical practice. This comprehensiveness and cohesiveness give mastery to the book.

The first 40 or more years of cardiac surgery and the first 25 years of "open-heart" operations are mileposts that have already fallen behind. We have thus witnessed a rapid stage of evolutionary progress in cardiovascular anesthesiology, which suggests that this is the perfect time to step back and to observe what has happened, what is known, and what is practiced. The authority whereby this book speaks so effectively involves the contributions made by its authors to what has happened and what is known, and, most importantly, to the application of this knowledge to a large ongoing single clinical practice. This very comprehensiveness and unification should also serve to expose any possible gaps in knowledge and any potential defects in techniques, thus revealing new challenges that must be addressed—new triumphs to be gained.

DWIGHT C. MCGOON

Preface

THIS BOOK represents a cooperative effort to provide clinicians with a detailed perspective on anesthesia for cardiovascular surgery. The chapters are deliberately designed to be read separately, and since they were prepared by several authors, some reiteration was inevitable. The writing style of each author was not altered, which hopefully will make reading more interesting.

One of the major problems was what to include and what to omit in a book of this type. It is our belief that a clear understanding of the pathophysiologic derangements produced by the various types of heart disease and a familiarity with the physiologic changes accompanying anesthesia and surgery undoubtedly are the most important factors for optimal anesthetic management. Therefore, an attempt was made to include pathologic and pathophysiologic alterations, as well as surgical procedures used. We concentrated our efforts on providing comprehensive knowledge on subjects that are not readily available in a composite published form. The chapters on radiology, anesthesia for closed cardiac operations, diagnostic procedures, abdominal and thoracic aortic aneurysms, carotid artery surgery, myocardial preservation, renal function, and blood in cardiovascular anesthesia are examples of such topics.

Surgery for congenital heart disease has experienced great progress during the last ten years, and it stands as a subspecialty among general cardiac surgery. Providing anesthesia for these patients also presents a challenge to the anesthesiologist. Therefore, a special emphasis was placed on this subspecialty.

Last but not least, postoperative care of the cardiovascular surgical patient remains one of the most important aspects of the entire surgical undertaking. Proper care can make the difference in the outcome of the patient. Without a section on that subject, a book of this type would be incomplete.

The methods discussed reflect the current practice in our institution. They have worked well for us in a large-volume practice, and no other claim is attached to them. They are by no means beyond challenge. Up-to-date options from other institutions also are discussed whenever appropriate.

We are greatly indebted to many colleagues from different disciplines at our institution who read and had constructive comments on many of the manuscripts. We also express our thanks to Dr. Marc Shampo, Virginia Dunt, Betty Calkins, and Mary Schwager of the Section of Publications, to Floyd Hosmer of the Section of Medical Graphics, and to members of the Section of Photography. Also our appreciation goes to our secretaries Ann Tvedt, Donna Huntley, and Jeanne Halbach for the countless hours that they spent in preparing the manuscripts.

A promise was made to complete this project in a few months, yet it has taken almost two years. We appreciate the forebearance and continuous support of our publishers.

The greatest reward for the contributors and editor alike will be if a reader finds this book understandable and informative.

SAIT TARHAN

1 / Preoperative Assessment of the Patient

SAIT TARHAN
JOSEPH M. MESSICK, JR.
RONALD J. FAUST

OPEN-HEART surgery has entered the third decade of its existence. New techniques and knowledge of pathophysiology of the heart have made possible the surgical correction of numerous cardiac problems.

PREOPERATIVE EVALUATION

Preanesthetic evaluation of the patient provides a guide for anesthetic management, supportive techniques, and postoperative care. Regardless of age and physical condition, a patient who is a candidate for cardiac surgery (or major vascular surgery) should be evaluated carefully because the organ that is primarily responsible for maintaining satisfactory hemodynamics is the one that will be most affected by the surgery.

History

Factors such as age, sex, cigarette smoking, high blood pressure, high cholesterol level, diabetes, arrhythmias, and ischemic heart disease may adversely affect the outcome of the surgery. Pulmonary function also should be checked preoperatively. Pulmonary status usually can be evaluated by means of clinical signs, roentgenograms of the chest, and data on blood gases. Ventilatory function may be impaired by pulmonary edema, chronic bronchitis, and emphysema. The status of the pulmonary vascular tree is important. The cardiac disease process may have produced changes leading to pulmonary hypertension.

The clinical manifestations of heart failure differ substantially in adults and children. Heart disease in children usually is due to congenital causes, so the mechanism of adaptation is deployed gradually in a heart with a healthy myocardium, while an adult myocardium is less able to adapt itself to the burdens of ongoing disease. However, the terminal phase in both types of heart failure is similar.

Breathlessness is the most common symptom of heart failure, yet the fact that it is not a reliable indicator of the extent of the failure is rarely stressed.

Although consideration of symptoms is essential for a correct diagnosis, classification of these patients on the basis of symptoms alone may be misleading. Symptoms may be absent despite serious anatomical or physiologic abnormalities, and an evaluation based on symptoms alone might not indicate the need for medical or surgical intervention.[11] For example, an interatrial septal defect that is producing no symptoms may cause physiologic abnormalities sufficient to warrant surgical treatment. Further, symptoms may appear only after the heart and lungs have undergone significant changes, which can prevent effective treatment of the underlying defect.[11]

Besides being concerned with the degree of physical activity that may be undertaken, one also is concerned that the patient receive optimal therapy. Generally, some therapies may alter the symptoms and the course of the disease only briefly, while others may change the course fundamentally. The lack of usefulness of previous classifications has been admitted by the Criteria Committee of the New York Heart Association,[11] and a new, refined classification has been published (Table 1–1). It is based on (1) cardiac status (reflecting etiologic, anatomical, and physiologic diagnosis) and (2) prognosis (assessment of the potential effects of optimal current medical and surgical therapies).

TABLE 1–1.—Major Changes Made by Criteria Committee of New York Heart Association*

CARDIAC STATUS	PROGNOSIS
Uncompromised	Good
Slightly compromised	Good with therapy
Moderately compromised	Fair with therapy
Severely compromised	Guarded despite therapy

*From Criteria Committee of the New York Heart Association.[11] Used by permission.

Physical Examination

The clinical value of the physical examination of the patient with a failing heart varies with the extent of the failure. In early left ventricular failure, only physical exercise may reveal the problem. In this instance, examining the patient at rest would not indicate the degree of physiologic cardiac impairment actually present. For example, in a patient with acute severe left ventricular failure due to myocardial infarction, the only abnormal physical sign may be a left ventricular diastolic gallop rhythm.[53] Some patients with this type of failure may also have pulmonary edema. When heart failure develops more slowly, however, secondary mechanisms may increase the blood volume, which in turn may produce such classic signs as pulmonary fine rales, hydrothorax, increased jugular venous pressure, distention of the liver, peripheral edema, and ascites. In left ventricular failure, clinical signs vary more with the rate of development of the failure than with its severity[30] and are of little use as a measure of its severity, and their absence is of no predictive value.

Radiologic Findings

Radiographically, the size and shape of the heart may vary with the type of heart disease. Lung changes are common in all forms of left heart failure. Signs of pulmonary venous hypertension are reflected in opacification of the veins in the upper lobes and often as peripheral horizontal linear opacities in the basal segments (Kerley B lines).[37]

Data From Cardiac Laboratory

Another method used to evaluate cardiac function in human subjects is cardiac catheterization. By knowing cardiac output and ventricular filling pressure, one can derive a reliable index of cardiac function. An increase in filling pressure, while output is maintained, often is the initial change in heart failure.[61] Measurements of changes in cardiac output alone without knowledge of ventricular filling pressure cannot be reliably interpreted in terms of cardiac function. In general, since ventricular filling pressure reflects end-diastolic volume,[61] measurement of left ventricular filling pressure alone is probably the most sensitive and readily available single method of detecting early left ventricular failure. The clinical applicability of this method is considerably enhanced by the close agreement among left ventricular diastolic, left atrial, and pulmonary wedge pressures.[61] A cardiac catheter has been designed that can be inserted percutaneously and easily positioned without fluoroscopy. With this balloon-tipped, flow-directed catheter, one can measure the pulmonary capillary wedge pressure, a reliable indirect assessment of left ventricular filling pressure.[39, 61, 66]

Caution must be exercised in the clinical application of pulmonary capillary wedge pressure measurements. Such measurements are most sensitive in early left ventricular failure. In chronic advanced heart failure, however, significant further increases in pressure are difficult to interpret. In this situation, other measures, such as radiographic heart size, are probably more quantitative.[61]

At the present time, there is no simple way to measure the discrete properties of mechanical behavior of the myocardium in intact man. Suggested noninvasive methods include the following: systolic time intervals derived from simultaneous records of ECG, phonocardiogram, and carotid pulse; echocardiography; apex cardiography; and impedance cardiography. In the hands of skilled investigators, each of these methods has been shown to give an estimate of a particular physiologic variable of left ventricular function, yet they are limited in their wider clinical applications.[61]

Correct interpretation of the data from the cardiac laboratory has a significant impact on the time and type of the operation and on the patient's prognosis.

Aortic Valve Disease

An important but unresolved problem in the management of patients with chronic aortic valvular disease is the determination of the proper timing of operative intervention.[31] If a patient is incapacitated by his cardiac disease, the decision is easy. Laboratory data can help in deciding the timing in borderline cases. Long-term survival is inversely correlated with the level of left ventricular end-diastolic pressure in patients with aortic regurgitation. The survival rate also is lower for patients with elevated pulmonary artery pressure and left atrial pressure and for patients with greatly elevated left ventricular pressure.[31]

Mitral Valve Disease

When surgery is considered in patients with pure or predominant mitral stenosis, information should be obtained regarding the presence and severity of valvular calcification. Valve mobility increases in the pure commissural type of mitral stenosis, which has little involvement of cusps compared with the mobility in stenosis associated with fibrocalcific disease of the valve cusps. This factor may make the difference in the surgeon's decision between valve replacement and valvotomy. Recent reports indicate that echocardiographic evidence of absence of calcification in the mitral valve is the most reliable indication for mitral commissurotomy, while heavy valve calcification or poor cusp mobility requires valve replacement.[44] Surgical treatment of mitral valve disease reportedly leads to a higher survival rate than medical treatment. Improvement is particularly significant among patients with mixed stenosis and regurgitation and moderate impairment of ejection fraction.[28]

Coronary Artery Disease

Coronary cineangiograms from the catheterization laboratory are important in the surgeon's preoperative evaluation of a patient with ischemic heart disease. Correct interpretation of the cineangiogram determines how many bypass grafts should be performed and where the distal anastomosis will be placed. The prognosis is different for single-, double-, or triple-vessel disease; the original report by Favaloro[21] on this subject showed that surgical treatment was followed by definite improvement in patients with double- and triple-vessel disease. This report has been confirmed by many cardiovascular centers. Some critics challenge the indications for surgery in patients with single-vessel obstructive disease. Nevertheless, it has been recommended that patients with proximal obstruction of a large left anterior descending coronary artery or with a single obstruction of a right coronary artery should undergo operation.[21] There have been reports that the perioperative myocardial infarction rate is extremely high among patients with left main coronary artery disease, and many investigators recommend that these patients also undergo operation.[38]

Other data predictive of surgical mortality among patients with coronary artery disease are end-diastolic volume, ejection fraction, and left ventricular end-diastolic pressure. Those patients whose end-diastolic volume is 103 ml/sq m or more and whose ejection fraction is 33% or less and those whose left ventricular end-diastolic pressure is 18 mm Hg or more have significantly increased surgical mortality.[27]

PULMONARY DYSFUNCTION

While the effects of acute heart failure on the lung are reversible, chronic congestive failure causes permanent morphologic damage and persistent abnormalities of pulmonary function. These effects are predominantly vascular. Passive congestion, such as that due to ventricular failure or mitral stenosis, hypoperfusion (as in right ventricular outflow tract obstruction), or hyperperfusion from left-to-right shunting, causes changes in the pulmonary vasculature. The degree of respiratory failure caused by passive congestion is related to the amount of water accumulated in the lung. Pulmonary edema leads to hypoxemia, as well as to an alteration in lung mechanics. A left-to-right shunt has a minimal effect on respiratory function early in life, although eventually there will be severe vascular deformities of the lung and limitations of appropriate perfusion.[40] Although congenital defects with right-to-left shunting are associated with hypoxemia, they do not affect the lung's mechanics as much. Pulmonary hypoperfusion secondary to severe right ventricular outflow tract obstruction, such as in tetralogy of Fallot, is associated with no specific ventilatory impairment.

Abnormalities in pulmonary function of patients with mitral stenosis have been reported. Dyspnea and shortness of breath with exercise are the most frequent symptoms. In addition, orthopnea, acute episodic dyspnea, chronic cough, recurrent pulmonary infections, wheezing, and hemoptysis may be present. These symptoms suggest that disease of the lung, together with abnormalities in pulmonary function test results, may lead the clinician to make an erroneous diagnosis of primary pulmonary disease unless he is aware of the impact of increased left atrial pressure on pulmonary function. Because of the long duration of increased left atrial pressure, the entire pulmonary vascular bed undergoes extensive pathologic changes. The main and large pulmonary arteries usually are dilated. The arterioles and small arteries show thickening of the media, with intimal proliferation. The lungs of patients with mitral stenosis may be stiffer than normal, with reduced compliance and an increased work of breathing. Increased left atrial pressure may be reflected back through the pulmonary circuit and may increase the capillary hydrostatic pressure, causing interstitial edema in the terminal bronchioles and alveoli. Bronchial mucosa may be engorged with fluid and dilated blood vessels, manifested symptomatically as wheezing, chronic cough, and hemoptysis. Increased pulmonary water may be a major contributor to the physiologic changes seen in mitral stenosis. The water may be localized in the vascular compartment or in the interstitial spaces.[10]

Several studies have documented similarly increased pulmonary water content in patients with elevated left ventricular end-diastolic pressure due to myocardial infarction.[26] The initial accumulation of fluid occurs in the dependent zones of the lung. Fluid accumulates around extra-alveolar blood vessels and compresses them, adversely affecting the perfusion in the dependent zones, with a progressive shift of perfusion to the upper or nondependent lung fields. This change in perfusion is seen in patients with mitral stenosis and in patients with myocardial infarction.[1, 36] Reduction of regional ventilation may be due to peribronchial edema, resulting in narrowing of small airways. Again, this effect would predominate in dependent zones and result in a progressive shift of ventilation to nondependent areas.

It is difficult to predict whether the pulmonary function of an individual patient will improve after commissurotomy or placement of a new valve. The degree of irreversibility is related to the duration and magnitude of the elevated venous pressure that result in fixed pathologic changes.[10] Vascular engorgement and interstitial edema caused by cardiac insufficiency, whether the insufficiency is due to mitral stenosis or to a failing heart, would profoundly influence ventilation during and after surgery.

HYPERTENSION

High blood pressure is a common health problem. Ten to twelve percent of the total surgical population may have high blood pressure or be receiving antihypertensive treatment.[23] Major complications associated with high blood pressure are coronary heart disease, angina, and myocardial infarctions. The incidence of these complications is twice as high in hypertensive patients as in persons with normal blood pressure.[34] Congestive heart failure, cerebrovascular disease, and cerebral atherosclerosis occur more frequently in the presence of untreated high blood pressure.[3] The increased systemic vascular resistance present in most forms of high

TABLE 1–2.—Classification of Antihypertensive Agents*

Diuretics
  Thiazide type
  Loop diuretics—furosemide, ethacrynic acid
  Potassium-sparing agents—spironolactone, amiloride, triamterene
Sympathetic inhibitors
  Central action—clonidine
  Ganglion blocking agents—trimethaphan, pentolinium, pempidine
  Blockade of neuroeffector transmission— guanethidine, bethanidine, debrisoquin, reserpine
  Combined central and peripheral action—methyldopa
  Adrenergic receptor blocking agents
    α-Adrenergic receptor blockade—phentolamine, phenoxybenzamine (presynaptic and postsynaptic blockade); prazosin (postsynaptic blockade)
    β-Adrenergic receptor blockade—nonselective (combined $β_1$ and $β_2$ blockade); cardioselective (predominantly $β_1$ blockade)
    Combined α- and β-adrenergic receptor blockade— labetalol
  Undefined action—monoamine oxidase inhibitors (pargyline)
Direct-acting vasodilators
  Arterial—hydralazine, diazoxide, minoxidil
  Arterial and venous—sodium nitroprusside
Angiotensin II analogues and converting enzyme inhibitors—saralasin, compound SQ20881

*From Wollam et al.[72] Used by permission of ADIS Australasia Pty.

blood pressure increases the work load of the left ventricle, leading to an augmentation of the left ventricular diastolic volume and eventually to left ventricular hypertrophy. Myocardial oxygen consumption is increased.[51] Therefore, patients suffering from high blood pressure frequently have a high incidence of myocardial ischemia.

Many patients who are to undergo surgery are receiving antihypertensive medication (Table 1–2). Antihypertensive drugs may cause some circulatory imbalance in hypertensive patients during anesthesia and surgery. Several early reports indicated that bradycardia and hypotension were common findings among patients who received antihypertensive agents, especially patients treated with rauwolfia alkaloids or reserpine.[8]

The introduction of newer antihypertensive agents, such as guanethidine, bethanidine, ganglionic blockers, and β-adrenergic receptor blockers created increased concern because of their greater effect on cardiovascular homeostasis (Table 1–3). For several years it was advocated that the use of such drugs be discontinued prior to surgery. The observation that cardiovascular accidents occurred more frequently when the antihypertensive agents were discontinued led to the current practice of maintaining antihypertensive therapy preoperatively.[23, 29] Drug interactions between antihypertensive and anesthetic agents can occur and should be considered. Both treated and untreated hypertensive patients may have cardiovascular instability during induction. In hemodynamic studies of hypertensive patients before and during induction of anesthesia, large variations in heart rate, arterial pressure, cardiac output, and systemic vascular resistance have been found.[51] No induction agent has been found to be completely satisfactory in this regard.[47] The skill of the anesthesiologist seems to be more important than the use of particular pharmacologic agents. The only agent found to be unsuitable has been ketamine, because of its tendency to cause hypertension even in normotensive patients.[47]

Ideally, the anesthetic agents chosen for induction and maintenance should have minimal effects on circulatory homeostasis. The patient's cardiovascular status should be monitored carefully, and any patient with warning signs of an adverse pharmacologic effect should be treated early. Although pharmacologic interactions between antihypertensive agents and anesthetic agents are important, it has become increasingly evident that problems of anesthesia and hypertension more often stem from ischemic heart disease and cerebrovascular disease than from interactions of these drugs.[23] Increased blood pressure and afterload can easily increase myocardial oxygen consumption and result in ischemia and infarction.

ELECTROLYTE DISTURBANCES

A number of electrolytes contribute to the genesis of the transmembrane action potential. Experimentally, potassium, calcium, sodium, and magnesium ions have had a role in producing arrhythmias.[22] However, in a clinical setting, altered concentrations of potassium are responsible for the vast majority of such arrhythmias. Within the ranges of levels encountered in clinical disorders, the serum potassium concentration can alter the electrophysiologic properties of the heart. Therefore, knowledge of potassium levels before surgery is important, and the level has considerable influence on the condition of the patient during and after surgery.

Hypokalemia

Potassium depletion in human subjects is most commonly due to continuous treatment with diuretics. Body potassium is mainly located within the cells; less than 3% is in the extracellular fluid.[17] Therefore, the level of plasma potassium reflects only indirectly the whole-body potassium status of the patient. Diuretics reduce the total body potassium level, not just the level of extracellular potassium. One study noted that a reduction of serum potassium concentration of 1 mEq/L was associated with a reduction of about 20% in the total body potassium value.[17] When plasma potassium concentration was 3.5 mEq/L or more, the total body potassium level usually was not reduced more than 10%.

Hypokalemia induces ectopic rhythms in many different experimental and clinical situations. In the clinical setting, a wide range of atrial junctional and ventricular arrhythmias appears.[12] Hypokalemia also enhances digitalis-induced arrhythmias. The loss of intracellular potassium due to heart failure may predispose to digitalis toxicity, which may explain the severely diseased heart's increased sensitivity to digitalis.

TABLE 1–3.—CONTRAINDICATIONS AND SIDE EFFECTS OF ANTIHYPERTENSIVE AGENTS*

DRUG	SIDE EFFECTS		CONTRAINDICATIONS‡
	INNOCUOUS, BUT SOMETIMES ANNOYING	HARMFUL OR POTENTIALLY HARMFUL	
Oral thiazide diuretics	Dry mouth, unpleasant taste, weakness, muscle cramps, hyperuricemia (sometimes with gout), gastrointestinal disturbances	Hypokalemia, hyponatremia,† hyperglycemia, hypercalcemia,† azotemia,† rash,† photosensitivity,† purpura,† marrow depression,† lithium toxicity† (patients receiving lithium therapy)	Persistent anuria-oliguria, advanced renal failure, hyponatremia
Spironolactone	Drowsiness, hirsutism, menstrual irregularities, gynecomastia, dry mouth, unpleasant taste, gastrointestinal disturbances	Hyperkalemia,† hyponatremia†	Renal failure, hyperkalemia, hyponatremia
Propranolol§	Bradycardia, weakness, lethargy, gastrointestinal disturbances	Congestive heart failure (only in patients with diminished cardiac reserve), bronchospasm† (in patients with asthmatic propensity), hypoglycemia† (propranolol can mask the warning symptoms in insulin-dependent diabetics), aggravation of arterial insufficiency† (in patients with peripheral occlusive arterial disease), nightmares,† insomnia,† hallucinations,† depression,† hyperglycemia, hyperosmolar coma,† abnormal liver function tests† (rare), allergic reactions† (rare), leukopenia† (rare), thrombocytopenia† (rare)	Bronchial asthma, second- or third-degree heart block, congestive heart failure (unless due to an arrhythmia amenable to therapy with propranolol or controlled hypertension), "brittle" diabetes mellitus

Drug	Side effects	Contraindications
Reserpine	Bradycardia, lethargy, lassitude, impotence, diarrhea, nasal congestion	Depression (past or present), active peptic ulcer, parkinsonism
Methyldopa	Drowsiness, lethargy, dry mouth, impotence, positive direct Coombs' test, nasal congestion	Depression,† activation of peptic ulcer,† parkinsonian state† Abnormal liver function test results, hepatitis,† drug fever,† hemolytic anemia,† retroperitoneal fibrosis,† rash,† orthostatic hypotension, depression† Positive Coombs' test, hemolytic anemia, hepatic disease
Guanethidine	Bradycardia, exercise hypotension, diarrhea (especially after meals), weakness, retrograde ejaculation or impotence, nasal congestion	Orthostatic hypotension (potentially harmful in patients with cerebral or myocardial ischemia and advanced renal insufficiency), drug sensitivity (rare)† Interacts with tricyclic antidepressants, sympathomimetic amines
Clonidine	Dry mouth, drowsiness, lethargy, impotence, gastrointestinal disturbances, constipation	"Rebound hypertension" when abruptly discontinued, parotid pain† (rare) None‡
Hydralazine	Tachycardia,‖ palpitation,‖ headache,‖ flushing,‖ nasal congestion, gastrointestinal disturbances	Aggravation of angina,†‖ precipitation of congestive failure in patients with myocardial disease,† lupus-like syndrome,† drug fever,† rash,† psychosis,† marrow suppression,† Symptomatic arteriosclerotic heart disease (unless used with propranolol), congestive heart failure
Prazosin	Headache, palpitation, drowsiness, dizziness, nausea	Sudden collapse and loss of consciousness (usually after initial dose; minimize by using low first dose) None‡

*From Wollam et al.[72] Used by permission of ADIS Australasia Pty.
†Usually requires cessation of therapy, at least temporarily.
‡Hypersensitivity is obviously a contraindication to any drug and will not be repeated for each.
§Some of these side effects are modified or absent with other β-adrenergic blocking agents due to differences in pharmacologic properties (CNS effects and aggravation of arterial insufficiency are more common with propranolol than with other β-adrenergic blockers).
‖These side effects are often minimized or prevented by the coadministration of a β-adrenergic blocker.

Generally, the clinical syndrome of hypokalemia does not occur until the level of serum potassium has decreased below 2.5 mEq/L. The predominant sign is weakness affecting most muscles. The ECG typically shows prolongation of the QT interval and sagging of the ST segment. On occasion, a low-amplitude V wave is seen, and it is believed that this is an indication of an afterpotential following an action potential[64] (Fig 1–1). Metabolic alkalosis also may develop because of potassium loss. Since hydrogen ions replace the potassium ions intracellularly, intracellular acidosis may accompany an extracellular alkalosis.[64]

Hypokalemia requires treatment. Preoperative oral therapy effectively increases the total body potassium level and is preferable to parenteral therapy because it avoids a large or sudden increase in the serum potassium level. The dose of oral potassium probably should be increased for at least one month before cardiac surgery.[70]

Intravenous therapy may be required either before or during operation. The rate of infusions containing potassium ions should not exceed 20 mEq/hour, and the daily intake of potassium should not normally exceed 500 mEq.[64] If potassium-containing solutions are given in superficial veins, severe skin reactions can occur because of the sclerosing action. The patient's ECG should be monitored. Rapid administration of potassium to human beings may result in ventricular ectopy.[22] The ectopy is accompanied by evidence of potassium-induced depression of conduction, suggesting that the mechanism of ectopy is reentry rather than automaticity.[22] However, in animals, ectopic arrhythmias can be suppressed by the administration of potassium.[22] This antiarrhythmic effect is somewhat more predictable when ectopy is due to digitalis.[22]

Hyperkalemia

The effects of hyperkalemia on the heart are seen at the level of 7 mEq/L, when dysrhythmias start to occur. When this level is exceeded, there is the added risk of decreased cardiac output and ventricular fibrillation.[64] The ECG changes of hyperkalemia are characterized by the high, tent-shaped T waves (Fig 1–2).

Causes of hyperkalemia are multiple. Renal failure of various origins is associated with an increased serum potassium level. Adrenal underactivity and inadequate production of mineralocorticosteroids can cause hyperkalemia. Therapeutic agents such as spironolactone, which act by inhibiting potassium ion exchange, can produce hyperkalemia.

Rapid transfusion of older banked blood (potassium concentration can reach 30 mEq/L) can cause high levels of serum potassium, especially in hypovolemic hypotension and after tissue damage and hypoxia.[64]

The dangers of hyperkalemia are related to the high level of serum potassium and not to the amount of total body potassium.[4] High serum levels of potassium can be reduced by causing the ion to move into the cells. This move can be accomplished with the infusion of insulin and 10% glucose (1 L with 50 units of insulin). Glucose and insulin induce potassium ions to move into the cells. An infusion of sodium bicarbonate (150 to 300 mEq) also can lead to temporary re-

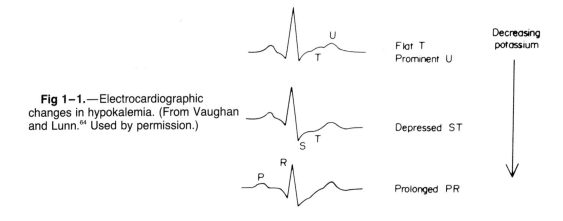

Fig 1–1.—Electrocardiographic changes in hypokalemia. (From Vaughan and Lunn.[64] Used by permission.)

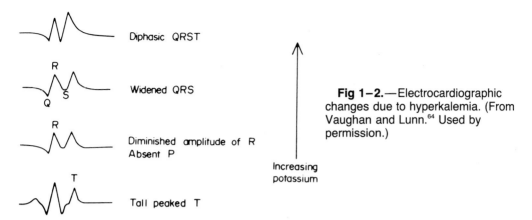

Fig 1-2.—Electrocardiographic changes due to hyperkalemia. (From Vaughan and Lunn.[64] Used by permission.)

distribution of serum potassium. Another compound used to counteract potassium is calcium lactate.[64] Calcium ion opposes the action of the potassium ion on the myocardium.

Serum Digitalis

Most patients who are to undergo cardiac surgery are maintained on a regimen of digitalis. However, clinical experience has suggested that the same persons exhibit increased sensitivity to digitalis during the early postbypass period.[43] Data from experimental animals and human subjects indicate that the concentration of myocardial digoxin is unchanged or slightly decreased at the end of cardiopulmonary bypass.[42] In most patients, the lowest serum levels do not occur until one to three hours after cessation of bypass.[43] This manifestation probably reflects the fluid and metabolic readjustments that continue for some time after a normal circulatory mechanism has been restored. The serum digoxin level then gradually increases to the preoperative value or exceeds it, although no more drug is administered.[43] In one study,[43] peak rebound value of serum digitalis occurred an average of 13 hours after bypass, and arrhythmias occurred at or near the peak of rebound and subsided as the peak was passed. The mean serum digoxin level at the time of arrhythmias was 1.3 ± 0.2 (SD) ng/ml, a significantly higher ($P<.001$) value than the 0.07 ± 0.003 ng/ml noted in patients without arrhythmias. The occurrence of arrhythmias could not be correlated with any other circumstances, such as electrolyte levels, blood gas values, or cardiac size. Yet, in a control group of 77 patients with ECG evidence of digoxin toxicity, the mean digoxin level was 3.1 ± 0.9 (SD) ng/ml. The study[43] concluded that myocardial sensitivity to the toxic effects of digitalis was increased during the first 24 hours after cardiopulmonary bypass. This conclusion was reached because (1) arrhythmias occurred at serum levels of digitalis lower than those observed in patients with toxic effects due to the drug who had not undergone cardiopulmonary bypass, (2) the arrhythmias subsided as the serum level declined, and (3) the levels were higher in patients who had arrhythmias after bypass than in those who did not.

Studies have shown that potassium salts protect the myocardium from digitalis toxicity, possibly by influencing myocardial glycoside binding, and conversely, that digitalis protects against the toxic manifestations of hyperkalemia.[52]

Calcium

Studies of calcium in myocardial function have shown that this ion increases myocardial contractility and excitability. Calcium also may potentiate the development of digitalis toxicity. Thus, calcium-chelating agents have been recommended for the treatment of digitalis toxicity, but their therapeutic benefits are often transient.[59]

Magnesium

Hypomagnesemia facilitates digitalis toxicity, and in these instances, the use of magnesium sulfate can abolish the arrhythmias promptly and permanently.[52] However, rather than using magnesium sulfate empirically as an antiarrhythmic agent, the serum levels of both potassium and magnesium should be determined in all patients with digitalis toxicity. If hypomagnesemia is present, the recommended corrective therapeutic dose is 7 to 15 ml of 25% magnesium sulfate, administered slowly intravenously under ECG monitoring.[52]

Antiarrhythmic Agents

Various antiarrhythmic drugs, including lidocaine, phenytoin, procainamide, quinidine, and propranolol, may be given to suppress ventricular ectopic beats when they are caused by digitalis toxicity. Occasionally, rapid overdrive pacing may be used for temporarily suppressing dangerous ventricular irritability in patients with digitalis intoxication.[35]

DRUGS TAKEN BEFORE SURGERY

Some of the various drugs that patients may be receiving before surgery may have serious effects on the management of the patient during and after surgery. The most important agents are discussed below briefly.

β-Adrenergic Blocking Drugs

β-Adrenergic blocking drugs are given frequently, especially to patients with hypertension, coronary artery disease, or idiopathic hypertrophic subaortic stenosis. To date, propranolol is the most widely used β-adrenergic blocker in the United States. Because of its cardiac-depressant action, some investigators have advocated that patients with coronary artery disease who are undergoing coronary artery surgery and taking propranolol should discontinue the use of the medicine two weeks[65] to 48 hours[20] before surgery. However, the abrupt discontinuation of the drug by patients with angina who have been receiving long-term propranolol therapy has caused an increase of angina, new arrhythmias, myocardial infarction, or sudden death.[2, 14, 41] Recent studies have shown that the continuation of propranolol therapy has no adverse effects on cardiac resuscitation or on the course of recovery. Therefore, the drug could be given to the patient up until 6 to 12 hours before operation[54] (see chap. 8). We now give it until surgery, without any adverse effects.

Diuretics

The adverse effects of diuretics can be grouped into two categories: (1) intravascular volume depletion and (2) metabolic abnormalities. Probably the most commonly used diuretics today are furosemide and ethacrynic acid. Despite their biochemical dissimilarities, the clinical effects of these drugs are almost identical.[46] These diuretics reduce left ventricular preload, with depletion of intravascular volume. Furosemide, by direct action on venous tone, also can increase venous capacitance. The most important metabolic effect of diuretics is hypokalemia, which can have profound effects on patients receiving digitalis and can cause cardiac rhythm disturbances. Diuretics are discussed in chapter 16.

Monoamine Oxidase Inhibitors

Monoamine oxidase inhibitors are a heterogeneous group of drugs that can block the oxidative deamination of naturally occurring monoamines. Although these agents are still used in the treatment of depression and certain phobic anxiety states,[25] they are seldom used now for the treatment of hypertension because of their potentially dangerous side effects. Newer sympatholytic agents with fewer side effects are available. The only commercially available product to treat hypertension is pargyline.[72] It is a potent antihypertensive drug that, like guanethidine, selectively blocks sympathetic transmission by preventing the release of norepinephrine at the neuroeffector junction.[72] Like other monoamine oxidase inhibitors, pargyline causes norepinephrine to accumulate within the sympathetic nerve terminal as degradation by monoamine oxidase is greatly reduced. Such an accumulation may result in a potentially fatal drug interaction with agents such as tyramine, ephedrine, or amphetamines. These drugs may release stores of norepinephrine, producing a severe hypertensive crisis.[72] In certain instances, fatal intracranial bleeding has occurred. Such episodes also may be encountered when monoamine oxidase inhibitors are used with sympathomimetic amines, methyldopa, dopamine, and tryptophan.[25] To treat such a crisis, a short-acting α-adrenergic blocking agent such as phentolamine is recommended.[72]

Monoamine oxidase inhibitors also interfere with detoxification mechanisms of certain drugs. They prolong and intensify the effects of CNS depressive agents, such as barbiturates, and potent analgesics, such as meperidine, and other narcotic drugs. A serious hyperpyrexic reaction also occurs after the concomitant use of meperidine.[25] Therefore, the use of monoamine oxidase inhibitors should be discontinued at least two weeks before surgery.[7]

Anticoagulants

Because as many as a million patients in the United States receive anticoagulants,[18] an anesthesiologist frequently will encounter such a patient in the operating room. Two of the anticoagulants, heparin and warfarin, are commonly used. Because of its immediate action and the rapidity with which its effect can be reversed, heparin is the anticoagulant of choice when a rapid or highly controllable anticoagulant is necessary. However, heparin must be given intravenously by continuous drip or intermittently every 2 to 8 hours to remain effective. The effect of warfarin, given either orally or parenterally, is usually accomplished in 12 hours. The effective dose of warfarin varies among patients because of differences in nutritional states, such as vitamin K intake, genetic factors, and rate of synthesis of clotting factors.[9] Discontinuing the use of anticoagulants preoperatively in cardiac patients does not seem to increase the risk of thromboembolization.[62] Heparin can be neutralized rapidly by protamine.

Three options can be used to reverse warfarin's effect: (1) vitamin K, (2) fresh-frozen plasma transfusions, and (3) concentrates of factors II, III, IX, and X. Vitamin K is the specific antidote for warfarin. However, after the oral or intravenous administration of vitamin K, from 3 to 6 hours are required before the prothrombin time is reduced.[73] The dose of vitamin K varies with the patient. If the level of anticoagulation is to be reduced gradually until treatment can be discontinued, only small doses of vitamin K (0.5 to 1.0 mg) should be used to ensure that the patient does not abruptly become relatively refractory to warfarin. However, complete reversal of the effect of warfarin may require as much as 50 mg of vitamin K.[74]

The use of fresh-frozen plasma, a second method of reversing warfarin-induced anticoagulation, is usually effective immediately. There is no precise formula for calculating the amount of plasma to accomplish this reversal, but 2 to 3 units of fresh-frozen plasma usually will bring an elevated prothrombin time to within normal limits. Because the vitamin K-dependent factors in the prothrombin complex (factors II, VII, IX, and X) are all present in stored whole blood, this component also will correct the hemostatic problem in a patient receiving warfarin therapy if transfusion of red cells is necessary. Because of the high risk of hepatitis, concentrates of factors II, VII, IX, and X are indicated only in a patient with warfarin-induced clotting deficiency who cannot tolerate the increased volume inherent in a fresh-frozen plasma transfusion or who cannot wait for a vitamin K infusion to correct the coagulation status.

BLEEDING DISORDERS

The most important information for the diagnosis of a bleeding disorder comes from a carefully taken history and a carefully performed physical examination. It is important to discover a significant, yet minor, bleeding diathesis before surgery, because intraoperative bleeding may be excessive and because suitable preoperative preparation is often successful in minimizing the chance of hemorrhage.

The questions should be specific in the taking of a history. Information regarding previous trials of hemostatic adequacy is helpful in the evaluation of these patients, particularly if they have undergone a major surgical procedure.[45g] Also, bleeding associated with circumcision, tonsillectomy, or dental extraction may point to a significant problem. Type of bleeding, patient age, family history, and careful investigation of drug intake also will be of diagnostic help. Generally, the physical examination itself is not diagnostic in most bleeding disorders. Its importance lies in the exclusion of some primary disease that may be causing the hemorrhagic diathesis.[45g]

Clinically, patients may be divided into three main groups: (1) those with severe bleeding tendency, (2) those with possible bleeding tendency, and (3) those with no bleeding tendency. Screening tests must be performed in any patient with a suspected bleeding tendency. Such tests must evaluate all phases of the hemostatic mechanism, that is, vascular function, platelets, and coagulation factors (see chap. 20). In most inherited coagulation problems, the abnormality will involve only one part of the hemostatic mechanism, whereas in acquired disorders there may be multiple hemostatic defects. Screening and diagnostic tests must be tailored according to the abnormality suggested by the history and physical examination.

The Ivy bleeding time is often used as a reliable test of both capillary and platelet functions. A platelet count is easily obtainable and will rule out a thrombocytopenic state but will not detect abnormal platelet function (as will the bleeding time). A partial thromboplastin time is a reliable screening test for deficiencies of all the procoagulants of the coagulation cascade except factors VII and XIII and platelet factor 3. The prothrombin time (Quick test) will detect a deficiency of factor VII; and, like the partial thromboplastin time, it measures factors V and X, prothrombin, and fibrinogen.[45a] Thus, the prothrombin time is a reliable measure of the "extrinsic" part of the coagulation system. The partial thromboplastin time measures the adequacy of the intrinsic factors (factors XII, XI, IX, and VIII), as well as others farther down the clotting chain. The incidence of coagulopathies differs much among the population of the United States. The incidence of classic hemophilia (factor VIII deficiency) is one per 10,000, which is about ten times the incidence of Christmas disease[45g] (factor IX deficiency). Hemophilia was recognized before any of the clotting factors were discovered but reflects a deficiency of a specific coagulant (factor VIII) with definable properties, which is also a relatively recent discovery.[45b]

In patients with milder bleeding problems, the presence of hemophilia B, factor IX deficiency, or von Willebrand's disease should be suspected. In von Willebrand's disease, a prolonged bleeding time, factor VIII level less than 50% of normal, and decreased adhesiveness of platelets are regularly found.[45c] An "overresponse" to factor VIII transfusion often produces higher-than-predicted levels of this factor after transfusion. The disease in both mild and severe forms tends to occur equally in both sexes and is inherited directly. Bleeding is mainly from the skin and mucous membranes. Epistaxis is the most common symptom.

Platelet Abnormalities

Platelets are the main factors in hemostasis. A decrease in their number (thrombocytopenia) or an abnormality of their function (thrombopathy, thrombasthenia) will result in abnormal bleeding. However, increases in their number (thrombocythemia) also can cause hemorrhage. Thrombocytopenia is most commonly seen in hemorrhagic diatheses.[45d] Intracerebral bleeding in thrombocytopenia is much more common than in deficiencies of coagulation factors.[45d] If the number of platelets is less than 100,000/cu mm in a patient undergoing surgery, significant bleeding is a real danger (see chap. 20). However, hemostasis is dependent on the adhesiveness of the platelets.[45d] Therefore, bleeding may occur at platelet counts considerably higher than 50,000/cu mm if circulating platelet function is abnormal. A decreased platelet count is the most important laboratory manifestation of thrombocytopenia. There also may be prolongation of the bleeding time. The bleeding time will be prolonged if there is thrombocytopenia or abnormal platelet function.[45d]

Various Drugs, Including Aspirin

Chlorpromazine, phenylbutazone, sulfinpyrazone, and certain antihistamines inhibit the release of adenosine diphosphate from platelets and thus inhibit the second wave of aggregation.[16, 68, 69] Ingestion of as little as 1.3 gm of aspirin lengthens the bleeding time and inhibits the platelet aggregation[69] by epinephrine and collagen.[5, 75] Aspirin inhibits cyclo-oxygenase, an essential enzyme in the production of platelet prostaglandin G_2. The effect of aspirin lasts virtually the entire life of the platelets, suggesting that damage is permanent.[45d] The bleeding time will return to normal as new populations of platelets are produced. Because the normal life span of platelets is 9 to 11 days, at least 5 days are required for the bleeding time to return to normal after the use of aspirin is discontinued. (The use of aspirin should be discontinued preferably a week before surgery.) Aspirin also will increase the bleeding time to a greater extent in patients with von Willebrand's disease.[48]

Vitamin K Deficiency

Evidence is convincing that the active forms of prothrombin and factors VII and X tend to disappear during vitamin K deficiency, thereby causing a characteristic abnormality of the blood clotting mechanism and a bleeding tendency.[45e] Since three of the four vitamin K-dependent factors (factors II, VII, and X) affect the prothrombin time, a prolonged prothrombin time is the first clue to a vitamin K deficiency. When the deficiency is severe, whole blood clotting time, plasma clotting time, and partial thromboplastin time also become prolonged.[45f] The platelet count and concentration of fibrinogen remain normal.

CARDIOVASCULAR SURGERY AND HEMATOLOGIC DISORDERS

In a study at our institution[13] involving 11 open-heart surgical patients with inherited hemoglobinopathies, RBC dyscrasias, or coagulopathies, there were no early or late deaths and no evident complications resulting from hematologic defects (Tables 1–4 and 1–5). The study concluded that thalassemia minor and elliptocytosis should not cause any problems during cardiac surgery. (If hemolytic activity is obvious, splenectomy is the treatment of choice for elliptocytosis.) However, attention should be paid to the sickle cell trait, glucose-6-phosphate dehydrogenase deficiency, spherocytosis, and von Willebrand's disease. Suggestions for guidelines for patients with hematologic disorders were summarized by deLeval et al.[13] as follows (used with permission):

1. Screening tests for sickle cell trait and glucose-6-phosphate dehydrogenase deficiency should be performed on all black patients before operation.
2. If the sickle cell trait is present, hypoxia or acidosis must be avoided. Intracardiac prosthetic valves also should be avoided if possible.
3. Patients with glucose-6-phosphate dehydrogenase deficiency should not receive drugs that may induce hemolytic crises (for example, antipyretics, analgesics such as aspirin, phenacetin, quinidine, menadiol sodium diphosphate, chloramphenicol, sulfonamides, nitrofurans).
4. Splenectomy should be performed before cardiac surgery in patients with spherocytosis, and prosthetic valves should be avoided whenever possible since mechanical fragility of spherocytes is increased.
5. Coagulation studies should be performed on all patients who have reported bleeding tendencies. Patients with von Willebrand's disease should receive cryoprecipitate before and after operation.

DIABETES

The onset of clinically evident cardiac disease frequently is observed years after the onset of diabetes. Patients without a prior diabetic history may exhibit glucose intolerance at the onset of a myocardial infarction.[56] Patients with decreased cardiac function also may have a similar intolerance.[19] These incidents may be secondary to chronic alterations in pancreatic β cells precipitated by circulatory or neurohumoral responses to cardiac dysfunction.[50] The primary effects of diabetes on the heart and its vasculature may be significantly affected by associated hyperlipidemia, obesity, or hypertension. The onset of hypertension in diabetic patients may occur late during the course of the disease, presumably secondary to atherosclerosis.[50] Even diabetic patients whose diabetes is well controlled, without ketosis, and who are in good clinical status with no significant obstructive coronary or valve disease, exhibit significant reduction of stroke volume index and elevation of left ventricular end-diastolic pressure when compared with control subjects of similar age.[50] If afterload is increased (for example, by the use of angiotensins) to an end-diastolic pressure of 15–18 mm Hg above control, diabetic patients may demonstrate a significant increase in left ventricular end-diastolic pressure (compared with a small increase of left ventricular end-diastolic pressure in normal subjects).[49] These data are considered consistent with the responses of a preclinical cardiomyopathy.[49] These factors must be considered in patients with long-standing diabetes who are to undergo surgery.

The incidence of silent myocardial infarction is higher in diabetic than in nondiabetic patients. Friedberg[24] reported this during the late 1950s, and the observation subsequently has been documented and statistically confirmed.[63] Soler et al.[55] noted that 101 of 285 diabetic patients with myocardial infarctions were admitted directly to the ward and were not placed in coronary units. Infarctions were not suspected because heart failure and uncontrollable diabetes were the prominent symptoms. A painless myocardial infarction was considered to be due to myocardial anoxia (possibly hypoxia) from dif-

TABLE 1–4.—Data on Nine Patients With Blood Disorders Who Had Undergone Open-Heart Surgery*

DIAGNOSIS	CASE	RACE OR NATIONALITY	OPERATION†	DIAGNOSTIC TESTS	PREOPERATIVE HEMOGLOBIN, GM/DL	POSTBYPASS PLASMA HEMOGLOBIN, MG/DL	LAST FOLLOW-UP HEMOGLOBIN, GM/DL	POSTOPERATIVE COURSE
Thalassemia minor	1	Vietnamese	Repair VSD and PS	65% Hb A_2	9.2	<40	12.6	Well
	2	Italian	SE mitral valve replacement	7.4% Hb A_2	9.3	<40	11.9	Systemic emboli
	3	Italian	SE mitral valve replacement	7.3% Hb A_2	9.6	<40	10.2	Systemic emboli
Sickle cell trait	4	Black American	Aortic valve replacement with homograft	41% Hb S	13.5	<40	14.1	Well
	5	Black American	Repair of tetralogy of Fallot	41% Hb S	16.5	<40	14.7	Well
Glucose-6-phosphate dehydrogenase deficiency	6	Black American	SE aortic valve replacement	Glucose-6-phosphate dehydrogenase test positive; glucose-6-phosphate dehydrogenase activity decreased	8.9	<40	13.8	Well
Spherocytosis	7	French	Mitral and tricuspid valve replacement; BC prosthesis	Microspherocytes; increased osmotic fragility	13.5	<40	13.5	Well
Elliptocytosis	8	White	SE mitral valve replacement	Marked elliptocytosis	12.6	<40	12.9	Cerebral emboli
	9	Scandinavian	SE mitral and tricuspid valve replacement	Marked elliptocytosis	10.0	<40	10.5	Well

*From deLeval et al.[13] Used by permission.
†VSD, ventricular septal defect; PS, pulmonary stenosis; SE, Starr-Edwards prosthetic valve; BC, Braunwald-Cutter prosthetic valve.

TABLE 1–5.—PREOPERATIVE LABORATORY DATA ON TWO PATIENTS WITH VON WILLEBRAND'S DISEASE WHO HAD UNDERGONE OPEN-HEART SURGERY*

LABORATORY DATA	NORMAL	CASE 1	CASE 2
Bleeding time (Duke), min	1 to 5	28	. . .
Bleeding time (Ivy), min	1 to 6	14½	9
Platelets/cu mm	130,000–370,000	107,000	150,000
Platelet aggregation (ristocetin)	. . .	. . .	Reduced
Platelet retention, %	70	4	50
Factor VIII, %	54–146	24	64
Factor VIII–related antigen, %	. . .	. . .	36
Ristocetin–von Willebrand factor, %	80	. . .	41

*Modified from deLeval et al.[13]

fuse changes in the small myocardial vasculature.[24] When so little healthy heart muscle is left, coronary artery occlusion loses its impact. Later, it was proved that intrinsic cardiac autonomic neuropathy was responsible for the blocking of reception and conduction of pain.[6]

Patients with diabetes of juvenile or adult onset should undergo surgery only if their diabetic status is well controlled. The methods for this control are outside the realm of this chapter and can be found in any general medical text. One fact, however, still remains. The reduced incidence of ketoacidosis and infection since the advent of insulin therapy unfortunately has not been associated with a notable improvement in cardiovascular morbidity and mortality in diabetic patients.[24] Insulin use in a more physiologic mode early in the course of the disease and the regulation of other hormones that affect carbohydrate metabolism have been proposed as means of preventing or delaying cardiovascular complications.[24]

CIGARETTE SMOKING

Smoking is a principal cause of chronic bronchitis and emphysema, which in turn are the chief causes of pulmonary heart disease and aggravate other types of heart disease. The contribution of cigarette smoking to the development of myocardial infarction and mortality from coronary heart disease has been confirmed.[33] It is estimated that cigarette smoking is responsible for 325,000 premature deaths each year. Thirty-seven percent of these deaths are due to coronary heart disease.[33] Nicotine and carbon monoxide have been incriminated as the most harmful by-products of smoking. Because of its affinity for hemoglobin and myoglobin, carbon monoxide interferes with transport and tissue utilization of oxygen. Anoxic damage to the arterial lining may be induced, which accelerates atherogenesis in the presence of hyperlipidemia.[32] Nicotine mobilizes catecholamines, which constrict small blood vessels, aggravating occlusive peripheral arterial disease. Nicotine also increases blood pressure, cardiac rate and work load, and myocardial irritability. These abrupt increases in cardiac work and oxygen consumption in an ischemic heart further penalized by curtailed oxygen transport may cause disastrous electrical instability, leading to ventricular fibrillation and sudden death.[32] In addition to these acute effects, chronic persistent structural atheromatous changes caused by anoxic damage to the arterial intima occur. These dual effects are dose-related.[32] Therefore, cigarette smoking should be discontinued as early as possible before surgery.

REOPERATIONS

As the number of cardiac operations increases, the number of reoperations necessary also increases. Any cardiac operation carries a significant risk if a patient is subjected to a second cardiac operation. This risk may be increased for several reasons, as follows. There are well-known technical difficulties arising from obliteration of the pericardium. Bleeding from adhesions between the heart and the surrounding tissues makes freeing the heart more difficult. Bleeding from the adhesions can be profuse, requiring more blood transfusions than usual. The cardiac wall or coronary artery can be damaged accidentally during division of the sternum. Difficult dissection may require excessive handling of the heart, therefore causing arrhythmias or reduced cardiac output and blood pressure. In spite of these problems, the technical difficulties do not seem to increase the operative mortality.[58, 60, 71] However, the hospital mortality among these patients is reported to be three times greater than that of patients who are undergoing their first cardiac operation[71] (22% vs. 8%). This high rate is due to myocardial failure, which is attributed to the more advanced diseases in these patients,[71] comprising mainly the myocardial disease itself and changes brought about by the pulmonary vasculature from the original cardiac problems.[71]

In one study of valve reoperations, a clear distinction was made between early and late reoperations after an initial prosthetic valve replacement.[60] The usual indication for early reoperations was prosthetic infection or paravalvular leak. Late reoperations were performed more often on patients who had either emboli or obstructive gradients.

Prosthetic infection occurs most frequently within six weeks of the original valve replacement.[15] A paravalvular leak tends to occur during the early postoperative period[67] and requires immediate reoperation. However, an embolism is usually managed by a strict anticoagulation program, unless repeated episodes of emboli force consideration of surgery, which is usually a late reoperation.[57]

A thrombus or prosthetic infection can occlude the orifice of the valve and is usually a late occurrence.[53] Both prosthetic infection and stenosis have grave indications.[60] Prosthetic infections are difficult to eradicate and frequently may result in multiple organ failure; the reoperative mortality is still close to 50%.[60]

The principal determinants of survival after reoperation seem to be the indication for reoperation and the clinical status of the patient. The preoperative classification of the patient can give a general indication of survival after surgery. Patients in class II of the New York Heart Association classification, particularly those with paravalvular fistula, have a good survival rate.[58]

REFERENCES

1. Al Bazzaz F.J., Kazemi H.: Arterial hypoxemia and distribution of pulmonary perfusion after uncomplicated myocardial infarction. *Am. Rev. Respir. Dis.* 106:721, 1972.
2. Alderman E.L., et al.: Coronary artery syndromes after sudden propranolol withdrawal. *Ann. Intern. Med.* 81:625, 1974.
3. Baker A.B., Resch J.A., Loewenson R.B.: Hypertension and cerebral atherosclerosis. *Circulation* 39:701, 1969.
4. Black D.A.K.: The biochemistry of renal failure. *Br. J. Anaesth.* 41:264, 1969.
5. Bowie E.J.W., Owen C.A. Jr.: Aspirin, platelets, and bleeding, editorial. *Circulation* 40:757, 1969.
6. Bradley R.F., Schonfeld A.: Diminished pain in diabetic patients with acute myocardial infarction. *Geriatrics* 17:322, 1962.
7. Cascorbi, H.F.: Perianesthetic problems with nonanesthetic drugs. Read before the 29th annual refresher course lectures of the American Society of Anesthesiologists Annual Meeting, Chicago, October 21 to 25, 1978, no. 212, p. 3.
8. Coakley C.S., Alpert S., Boli J.S.: Circulatory responses during anesthesia of patients on rauwolfia therapy. *J.A.M.A.* 161:1143, 1956.
9. Coon W.W., Willis P.W. III: Some aspects of the pharmacology of oral anticoagulants. *Clin. Pharmacol. Ther.* 11:312, 1970.
10. Cortese D.A.: Pulmonary function in mitral stenosis. *Mayo Clin. Proc.* 53:321, 1978.
11. Criteria Committee of the New York Heart Association: *Nomenclature and Criteria for Diagnosis of Diseases of the Heart and Great Vessels*, ed. 8. Boston, Little, Brown & Co., 1979, p. 290.
12. Davidson S., Surawicz B.: Ectopic beats and atrioventricular conduction disturbances: In patients with hypopotassemia. *Arch. Intern. Med.* 120:280, 1967.
13. DeLeval M.R., et al.: Open heart surgery in patients with inherited hemoglobinopathies, red cell dyscrasias, and coagulopathies. *Arch Surg* 109:618, 1974.
14. Diaz R.G., et al.: Myocardial infarction after propranolol withdrawal. *Am. Heart J.* 88:257, 1974.
15. Dismukes W.E., et al.: Prosthetic valve endocarditis: Analysis of 38 cases. *Circulation* 48:365, 1973.
16. Doery J.C.G., Hirsh J., de Gruchy G.C.: Aspirin: Its effect on platelet glycolysis and release of adenosine diphosphate. *Science* 165:65, 1969.
17. Edmonds C.J., Jasani B.: Total-body potas-

sium in hypertensive patients during prolonged diuretic therapy. *Lancet* 2:8, 1972.
18. Ellison N., Ominsky A.J.: Clinical considerations for the anesthesiologist whose patient is on anticoagulant therapy. *Anesthesiology* 39: 328, 1973.
19. Ettinger P.O., et al.: Glucose intolerance in nonischemic cardiac disease: Role of cardiac output and adrenergic function. *Circulation* 43:809, 1971.
20. Faulkner S.L., et al.: Time required for complete recovery from chronic propranolol therapy. *N. Engl. J. Med.* 289:607, 1973.
21. Favaloro R.G.: Direct myocardial revascularization: A ten year journey; myths and realities. *Am. J. Cardiol.* 43:109, 1979.
22. Fisch C.: Relation of electrolyte disturbances to cardiac arrhythmias. *Circulation* 47:408, 1973.
23. Foëx P., Prys-Roberts C.: Anaesthesia and the hypertensive patient. *Br. J. Anaesth.* 46:575, 1974.
24. Friedberg C.K.: *Diseases of the Heart*, ed. 2. Philadelphia, W.B. Saunders Co., 1956, p. 51.
25. Goodman L.S., Gilman A.: *The Pharmacological Basis of Therapeutics*, ed. 5. New York, Macmillan Publishing Co., 1975, p. 180.
26. Hales C.A., Kazemi H.: Pulmonary function after uncomplicated myocardial infarction. *Chest* 72:350, 1977.
27. Hammermeister K.E., Kennedy J.W.: Predictors of surgical mortality in patients undergoing direct myocardial revascularization. *Circulation* 50(suppl. 2):112, 1974.
28. Hammermeister K.E., et al.: Prediction of late survival in patients with mitral valve disease from clinical, hemodynamic, and quantitative angiographic variables. *Circulation* 57:341, 1978.
29. Hansson L., Hunyor S.N.: Blood pressure over-shoot due to acute clonidine (Catapres) withdrawal: Studies on arterial and urinary catecholamines and suggestions for management of the crisis. *Clin. Sci. Mol. Med.* 45(suppl.):181, 1973.
30. Harlan W.R., et al.: Chronic congestive heart failure in coronary artery disease: Clinical criteria. *Ann. Intern. Med.* 86:133, 1977.
31. Hirshfeld J.W. Jr., et al.: Indices predicting long-term survival after valve replacement in patients with aortic regurgitation and patients with aortic stenosis. *Circulation* 50:1190, 1974.
32. Kannel W.B., et al.: Report of the Ad Hoc Committee on Cigarette Smoking and Cardiovascular Diseases for Health Professionals. *Circulation* 57:404A, 1978.
33. Kannel W.B., et al.: American Heart Association Report of Ad Hoc Committee on Cigarette Smoking and Cardiovascular Diseases. *Circulation* 57:406A, 1978.
34. Kannel W.B., Schwartz M.J., McNamara P.M.: Blood pressure and risk of coronary heart disease: The Framingham study. *Dis. Chest* 56:43, 1969.
35. Kastor J.A.: Digitalis intoxication in patients with atrial fibrillation. *Circulation* 47:888, 1973.
36. Kazemi H., et al.: Distribution of pulmonary blood flow after myocardial ischemia and infarction. *Circulation* 41:1025, 1970.
37. Kostuk W., et al.: Correlations between the chest film and hemodynamics in acute myocardial infarction. *Circulation* 48:624, 1973.
38. Langou R.A., et al.: Incidence and mortality of perioperative myocardial infarction in patients undergoing coronary artery bypass grafting. *Circulation* 56(suppl. 2):54, 1977.
39. Lappas D., et al.: Indirect measurement of left-atrial pressure in surgical patients—pulmonary-capillary wedge and pulmonary-artery diastolic pressures compared with left-atrial pressure. *Anesthesiology* 38:394, 1973.
40. Laver M.B., Hallowell P., Goldblatt A.: Pulmonary dysfunction secondary to heart disease: Aspects relevant to anesthesia and surgery. *Anesthesiology* 33:161, 1970.
41. Miller R.R., et al.: Propranolol-withdrawal rebound phenomenon: Exacerbation of coronary events after abrupt cessation of antianginal therapy. *N. Engl. J. Med.* 293:416, 1975.
42. Molokhia F.A., et al.: Constancy of myocardial digoxin concentration during experimental cardiopulmonary bypass. *Ann. Thorac. Surg.* 11:222, 1971.
43. Morrison J., Killip T.: Serum digitalis and arrhythmia in patients undergoing cardiopulmonary bypass. *Circulation* 47:341, 1973.
44. Nanda N.C., et al.: Mitral commissurotomy versus replacement: Preoperative evaluation by echocardiography. *Circulation* 51:263, 1975.
45. Owen C.A. Jr., Bowie E.J.W., Thompson J.H. Jr.: *The Diagnosis of Bleeding Disorders*, ed. 2. Boston; Little, Brown & Co., 1975, pp. 112(a), 155(b), 194(c), 226(d), 266(e), 272(f), and 368(g).
46. Plumb V.J., James T.N.: Clinical hazards of powerful diuretics: Furosemide and ethacrynic acid. *Mod. Concepts Cardiovasc. Dis.* 47:91, 1978.
47. Prys-Roberts C., et al.: Studies of anaesthesia in relation to hypertension: II. Haemodynamic consequences of induction and endotracheal intubation. *Br. J. Anaesth.* 43:531, 1971.
48. Quick A.J.: Salicylates and bleeding: The as-

pirin tolerance test. *Am. J. Med. Sci.* 252:265, 1966.
49. Regan T.J., et al.: Evidence for cardiomyopathy in familial diabetes mellitus. *J. Clin. Invest.* 60:885, 1977.
50. Regan T.J., et al.: The myocardium and its vasculature in diabetes mellitus: Parts I and II. *Mod. Concepts Cardiovasc. Dis.* 47:71, 75, 1978.
51. Sarnoff S.J., et al.: Hemodynamic determinants of oxygen consumption of the heart with special reference to the tension-time index. *Am. J. Physiol.* 192:148, 1958.
52. Seller R.H.: The role of magnesium in digitalis toxicity. *Am. Heart J.* 82:551, 1971.
53. Shepherd R.L., et al.: Hemodynamic confirmation of obstruction to left ventricular inflow by a caged-ball prosthetic mitral valve: Case report. *J. Thorac. Cardiovasc. Surg.* 65:252, 1973.
54. Slogoff S., Keats A.S., Ott E.: Preoperative propranolol therapy and aortocoronary bypass operation. *J.A.M.A.* 240:1487, 1978.
55. Soler N.G., et al.: Myocardial infarction in diabetics. *Q. J. Med.* 44:125, 1975.
56. Sowton E.: Cardiac infarction and the glucose-tolerance test. *Br. Med. J.* 1:84, 1962.
57. Starr A., et al.: Late complications of aortic valve replacement with cloth-covered, composite-seat prostheses: A six-year appraisal. *Ann. Thorac. Surg.* 19:289, 1975.
58. Stewart S., DeWeese J.A.: The determinants of survival following reoperation on prosthetic cardiac valves. *Ann. Thorac. Surg.* 25:555, 1978.
59. Surawicz B., et al.: Treatment of cardiac arrhythmias with salts of ethylenediamine tetraacetic acid (EDTA). *Am. Heart J.* 58:493, 1959.
60. Syracuse D.C., Bowman F.O. Jr., Malm J.R.: Prosthetic valve reoperations: Factors influencing early and late survival. *J. Thorac. Cardiovasc. Surg.* 77:346, 1979.
61. Taylor S.H.: Heart failure—I. *Recent Adv. Cardiol.* 7:369, 1977.
62. Tinker J.H., Tarhan S.: Discontinuing anticoagulant therapy in surgical patients with cardiac valve prostheses: Observations in 180 operations. *J.A.M.A.* 239:738, 1978.
63. Vaisrub S.: Painless myocardial infarction in diabetes, editorial. *J.A.M.A.* 239:1790, 1978.
64. Vaughan R.S., Lunn J.N.: Potassium and the anaesthetist: A review. *Anaesthesia* 28:118, 1973.
65. Viljoen J.F., Estafanous F.G., Kellner G.A.: Propranolol and cardiac surgery. *J. Thorac. Cardiovasc. Surg.* 64:826, 1972.
66. Walston A. II, Kendall M.E.: Comparison of pulmonary wedge and left atrial pressure in man. *Am. Heart J.* 86:159, 1973.
67. Weldon C.S., Ferguson T.B.: The elimination of periprosthetic leaks as a complication of mitral valve replacement. *Ann. Thorac. Surg.* 18:447, 1974.
68. Weiss H.J., Aledort L.M.: Impaired platelet/connective-tissue reaction in man after aspirin ingestion. *Lancet* 2:495, 1967.
69. Weiss H.J., Aledort L.M., Kochwa S.: The effect of salicylates on the hemostatic properties of platelets in man. *J. Clin. Invest.* 47:2169, 1968.
70. White R.J.: Effect of potassium supplements on the exchangeable potassium in chronic heart disease. *Br. Med. J.* 3:141, 1970.
71. Wisheart J.D., Ross D.N., Ross J.K.: A review of the effect of previous operations on the results of open-heart surgery. *Thorax* 27:137, 1972.
72. Wollam G.L., Gifford R.W. Jr., Tarazi R.C.: Antihypertensive drugs: Clinical pharmacology and therapeutic use. *Drugs* 14:420, 1977.
73. Wright I.S.: Anticoagulant therapy—practical management. *Am. Heart J.* 77:280, 1969.
74. Zieve P.D., Solomon H.M.: Variation in the response of human beings to vitamin K_1. *J. Lab. Clin. Med.* 73:103, 1969.
75. Zucker M.B., Peterson J.: Inhibition of adenosine diphosphate-induced secondary aggregation and other platelet functions by acetylsalicylic acid ingestion, *Proc. Soc. Exp. Biol. Med.* 127:547, 1968.

2 / Radiology

ANTHONY W. STANSON
W. EUGENE MILLER

THE PRESENT chapter is not intended to supply a core curriculum for the interpretation of chest roentgenograms but rather to provide an appreciation of the general appearances of normal and pathologic roentgenographic entities that may be encountered before and after cardiovascular surgery.

THE PREOPERATIVE CHEST ROENTGENOGRAM

Different diseases can have similar roentgenographic appearances and thus can be confusing not only to the anesthesiologist but also to the radiologist.[1, 2] Often the radiologist cannot give a definite diagnostic impression and can supply only a short differential selection. Therefore, some clinical information should be provided on the roentgenogram request card. With such information, the radiologist then would be the one most able to reach a diagnosis and to proceed with any necessary additional films and special diagnostic procedures. Although the words "routine preoperative chest" may be stated on the request card, the patient is not having routine surgery. There is a specific reason why the patient is having surgery, and that type of information and the pertinent medical history can be helpful to the radiologist. For a vast majority of patients, the chest findings are negative and accurate information on the clinical presentation seems to be immaterial. However, the radiologist is interested in providing as thorough an interpretation as possible, and often additional information supplies that opportunity. In cardiovascular surgery, the medical justification of routine preoperative chest radiography is controversial, and the detection rate of significant positive findings on a preoperative chest film is extremely small.[3]

Negative Chest Findings

In the average practice of radiology, roentgenograms of the chest comprise much of the work, and the results of most of these examinations are within normal limits (Fig 2–1). The normal range is from the finding of no identifiable abnormality to the finding of features that reflect chronic processes with no clinical significance.

Pulmonary calcified granulomas, single or multiple, in a wide range of sizes from 1 mm in diameter to 2 or 3 cm, are commonly seen and are rarely of clinical significance. Some of these are associated with ipsilateral hilar lymph node calcification or paratracheal node calcification. If the calcific deposits are central, concentric, or homogeneous, they can be assumed to be simple granulomas. Often, on posteroanterior views, such granulomas do not appear to be calcified, and tomograms (at lower kilovoltage) are necessary to detect the calcification and to distinguish these harmless calcified granulomas from pulmonary nodules of other sources.

Old healed rib fractures often leave residual deformities of the bone, as well as some underlying pleural thickening. These films are rarely confusing.

Pleural thickening over the apical caps of the lungs can be confused with Pancoast's tumors in this region. The lesion is usually benign if the contour of the pleural thickening conforms to the basic curvature of the apical portion of the lung and is not more than a few millimeters thick.

At the apex, small blebs can be present, especially in the older population. These are not to be confused with apical cavitary tuberculosis.

Prominent nipple shadows should not be confused with pulmonary nodules. A stereoscopic

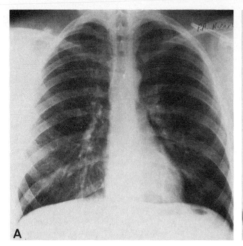
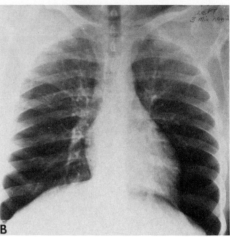
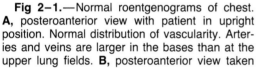

Fig 2–1.—Normal roentgenograms of chest. **A,** posteroanterior view with patient in upright position. Normal distribution of vascularity. Arteries and veins are larger in the bases than at the upper lung fields. **B,** posteroanterior view taken while subject was hanging by the knees from a bar above the film holder. Note reversal of flow pattern, with larger upper lung vessels, showing influence of gravity on pulmonary blood flow.

view of the chest can readily establish the difference. Similarly, large moles or other cutaneous nodules also can cast shadows that have the appearance of pulmonary nodules. Redundant folds of skin projected over the lateral chest margin should not be confused with a pneumothorax. Nonpendulant breast tissue on the posteroanterior film can mimic pulmonary infiltrates.

Another area of confusion arises from unusual pulmonary fissures, including the azygous lobe seen at the right apex and the accessory lower lobe fissure, which sometimes can tent up the hemidiaphragm.

A prominent pulmonary outflow tract and a main pulmonary artery segment in a young, thin woman are not to be confused with the abnormality of pulmonary valvular disease or pulmonary arterial hypertension. Also, there can be a wide range of widening of the superior mediastinum that is completely acceptable because of normal vascular shadows. The apical portion of the heart may be prominent, secondary to a large pleural fold or apical fat pad. Similarly, in the right cardiophrenic angle, prominent fat pads and pleural folds can be present.

Certain radiographic technical features also must be considered, including proper positioning of the chest. A few degrees of rotation to the right or to the left can cause rather striking changes in the mediastinal silhouette, which can be confusing to the inexperienced observer. Films must be taken while the subject is in deep inspiration so as not to cause artifactual clouding of the lung bases. Shallow inspiration obscures the lower lung fields behind the diaphragm and gives a false impression of cardiomegaly. Similarly, respiration must be suspended during filming so as not to cause blurring of the pulmonary structures, which could make pulmonary nodules or infiltrates difficult to detect. In the posteroanterior view, the shoulders must be rolled forward to remove the scapula from the lung fields. When a portable film technique is required, the view generally will be anteroposterior and the distance from the patient to the x-ray tube will be considerably shorter than that in the posteroanterior view taken in the nonportable situation. Consequently, the heart size and mediastinal structures will be magnified. Also, the patient may have more difficulty depressing the diaphragm with inspiration while in the recumbent or semierect position. These considerations are important when standard films are compared with films taken at the bedside or in the intensive care unit.

The radiographic factors of milliamperage and kilovoltage must be well balanced to achieve optimal enhancement of soft tissues at the expense of bone.

Apparently Positive Chest Findings

False-positive findings may be encountered after an operation or in certain congenital conditions. The best example is previous pneumonectomy in which the entire hemithorax is opaque. In this situation, the history is important. The mediastinum should be shifted toward the involved side, and there is compensatory overinflation of the remaining lung. When lobectomy has been done, the mediastinum will shift somewhat toward the side of surgery, and there is elevation of the hemidiaphragm and compensatory overinflation of the remaining lung on that side. This feature will be present as an alteration of the hemithorax, and the history is important to make the proper correlation. After thoracotomy, many patients have blunting of a costophrenic angle, which can be due to fluid or thickened pleura. Postoperative changes of ribs are not to be confused with destructive metastatic lesions.

Rib fractures from previous trauma can result in pleural thickening, pleural adhesions, and irregularities of the ribs. An abnormally high hemidiaphragm may be related to previous damage to a phrenic nerve. In a small percentage of the population, the left hemidiaphragm will be higher than the right normally.

Congenital conditions include an elevated hemidiaphragm (eventration) or hypoplasia of the right or left pulmonary artery, with subsequent decreased volume of that side of the thorax and compensatory overinflation of the opposite lung. The diaphragm also can be elevated on the involved side, with a shift of the mediastinum toward the hypoplastic lung. Another mediastinal abnormality that is not clinically significant includes abnormal positions of the cardiac shadow that, within reasonable limits, can appear to be similar to dextrocardia or mesocardia. A small percentage of the population will also have a right-sided aortic arch without associated congenital heart disease.

From a radiographic standpoint, there are technical reasons why the appearance of the film can be unusual. Failure of deep inspiration can cause considerable clouding of the lung fields with an appearance similar to congestive heart failure. The heart shadow can have a false appearance of being large, and lung markings can appear to be crowded, such that they have an appearance of focal areas of atelectasis or even pneumonitis. Rotation of the chest can cause mediastinal shadows to project in unusual locations, simulating mass lesions.

Apparently Negative Chest Findings

Most chest films that appear to be normal at first glance are so; however, all films deserve review to ensure that some subtle finding is not present (Fig 2-2). A small pneumothorax is easily missed, and its detection necessitates careful observation of the apices of the lung field and laterally along the upper lobe region. Also, pulmonary nodules can be difficult to see behind the heart shadow, behind curvatures of the diaphragm, and especially in the perimeter of the lung field adjacent to the axillary margins of the ribs. Early presentation of pneumonitis, especially in the right middle lobe, also can be difficult to identify in the posteroanterior view without help from the lateral view. Overexposed films can mask lung nodules of low density and early areas of pneumonitis.

A multitude of diseases seen initially with an early opaque lung pattern can be present and, without previous experience in interpretation, can be difficult to fully appreciate. Such condi-

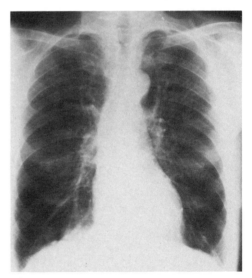

Fig 2-2.—Lungs appear to be clear; however, there is considerable overexpansion, with some prominence of central bronchovascular markings. This patient has emphysema. Prominent 1-cm nodules in each midlung field are nipple shadows, which can be confusing at times. Stereoscopic pair of films or repeat film with nipple markers can resolve the situation.

tions include infiltrates, atelectasis, masses, pleural diseases, cysts, and vascular patterns and abnormalities of the lungs.

Infiltrates

Infiltrates in the lung cover a wide range of diseases and presentations (Fig 2–3). Involved may be a subsegment, the entire lobe, or even the entire lung, either unilaterally or bilaterally. Infiltrates are usually caused by pneumonitis. However, certain tumors, such as lymphoma and alveolar cell carcinoma, can have a similar appearance. Lung contusion resulting from chest trauma and aspiration also can be seen initially as an infiltrate. Certain infiltrates are difficult to distinguish from fibrosis or congestive failure in a nonuniform pattern. In such instances, previous films, as well as follow-up films, should be obtained for comparison.

Because of the recent refinements in diagnostic techniques and interpretation of the location and nature of lung infiltrates, if such an infiltrate is encountered, it is best to consult the radiologist.

Atelectasis

Atelectasis may involve an entire lung or a lobe, segment, or subsegmental area and sometimes may involve subsegments so small as to produce no more than a short discoid mark in the lung field (Fig 2–4). Segmental areas of atelectasis or even lobar atelectasis can be missed entirely on a chest film, unless one is aware of certain signs and has experience in their interpretation. One common site for atelectasis is the small subsegmental areas of the lung bases of hospitalized patients. These patients usually are asymptomatic, and the presence of atelectasis presumably is related to collections of secretions in the bronchi of the posterior bases in patients recuperating from various illnesses and surgical procedures. Sometimes if multiple or large areas of lung are involved, the patient has a fever. These areas are not difficult to identify on the film, and when they are large, they may be confused with pulmonary infarction. Classically, the pulmonary infarction abuts the pleural surface, has a wedge-shaped appearance, and may be associated with cough, fever, and pleuritic pain. Evaluation of atelectasis is sometimes a complex diagnostic problem.

Masses

Mass lesions in the chest can be related to the lung, the pleura, the bones, the soft tissues of the thorax, the vascular structures, the diaphragm, the mediastinum, and the heart. Most masses are readily apparent on film (Fig 2–5). However, some are more difficult to see and others are difficult to evaluate, even when they are easily detected.

The three main reasons for not detecting a mass lesion on a chest film are (1) the lesion is hidden behind or adjacent to normal structures and cannot be distinguished from them, (2) the lesion is misinterpreted as a normal structure, and (3) the lesion is just overlooked.

In the mediastinal area, smaller masses may be either hidden or difficult to distinguish from normal mediastinal shadows. Multiple views, as well as fluoroscopy and sometimes even tomography, may be necessary to make a diagnosis. In the middle of the lung fields, an additional problem exists—that is, smaller masses may be of such low density as to be obscured by overlying ribs or just not visible without the benefit of altering technical factors of the filming process, obtaining stereoscopic views, or performing tomography. Smaller mass lesions can be situated behind the dome of the diaphragm. Some of

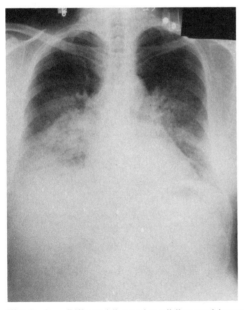

Fig 2–3.—Diffuse bilateral perihilar and lower lobe infiltrates. High-altitude pulmonary edema.

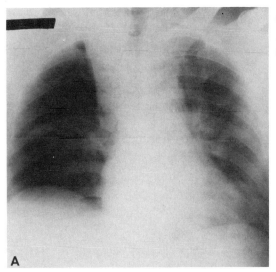 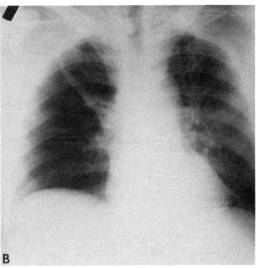

Fig 2–4.—**A,** right upper lobe atelectasis with compensatory hyperinflation of right lower and middle lobes. Focal or plate-like atelectasis of left lower lobe. **B,** almost complete reexpansion of right upper lobe, but residual subsegmental atelectasis remains.

these lesions can best be seen with lateral or oblique views, and tomography may be necessary to further evaluate them.

Some mass-like lesions represent collections of fluid. They can be found in the minor or major fissures and are sometimes referred to as phantom tumors. These lesions probably are collections of fluid adjacent to an area of lung that has less compliance (more easily displaced by fluid). Artifacts also can be considered phantom nodules over the lungs. Some artifacts are produced during the handling and processing of the films, whereas others are caused by patients' clothing, braided hair, foreign bodies worn around the neck, and at times by superficial skin lesions such as large moles, which cast confusing shadows. Comparison films, as well as additional views and tomography, must be used aggressively for further evaluation of most mass lesions in the chest.

Pleural Diseases

Pleural diseases that can be readily recognized roentgenographically include effusion, unilateral thickened pleura, local masses, pleural calcification, and pneumothorax (Fig 2–6).

A small amount of pleural fluid is seen as blunting of the costophrenic angle laterally on the posteroanterior view or posteriorly on the lateral view in the costophrenic sulci, where even a few milliliters of fluid can be detected. The fluid is frequently not seen when it conforms to the curvature of the diaphragm and mimics an elevated diaphragm. This feature is referred to as subpulmonic pleural effusion. Lateral decubitus views are necessary to demonstrate the presence of free pleural fluid and also to differentiate the presence of free fluid, which

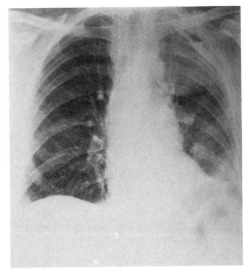

Fig 2–5.—Large density in left apex is loculated pleural effusion. Additional pleural effusion can be identified in left costophrenic angle.

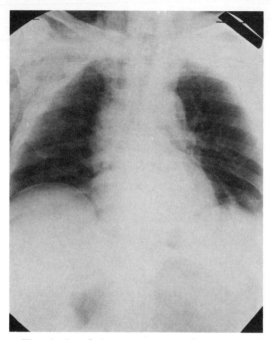

Fig 2–6.—Subcutaneous emphysema and pneumomediastinum. Mediastinal air outlines heart.

is due to active pleural disease, from unilateral thickened pleura, which will not change shape on decubitus views and is usually a residual from previous infections. However, pleural adhesions may not allow fluid to shift enough to distinguish between the trapped fluid and the underlying parenchymal lung disease. Careful radiographic technique and additional views usually allow the radiologist to determine which is present. Fluid can completely fill a pleural cavity and cause complete opacification and secondary compression of the lung.

Pleural masses may be single or multiple and may be seen radiologically as a mass with a broad base against the chest wall, with an obtuse angle between the pleura and the mass. Such masses can be one of many entities, including benign tumors of the pleura (mesotheliomas), rib tumors, or other chest-wall tumors protruding into the lung. When they are multiple, they may represent pleural metastasis. Lobulated pleural fluid or empyema also can have this appearance. Unilateral pleural calcifications are almost always due to previous hemothorax or pyothorax and do not represent active disease.

Cysts

Some cysts are filled with fluid and are seen as masses, whereas others are completely lucent, and some have fluid levels (Fig 2–7). Bronchogenic cysts or hydatid cysts are examples of fluid-filled cysts that usually present as masses. Communicating bronchogenic cysts, infectious cysts, cavitating neoplasms, lung abscesses, and pulmonary sequestrations are examples of cysts and cyst-like lesions that can have fluid levels. Besides fluid, fragments of tumor or secondary infective so-called fungus balls can be present in cavitated tumors. Fungus balls also can be present in cyst-like lesions in postinflammatory conditions. Certain inflammatory conditions have a propensity to develop cyst-like lesions or cavitation. This feature is true of tuberculosis, in which air-fluid levels or cysts may be seen in the involved segments, usually the upper lobes. Cyst-like lesions can also be seen in infections of *Aspergillus* and staphylococcal pneumonitis, especially in children. Both primary and secondary neoplasms can cavitate. Usually, these are squamous cell lesions and may be as small as 1 cm or as large as several centimeters in diameter. Obvious internal irregularity of the internal cyst wall with nodule-like

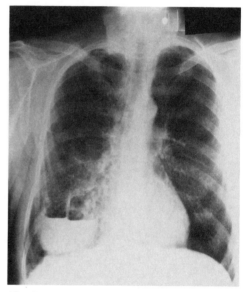

Fig 2–7.—Biloculated cyst in right lung base with air-fluid levels. There is hemorrhage into emphysematous bullae, probably secondary to anticoagulation.

filling defects within its lumen is more likely to be a tumor or an inflammatory process rather than some simple cyst. Simple cysts or bronchogenic cysts are usually smooth internally, with or without fluid or air-fluid levels. Sometimes air-filled cysts can be confused with emphysematous bullae or blebs or even loculated areas of pneumothorax. In certain patients with severe emphysema and scattered areas of pleural adhesions, large bullae may be impossible to distinguish from loculated pneumothorax.

ANGIOGRAPHY

Vascular Patterns and Abnormalities of the Lungs

In the normal upright chest, the arteries and veins of the lower lobes are larger and more prominently displayed than are their counterparts in the upper lobes (see Fig 2–1). This feature is present primarily because of the gravitational influence of the additional height from the low lung fields to the apex of the lung. This hydrostatic pressure can be measured directly on the roentgenogram. In the resting upright subject, very little flow goes through the upper pulmonary arteries and veins. This area acts as a reservoir for situations that demand increased circulation and ventilation. During exercise, flow increases in all areas of the lungs, and that in the upper and lower pulmonary arteries and veins will be increased equally. In the presence

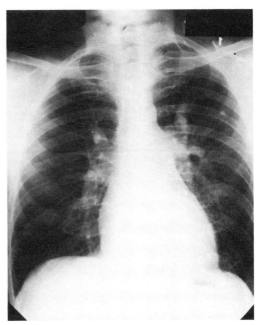

Fig 2–9.—Pulmonary arterial hypertension secondary to chronic left-to-right shunt (atrial septal defect). Note marked enlargement of central pulmonary vessels, with rapid tapering in middle third and virtual absence of vascular shadows beyond. Heart is somewhat enlarged.

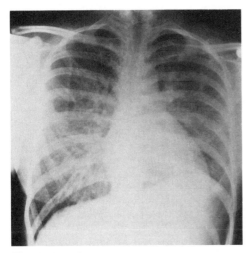

Fig 2–8.—Pulmonary edema secondary to head injury. Note symmetric involvement and obliteration of hilar shadows.

of a left-to-right shunt, the demand for the pulmonary arteries to accept blood flow is increased, and initially, this blood flow goes to the upper lobes; subsequently, the upper and lower lobes demonstrate equal distribution. In congestive failure in the upright patient, because the hydrostatic pressure is greater in the lower lobes, this area is the first to display interstitial edema as the pulmonary venous pressure increases and the oncotic pressure is overcome.[4] Therefore, there is a secondary constriction of the arteries and veins of the lower lobe, with shunting of the flow to the upper lobes, where the hydrostatic pressure is very low, and edema will appear in these regions only after significant levels of venous hypertension have been reached.

An additional pulmonary flow pattern occurs in right-to-left shunts that bypass the lungs. The most notable example is that of tetralogy of Fallot, in which there is stenosis of the subvalvular pulmonary region and a right-to-left shunt through a ventricular septal defect. There are other anatomical patterns of disease that result

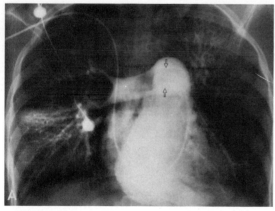
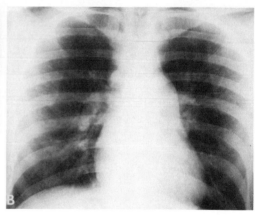

Fig 2–10.—Pulmonary embolism. **A,** pulmonary angiogram shows large thrombus within proximal lumen of right main pulmonary artery *(arrows)*, with additional large thrombus over saddle of right upper and lower lobe pulmonary arteries. There is decreased arterial perfusion to right upper lobe and left lower lobe. Thrombus within left lower pulmonary artery is not seen in this view. **B,** anteroposterior view shows decreased vascularity in right upper lobe and left base when compared with their respective opposite sides. Central pulmonary arteries are prominent bilaterally.

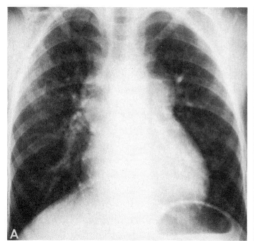
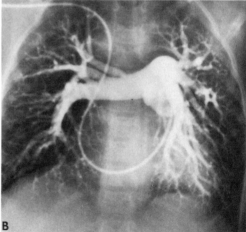
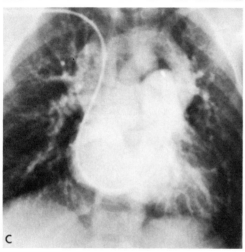

Fig 2–11.—Total anomalous pulmonary venous return. **A,** posteroanterior view of chest. Note prominent mass-like lesion in superior mediastinum and dilatation of pulmonary arteries and veins in uniform distribution throughout lungs. Pulmonary vascularity reflects a high-flow state, presumably from left-to-right shunt. Pattern of mediastinum is consistent with so-called "snowman" sign of total anomalous pulmonary venous return through left vertical vein. **B,** pulmonary angiogram demonstrates uniform dilatation of pulmonary arteries. **C,** venous phase shows ascending left vertical vein draining virtually all of pulmonary venous return into left innominate vein (left-to-right shunt), causing bulge of superior vena cava on right side of superior mediastinum.

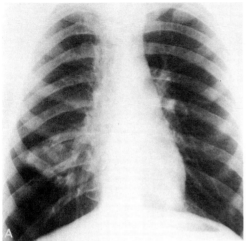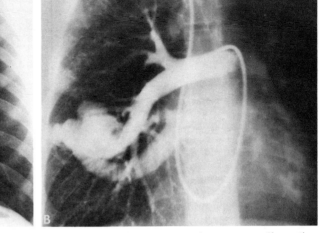

Fig 2-12.—**A,** posteroanterior view of chest shows large serpiginous vascular structure in right midlung. **B,** right pulmonary angiogram demonstrates huge arteriovenous malformation and fistulous communication with pulmonary vein.

in this same phenomenon. In agenesis of the left or right pulmonary artery, that particular lung demonstrates decreased flow. Furthermore, in certain types of postoperative shunts, such as the Blalock anastomosis of the subclavian artery to pulmonary artery, the ipsilateral side demonstrates a high flow while the contralateral side may persist in a low flow state (Figs 2–8 through 2–19).

Coronary Angiography

Coronary arterial bypass graft surgery is a relatively common cardiac surgical procedure (Figs

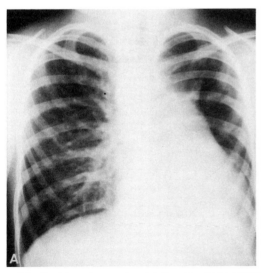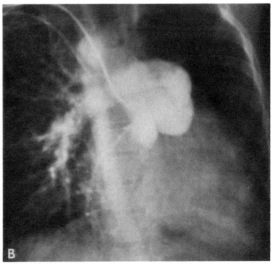

Fig 2-13.—Agenesis of left pulmonary artery and truncus arteriosus. **A,** posteroanterior view of chest. Prominent pulmonary arteries in right lung are compatible with high flow or left-to-right shunt. Left lung has smaller volume. Mediastinum is shifted to left, and arterial pattern is not prominent. Cardiac silhouette is prominent at level of pulmonary outflow tract. Heart is also enlarged. **B,** aortic root angiogram shows truncus arteriosus type I or II, with agenesis of left pulmonary artery and right aortic arch.

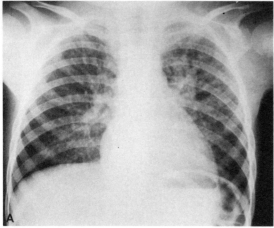
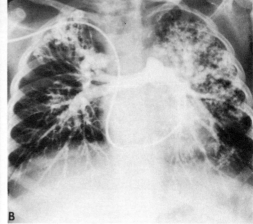

Fig 2–14.—Diffuse-type arteriovenous malformation. **A,** posteroanterior view of chest shows prominent arterial pattern, mostly in upper two thirds of lung fields. Appearance of left upper lung field suggests some type of infiltrate. Left ventricular outline is prominent. **B,** pulmonary angiogram demonstrates diffuse arteriovenous malformations in both upper lungs and scattered areas in midlung and left lower lobe, which accounts for nonhomogeneous appearance of prominent vascularity.

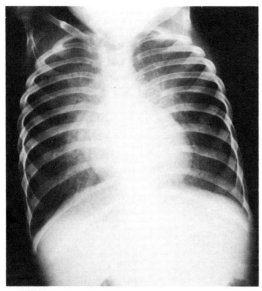

Fig 2–15.—Congenital stenosis of pulmonary veins. Central pulmonary edema is present bilaterally, with sparing of outer third of lung fields. This feature helps make differential diagnosis between respiratory distress syndrome and edema.

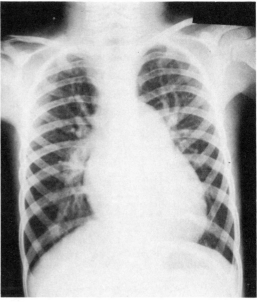

Fig 2–16.—Ventricular septal defect and pulmonary arterial hypertension. Note prominent pulmonary arterial flow pattern, with rapid tapering of vessels in middle third of each lung associated with cardiomegaly and prominent pulmonary outflow tract.

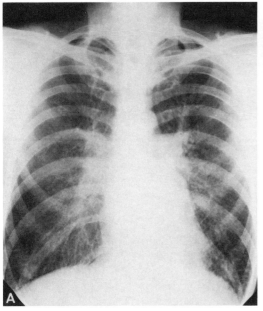
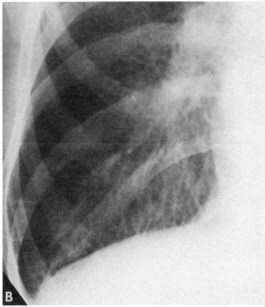

Fig 2–17.—Chronic interstitial edema and mitral valve stenosis. **A,** posteroanterior view of chest shows diffuse interstitial pattern throughout lungs. Left atrial appendage is prominent along left heart border. **B,** localized view of right lower lung field shows horizontal lines (Kerley B lines) at costophrenic angle, which represent fluid in interstitial septa.

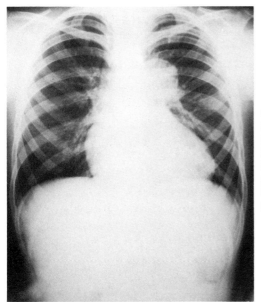

Fig 2–18.—Left pulmonary artery aneurysm secondary to pulmonary valve stenosis. Large mass adjacent to left hilum is pulmonary artery aneurysm mostly involving left pulmonary artery. Left pulmonary artery is in direct path of nozzle-like effect of blood streaming through stenotic pulmonary valve. This effect is almost never seen in subvalvular stenosis because of longer zone of stenosis.

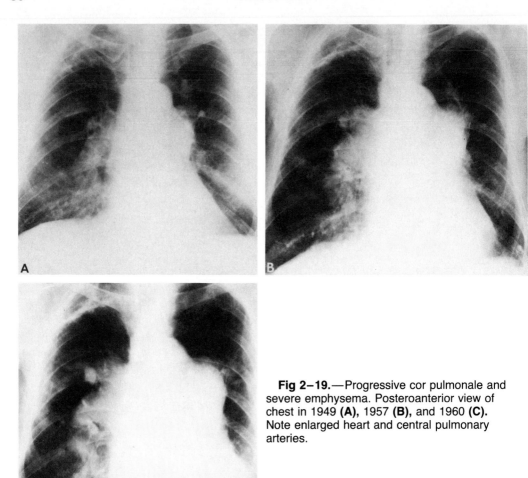

Fig 2–19.—Progressive cor pulmonale and severe emphysema. Posteroanterior view of chest in 1949 **(A)**, 1957 **(B)**, and 1960 **(C)**. Note enlarged heart and central pulmonary arteries.

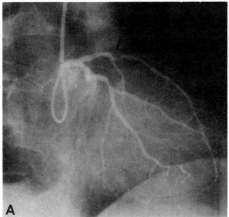
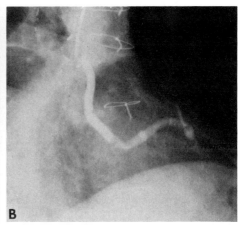

Fig 2–20.—Isolated left anterior descending coronary artery stenosis. **A,** right anterior oblique view of left coronary artery injection. Note stenosis of left anterior descending artery *(arrow)*. There is also a high-grade stenotic lesion in circumflex artery just proximal to first major obtuse marginal branch. **B,** bypass graft from aorta to distal left anterior descending artery. Note antegrade and retrograde filling of left anterior descending artery.

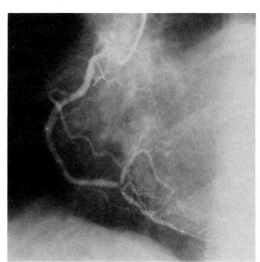

Fig 2–21.—Left anterior oblique view of right coronary artery injection. Stenosis is present at distal-most right coronary artery, involving proximal posterior descending branch.

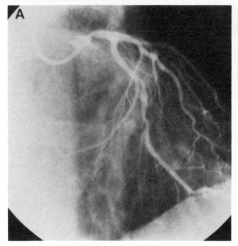 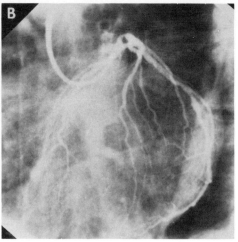

Fig 2–22.—Ostial stenosis of left coronary artery. **A,** right anterior oblique view. Note 75% focal stenosis at origin of artery. **B,** left anterior oblique view. Again, stenosis is identified. Because of position of catheter with its tip at area of stenosis, catheter spasm also must be included as cause of stenosis.

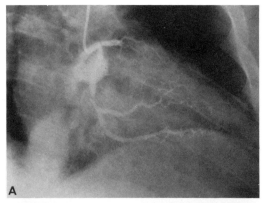
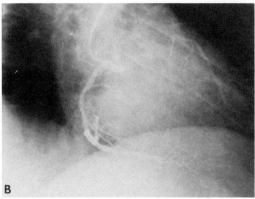

Fig 2–23.—Occluded left anterior descending artery. **A,** right anterior oblique view of left coronary artery injection. Abrupt occlusion of left anterior descending artery about 2 cm from its origin. Note high-grade stenosis in distal main circumflex coronary artery and at proximal second main marginal branch. **B,** right anterior oblique view of right coronary artery injection. Note septal perforating arteries that refill the distal left anterior descending artery from the right coronary artery.

2–20 through 2–23). The most frequent indication is arteriosclerotic disease, and generally obstructive lesions need to be bypassed. Occasionally, aneurysms or fistulas of the coronary arteries may be the initial problem. The chest film gives no specific clue to coronary artery disease, although disease may be suspected because of generalized arteriosclerosis that may be evidenced by calcification of the aorta or of the brachiocephalic vessels—findings that can be seen on the chest film. At fluoroscopy, calcification of the coronary arteries can be seen, although it is an unreliable sign of significant stenosis of the coronary arteries. Sequelae of myocardial infarction may be demonstrated on a chest film or on fluoroscopy as aneurysms or akinetic segments of the left ventricle. The coronary angiogram is essential in outlining the anatomic presentation of the arterial disease necessary for establishing the indications for surgery and planning the surgical approach.

REFERENCES

1. Felson B.: *Chest Roentgenology*. Philadelphia, W.B. Saunders Co., 1973.
2. Fraser R.G., Paré J.A.P.: *Diagnosis of Diseases of the Chest: An Integrated Study Based on the Abnormal Roentgenogram*. Philadelphia, W.B. Saunders Co., 1970, vols. 1 and 2.
3. Kerr I.H.: The preoperative chest x-ray. *Br. J. Anaesth*. 46:558, 1974.
4. Kostuk W., et al.: Correlations between the chest film and hemodynamics in acute myocardial infarction. *Circulation* 48:624, 1973.

3 / Preoperative Medication

SAIT TARHAN
FROUKJE M. BEYNEN

BECAUSE patient apprehension before surgery is disturbing emotionally and should be controlled, premedication should provide a patient who is comfortably sedated, free from apprehension, and able to cooperate in the preliminary preparations for anesthesia. Different drugs and drug combinations can be chosen to accomplish this effect. However, a preoperative visit by the patient's anesthesiologist also may be important. The confidence developed through this association can be augmented by mild doses of depressant drugs to achieve the desired state of sedation.

There is no general agreement or specific indication for the selection of preoperative medications. The choices are many: sedatives, narcotics, potentiating agents, tranquilizers, and vagolytic agents. Premedication often consists of two or more compounds from different pharmacologic groups. There is no standard procedure to evaluate the efficacy of this premedication. Visually evoked responses, catecholamine excretion, blood pressure, pulse, and respiration have been used as objective measures of sedation and apprehension,[2] yet the results have been difficult to correlate with clinical behavior. Arbitrarily chosen dosages determined from common clinical practice have been used for the administration of different drugs. Recently, it has been claimed that none of the drugs used as premedication at any dose level has any significant effect when compared with a placebo.[2] However, these studies also may have been affected by the lack of sensitivity for demonstrating changes in apprehension and anxiety.[3] In spite of these recent publications, the practice of premedication continues, and the common belief still holds that premedication allays anxiety, decreases respiratory secretions, assists anesthesia, provides some analgesia during surgery,[9] and makes the operating room experience more pleasant for the patient and the work of the anesthesiologist a little easier. Some anesthesiologists believe that possible undesirable depressant effects of preoperative drugs in patients with diminished cardiac responses are more than compensated for by the beneficial situation of having calm, sedated patients for the induction of anesthesia, and consequently, they favor having a properly sedated patient before open-heart surgery.

Our practice is to premedicate the patient routinely, on the assumption that any patient who is to undergo cardiac surgery has considerable anxiety. Some of these patients may need multiple monitoring and infusion lines before induction. Some patients with angina or hypertension cannot be optimally controlled by medical management, and anxiety may add further stress to their underlying problem. Effects of increased anxiety on the heart rate and blood pressure are known. The heart rate and blood pressure are also the determinants of myocardial oxygen consumption.[5] Therefore, a high level of anxiety before surgery in patients with compromised coronary heart disease may be detrimental.

Sudden death of patients awaiting coronary artery surgery has been described.[8] It occurs among patients who have a high degree (90%) of narrowing of major coronary arteries supplying large portions of the left ventricular myocardium. The precise reasons for myocardial infarction in these patients have not been determined. The role of expectations and the anxiety of approaching surgery in causing increased heart rate and blood pressure could be partly responsible.

PREMEDICANT DRUGS

Depending on the clinical experiences and favored routine, the anesthesiologist may order a sedative, a tranquilizer, an analgesic drug, or a vagolytic agent as premedication, and any combination of these drugs could provide satisfactory results as long as the anesthesiologist is familiar with the effects and side effects of the agent.

Morphine

Of the narcotic-analgesic drugs used for premedication, our choice is morphine sulfate with a sedative-class drug (pentobarbital). The following are the properties of morphine and of the entire narcotic-analgesic drug group[12]:

1. They depress response to discrete stimuli more than they depress overall level of consciousness (in contrast to the sedatives).
2. They depress carbon dioxide response even in the conscious patient. However, they rarely produce apnea or unconsciousness unless (a) the patient is very old or chronically ill, (b) massive doses are used, or (c) other sedative drugs are used simultaneously.
3. They can produce either dysphoria or euphoria, depending on (a) which drug is chosen, (b) how the patient responds to narcotics in general and to the narcotic being used in particular, and (c) whether scopolamine or diazepam is also given.
4. They are much more likely than sedative-group drugs to cause postural hypotension or bradycardia or both.
5. Their effects are completely reversed by naloxone.

For adults, pentobarbital is given orally (dose, 2 mg/kg; maximum, 100 mg) two hours before operation; and morphine is administered intramuscularly (dose, 1 mg/5 kg; maximum, 10 mg) one hour before operation. Pentobarbital provides sedation that is dose-dependent and can easily progress to hypnosis. It may produce amnesia, and the drug does not depress the carbon dioxide response until sleep occurs.[12] The drug often continues to produce sleepiness in the recovery room. However, this effect after a long cardiac procedure may not be as pronounced as the effect after shorter procedures.

Studies have shown that a combination of barbiturate and narcotic (morphine) for preoperative medication is safe and results in no marked deleterious cardiovascular or respiratory effects.[9] Morphine's sedative anxiety-reducing and analgesic actions are satisfactory in terms of not depressing the respiration with the dosage of 0.14 mg/kg.[9]

Morphine sulfate has been used for years to treat patients with heart disease. It is also an important drug in the therapy of acute pulmonary edema due to left heart failure and was the first drug to be introduced as a preoperative medicant. It is believed to possess definite advantages—for instance, relief of pain and decreasing anxiety.[3]

Morphine also is frequently used for pain relief in patients with acute myocardial infarction. Clinical experience suggests that no major adverse cardiac effects occur when this drug is properly used in patients with cardiac disease. However, some recent studies have shown that its administration to dogs caused some increase in coronary vascular resistance and a decrease in coronary blood flow.[7] In one study involving dogs, the decrease in coronary blood flow was 28%, with an increase of 31% in vascular resistance 15 minutes after the administration of the drug, yet the dosage of morphine in that experiment was 2.0 mg/kg body weight,[14] approximately the equivalent of the morphine dosage used for anesthesia for cardiac surgery. However, another study done on human subjects with morphine sulfate at a dosage of 0.2 mg/kg[7] (dosage used for premedication) revealed a minimal (8%) increase in coronary blood flow and a significant (11%) decrease in coronary vascular resistance 15 minutes after morphine administration (Fig 3–1). Although there was a slight increase in heart rate (3.1 beats per minute) at 15 minutes and a reduction in arterial pressure, neither was significant.

Clinical implications of the results of this study are clear. Unlike dogs, patients, including those with coronary artery disease, do not respond to the administration of morphine by the constriction of coronary arteries. Because morphine in premedicating doses does not significantly alter myocardial oxygen requirements or coronary blood flow,[7] one can conclude that the drug is safe as a premedication for patients who are to undergo cardiac surgery, even for those with coronary artery disease.

Diazepam

Diazepam, both by the parenteral and oral routes, has been widely used as a premedicant drug. It is useful in inducing anesthesia and am-

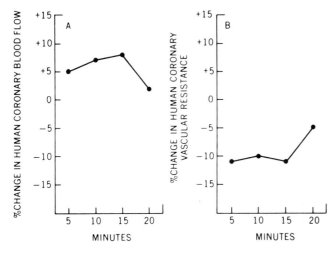

Fig 3–1.—Percentage of change in coronary blood flow and coronary vascular resistance in ten cases 5, 10, 15, and 20 minutes after administration of morphine. (From Leaman, et al.[7] Used by permission.)

nesia during direct-current cardioversion.[15] The drug also is prescribed frequently for the management of patients with angina. Because the anginal pain is often related to stressful stimuli, the beneficial effects of this tranquilizing drug are believed to be mediated through its action on the psyche.[1] Diazepam also has been advocated as an acceptable alternative to morphine-barbiturate combinations as a premedication if it is given orally in doses of 20 mg.[9] However, there is still controversy about its effect on ventilation. One study reported no circulatory or respiratory depression with diazepam at doses of 10 or 20 mg orally.[9] However, a different study[1] using diazepam intravenously, 0.1 mg/kg body weight, with blood gas and hemodynamic studies repeated five and 15 minutes after the injection, revealed that the $Paco_2$ was increased and the Pao_2 and pH decreased in five minutes but that the values returned to near control levels after 15 minutes. The heart rates of these patients were not altered, but the aortic pressure decreased significantly (average 7 to 8 mm Hg in mean aortic pressure). The patients with a low aortic basal pressure usually showed no decrease after diazepam administration. The particular interest in this study was the consistent decrease in left ventricular end-diastolic pressure. This substantial decrease was more obvious when basal left ventricular end-diastolic pressure was elevated in some of the patients who had significant coronary artery disease.[1]

Tension-time index and myocardial oxygen consumption also were significantly decreased.[1] The decrease in left ventricular end-diastolic pressure possibly was due to a decrease in afterload or in venous return or in both. The combination of these effects could reduce intracavitary volume, myocardial wall tension, and left ventricular myocardial oxygen consumption.[1] Therefore, the data suggest that, in addition to the sedative effects of diazepam, there is a nitroglycerin-like action on the coronary and systemic circulations.[1] The study concluded that diazepam was the agent of choice in sedating patients who have heart disease.[1] The drug causes minimal depression of respiration, has negligible side effects, and can improve cardiac function.

Topical Nitroglycerin

During the past few years, topical nitroglycerin has enjoyed a revival as a therapeutic agent, especially for patients with unstable or nocturnal angina. It provides sustained, gradual absorption as a prophylactic agent for the prevention of angina pectoris, and it is as effective as sublingual nitroglycerin.[10] Effects on blood pressure, heart rate, and left ventricular end-diastolic diameter are similar to those of oral nitroglycerin. A typical response to sublingual nitroglycerin is a slight decrease in heart rate and blood pressure[10] and a significant decrease in the end-diastolic diameter within the first 15 minutes of administration of the drug; these effects persist for less than one hour (Fig 3–2). In contrast, topical nitroglycerin produces a gradual change in the same measurements, and these changes increase for up to one hour and can be maintained for as

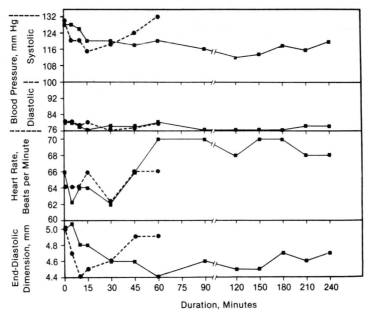

Fig 3–2.—Effects of sublingual nitroglycerin (circle and dotted line) and topical nitroglycerin (square and solid line) on systolic and diastolic blood pressure, heart rate, and left ventricular end-diastolic dimension. (From Miner and Conti.[10] Used by permission.)

long as four hours. We find that topical nitroglycerin application is a useful adjunct to the premedication of coronary patients. If the drug is applied one or one and a half hours before surgery in combination with other premedication, it may act as a prophylactic agent in preventing angina[10] during the preoperative period and induction of anesthesia.

Nitroglycerin ointment is available as 2% glycerol trinitrate in a lanolin base. The ointment is squeezed onto a premeasured strip of paper (1.3 to 5 cm), which is then placed on the skin and secured with an adhesive. The usual dosage ranges from 1.3 to 5 cm every four hours, although higher dosages have been used in patients with recurrent angina.[10]

Patients who take nitroglycerin sublingually may have a reduction in their Pa_{O_2}.[6] The same problem also may exist with the application of nitroglycerin ointment. Therefore, increased oxygen concentration by mask should be provided to patients who receive nitroglycerin ointment before surgery.

Anticholinergic Drugs

Patients are commonly given anticholinergic drugs to prevent bradycardia and to reduce respiratory tract secretions. Bradycardia is usually the result of vagal reflex or the pharmacologic effects of repeated doses of succinylcholine or of an anesthetic overdose or a combination of these.

Vagal reflex and succinylcholine-induced bradycardias are most common among children and young adults, and anesthetic-induced bradycardia is most common in old and very sick patients.

Few patients have important problems with airway secretions, because the anesthetic agents usually do not intensify the problem. Thus, the use of an antisialagogue drug is questioned by some. Patients who smoke or who are obese may be more likely to have secretions, and these can be treated as they occur, rather than exposing all patients to an unneeded drug.[12]

Some anesthesiologists believe that a parasympatholytic drug, usually atropine, should be administered routinely to the patient, especially to a child, to counteract the increase in vagal tone; the intramuscular route is used most often, and the drug is given 45 minutes before the induction of anesthesia. Others advocate the intravenous use of atropine just before the intravenous administration of succinylcholine to avoid the frequent occurrence of succinylcholine-induced bradyarrhythmias.

Our group does not use anticholinergic drugs in the premedication schedule. Our experience over the years has shown that bronchial secretions are not a problem, because belladonna drugs are omitted from premedication. However, use of the anticholinergic drugs may cause an undesirable increase in heart rate.[11] If a vagolytic drug is needed during anesthesia, atropine can be given intravenously in small, controlled increments, until the desired effect is achieved.

PREMEDICATION OF PATIENTS WITH CORONARY ARTERY DISEASE

Since the anxiety of patients awaiting surgery for coronary heart disease can cause increases in heart rate and blood pressure[5] and can provoke an angina attack, this group of patients may require heavier sedation than other types of cardiac surgical patients. This goal can be accomplished by the use of several different combinations of drugs. The choices of drugs are no different, however, than those for patients with valve replacement—only the dosage of the drugs changes.

PREMEDICATION OF CHILDREN

There are few standard rules regarding premedication of pediatric patients. Many different combinations of drugs can be given, and there is no unanimity of opinion regarding the type of sedative drug that should be used as premedication. However, whatever is given should be individualized, depending on the degree of apprehension of the child. Advance planning of the anesthetic also may be considered in selection of premedication.

Infants with congenital heart disease generally tolerate premedication well, and medication that is carefully chosen and given in proper dosages usually allows lesser amounts of anesthetic agents to be used during surgery. To achieve a sufficient preoperative sedation is especially important in cyanotic children. A quiet, smooth induction in a child already half asleep prevents an increase in the cyanosis that so readily may happen in a crying, straining child.

Small doses of droperidol (Table 3–1) can provide reliable sedative action and may potentiate the effects of other premedicant drugs given simultaneously, such as promethazine or diazepam, and with the dosages shown in Table 3–1, there are no significant observable depressant effects of those drugs on the cardiovascular or respiratory system.[13]

TABLE 3–1.—INTRAMUSCULAR PREMEDICATIONS FOR PEDIATRIC CARDIAC PATIENTS*

AGENT	DOSE
Atropine	0.005 to 0.01 mg/kg body weight
Droperidol	0.5 mg/3 to 5 kg body weight (maximum, 5 mg)
Promethazine	1 mg/kg body weight
Diazepam	0.2 mg/kg body weight

*Data from Santoli et al.[13]

Optimal sedation is especially needed in patients in whom an increased sympathetic tone followed by increased contractility of the myocardium may endanger the outflow of blood from the ventricle—that is, patients with muscular subaortic stenosis, tetralogy of Fallot, pulmonary valvular stenosis, and infundibular right ventricular hypertrophy.[4]

Patients with valvular stenosis, especially mitral valve stenosis, also require good sedation, because the sympathetic overtones cause tachycardia. This rapid heart rate in turn causes the diastolic filling time of the left ventricle to be shortened, and as a result, cardiac output is reduced.

Our premedication schedule for children consists of pentobarbital given rectally (dose, 4 mg/kg) and morphine given intramuscularly according to weight (0.2 mg/kg); however, children who weigh less than 10 kg generally do not receive morphine.

REFERENCES

1. Côté P., Guéret P., Bourassa M.G.: Systemic and coronary hemodynamic effects of diazepam in patients with normal and diseased coronary arteries. *Circulation* 50:1210, 1974.
2. Forrest W.H. Jr., Brown C.R., Brown B.W.: Subjective responses to six common preoperative medications. *Anesthesiology* 47:241, 1977.
3. Halpern L.M.: Rational choice of preoperative medication: The Emperor's new clothes? editorial. *Anesthesiology* 47:239, 1977.
4. Janssen P.J.: Anesthesia for corrective open-heart surgery of congenital defects beyond infancy. *Int. Anesthesiol. Clin.* 14:205, 1976.
5. Jobes D.R.: Anesthesia for cardiac surgery. *Surg. Clin. North Am.* 55:893, 1975.

6. Kopman E.A., et al.: Arterial hypoxemia following the administration of sublingual nitroglycerin. *Am. Heart J.* 96:444, 1978.
7. Leaman D.M., et al.: Effects of morphine sulfate on human coronary blood flow. *Am. J. Cardiol.* 41:324, 1978.
8. Lewis B.S., Gotsman M.S.: Sudden death in patients awaiting coronary artery surgery. *Thorax* 29:209, 1974.
9. Lyons S.M., Clarke R.S.J., Vulgaraki K.: The premedication of cardiac surgical patients: A clinical comparison of four regimens. *Anaesthesia* 30:459, 1975.
10. Miner J.A., Conti C.R.: Topical nitroglycerin for ischemic heart disease. *J.A.M.A.* 239:2166, 1978.
11. Moffitt E.A.: Anesthesia and supportive care during operation, in Ellis F.H. Jr. (ed.): *Surgery for Acquired Mitral Valve Disease*. Philadelphia, W.B. Saunders Co., 1967.
12. Ominsky A.J.: Preanesthetic medication: An obsolete practice? Read before the annual meeting of the American Society of Anesthesiologists, Chicago, October 21 to 25, 1978.
13. Santoli F.M., Pensa P.M., Azzolina G.: Anesthesia in open-heart surgery for correction of congenital heart diseases in children over 1 year of age. *Int. Anesthesiol. Clin.* 14:165, 1976.
14. Vatner S.F., Marsh J.D., Swain J.A.: Effects of morphine on coronary and left ventricular dynamics in conscious dogs. *J. Clin. Invest.* 55:207, 1975.
15. Vinge L.N., Wyant G.M., Lopez J.F.: Diazepam in cardioversion. *Can. Anaesth. Soc. J.* 18:166, 1971.

4 / Anesthetic Agents and Anesthesia for Cardiac Surgery

CARL R. NOBACK
HUGO S. RAIMUNDO

SEVERAL anesthetic techniques have been advocated for the induction and maintenance of anesthesia for patients undergoing open- and closed-cardiac surgery. In the vast majority of patients, however, anesthesia is induced by use of a rapid-acting barbiturate, followed by the use of a muscle relaxant to facilitate tracheal intubation and produce skeletal muscle relaxation. Analgesia and amnesia are maintained by inhalation or intravenous administration of anesthetics, or both, so that the level of anesthesia suited to the condition of the patient and the needs of the procedure is achieved.

In addition to the usual factors to be considered in the planning of the anesthetic management (for example, previous anesthetic experiences, drug intake, associated pulmonary disease), particular attention should be paid to the status of the ventricular function and the pathophysiologic changes produced by the underlying cardiac disease. With this background knowledge and appropriate monitoring, one can use different anesthetic drugs and adjust the cardiovascular hemodynamics to safely achieve the anesthetic goals.

CARDIOVASCULAR EFFECTS OF ANESTHETIC DRUGS AND NEUROMUSCULAR BLOCKING AGENTS

Some features of drugs are particularly pertinent to the conduct of anesthesia for cardiovascular surgery. A patient's specific disease, previous drug therapy, or previous surgery may alter the dosage of a drug required for a given effect, or even alter the effect itself. Merin[52] addressed himself to this point when he said:

. . . the only safe way to anesthetize such [patients with diseased hearts] is to adjust the concentration (dose) of whatever anesthetic is used to be comparative with effective ventricular function as determined by the best available monitor(s).

Inhalational Anesthetics

Nitrous Oxide

The dose-effect relationship of nitrous oxide for healthy subjects has been reported: a 20% dose is equivalent to 14 mg of morphine, 40% results in an inability of the patient to cooperate, 60% results in nearly complete amnesia, 80% results in unconsciousness, and 100% results in lack of movement to surgical stimulation (minimum alveolar concentration [MAC][34]). The presence of systemic disease may significantly alter these relationships. The direct effect of nitrous oxide on the myocardium is a depression of contractility.[46] Additionally, nitrous oxide produces signs of increased sympathetic nervous system activity by its action on the suprapontine region of the brain.[29, 54] These signs include peripheral vascular constriction and increased serum levels of norepinephrine.[64] Eisele and Smith[20] substituted 40% nitrous oxide in oxygen for 40% nitrogen in oxygen and showed a decrease of 15% to 20% in cardiac output secondary to decreases in heart rate and contractility. Concomitantly, an increase of 20% in systemic vascular resistance was observed. The net effect on systolic blood pressure was negligible. They also demonstrated elevated levels of circulating catecholamines, especially norepinephrine. Thus, inhalation of 40% nitrous oxide can depress ventricular function in patients without coronary artery disease. In a follow-up study,

Eisele et al.[22] demonstrated that the inhalation of 40% nitrous oxide (after coronary angiography) by patients with coronary artery disease depressed arterial pressure 5% and decreased differential left ventricular pressure (dp/dt) by 14%, with an increase of 21% in left ventricular end-diastolic pressure in patients with impaired left ventricular function.

Nitrous oxide is not a "complete" anesthetic by itself, and, as such, it must be supplemented with other drugs: oxygen, muscle relaxants, and other anesthetics. The weak sympathetic stimulatory and cardiovascular effects of nitrous oxide are still evident when it is combined with other anesthetics in healthy volunteers[34] (Table 4–1); the addition of nitrous oxide to halothane-oxygen anesthesia results in less myocardial depression than that of halothane-oxygen alone.[79] This effect was shown to be in part due to the sympathetic stimulatory effects of nitrous oxide, because the halothane concentration was held constant. An addition of 60% nitrous oxide to 0.55% end-tidal halothane in patients undergoing surgery for aortic and mitral valvular replacements produced no change in mean arterial pressure, right atrial pressure, left atrial pressure, pulmonary artery pressure, heart rate, cardiac index, stroke volume index, systemic vascular resistance, or pulmonary vascular resistance.[79] Stoelting et al.,[79] therefore, recommended 60% nitrous oxide as a useful adjunct to low end-tidal halothane concentrations for valve replacement surgery.

The results are different when nitrous oxide is added to inflow concentrations of enflurane of between 2% and 3%. When the concentration of nitrous oxide reached or exceeded 20%, Bennett et al.[2] demonstrated significant dose-related decreases in cardiac output, stroke volume, and mean arterial pressure. The cardiac depressant effects of nitrous oxide are even more noticeable when it is added to narcotic anesthesia.[92] Stoelting and Gibbs[78] reported that the addition of nitrous oxide to morphine in patients with both valvular disease and ischemic heart disease resulted in a decrease in stroke volume of between 20% and 25%.

Hug[34] noted three actions of nitrous oxide: (1) because it decreases the dosage requirements of other drugs, it limits the cardiovascular effects of these drugs; (2) in the presence of a stable dose of a general anesthetic (particularly halothane), it tends to increase blood pressure by increasing systemic vascular resistance; and (3) the direct cardiac depressant action of nitrous oxide may be masked by cardiac depression induced by volatile anesthetics. This accompanying depressant action may severely limit or preclude the use of nitrous oxide in critically ill patients. If undesirable hypotension occurs during its administration, the inspired concentration of nitrous oxide may be decreased or eliminated completely. Normalization of the blood pressure should be evident within one or two minutes.

Halothane

The potential dose-dependent depression of cardiac function of halothane limits its use as a sole anesthetic agent. In critically ill patients, concentrations of halothane less than 1 MAC can produce anesthesia and potentiate the relaxant effects of nondepolarizing blocking agents.[55] Mechanisms of cardiovascular depression include direct action on cardiac and vascular smooth muscles and depression of the sympathetic nervous system. The primary effect is to inhibit the intensity with which contractile elements generate tension, and a secondary effect is to shorten the duration of the active state of contraction.[5] These effects are accomplished by

TABLE 4–1.—CARDIOVASCULAR CHANGES WITH NITROUS OXIDE AND AFTER ITS ADDITION TO PREEXISTING GENERAL ANESTHETICS

	EFFECT			
MEASUREMENT	NITROUS OXIDE	NITROUS OXIDE–HALOTHANE	NITROUS OXIDE–ENFLURANE	NITROUS OXIDE–MORPHINE
Blood pressure	None	Increased	None	None
Heart rate	Decreased	None	Decreased	Decreased
Cardiac output	Decreased	None	Increased	Decreased
Systemic vascular resistance	Increased	Increased	None	Increased
Central venous pressure	Increased	Increased	None	Increased

an inhibition of the release of membrane-bound calcium involved in excitation-contraction coupling.[5] Halothane has been shown to cause a dose-related depression of isometric (isovolemic) contraction (documented by the use of a strain-gauge arch sewn to the ventricular epicardium[48]) and of isotonic performance (documented by repeat cardiac output determinations[18]). The depression of contractility slowly recovers as the duration of anesthesia progresses,[58] but the amplitude of the I-J wave of the ballistocardiogram does not recover, as does cardiac output.[19] Elevation of the blood pressure during halothane anesthesia does not reverse the depression of ventricular function, thus indicating that cardiac depression is an important part of the mechanism for hypotension.[23] Eger et al.[18] showed a dose-dependent decrease in cardiac output (to 50% of control with 2% halothane) due to equal decreases in stroke volume and contractility. No change was seen in heart rate, but right atrial pressure increased and mean blood pressure decreased along with cardiac output. Theye and Michenfelder[85] determined that total-body and myocardial oxygen consumption decreased along with cardiac output. In patients undergoing coronary artery bypass grafting, halothane for induction decreased the cardiac index by 28%, mean arterial pressure by 22%, and heart rate by 10%.[49]

The depressant effects of halothane may be reversed by intravenously administered calcium, noncatecholamine-containing sympathomimetic agents (ephedrine or mephenteramine), administration of 100% oxygen and hyperventilation to hasten pulmonary excretion, augmented venous return, and anticholinergic agents to treat bradycardia.[34] In certain circumstances, however, the negative inotropic effect of halothane may prove, within limits, to be beneficial. With the fixed coronary blood flow of coronary atherosclerosis, halothane may blunt the increase in myocardial work and oxygen demand that occurs with sympathetic stimulation. Severe decreases in arterial pressure can decrease flow and myocardial oxygen supply. The use of halothane in patients with congestive heart failure is relatively contraindicated.

Cardiac output may additionally be altered by rhythm disturbances, the most common of which are bigeminy, nodal rhythms, and junctional and premature ventricular contractions.[34] Rhythm disturbances are in part due to the effect of halothane in sensitizing the myocardium to circulating catecholamines. Therefore, the dose of exogenous epinephrine should be limited, except for resuscitation purposes, to approximately 1 µg/kg in ten minutes, not to exceed 4 µg/kg/hour.[36]

Although adrenergic blocking agents may increase the sensitivity of the patient to the cardiovascular depressant actions of halothane, treatment with propranolol should be continued up to the time of surgery. The continued presence of propranolol seems to decrease the incidence of severe perioperative dysrhythmias, tachycardia, and hypertension.[41] Continuation of therapy with cardiac glycosides perioperatively is also favored, as it has been demonstrated in dogs that digoxin can antagonize or reverse the cardiovascular depressant effects of halothane.[62]

Enflurane

At equivalent MAC, enflurane produces greater muscular relaxation than does halothane and potentiates nondepolarizing muscle relaxants to a greater degree.[27] Myocardial contractility is decreased in a dose-related fashion, as with halothane; however, the magnitude of depression is greater with enflurane, contrary to early reports. In isolated papillary muscles of the cat exposed to equal MAC of a given anesthetic, Brown and Crout[5] determined the following order of depressant activity, from most to least depressant of contractility:

enflurane > halothane > methoxyflurane > cyclopropane > diethyl ether

In general, heart rate increases and systemic vascular resistance decreases because of decreased activity of the sympathetic nervous system and a direct depressant action on contractile elements, similar to that of halothane. Calverley et al.[6] found that 1 MAC of enflurane decreased cardiac output 26%, stroke volume 40%, systemic vascular resistance 15%, and blood pressure 36%, while heart rate increased 22%. A value of 1.5 MAC of enflurane further decreases stroke volume but not blood pressure or cardiac output. A value of 2 MAC of enflurane could not be achieved without producing profound hypotension. The therapeutic index of enflurane is therefore low, and there is little margin of safety.

The sympathomimetic response seen when

nitrous oxide is added to halothane is not evident when it is added to enflurane.[65] Thus, nitrous oxide offers little protection against the cardiovascular depressant actions of enflurane. As with halothane, the depressant activity may be beneficial in patients with fixed coronary blood flow (presuming coronary perfusion pressure is maintained), because myocardial blood flow decreases in parallel with decreased myocardial work and myocardial oxygen demand.[53]

Sensitization to catecholamines is less with enflurane than with halothane, and dysrhythmias, when they occur, are less severe.[40] In contrast to halothane, enflurane use is associated with cardiovascular instability in patients receiving chronic therapy with propranolol. Horan et al.[33] found greater hemodynamic changes with enflurane when equal anesthetic doses of halothane and enflurane were administered to dogs undergoing propranolol treatment. More impairment of contractility was noted, and loss of blood was tolerated less well; therefore, the concentration of enflurane should be limited in patients receiving propranolol chronically.

In our anesthetic practice, we no longer use other inhalational agents.

Intravenous Anesthetics

Sodium Thiopental (Pentothal)

Thiopental was introduced to anesthetic practice by Lundy in 1934 and has since become the most widely used ultra-short-acting barbiturate for the induction of anesthesia and serves as the prototype of its class. Its cardiovascular effects are dose-related and proportional to the circulating plasma levels. In the patient with a compromised myocardium, the usual large intravenous boluses for induction may produce excessive cardiac depression.

Thiopental is a direct cardiac depressant,[57] and decreased myocardial function is shown by a prolonged preejection period, decreased left ventricular ejection time, and an increased ratio of preejection period to left ventricular ejection time in patients with or without cardiovascular disease.[13] A dose of 4 mg/kg may depress the cardiac index by 10% to 25% and stroke volume by 35%, while heart rate may increase.[47, 86] With thiopental use, the heart rate may increase 19% (36% during intubation), with increases of 30% in cardiac index and of 23% in systolic blood pressure.[86] Venous capacitance may be increased because of decreased sympathetic tone[63] and increased peripheral pooling. The observed decrease in cardiac output may be due to any combination of the following[34]: (1) direct depression of cardiac contractility, (2) decreased filling pressure due to peripheral pooling, and (3) decreased sympathetic outflow from the CNS. The degree of hypotension is reduced by compensatory increases in heart rate and peripheral vascular resistance (32%).[8] The speed of injection influences the degree of hypotension. With slow infusions, there is time for compensatory mechanisms to become effective. Decreases in arterial pressure are seen within 90 seconds, and recovery begins by three minutes.[26] The desired depth of anesthesia can be reached with incremental doses of 0.5 to 1 mg/kg, and the magnitude of cardiac changes is minimized.

In patients with poor left ventricular function, thiopental may induce further impairment of contractility. The drug selected for induction should produce little or no cardiac depression (for example, fentanyl or diazepam). The existence of fixed coronary flow with good left ventricular function may be an indication for thiopental, as myocardial oxygen consumption will be decreased by the negative inotropic effects, if it is assumed that the compensatory tachycardia is blocked (for example, by propranolol).

Diazepam

Induction as well as anesthesia may be accomplished with diazepam. Although most patients may tolerate as much as 1 mg of diazepam per kilogram of body weight, some patients experience depression of respiratory and cardiovascular function when much lower doses are used.[34] Low doses of diazepam (0.13 mg/kg) have little effect on cardiac output, while large doses (0.77 mg/kg) decrease stroke volume by 30%.[60] A decrease in cardiac output secondary to the decrease in stroke volume is noted, and this is associated with a decrease of between 5% and 20% in arterial pressure.[34]

The cardiac depressant effects of diazepam are more evident when the drug is used with a narcotic. A dose of 5 mg of diazepam after morphine administration (2 mg/kg) produced decreases in heart rate and mean arterial pressure, with an increase in peripheral vascular resistance.[70] A second dose of diazepam further reduced systolic blood pressure. After 50 μg of fentanyl per kilogram, 10 mg of diazepam decreased stroke volume, cardiac output, blood pressure, and peripheral vascular resistance and increased central venous pressure with no change in heart rate.[68] Thus, cardiovascular depression can be seen when diazepam is given after morphine and fentanyl.

Increases in coronary blood flow have been noted after the administration of diazepam, and the increase was greater in patients with coronary artery disease than in normal subjects.[35] Diazepam also decreases left ventricular end-diastolic pressure by as much as one third in patients whose values were increased previously.[11] Decreases in myocardial oxygen consumption and left ventricular stroke work also have been found after the administration of diazepam. Small incremental doses (2.5 to 5 mg) intravenously, titrated to effect, are advocated for induction.

Droperidol

The concept of neuroleptanalgesia was introduced by de Castro and Mundeleer[14] in 1959. In 1966, Foldes et al.[28] used the term "neuroleptanesthesia" to describe the addition of nitrous oxide to droperidol and fentanyl, and it is in this context that droperidol is often used. Droperidol (dehydrobenzperidol) is a butyrophenone, and, like other major tranquilizers, can produce a neuroleptic state that is characterized by suppression of affect, slowing of motor function, and an outwardly calm appearance. The half-life of droperidol is 2 to 3 hours, and its duration of effect is 6 to 12 hours; the usual pharmacologic agents do not reverse its effect. In addition to its tranquilizing properties, droperidol has an antiemetic effect, reduces total-body oxygen consumption by 25% with a 10-mg dose, and suppresses temperature-regulating mechanisms.[34] Because its effect on sedation is variable, droperidol should be used with other drugs to provide anesthesia.

After the administration of droperidol, hypotension may occur on the basis of depression of the central nervous system and α-adrenergic blockade. The intravenous injection of 0.15 mg of droperidol per kilogram produces a transient decrease in arterial pressure.[89] Direct aortic injection produces an immediate decrease in blood pressure because of α-adrenergic blockade. Muldoon et al.[56] showed that concentrations of droperidol that are α-adrenergic blocking do not depress myogenic contractility. Injection of 2.5 mg of droperidol after 2 mg of morphine per kilogram increased heart rate and cardiac output, with a decrease in peripheral vascular resistance.[70] These changes were not present after five minutes. In one study, a dose of 5 mg of droperidol injected into patients receiving an enflurane-nitrous oxide-oxygen anesthetic decreased systemic vascular resistance and blood pressure and increased heart rate and total blood flow.[66] The changes were maximal in five minutes and returned to control in 15 minutes. Thus, small amounts of droperidol produce significant, although transient, decreases in blood pressure and systemic vascular resistance, similar to the changes seen with halothane and morphine.

Injection of droperidol into the oxygenator during cardiopulmonary bypass decreases blood pressure, and when the droperidol effect is maximal, the pressor response to epinephrine and norepinephrine is suppressed.[89] This effect suggests that droperidol may be a generalized adrenergic blocking agent, in addition to its α-adrenergic blockade. Droperidol also has an antiarrhythmic effect. Long et al.[43] found that 0.2 mg/kg doubled the arrhythmic threshold for epinephrine-induced dysrhythmias. Low doses of droperidol (250 μg/kg) prevented epinephrine-halothane–induced arrhythmias in cats without inhibiting the increase in blood pressure—an activity independent of α-adrenergic blockade.[3] Induction of ventricular fibrillation by coronary occlusion also was prevented. Similar to quinidine, droperidol lengthens the effective refractory period.[3] This effect is not reduced by doses of norepinephrine sufficient to induce positive inotropic effects.

The effects of droperidol in cardiac patients were summarized by Ferrari et al.,[25] who found that 0.25 to 0.5 mg/kg decreased systemic vascular resistance, central venous pressure, and arterial pressure without negative inotropic effects. Thus, droperidol may be useful in the digitalized patient with congestive heart failure or in the patient with congestive heart failure who is likely to develop arrhythmia.

Narcotic Agents

Narcotics are not anesthetics, and although anesthesia and apnea may be induced, unconsciousness may not be rendered. Supplementation of these drugs with depressants of the CNS and muscular relaxants is common and reduces the risk of intraoperative awareness, decreases skeletal muscle rigidity, provides surgical relaxation, and decreases the required dose of the narcotic.

MORPHINE.—In 1965, Lowenstein[44] introduced the practice of intravenously administering large doses of morphine (0.5 to 3 mg/kg) for cardiac surgery. Subsequent studies showed that 1 mg/kg intravenously did not affect cardiac output, systemic vascular resistance, blood pressure, central venous pressure, or heart rate in healthy patients but decreased systemic vascular resistance and increased cardiac output in patients with aortic valve disease.[52]

Hypotension may occur after the administration of morphine and may be secondary to bradycardia, release of histamine, or depression of the sympathetic nervous system.[34] Bradycardia may be secondary to increased vagal activity and is corrected by the use of an anticholinergic agent. Release of histamine is variable in incidence and severity, and its consequences are minimized by the slow injection of morphine and by circulatory support. Assisted ventilation during induction to prevent the accumulation of carbon dioxide is desirable. Hypotension secondary to sympathetic depression may be overcome by vasopressors or intravenously administered fluids (or both). The use of morphine increases the intraoperative requirements for intravenous fluids and transfusions.[69]

Morphine neither directly depresses myocardial and vascular smooth muscle nor sensitizes the heart to catecholamines nor predisposes to arrhythmias.[34] The net hemodynamic effect is dependent on the circulating blood volume—if the volume is below a certain threshold value, the decreased resistance and increased capacitance may stimulate baroreceptors and produce a catecholamine-induced vasoconstriction, with a secondary decrease in cardiac output.[45] The myocardial depressant and sympathomimetic effects of nitrous oxide are evident when it is added to morphine. Martin et al.[50] observed decreased cardiac output and increased systemic vascular resistance when nitrous oxide was added to morphine. In patients with coronary artery disease, the addition of 60% nitrous oxide decreased blood pressure by 25% and cardiac output by 17%.[78] Prior administration of barbiturates may invalidate the assumption of relatively benign cardiac effects of morphine. Stoelting[75] found that, after induction with 4 mg of thiamylal per kilogram, the administration of 1 mg of morphine per kilogram resulted in a decrease of 16% in mean arterial pressure, a decrease of 42% in cardiac index, and an increase of 35% in systemic vascular resistance. Morphine, when used judiciously and combined with drugs that minimally depress the heart, is an excellent anesthetic for cardiac surgery.

MEPERIDINE.—Meperidine is approximately one tenth as potent as morphine and has a shorter duration of action. Hypotension may occur owing to a negative inotropic effect, decreased systemic vascular resistance, and decreased venous return secondary to increased capacitance or bradycardia.[34] Meperidine has a direct depressant effect on contractility that is approximately 200 times greater than that of morphine.[82] In anesthetized patients, bradycardia and decreases in systolic blood pressure may be observed.[24] Meperidine in a dose of 2 mg/kg in dogs decreased cardiac output by 30%, secondary to decreases in stroke volume and heart rate; however, systemic vascular resistance and pulmonary vascular resistance were significantly increased.[31] The initial dose is 1 to 3 mg/kg, supplemented with approximately 0.5 mg/kg as needed.

FENTANYL.—Fentanyl is approximately 100 times more potent than morphine and 1,000 times more potent than meperidine, and has a shorter duration of action, at least after a single dose. Its onset of action is almost immediate, and the effects of a single dose are dissipated within 30 minutes.[51] Compared with the effect with morphine administration, histamine release is negligible, and there is less increase in venous capacitance. The primary cardiac effect is bradycardia, which is prevented by the use of atropine[21] and minimized by slow infusion, especially during induction.[68] Equal analgesic doses of morphine and fentanyl decrease heart rate similarly, but the decrease in blood pressure is much less with fentanyl.[51] No negative inotropic effect is evident, and sympathetic responses with associated tachycardia and hypertension are suppressed.[34]

Fentanyl in doses of 20 µg/kg decreased heart rate and blood pressure but did not change stroke volume, cardiac output, central venous pressure, or peripheral resistance.[68] No further changes were seen when the dosage was increased from 20 to 50 µg/kg. At a dose of 10 µg/kg, no significant circulatory changes were seen. Unresponsiveness was observed at a dose of approximately 11 µg/kg. The total dose for mitral valve replacement averaged 74 µg/kg.[68]

Tarhan et al.,[84] using droperidol and fentanyl in a ratio of 50:1 for analgesia and sedation during coronary angiography, observed a decrease of 11% in systemic vascular resistance, a decrease of 9% in mean arterial pressure, a decrease of 11% in total-body oxygen consumption, and no change in cardiac index. Stoelting et al.,[80] using fentanyl (10 µg/kg) or fentanyl (10 µg/kg) and droperidol (100 µg/kg), found minimal changes in circulatory dynamics in adults with acquired valvular disease. An increase in central venous pressure was noted during infusion of the drug; the pressure decreased to awake levels after controlled ventilation and skeletal muscle relaxation. They believed that this reflected thoracoabdominal muscular rigidity rather than a circulatory response. The addition of 60% nitrous oxide after either of the above regimens significantly decreased mean arterial pressure, heart rate, and cardiac index.

Fentanyl has a large therapeutic index, and its major cardiovascular effect (bradycardia) is easily corrected. Vascular tone is preserved better than with morphine. Cardiovascular depressant effects of adjuvant drugs (for example, nitrous oxide) are rarely seen. Thus, fentanyl is an entirely reasonable choice for cardiac anesthesia.

Ketamine

Ketamine is a cardiovascular stimulant and increases blood pressure, heart rate, and cardiac output. Its stimulatory effects follow the course of its anesthetic effects. Coppel and Dundee[10] showed that the stimulatory response to ketamine had dissipated by 16 minutes after injection and that subsequent injections did not produce a further increase in pressure. The mechanism of stimulation is complex and includes increased sympathetic outflow and impairment of baroreceptor reflexes. Tweed et al.[87] showed that a dose of 2 mg/kg produces an increase of 30% in mean arterial pressure, heart rate, and cardiac index, thus enhancing myocardial contractility. This increase is associated with increased cardiac work and an increase in myocardial oxygen consumption. Therefore, ketamine should not be used in patients with coronary artery disease and should be administered with caution to patients with severe myocardial disease of any type. Increases in pulmonary artery pressure and pulmonary blood flow also are seen with ketamine, but these increases are related to the increased cardiac output rather than to a change in the pulmonary vasculature.[30]

Because it increases cardiac output without a large decrease in systemic vascular resistance, ketamine may be a desirable agent in patients with hypovolemia, hemorrhage, or shock (as in traumatic injury to the heart or great vessels). When an increase in mean arterial pressure is undesirable, the use of ketamine is contraindicated. Ketamine also may be of value as an induction agent for patients with constrictive pericarditis.[38] These patients have a low cardiac output and increased central venous pressure due to the pericardial restriction. The minimal depressant actions of diazepam are accentuated in these patients, while ketamine may help maintain circulatory dynamics.[38] The induction of a pediatric cardiac patient who has a right-to-left shunt may proceed more rapidly with ketamine than with inhalational agents.[59] Ketamine is seldom used in our clinical practice.

Neuromuscular Blocking Agents

Succinylcholine

Small and inconsistent hemodynamic effects are seen after the administration of succinylcholine.[32] Bradycardia may occur and is more common with halothane anesthesia.[90] The presence of hyperkalemia or conditions that may result in hyperkalemia with succinylcholine administration (burns, tetanus, upper motor neuron disease, and so forth) predisposes to the development of arrhythmias.

d-Tubocurarine

Intravenously administered d-tubocurarine produces a dose-related hypotension due to a decrease in systemic vascular resistance. The decrease in systemic vascular resistance is based on the release of histamine. Another action of d-tubocurarine is blockade of the sympathetic ganglia.[17] Halothane and hypovolemia enhance the hypotensive effects of d-tubocurarine,[7, 73] which are readily corrected by the administration of fluids or vasoconstrictors.

Pancuronium

Pancuronium is the most potent clinically available neuromuscular blocker. Its cardiac actions include an increase in heart rate and, therefore, result in secondary increases in cardiac output and systolic blood pressure, while systemic vascular resistance remains unchanged. When boluses of pancuronium are given rapidly, tachyarrhythmias tend to develop. This effect is not a problem with the slow intravenous administration. Histamine release is not seen with pancuronium.[15] When pancuronium is added to enflurane anesthesia, a decrease of 10% in cardiac index and a decrease of 20% in stroke volume can be demonstrated.[39] This result contrasts with the effect of administering pancuronium during halothane, in which an increase in cardiac index is seen with an increase in heart rate.[71]

Gallamine

Gallamine produces tachycardia by vagal blockade and releases norepinephrine limited to the cardiac sympathetic nerves.[4] Associated with the tachycardia is an increase in cardiac output and systolic blood pressure, with a decrease in systemic vascular resistance.[72] Because of this effect, the use of gallamine is limited to treatment before intubation using succinylcholine.

Metocurine

Metocurine promises to be the most useful neuromuscular blocker for cardiac anesthesia. It was first synthesized by King[37] in 1934 as a trimethylated derivative of d-tubocurarine, and its chemical name is dimethyl tubocurarine. Metocurine was introduced into clinical practice in 1948 by Stoelting, Graf, and Vieira[81] and Wilson, Gordon, and Raffan.[91]

Metocurine has an ED_{50} and an ED_{95} for twitch inhibition of 0.13 and 0.28 mg/kg, respectively.[61] The potency ratio of metocurine is 0.25 compared with pancuronium and 1.8 compared with d-tubocurarine (Table 4–2). Recovery to 25% of control twitch height takes approximately 82 minutes.[61] No changes in heart rate or mean arterial pressure are seen until the dose reaches 0.4 mg/kg; then the rate increases by 18% and the mean arterial pressure decreases by 6%, suggestive of histamine release (which was shown in 6 of 18 patients[61]). Cardiac muscarinic receptors are not blocked.

TABLE 4–2.—COMPARATIVE POTENCIES AND TIMES TO RECOVERY OF 25% OF ORIGINAL TWITCH HEIGHT*

AGENT	ED_{95}, MG/KG	RECOVERY OF 25% TWITCH HEIGHT	
		DOSE, MG/KG	TIME, MIN
Metocurine	0.28	0.3	82.4
d-Tubocurarine	0.51	0.6	80.5
Pancuronium	0.07	0.1	99.3

*Data from Savarese et al.[61]

During deep levels of enflurane–nitrous oxide–oxygen anesthesia, modest doses sufficient to abolish thumb adduction have little influence on cardiovascular dynamics.[67] Anesthetic technique alters the dose required: Savarese et al.[61] reported 0.28 mg/kg as the ED_{95} for morphine–thiopental–nitrous oxide, Stoelting[73] reported 0.2 mg/kg as the ED_{95} for halothane–nitrous oxide–oxygen, and Stanley[67] reported 0.12 mg/kg as the ED_{95} for deep enflurane–nitrous oxide–oxygen anesthesia. Enflurane anesthesia seems to potentiate the action of metocurine. In the presence of propranolol treatment, 0.35 mg of metocurine per kilogram produced a decrease of 20% in systemic vascular resistance. This effect resulted in an increase of 26% in cardiac output, with a corresponding increase in stroke volume to maintain coronary perfusion pressure. No change was seen in mean arterial pressure, heart rate, or central venous pressure.[93] Because of the minimal effects on cardiovascular dynamics, metocurine may be the relaxant of choice for cardiac anesthesia.

INDUCTION OF ANESTHESIA

Induction of the Adult Patient

Patients with cardiac disease tolerate much less depression of their circulation than do normal, healthy subjects. Fortunately, the depth of anesthesia required by most cardiac patients undergoing open-heart surgery is also much less than that needed for a patient without cardiac disease.[83] Occasionally, patients undergoing cardiac surgery are critically ill, and a successful outcome for such patients demands scrupulous attention to every detail of their perioperative management. This approach has been helpful in the development of anesthetic techniques that are suited to all critically ill patients undergoing noncardiac operations and fulfilling the classic triad of anesthetic goals: analgesia, amnesia, and skeletal muscle relaxation. Induction of anesthesia in the operating room is greatly facilitated by appropriate preoperative medication (see chap. 3).

In the management of the adult patient undergoing elective cardiac surgery, monitoring of the vital signs should begin as soon as the patient arrives in the operating room. A blood pressure cuff is applied to either one of the upper extremities, and the initial pressures are obtained. If the patient has had previous bilateral Blalock-Taussig shunts, the blood pressure cuff should be applied to one of the lower extremities. Electrocardiographic leads are attached, and the ECG is displayed continuously on an oscilloscope throughout the procedure. The V_5 lead is monitored to provide early indication of ventricular ischemia. In each upper extremity, intravenous routes are established with large-bore 14- or 16-gauge Teflon catheters. After testing for the adequacy of collateral circulation by means of a modified Allen test, an 18- or 20-gauge Teflon catheter is inserted percutaneously into the radial artery under local anesthesia. Generally, the use of the artery on the side of a previous brachial arteriotomy for cardiac angiography is avoided. The femoral artery can alternatively be cannulated percutaneously with a 10- or 15-cm Teflon catheter or with a long catheter advanced into the thoracic aorta by means of the Seldinger technique.[88] Catheterization of the femoral artery is usually done with the patient anesthetized, but can be done under local anesthetic infiltration if necessary. After intubation in patients without compromised left ventricular function and before intubation in patients with left ventricular dysfunction, a central line is established using either the internal jugular vein or external jugular vein, with a modified Seldinger and J-wire technique. A Swan-Ganz catheter, if necessary, is also inserted at this time. If a Swan-Ganz catheter is used, a Cordis introducer sheath is used because the side port allows an additional infusion site.

With these preliminary steps accomplished, the induction of anesthesia can begin. Small incremental doses of thiopental (50 to 75 mg), as needed and as tolerated, are given slowly until the lid reflex is obtunded. Critically ill patients usually require small doses of thiopental to achieve hypnosis, thus decreasing the chances of significant myocardial depression so well known to all anesthesiologists.[16]

Next, the trachea is intubated with a low-pressure cuff endotracheal tube. In our current practice, this is preceded by an intravenous injection of pancuronium (0.08 to 0.1 mg/kg) during the induction with thiopental, and three to five minutes are allowed to elapse before intubation is attempted. Succinylcholine (1.5 mg/kg) or metocurine (0.35 mg/kg) may be used intravenously, depending on the clinical situation. Before endotracheal intubation, 2 to 4 ml of 4% lidocaine is applied topically to the trachea to attenuate the circulatory changes produced by direct laryngoscopy and tracheal intubation.[74,76] Less frequently, sodium nitroprusside, administered either in a single rapid intravenous injection (1 to 2 μg/kg) or in an intravenous drip, has been used to achieve the same purpose.[77]

After intubation, the patient is mechanically ventilated to keep the $PaCO_2$ between 35 and 40 mm Hg. There are different techniques for the maintenance of anesthesia. Generally, to achieve the anesthetic goals for cardiac surgery in a given patient, we use nitrous oxide–oxygen (50:50) supplemented with a volatile anesthetic (halothane or enflurane), an intravenous narcotic (meperidine, morphine, or fentanyl), or an intravenous tranquilizer (droperidol or diazepam).

The choice of anesthetic agent for a specific patient should reflect the patient's status, the disease, and the known drug effects. Either inhalation agent, halothane or enflurane, may be used in patients with fixed coronary flows or in patients in whom a mild decrease in contractility would not be disastrous. Narcotic techniques are more appropriate for patients with limited cardiac reserve. In these patients, fentanyl may offer advantages over morphine, because the risk of histamine release is much less and a negative inotropic effect is not evident.[34] Usual induction techniques should be altered before the use of a narcotic, because barbiturate induction followed by morphine administration may result in significant decreases in mean arterial pressure, cardiac index, and stroke volume index while increasing systemic vascular resistance.[75]

The choice of narcotic supplement should be carefully considered, because the addition of nitrous oxide to morphine may produce significant cardiovascular depression.[78] Scopolamine, 0.5 mg intravenously, may increase heart rate, stroke volume, cardiac output, and blood pressure during morphine-nitrous oxide anesthesia.[1] At the same time, central venous pressure and peripheral vascular resistance may decrease. Scopolamine may be a more effective supplement than nitrous oxide during high-dose morphine anesthesia; however, diazepam or droperidol also can be used safely as a supplement.[70]

The choice of muscle relaxant should receive equal consideration. While the use of succinylcholine in the acutely hypotensive patient allows reflex sympathetic stimulation and an increase in blood pressure, these effects are totally undesirable in the patient with fixed coronary flows or minimal cardiac reserve. Pancuronium may be useful in the patient in whom bradycardia is a problem; however, the increase in rate may severely increase myocardial oxygen consumption. The hypertensive patient could benefit from the histamine release associated with d-tubocurarine, but a stroke or heart failure may occur in the patient with borderline compensation. For patients unable to tolerate a change in their hemodynamic state, metocurine may be the agent of choice.

There is no universal anesthetic or relaxant, and thus no panacea for cardiac anesthesia. The selection of agents for a specific patient involves clinical judgment and acumen, as well as a detailed knowledge of the hemodynamic effects of the particular drugs. When these factors are considered, one can follow the dictum of *primum non nocere* and make active interventions to improve the patient's status.

Induction of the High-Risk Cardiac Patient

"High-risk" patients usually are so critically ill that most of them will not tolerate the usual stress of anesthetic induction and may not be able to maintain their hemodynamic homeostasis until cardiopulmonary bypass is instituted. These patients usually have a combination of intractable heart failure and advanced pulmonary, renal, or hepatic disease.[12]

Once the patient arrives in the operating room, the usual monitoring is started. Under local anesthesia, intravenous, intra-arterial, and central venous lines are established. Small increments of sedative drugs (diazepam) or narcotics (morphine, meperidine, or fentanyl) are given concurrently. After the skin is prepared, the patient is draped, the instrument tables are brought into position, and the appropriate lines are connected to the cardiopulmonary bypass machine. Under local anesthesia, the right femoral vessels are exposed. The patient is fully heparinized, and a long venous cannula and the usual short arterial cannula are inserted. If needed, the opposite femoral vein may be cannulated and connected to the venous line to improve venous drainage. After these preparations, cardiopulmonary bypass may be instituted at any time, depending on the condition of the patient.

In these critically ill patients with precarious hemodynamics, cardiopulmonary bypass should be instituted and anesthesia simultaneously induced with thiopental (300 to 500 mg) or diazepam (20 to 40 mg) followed by succinylcholine (100 to 150 mg) and tracheal intubation without undue rush, because the cardiopulmonary functions already have been bypassed. The required amnesia-analgesia and adequate skeletal muscle relaxation then can be established. Although most cardiac patients require relatively light planes of anesthesia, this special group of high-risk patients requires mainly adequate paralysis with amnesia-analgesia and great efforts at resuscitation. In recent years, we have used intra-aortic balloon support before the induction of anesthesia in selected patients to maintain myocardial blood flow and to decrease afterload of a compromised ventricle.[9, 42] These measures should reduce the operative mortality and perioperative myocardial infarction rate.

REFERENCES

1. Bennett G.M., Loeser E.A., Stanley T.H.: Cardiovascular effects of scopolamine during morphine-oxygen and morphine-nitrous oxide-oxygen anesthesia in man. *Anesthesiology* 46:225, 1977.
2. Bennett G.M., et al.: Cardiovascular responses to nitrous oxide during enflurane and oxygen anesthesia. *Anesthesiology* 46:227, 1977.
3. Bertoló L., Novaković L., Penna M.: Antiarrhythmic effects of droperidol. *Anesthesiology* 37:529, 1972.

References

4. Brown B.R. Jr., Crout J.R.: The sympathomimetic effect of gallamine on the heart. *J. Pharmacol. Exp. Ther.* 172:266, 1970.
5. Brown B.R. Jr., Crout J.R.: A comparative study of the effects of five general anesthetics on myocardial contractility: I. Isometric conditions. *Anesthesiology* 34:236, 1971.
6. Calverley R.K., et al.: Cardiovascular effects of enflurane anesthesia during controlled ventilation in man. *Anesth. Analg.* 57:619, 1978.
7. Chatas G.J., Gottlieb J.D., Sweet R.B.: Cardiovascular effects of d-tubocurarine during fluothane anesthesia. *Anesth. Analg.* 42:65, 1963.
8. Conway C.M., Ellis D.B.: The haemodynamic effects of short-acting barbiturates. *Br. J. Anaesth.* 41:534, 1969.
9. Cooper G.N., et al.: Preoperative intra-aortic balloon support in surgery for left main coronary stenosis. *Ann. Surg.* 185:242, 1977.
10. Coppel D.L., Dundee J.W.: Ketamine anaesthesia for cardiac catheterisation. *Anaesthesia* 27:25, 1972.
11. Côté P., Guéret P., Bourassa M.G.: Systemic and coronary hemodynamic effects of diazepam in patients with normal and diseased coronary arteries. *Circulation* 50:1210, 1974.
12. Danielson G.K., Hasbrouck J.D., Bryant L.R.: Cannulation under local or regional anesthesia for the "salvage" cardiac patient. *J. Thorac. Cardiovasc. Surg.* 55:864, 1968.
13. Dauchot P.J., et al.: On-line systolic time intervals during anesthesia in patients with and without heart disease. *Anesthesiology* 44:472, 1976.
14. De Castro J., Mundeleer P.: Anesthésie sans barbituriques: La neuroleptanalgésie. *Anesth. Analg.* 16:1022, 1959.
15. Dobkin A.B., Arandia H.Y., Levy A.A.: Effect of pancuronium bromide on plasma histamine levels in man. *Anesth. Analg.* 52:772, 1973.
16. Dwyer E.M. Jr., Wiener L.: Left ventricular function in man following thiopental. *Anesth. Analg.* 48:499, 1969.
17. Eger E.: Hypotension and intravenous administration of d-tubocurarine. *Anesthesiology* 19:404, 1958.
18. Eger E.I. II, et al.: Cardiovascular effects of halothane in man. *Anesthesiology* 32:396, 1970.
19. Eger E.I. II, et al.: A comparison of the cardiovascular effects of halothane, fluroxene, ether and cyclopropane in man: A resumé. *Anesthesiology* 34:25, 1971.
20. Eisele J.H., Smith N.T.: Cardiovascular effects of 40 percent nitrous oxide in man. *Anesth. Analg.* 51:956, 1972.
21. Eisele J.H., et al.: Myocardial sparing effect of fentanyl during halothane anaesthesia in dogs. *Br. J. Anaesth.* 47:937, 1975.
22. Eisele J.H., et al.: Myocardial performance and N_2O analgesia in coronary-artery disease. *Anesthesiology* 44:16, 1976.
23. Etsten B.E., Shimosato S.: Influence of stress upon the performance of the heart during halothane and ether anesthesia. *Acta Anaesthesiol. Scand.*, suppl. 23, 1966, p. 242.
24. Faulkner S.L., Boerth R.C., Graham T.P. Jr.: Direct myocardial effects of precatheterization medications. *Am. Heart J.* 88:609, 1974.
25. Ferrari H.A., et al.: The action of droperidol and fentanyl on cardiac output and related hemodynamic parameters. *South. Med. J.* 67:49, 1974.
26. Fieldman E.J., Ridley R.W., Wood E.H.: Hemodynamic studies during thiopental sodium and nitrous oxide anesthesia in humans. *Anesthesiology* 16:473, 1955.
27. Fogdall R.P., Miller R.D.: Neuromuscular effects of enflurane, alone and combined with d-tubocurarine, pancuronium, and succinylcholine, in man. *Anesthesiology* 42:173, 1975.
28. Foldes F.F., et al.: A rational approach to neuroleptanesthesia. *Anesth. Analg.* 45:642, 1966.
29. Fukunaga A.F., Epstein R.M.: Sympathetic excitation during nitrous oxide-halothane anesthesia in the cat. *Anesthesiology* 39:23, 1973.
30. Gassner S., et al.: The effect of ketamine on pulmonary artery pressure: An experimental and clinical study. *Anaesthesia* 29:141, 1974.
31. Goldberg S.J., et al.: The effects of meperidine, promethazine, and chlorpromazine on pulmonary and systemic circulation. *Am. Heart J.* 77:214, 1969.
32. Graf K., Ström G., Wåhlin Å.: Circulatory effects of succinylcholine in man. *Acta Anaesthesiol. Scand.* 7(suppl. 14):1, 1963.
33. Horan B.F., et al.: Haemodynamic responses to enflurane anaesthesia and hypovolaemia in the dog, and their modification by propranolol. *Br. J. Anaesth.* 49:1189, 1977.
34. Hug C.C. Jr.: Pharmacology—anesthetic drugs, in Kaplan J.A. (ed.): *Cardiac Anesthesia*. New York, Grune & Stratton, 1979, p. 3.
35. Ikram H., Rubin A.P., Jewkes R.F.: Effect of diazepam on myocardial blood flow of patients with and without coronary artery disease. *Br. Heart J.* 35:626, 1973.
36. Johnston R.R., Eger E.I. II, Wilson C.: A comparative interaction of epinephrine with enflurane, isoflurane, and halothane in man. *Anesth. Analg.* 55:709, 1976.
37. King H.: Curare alkaloids: I. Tubocurarine. *J. Chem. Soc.*, 1935, p. 1381.

38. Kingston H.G.G., et al.: A comparison between ketamine and diazepam as induction agents for pericardiectomy. *Anaesth. Intensive Care* 6:66, 1978.
39. Klauber P.V., et al.: Cardiovascular haemodynamics during enflurane-pancuronium anaesthesia in patients with valvular heart disease. *Can. Anaesth. Soc. J.* 25:113, 1978.
40. Konchigeri H.N., Shaker M.H., Winnie A.P.: Effect of epinephrine during enflurane anesthesia. *Anesth. Analg.* 53:894, 1974.
41. Kopriva C.J., Brown A.C.D., Pappas G.: Hemodynamics during general anesthesia in patients receiving propranolol. *Anesthesiology* 48:28, 1978.
42. Langou R.A., et al.: Surgical approach for patients with unstable angina pectoris: Role of the response to initial medical therapy and intraaortic balloon pumping in perioperative complications after aortocoronary bypass grafting. *Am. J. Cardiol.* 42:629, 1978.
43. Long G., Dripps R.D., Price H.L.: Measurement of anti-arrhythmic potency of drugs in man: Effects of dehydrobenzperidol. *Anesthesiology* 28:318, 1967.
44. Lowenstein E.: Morphine 'anesthesia'—a perspective, editorial. *Anesthesiology* 35:563, 1971.
45. Lowenstein E., et al.: Cardiovascular response to large doses of intravenous morphine in man. *N. Engl. J. Med.* 281:1389, 1969.
46. Lundborg R.O., Milde J.H., Theye R.A.: Effect of nitrous oxide on myocardial contractility of dogs. *Can. Anaesth. Soc. J.* 13:361, 1966.
47. Lyons S.M., Clarke R.S.J.: A comparison of different drugs for anaesthesia in cardiac surgical patients. *Br. J. Anaesth.* 44:575, 1972.
48. Mahaffey J.E., et al.: The cardiovascular effects of halothane. *Anesthesiology* 22:982, 1961.
49. Mallow J.E., et al.: Hemodynamic effects of isoflurane and halothane in patients with coronary artery disease. *Anesth. Analg.* 55:135, 1976.
50. Martin W.E., et al.: Cited by Lowenstein E., et al.[45]
51. Maunuksela E.-L.: Hemodynamic response to different anesthetics during open-heart surgery. *Acta Anaesthesiol. Scand.*, suppl. 65, 1977, p. 1.
52. Merin R.G.: The function of the heart and effects of anesthetics and adjuvant drugs. *A.S.A. Refresher Courses in Anesthesiology* 6:81, 1978.
53. Merin R.G., Kumazawa T., Luka N.L.: Enflurane depresses myocardial function, perfusion, and metabolism in the dog. *Anesthesiology* 45:501, 1976.
54. Millar R.A., et al.: Central sympathetic discharge and mean arterial pressure during halothane anaesthesia. *Br. J. Anaesth.* 41:918, 1969.
55. Miller R.D., et al.: The dependence of pancuronium-and d-tubocurarine-induced neuromuscular blockades on alveolar concentrations of halothane and forane. *Anesthesiology* 37:573, 1972.
56. Muldoon S.M., et al.: Alpha-adrenergic blocking properties of droperidol on isolated blood vessels of the dog. *Br. J. Anaesth.* 49:211, 1977.
57. Price H.L., Helrich M.: The effect of cyclopropane, diethyl ether, nitrous oxide, thiopental, and hydrogen ion concentration on the myocardial function of the dog heart-lung preparation. *J. Pharmacol. Exp. Ther.* 115:206, 1955.
58. Price H.L., et al.: Evidence for β-receptor activation produced by halothane in normal man. *Anesthesiology* 32:389, 1970.
59. Radnay P.A., et al.: Ketamine for pediatric cardiac anesthesia. *Anaesthesist* 25:259, 1976.
60. Rao S., et al.: Cardiopulmonary effects of diazepam. *Clin. Pharmacol. Ther.* 14:182, 1973.
61. Savarese J.J., Ali H.H., Antonio R.P.: The clinical pharmacology of metocurine: Dimethyltubocurarine revisited. *Anesthesiology* 47:277, 1977.
62. Shimosato S., Etsten B.: Performance of digitalized heart during halothane anesthesia. *Anesthesiology* 24:41, 1963.
63. Skovsted P., Price M.L., Price H.L.: The effects of short-acting barbiturates on arterial pressure, preganglionic sympathetic activity and barostatic reflexes. *Anesthesiology* 33:10, 1970.
64. Smith N.T., et al.: The cardiovascular and sympathomimetic responses to the addition of nitrous oxide to halothane in man. *Anesthesiology* 32:410, 1970.
65. Smith N.T., et al.: Impact of nitrous oxide on the circulation during enflurane anesthesia in man. *Anesthesiology* 48:345, 1978.
66. Stanley T.H.: Cardiovascular effects of droperidol during enflurane and enflurane-nitrous oxide anaesthesia in man. *Can. Anaesth. Soc. J.* 25:26, 1978.
67. Stanley T.H.: Cardiovascular effects of metocurine during enflurane anesthesia in man. *Anesth. Analg.* 57:540, 1978.
68. Stanley T.H., Webster L.R.: Anesthetic requirements and cardiovascular effects of fentanyl-oxygen and fentanyl-diazepam-oxygen anesthesia in man. *Anesth. Analg.* 57:411, 1978.
69. Stanley T.H., et al.: The effects of high-dose

morphine on fluid and blood requirements in open-heart operations. *Anesthesiology* 38:536, 1973.
70. Stanley T.H., et al.: Cardiovascular effects of diazepam and droperidol during morphine anesthesia. *Anesthesiology* 44:255, 1976.
71. Stoelting R.K.: The hemodynamic effects of pancuronium and *d*-tubocurarine in anesthetized patients. *Anesthesiology* 36:612, 1972.
72. Stoelting R.K.: Hemodynamic effects of gallamine during halothane-nitrous oxide anesthesia. *Anesthesiology* 39:645, 1973.
73. Stoelting R.K.: Hemodynamic effects of dimethyltubocurarine during nitrous oxide-halothane anesthesia. *Anesth. Analg.* 53:513, 1974.
74. Stoelting R.K.: Circulatory changes during direct laryngoscopy and tracheal intubation: Influence of duration of laryngoscopy with or without prior lidocaine. *Anesthesiology* 47:381, 1977.
75. Stoelting R.K.: Influence of barbiturate anesthetic induction on circulatory responses to morphine. *Anesth. Analg.* 56:615, 1977.
76. Stoelting R.K.: Blood pressure and heart rate changes during short-duration laryngoscopy for tracheal intubation: Influence of viscous or intravenous lidocaine. *Anesth. Analg.* 57:197, 1978.
77. Stoelting R.K.: Attenuation of blood pressure response to laryngoscopy and tracheal intubation with sodium nitroprusside. *Anesth. Analg.* 58:116, 1979.
78. Stoelting R.K., Gibbs P.S.: Hemodynamic effects of morphine and morphine-nitrous oxide in valvular heart disease and coronary-artery disease. *Anesthesiology* 38:45, 1973.
79. Stoelting R.K., Reis R.R., Longnecker D.E.: Hemodynamic responses to nitrous oxide-halothane and halothane in patients with valvular heart disease. *Anesthesiology* 37:430, 1972.
80. Stoelting R.K., et al.: Hemodynamic and ventilatory responses to fentanyl, fentanyl-droperidol, and nitrous oxide in patients with acquired valvular heart disease. *Anesthesiology* 42:319, 1975.
81. Stoelting V.K., Graf J.P., Vieira Z.: Dimethyl ether of *d*-tubocurarine iodide as an adjunct to anesthesia. *Proc. Soc. Exp. Biol. Med.* 69:565, 1948.
82. Strauer B.E.: Contractile responses to morphine, piritramide, meperidine, and fentanyl: A comparative study of effects on the isolated ventricular myocardium. *Anesthesiology* 37:304, 1972.
83. Tarhan S., Moffitt E.A.: Anesthesia and postoperative care for cardiac surgery: Principles and practice, in Danielson G.K., Goldsmith H.S. (eds.): *Lewis' Practice of Surgery*, vol. 11: *Cardiovascular Surgery.* Hagerstown, Md., Harper & Row, 1974, chap. 19.
84. Tarhan S., et al.: Hemodynamic and blood-gas effects of innovar in patients with acquired heart disease. *Anesthesiology* 34:250, 1971.
85. Theye R.A., Michenfelder J.D.: Whole-body and organ Vo_2 changes with enflurane, isoflurane, and halothane. *Br. J. Anaesth.* 47:813, 1975.
86. Thomas B.: Clinical experience with four intravenous induction agents in cardiac surgery patients. *Acta Anaesthesiol. Belg.* 28:75, 1977.
87. Tweed W.A., Minuck M., Mymin D.: Circulatory responses to ketamine anesthesia. *Anesthesiology* 37:613, 1972.
88. White R.D., Tarhan S.: Anesthetic aspects of cardiac surgery: A review of clinical management. *Anesth. Analg.* 53:98, 1974.
89. Whitwam J.G., Russell W.J.: The acute cardiovascular changes and adrenergic blockade by droperidol in man. *Br. J. Anaesth.* 43:581, 1971.
90. Williams C.H., et al.: Effects of intravenously administered succinyldicholine on cardiac rate, rhythm, and arterial blood pressure in anesthetized man. *Anesthesiology* 22:947, 1961.
91. Wilson H.B., Gordon H.E., Raffan A.W.: Dimethyl ether of d-tubocurarine iodide as a curarizing agent in anaesthesia for thoracic surgery. *Br. Med. J.* 1:1296, 1950.
92. Wong K.C., et al.: The cardiovascular effects of morphine sulfate with oxygen and with nitrous oxide in man. *Anesthesiology* 38:542, 1973.
93. Zaidan J., et al.: Hemodynamic effects of metocurine in patients with coronary artery disease receiving propranolol. *Anesth. Analg.* 56:255, 1977.

5 / Monitoring During Cardiovascular Surgery

DUANE K. RORIE

BECAUSE patients who undergo cardiac surgery generally are very ill and because the derangements in normal physiology occurring before, during, and after surgery may be considerable, more extensive monitoring is needed for cardiac surgical patients than for patients undergoing most other types of surgery. Although monitoring must be done, there is controversy on the extent to which various monitoring devices are to be used in patients undergoing cardiovascular surgery. However, the greater availability and reliability of electronic monitoring devices during recent years has increased the monitoring capability available to anesthesiologists. The extent to which these devices are used depends principally on the needs of the patient and the benefits to be gained. When vital decisions are to be made about therapy or a course of action regarding the patient, there is no substitute for accurate information about the patient's condition.

Variables that are monitored in patients undergoing a cardiovascular operative procedure include (1) arterial pressure, (2) electrocardiographic findings, (3) central venous pressure, (4) temperature, (5) left atrial pressure, (6) cardiac output, (7) arterial blood gases, pH, and serum potassium, and (8) urinary output.

ARTERIAL PRESSURE

In patients undergoing cardiac surgery, the arterial pressure must be measured directly and continuously. The placing of an intra-arterial cannula and the flushing associated with its connection to the pressure transducer can be painful and distressing to an awake patient. Patient cooperation is needed during the cannulation. For these reasons, arterial measurements are made indirectly by means of an arm cuff before, during, and after the induction of anesthesia, until an intra-arterial cannula can be placed. This protocol is followed in all but a few very sick patients, in whom it may be desirable to use local anesthesia to place the cannula.

In children and in certain hypotensive or obese patients in whom Korotkoff's sounds are unclear or the oscillations of the manometer indicator are indistinct, a Doppler flowmeter can be positioned over the radial, ulnar, or brachial artery and can be used to detect the beginning of blood flow during deflation of a conventional cuff. This end point is considered to represent systolic pressure.

Direct Arterial Cannulation

Several arteries are available for cannulation. Because of accessibility, size, ease of cannulation, and lack of complications, the radial artery is nearly ideal. Most significant complications associated with radial artery cannulation are related to thrombosis during or after cannulation and the absence of adequate collateral circulation for supplying the hand if thrombosis occurs. No intra-arterial cannula should be placed without first determining the adequacy of collateral circulation. The clinical test first described to determine the adequacy of collateral circulation to the hand was the Allen test. This test or some modification of it should be done preoperatively, and the results should be recorded.

Collateral Circulation to the Hand

The ulnar and radial arteries, the major arteries supplying the hand, are the terminal branches of the brachial artery, which divides in the lower part of the antebrachial fossa. These branches reach the hand by coursing down the front of the radial and ulnar sides of the forearm. The radial artery, though usually smaller than the ulnar artery, appears to be the more direct continuation of the brachial artery. At the wrist, the radial artery lies just below the subcutaneous tissue in the interval between the flexor carpi radialis tendon medially and the lower part of the anterior border of the radius laterally, where its pulsations can be readily felt (Fig 5–1). Because of this superficial and readily accessible location, the radial artery is used extensively for intra-arterial pressure monitoring.

Just below the styloid process of the radius, the artery courses to the back of the hand to reach the space between the first and the second metacarpal bone (see Fig 5–1). The radial artery then passes palmward and crosses toward the ulnar side to form the deep palmar arterial arch. As the radial artery begins its course to the back of the hand, it gives off a superficial palmar branch, which typically joins the superficial palmar arterial arch lying between the palmar aponeurosis and the tendons of the flexor digitorum superficialis. The ulnar artery courses to the medial side of the wrist, crosses the flexor retinaculum, where it gives rise to the deep palmar branch, and then courses laterally to become the chief contributor to the superficial palmar arch. According to Coleman and Anson,[7] 80% of patients have a complete superficial volar arch; a complete deep volar arch is less variable than the superficial and is complete in 97% of patients. The caliber of the deep arch is usually inversely related to that of the superficial arch. Many connections usually exist between the superficial and the deep palmar arteries.

Allen Test

The Allen test is used to assess collateral blood flow to the hands in syndromes in which occlusive lesions in arteries distal to the wrist might be expected.[1] As originally described, the test requires that the patient close his hands as tightly as possible for one minute to squeeze the blood from the hands. At the end of this time, the examiner places one thumb over each radial artery, with the four fingers of each hand behind the patient's wrist, and compresses the wrist between the thumb and the fingers, thus occluding the radial arteries (the same process is later repeated while compressing the ulnar artery). The patient extends his fingers partially while compression of the radial arteries is maintained by the examiner. In patients with an intact collateral circulation, the pallor is quickly replaced by rubor of a higher degree than normal which gradually fades to the normal color. The time required for color to develop in the hand with normal circulation was not given by Allen; however, others have suggested that 5 or 6 seconds are adequate[16, 18] and that the radial artery should not be cannulated if circulation is not restored in 15 seconds.[3, 16]

Subsequently, false readings have been obtained if the hand is extended completely at the wrist or if the fingers are extended forcibly at the metacarpophalangeal and interphalangeal joints.[18] Thus, the test should be done with the hand halfway between flexion and extension at the wrist and with the fingers only partially extended. Although Allen did not describe the end point of the test in terms of positive or negative, the presence of inadequate collateral circulation to permit the pallor to be replaced by rubor in 5 or 6 seconds has become known as a positive Allen test.

Technique for Cannulation of Vessel

If a patient has recently undergone cardiac catheterization or angiography through a bra-

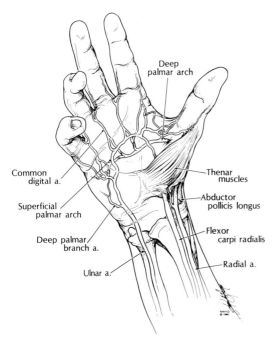

Fig 5–1.—Superficial palmar arch. Note that major contribution to this arch is from ulnar artery.

chial artery, the use of an artery in that arm for direct arterial pressure monitoring is generally avoided. When adequacy of collateral circulation to the hand has been established, radial artery cannulation can be undertaken. The hand is supinated, then dorsiflexed to approximately a 50-degree angle (Fig 5–2). With the hand in this position, the radial artery is palpated several centimeters proximal to the wrist in its position just below the subcutaneous tissue and anterior to the radius. The skin is prepared with an antiseptic solution. If the patient is awake, infiltration of the skin with local anesthetic is necessary. An 18-gauge skin punch is then used to make a hole in the skin over the radial artery, through which the arterial cannula is to be inserted. The skin hole minimizes fraying of the tip of the catheter as it passes through the skin. An 18- or 20-gauge nontapered Teflon catheter attached to a 2-ml glass syringe containing approximately 0.5 ml of heparinized saline is inserted through the skin hole toward the radial artery at an angle of approximately 30 degrees to the anterior surface of the wrist. When the artery is punctured, bright red blood is seen entering the syringe and pushing the plunger out. At this point, the needle and catheter together are advanced another 1 or 2 mm. This step is critical and improves the successful cannulation rate considerably by ensuring that the cannula's tip is within the lumen of the artery, where it readily threads up the artery instead of pushing the artery off the needle's tip. Once the needle and catheter together have been advanced sufficiently that the catheter's tip is within the artery, the needle is fixed and the cannula is advanced into the arterial lumen. The needle is withdrawn and the cannula is connected to the transducer.

After its insertion, the catheter is secured to the skin with a suture, an antibacterial ointment is applied to the puncture site, and the catheter and suture are enclosed in a sterile, occlusive dressing.

If one of the patient's hands has inadequate collateral circulation, the other hand should be examined. If it also has reduced collateral circulation, another artery should be selected. Options include the dorsalis pedis, femoral, or brachial artery. The brachial artery has been associated with a high incidence of postcatheterization obstruction. A femoral artery can be readily cannulated percutaneously with an 18-gauge, 10- or 15-cm Teflon catheter. However, it is more satisfactory to insert an 18-gauge Teflon catheter percutaneously into the femoral artery using the Seldinger technique[24] and advancing it into the thoracic aorta, because the catheter remains patent longer and is relatively trouble-free (Fig 5–3). This method is especially useful for withdrawing blood to determine the cardiac output dye-dilution curves during and after operation.

Regardless of the artery selected for cannulation, the incidence of thrombosis increases with increasing duration of cannulation. Further, the use of tapered cannulas appears to increase the incidence of thrombosis.[9] The incidence of obstruction due to thrombosis is greater in patients less than 5 years of age.[21]

Open-heart operations in children require cannulation of either the radial artery percuta-

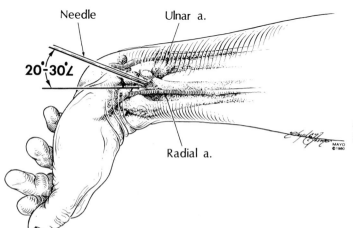

Fig 5–2.—Wrist position is shown for percutaneous radial artery cannulation.

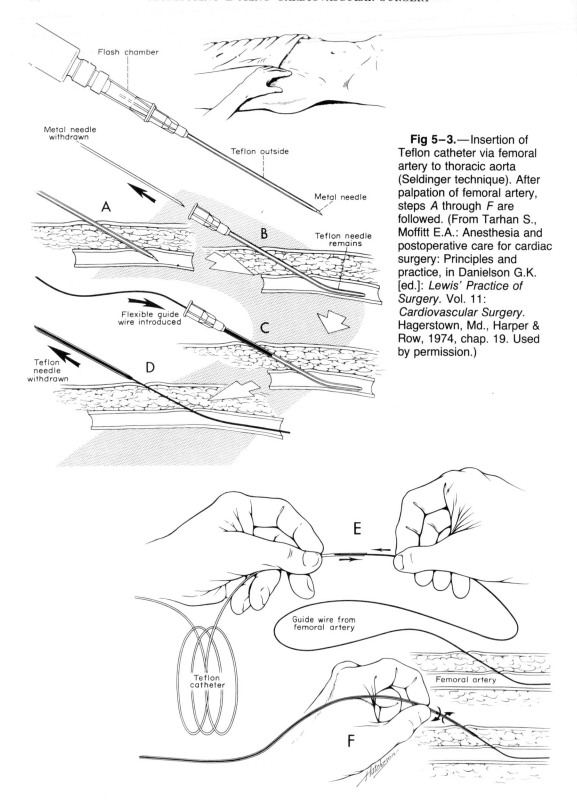

Fig 5–3.—Insertion of Teflon catheter via femoral artery to thoracic aorta (Seldinger technique). After palpation of femoral artery, steps A through F are followed. (From Tarhan S., Moffitt E.A.: Anesthesia and postoperative care for cardiac surgery: Principles and practice, in Danielson G.K. [ed.]: *Lewis' Practice of Surgery.* Vol. 11: *Cardiovascular Surgery.* Hagerstown, Md., Harper & Row, 1974, chap. 19. Used by permission.)

neously with a 20-gauge, 5-cm Teflon catheter or the femoral artery with an 18- or 20-gauge, 10-cm Teflon catheter. If percutaneous arterial cannulation is unsuccessful, a cutdown to either the radial or the femoral artery is done.

ELECTROCARDIOGRAM

Continuous monitoring of the ECG should be routine in all patients undergoing cardiovascular surgery. The continuous display of the ECG will permit instantaneous assessment of the electrical activity of the heart and may represent the earliest warning of the development of a serious problem.

The ECG can provide valuable information with respect to the detection of dysrhythmias and the efficacy of treatment directed at their correction. Although this function of continuous ECG monitoring is perhaps the most helpful, the ECG can be used to identify myocardial ischemia during anesthesia and surgery and thus may serve as an early indicator of inadequate oxygenation. It also may serve to warn the surgeon that a stitch has been placed within or perilously close to the atrioventricular conducting system.

The ECG is one of the first of the monitoring devices affixed to the patient in the operating room. As soon as the patient is on the operating table, ECG pads are attached on the lateral surface of the thighs and on the posterior surfaces of the shoulder or upper arm, and the appropriate leads are connected. Disposable adhesive ECG pads are highly satisfactory for placing the leads. It may be convenient to fix the ECG cable permanently to the undersurface of the operating table, so that the leads to the right and left legs are near the respective knees and the leads to the right and left arms are near the shoulders. A standard bipolar lead II, which measures differences in potential between the right arm and the left leg, is usually monitored. This lead is selected for monitoring because its axis parallels that between the sinoatrial and the atrioventricular nodes; hence, the P wave is larger and easier to identify, and the differentiation of ventricular from supraventricular dysrhythmias is enhanced. As has been emphasized by Kaplan and King,[19] myocardial ischemia of the inferior wall may be evidenced by ST-segment depression in lead II; however, the more common anterior or lateral wall ischemia may be missed. They suggested that ischemia of the anterior or lateral wall of the heart (indicative of disease of the left anterior descending or circumflex artery) can be best demonstrated by selecting a lead near the cardiac apex. They recommended that lead V_5 (left fifth interspace at the anterior axillary line) be used for this purpose. In our experience, a midline sternotomy incision does not preclude the attachment of lead V_5.

After the leads have been attached, the ECG configurations of each lead should be noted and a printout recording of the rhythm in each lead should be made before the induction of anesthesia. These printouts should be used as references to which changes in rhythm that may occur later can be compared.

Several reliable ECG monitors are available. Models that retain previous beats for the entire sweep across the screen permit instant comparison of current electrical activity with the previous four to six beats. As pointed out previously, a printout for permanently recording the rhythm is valuable, as is an audible signal coupled with the QRS complex.

CENTRAL VENOUS PRESSURE

A central venous pressure monitoring line can be placed either before the induction of anesthesia or shortly afterward. Knowledge of this pressure is useful in establishing the relationships among blood volume, right ventricular function, and venous tone before and after bypass; the line also can serve as a medication line and a route for obtaining mixed venous blood samples.

The monitoring of central venous pressure for the first 12 to 24 hours or longer after operation is an essential routine measure. If the central venous pressure line inserted at the onset of the operation is not satisfactory, a small polyethylene catheter can be inserted into the right atrium via its appendage after decannulation at the end of bypass and can be brought out through the body wall and attached to a pressure transducer (Fig 5–4).

The most common problem associated with the measurement of central venous pressure is the uncertainty as to the exact location of the catheter's tip. When the catheter is being positioned, it should be kept in mind that accurate readings can be made only if the tip is within

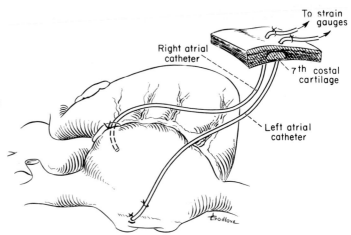

Fig 5–4.—Placement of polyethylene catheters before closure of chest for monitoring atrial pressures. (From McGoon D.C.: Technics of open-heart surgery for congenital heart disease. *Curr. Probl. Surg.*, April 1968, p. 17. Used by permission.)

the chest and that the most reliable central venous pressure is obtained when the tip of the catheter lies within the superior vena cava or right atrium. Mean right atrial pressure should be between 1 and 5 mm Hg.[6] When final position of the catheter is achieved, the pressure must fluctuate with respiration, and aspiration of blood from the catheter should be possible. The central venous pressure line is connected to a pressure transducer so that direct readings of central venous pressure are continuously available. Because pressures are usually low, particular care must be used to remove all air bubbles from the central venous pressure line, since these can dampen the transmission of pressure, resulting in falsely low readings.

A central venous pressure line can be inserted by catheterizing one of several different veins.

Basilic and Cephalic Veins

The basilic or cephalic vein can be used to introduce a central venous pressure line (Fig 5–5). Either route is associated with fewer potential complications than are the subclavian or jugular routes (pneumothorax, inadvertent arterial puncture). Of these two veins, the basilic is usually the better choice because, from the usual site of venipuncture in the antecubital fossa to the superior vena cava, the veins increase progressively in size. However, the presence of valves in the axillary vein frequently prevents passage of the catheter's tip beyond the axilla to the desired location in the superior vena cava or right atrium. This problem can occur despite maneuvers such as abduction of the arm to 90 degrees, which is often helpful in passing the catheter through these areas. The cephalic vein is typically smaller than the basilic and frequently increases little, if any, in size in its course up the arm. After reaching the shoulder, the vessel pierces the clavipectoral fascia in the deltopectoral triangle to empty into the axillary vein at an angle of approximately 90 degrees (Fig 5–6). Near its termination, the cephalic vein may bifurcate into two very small veins, one joining the external jugular vein and the other joining the axillary vein, or the cephalic vein may join the external jugular vein only.[27]

Variability in the subcutaneous veins of the upper extremity is well recognized. Occasionally, the cephalic vein is larger than the basilic vein, and when this is true, correct positioning of a central venous pressure line can be accomplished, sometimes with ease, through the cephalic vein.

In young children, veins in the lower extremity are often used; occasionally, cutdown to an ankle vein is necessary.

External Jugular Vein

The external jugular vein is frequently used to establish a central venous pressure line. As with the basilic and cephalic veins, when the external jugular vein is cannulated, it is often difficult to pass the catheter into the superior vena cava–right atrial position because of valves or tortuosity (or both) of the vessel.

The external jugular vein begins in the lateral region of the neck near the angle of the jaw and

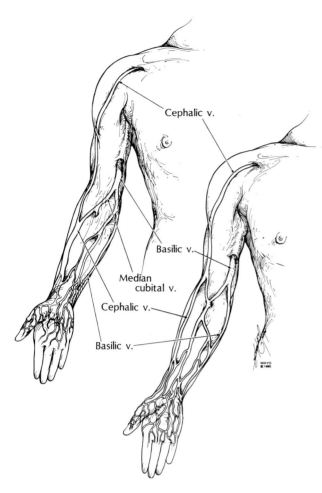

Fig 5–5.—Anterior view of superficial veins of upper limb. Note difference in arrangement and size of basilic and cephalic veins and tributaries to these veins.

descends in the neck to end in the subclavian vein on that side of the neck near the middle of the clavicle (Fig 5–7). At its termination, it is lateral to or in front of the scalene anterior muscle and is covered by platysma muscle, superficial fascia, and skin. In its upper two thirds, however, the vein is covered only by skin and superficial fascia.

The external jugular vein varies in size, depending on the number and size of other veins in the neck. It is occasionally double. In chronic heart failure, the vein appears to be enlarged, a fact that would seem to make cannulation and right atrial catheterization easier but that is not necessarily true because of an increase in tortuosity.

The external jugular has two pairs of valves, a lower one at its entrance into the subclavian vein and an upper one 4 cm above the clavicle. The valves do not prevent reflux of blood. Because of this factor, if the patient is placed a few degrees head-down or is asked to inspire deeply and then maintain the inspiration for a few seconds or to perform a Valsalva maneuver, the external jugular vein will become distended throughout. If the patient is asleep and intubated, a slight head-down position, combined with positive airway pressure, also will distend the vein. These maneuvers also will distend the internal jugular vein. Because of the more direct access that the vein provides to the superior vena cava, most clinicians prefer cannulation of the right external jugular vein.

Because of difficulties associated with advancing the catheter past obstructions in the external jugular vein and into the superior vena cava, a technique of first inserting a flexible angiographic wire guide has been described.[4] The

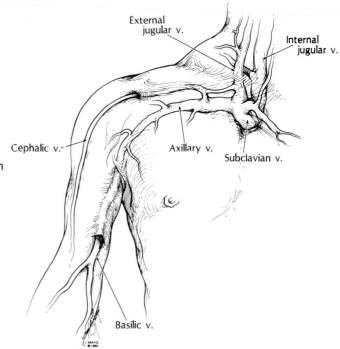

Fig 5–6.—Anatomy of venous plexus around the shoulder. Note sharp angle at which cephalic vein joins axillary vein, reduced size, and bifurcations often found near its termination.

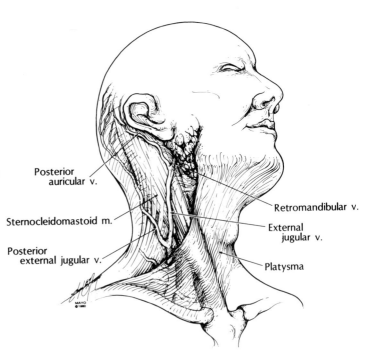

Fig 5–7.—Formation and course of external jugular vein in neck. Note that, in its lower third, the vein courses deep to the platysma muscle.

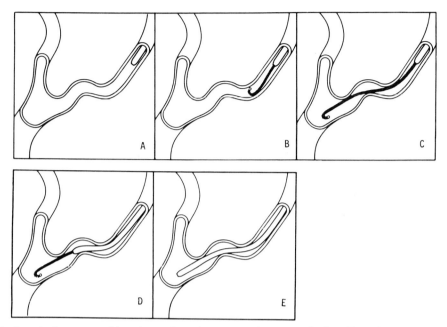

Fig 5-8.—J-wire external jugular catheterization technique. Steps are as follows: **A,** catheter in vein. **B,** J-wire advancing past first obstruction. **C,** J-wire completely inserted. **D,** catheter advancing over J-wire. **E,** catheter completely advanced; J-wire removed. (From Blitt et al.[4] Used by permission.)

technique is called the J-wire external jugular catheterization technique. To perform the technique, the patient is placed in a 30-degree head-down position, with the head turned away from the site of venipuncture. After sterile preparation of the neck, the external jugular vein is cannulated between the level of the cricoid cartilage and the clavicle with a 14- or 16-gauge, 14-cm Teflon catheter. The Teflon catheter is threaded a short distance off the needle into the external jugular vein. The needle of the intravenous placement unit is then removed, and the catheter is aspirated with a syringe to verify that it is in the vein. After verification of catheter placement, a 30.5-cm long, 0.89-mm diameter, flexible angiographic wire catheter guide with a 3-mm radius of curvature is inserted into the hub of the catheter (Fig 5–8). The J-wire or spring guide is advanced through the catheter until it is ascertained to be in the thorax. Insertion of the wire guide 20 to 25 cm is usually sufficient to ensure that it is in the thorax. After placement of the wire into the chest, the 14-cm catheter is threaded over the wire, until the hub of the catheter meets the skin. This position places the tip of the catheter in the superior vena cava. The wire is removed, an intravenous infusion line is attached, and the catheter is securely fastened to the neck. Antibacterial ointment and sterile dressings are then applied. The technique improves the rate of successful placement of the central venous pressure line through the external jugular vein.

For children, after induction of anesthesia, a central venous pressure cannula is inserted through an external jugular vein. This line is connected to a transducer, and central venous pressure is displayed continuously.

After successful cannulation of the external (or internal) jugular vein, precautions should be taken to minimize the risk of air embolism during the process of connecting the cannula to the transducer or manometer. These precautions can include head-down position, positive airway pressure, or, if the patient is awake, asking him to stop breathing until the catheter is attached to the transducer.

Internal Jugular Vein

Superficially, the internal jugular vein is represented by a broad band drawn from the lobule

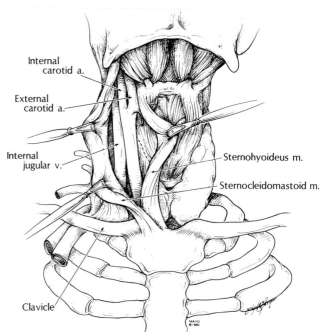

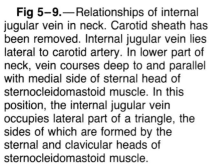

Fig 5–9.—Relationships of internal jugular vein in neck. Carotid sheath has been removed. Internal jugular vein lies lateral to carotid artery. In lower part of neck, vein courses deep to and parallel with medial side of sternal head of sternocleidomastoid muscle. In this position, the internal jugular vein occupies lateral part of a triangle, the sides of which are formed by the sternal and clavicular heads of sternocleidomastoid muscle.

of the ear to the medial end of the clavicle. The vein is a direct continuation of the sigmoid sinus and begins at the base of the skull in the posterior compartment of the jugular foramen. The vein runs within the carotid sheath downward through the neck. Being within the carotid sheath, the vein is closely related to the carotid arterial tree. Throughout the downward course in the neck, the internal carotid artery and the lower common carotid artery lie just medial to the internal jugular vein, with the vagus nerve lying between but posterior to the carotid artery and internal jugular vein. The internal jugular vein is overlapped by the upper part and covered by the lower part of the sternocleidomastoid muscle. The lower part of the internal jugular vein lies behind a depression that marks the interval between the sternal and the clavicular heads of the sternocleidomastoid (Fig 5–9). The internal jugular vein unites with the subclavian vein behind the sternal end of the clavicle to form the brachiocephalic vein. A pair of valves are located just above the termination of the internal jugular vein.

Several techniques have been proposed for locating and cannulating the internal jugular vein.[2, 8, 10, 20, 22] The variety of methods probably means that experience gained with a given technique is a more important determinant of successful cannulation than is the particular technique used. A useful technique is to outline, on the right side of the neck, the triangle formed by the sternal and clavicular heads of the sternocleidomastoid muscle and the clavicle (Fig 5–10). If difficulty is encountered in identifying the muscle, maneuvers such as asking the patient to make a maximal inspiratory effort, to turn his head to the left against force, or to extend his head will assist in outlining the right

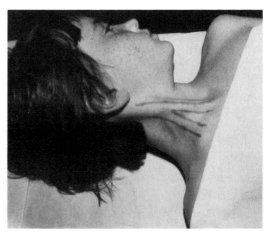

Fig 5–10.—Triangle formed by sternal and clavicular heads of sternocleidomastoid muscle.

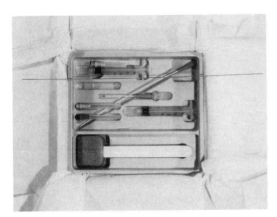

Fig 5-11.—Disposable internal jugular puncture kit.

sternocleidomastoid muscle. Once these landmarks are identified, the patient's head is turned to the left and he is placed in a 20-degree, head-down position. A disposable internal jugular puncture kit (Arrow International, Hill and George avenues, Reading, PA. 19610) is opened (Fig 5–11), the skin over the area of anticipated venipuncture is cleaned with antiseptic solution, and a drape is placed over the field. Lidocaine (1%) is drawn into a 3-ml syringe, and a skin wheal is made at the apex of the triangle formed by the two heads of the sternocleidomastoid muscle. The initial venipuncture is made with an 18-gauge, 4-cm catheter over a 20-gauge introducer needle on a 3-ml syringe (Fig 5–12). With the skin tensed, the needle is advanced at

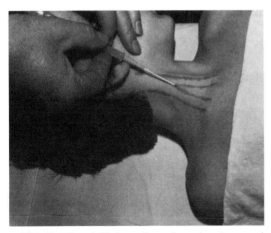

Fig 5-12.—Initial venipuncture locates and cannulates the internal jugular vein with 18-gauge, 4.0-cm catheter. Skin puncture is at apex of sternocleidomastoid triangle.

an angle of 30 degrees to the skin in a caudal direction, approximately parallel to the medial border of the clavicular head of the sternocleidomastoid muscle. Constant aspiration is maintained on the syringe as it advances toward the vein. The valves in the lower internal jugular vein do not prevent reflux of blood from the thoracic veins, and positive airway pressure or a Valsalva maneuver by the patient will greatly distend the vein.

After the vein has been located and catheterized, the introducer needle is removed and a 30.5-cm spring wire guide with flexible tip is threaded through the catheter and advanced into the superior vena cava. With the spring wire guide held in place, the 18-gauge catheter is removed and a 16-gauge, 15-cm catheter is placed over the spring wire guide, introduced into the internal jugular vein, and advanced into the superior vena cava. The spring wire guide is then removed, and the central venous pressure transducer line is attached. The precautions listed previously to avoid air embolism should be observed during attachment of a central venous pressure line to the catheter. An antibiotic ointment is applied to the puncture site, and the catheter is secured with tape.

Complications have been associated with internal jugular venipuncture. Some complications, such as neck tenderness, may be minor; others, more serious, include pleural puncture, nerve damage, thoracic duct injury, and bilateral vocal cord damage. A patient with damage to the ascending cervical artery resulting in fatal hemorrhage has been described.[28] The incidence of complications, however, appears to be small; one study reported only one complication in 500 patients,[10] whereas another reported three complications in 1,000 patients, all of whom were treated successfully.[17]

An open thorax also renders the esophagus an unsuitable location from which to monitor body temperature during surgery. The nasopharyngeal temperature is reported to be a more reliable guide to body-core and brain temperatures when the thorax is open than either the rectal or the upper esophageal temperature.[15] Placing a temperature thermistor in the nasopharynx is a reliable guide to body-core temperature and can be used routinely to monitor temperature at this location. The nasopharyngeal thermistor probe is always placed before heparin is given.

Because patients undergoing cardiopulmonary

bypass are cooled, some special problems with respect to uneven rewarming may occur after bypass.

After deep (15 to 18 C) or moderate (30 to 32 C) hypothermia, uneven rewarming of areas of the body may occur. The highly vascular and hence well-perfused areas may be brought back to near 37 C; the less well-perfused areas of the body (bone, cartilage, skin, and so forth) may return to only 33 or 34 C. These cooler areas, therefore, will cause a downward drift in body temperature after bypass. The decrease in body temperature due to uneven rewarming is enhanced by the increased loss of heat due to the open thorax.

The decrease in body temperature after bypass can be minimized by the use of external heating blankets, through which warmed fluid is circulated. They are placed on the operating table before the patient is positioned. Care must be taken to pad the blankets well, because a cold patient can be more easily burned than a warm patient.

LEFT ATRIAL PRESSURE

The effectiveness of the left ventricle in handling venous return must be evaluated continuously during withdrawal from cardiopulmonary bypass and during the immediate postoperative period. In making this assessment, knowing the left atrial pressure is helpful. Left atrial pressure can be measured during emergence from cardiopulmonary bypass by inserting a needle directly into the left atrium immediately before emergence. If problems with the left side of the heart are expected or if a need for left atrial pressures beyond emergence from cardiopulmonary bypass is anticipated, a catheter can be introduced directly through the atrial wall into the left atrial chamber and brought out of the chest wall before the thorax is closed and can be secured with a pursestring suture (see Fig 5–4). This catheter remains in the patient after operation.

Left atrial pressure is monitored continuously in patients whenever the mitral valve has been operated on or in patients with poor left ventricular function.

If avoidance of direct cannulation of the left atrium is desired, a Swan-Ganz balloon-tipped catheter may be introduced and the pulmonary capillary wedge pressure may be determined.[25]

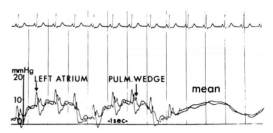

Fig 5–13.—Simultaneous recording of left atrial and pulmonary capillary wedge pressures demonstrates similarity of waveforms and near identity of mean pressures. (From Buchbinder et al.[6] Used by permission.)

This pressure (5 to 15 mm Hg) approximates the left atrial pressure.[12, 26] A simultaneous recording of left atrial and pulmonary capillary wedge pressures is shown in Figure 5–13.[6]

The Swan-Ganz catheter (Fig 5–14) is a flexible, flow-directed, balloon-tipped catheter.[25] Catheters of variable size (5 and 7 F) and number of lumina (two, three, or four) or with electrode leads for pacing are available commercially. The 5 F catheters are rarely used by anesthesiologists, except in pediatric cases. In essence, the catheter is designed to obtain hemodynamic pressures (most often, right atrial and pulmonary artery with pulmonary capillary wedge pressures) and, with specially equipped 7 F catheters, to determine cardiac output by thermodilution techniques. Additional pressures (that is, superior vena cava and right ventricular pressures) may be measured through the distal lumen as the catheter advances during insertion. Once the catheter is positioned in the pulmonary capillary wedge position, mixed venous blood may be withdrawn from this port.

A second lumen connects to the 1.5-ml capacity balloon at the catheter's tip. Inflation of this balloon either allows the catheter to advance to the point where the pulmonary artery diameter equals balloon diameter or impinges on the lumen of the pulmonary artery so that there is no further movement of the catheter. In either situation, the forward flow of blood through the pulmonary artery is obstructed and the distal lumen reads the pressure distal to it—the pressure in the valveless pulmonary capillaries (thus, "pulmonary capillary wedge pressure"). Because of the valveless nature of the pulmonary venous system, the wedge pressure, in the absence of pulmonary structural disease, represents left

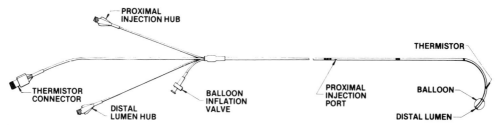

Fig 5–14.—Four-lumen Swan-Ganz balloon catheter designed to obtain hemodynamic pressures and to determine cardiac output by thermodilution technique. (Drawing courtesy of Edwards Laboratories, Santa Ana, Calif.)

atrial pressure. At the end of diastole, this pressure closely approximates left ventricular end-diastolic pressure, which may correlate with left ventricular end-diastolic volume.

A third lumen transmits the electrical signal from the thermistor positioned 4 cm proximal to the catheter's tip. The thermistor information processed through a computer allows the determination of cardiac output by thermodilution.

The fourth lumen, the proximal lumen, terminates 30 cm proximal to the catheter's tip and is positioned in the right atrium in most adults when the catheter's tip is in wedge position. It is through this lumen that the injectate necessary for cardiac output computation is delivered. Additional space within the catheter may be allotted to the electrodes necessary for endocardial atrioventricular sequential, atrial, or ventricular pacing.

The catheter is inserted percutaneously under sterile conditions, although a cutdown occasionally may be necessary. The most frequently used sites are the internal or external jugular veins and the subclavian or a cubital vein. The femoral vein may be used in patients with the superior vena cava syndrome. Use of the cephalic vein results in much more difficult placement than does use of the basilic vein. After cannulation of the vein, a flexible guide wire is passed through the cannula; the original cannula is then removed. After appropriate enlargement of the skin puncture site, an 8 F sheath of approximately 10-cm length, with a tapered vein dilator, is passed over the guide wire. After placement in the vein, the guide wire and dilator may be withdrawn, leaving the sheath. The catheter, which has had its pressure lumina connected to transducers, and the balloon (which has been checked for patency and the absence of leaks) is then passed through the sheath and threaded centrally. Placement is optimally performed by continuous monitoring of the pressures with electronic transduction and oscilloscopic display. When, as indicated by intracardiac pressures (Table 5–1) and waveform (Fig 5–15), the catheter is determined to be within the right atrium, the balloon is inflated with 0.8 ml of air (or carbon dioxide, if passage to the arterial system is considered possible). The flow of blood should carry the inflated balloon across the tricuspid valve and into the right ventricle. Difficulty may arise, particularly with tricuspid stenosis, that will force an alteration in balloon volume. Repeated attempts may be required. From the right ventricle, the catheter must pass the pulmonic valve to enter the pulmonary outflow tract. Again, difficulties may be encountered if valvular disease exists or if the ventricles are ejecting poorly or are massively dilated. Once the pulmonary outflow tract is entered, the catheter, because it is flow-directed, will go to the area with the greatest blood flow—generally to the right arterial tree. Reaching a wedge position may be difficult if the catheter's forward progress is obstructed by a bifurcation

TABLE 5–1.—Normal Intracardiac Pressures*

SITE	PRESSURE, MM HG	
	MEAN	RANGE
Right atrium	5	1–10
Right ventricle	25/5	15–30/0–8
Pulmonary artery		
Systolic	23	15–30
Diastolic	9	5–15
Pulmonary capillary wedge	10	5–15

*Adapted from Kaplan J.A.: *Cardiac Anesthesia*. New York, Grune & Stratton, 1979. Used by permission.

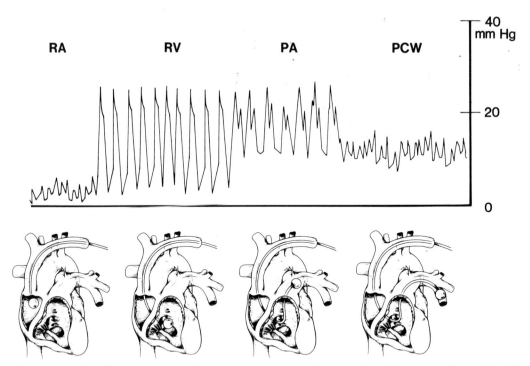

Fig 5–15.—Oscilloscope tracing of pressures encountered as tip of Swan-Ganz catheter traverses heart chambers and pulmonary arterial tree during insertion. *RA*, right atrium; *RV*, right ventricle; *PA*, pulmonary artery; *PCW*, pulmonary capillary wedge.

or if pulmonary hypertension or mitral regurgitation is present. Once the wedge position is reached, the pressure should be measured and the balloon should be deflated to avoid pulmonary infarction distal to the catheter's tip. Criteria that may be used to determine the wedge position include a change in configuration of the tracing on the oscilloscope from pulmonary artery pressure to left atrial pressure (see Fig 5–13) and a mean pressure less than mean pulmonary artery pressure. After placement, the catheter may advance if redundant length is available, particularly in the right ventricle, or if the diameter of the pulmonary artery changes. Repositioning of the catheter should be performed with the same sterile precautions that were used for insertion.

CARDIAC OUTPUT

Methods commonly used for measuring cardiac output during cardiac surgery include the dye-dilution[23] and thermodilution[5, 11, 13, 14] techniques. With the dye-dilution technique, a dye is injected into the circulation and the optical density of the blood is increased in specific wavelengths. The injection is made into one part of the circulation, and samples are removed at another site by continuous withdrawal through a cuvette that senses changes in the optical density at the wavelengths specific for the dye used. One of the more commonly used dyes is indocyanine green, which, when injected into the blood, increases optical density in the infrared range (± 810 nm). In this range, the optical densities of reduced hemoglobin and oxyhemoglobin are similar; thus, baseline variation is negligible.[23]

To measure cardiac output with the dye-dilution method, dye is injected into a central vein, such as the superior vena cava, and sampling is done in a peripheral artery. Before measurement of cardiac output, the densitometer is calibrated for known concentrations of dye in blood. Calibration requires that blood be withdrawn from the patient and reinfused and that the densitometer controls be adjusted for baseline. When the baseline is steady, two concentrations of dye (5 and 10 mg/L) in known volumes of blood are passed through the

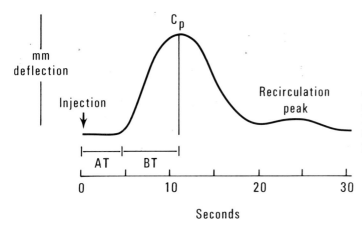

Fig 5-16.—Normal dye-dilution curve showing injection of dye, appearance time *(AT)*, buildup time *(BT)*, peak concentration *(C_p)*, and recirculation.

densitometer cuvette. From these samples, linearity in response can be confirmed, and the deflections for known concentrations of dye per milliliter of blood can be obtained.

The dye should be injected as a bolus. After injection, the optical densities of continuously withdrawn arterial blood samples are used to construct a concentration curve similar to that shown in Figure 5-16. This figure shows a peak concentration curve and a recirculation peak as a function of time. Cardiac output (CO) is calculated by dividing the amount (milligrams) of indicator injected *(I)* by the mean concentration *($\bar{c}$)* of the indicator during the period that the concentration curve is inscribed before recirculation:

$$CO = \frac{I \text{ (mg)}}{\bar{c} \text{ (mg/ml)} \times t \text{ (sec)}}$$

This computation will give cardiac output in milliliters per second. To measure in liters per minute, the equation would be:

$$CO \text{ (L/min)} = \frac{I \text{ (mg)} \times 60}{\bar{c} \text{ (mg/L)} \times t \text{ (sec)}}$$

The mean concentration of dye is obtained by dividing the sum of the heights of the curve above baseline every second from the beginning to the end of the peak concentration curve (assuming that the concentration decreases exponentially) by total observations (seconds) and comparing the mean deflection (obtained in the same way) produced by a known concentration of dye during calibration. Computers have been programmed to make these calculations and give instantaneous readout of cardiac output.

Dye-dilution curves also can be used to detect shunts and incompetent valves. The rapid recirculation curve noted with left-to-right shunt results in a curve that may show a sudden change in the downslope just beyond the peak (Figs 5-17 and 5-18). The earlier this change occurs, the larger is the left-to-right shunt. An early appearance of dye is indicative of a right-to-left shunt (Fig 5-19).

The level of right-to-left shunting also can be detected by sampling from a peripheral artery and selectively injecting dye into different chambers. If there is an atrial right-to-left shunt, normal curves will be seen with injections into the pulmonary artery or the right ventricle, but an early appearance will be noted in the right atrial or vena cava injection. Although these uses of the dye-dilution technique are mainly diagnostic and are not done during cardiac surgery, they can be used to evaluate completeness of closure of shunts.

At the Mayo Clinic, intraoperative double-sampling dye-dilution curves are commonly done after atrioventricular canal repair. Indocyanine green is injected into the left ventricle, and simultaneous sampling is done in the left atrium and aorta. This technique permits an evaluation of the mitral valve for insufficiency while the chest is open so that a prosthetic mitral valve can be inserted if required.

A variation of the dye-dilution technique that is being used more frequently measures cardiac output by thermodilution.[5, 11, 13, 14] The principle is identical to that used in dye-dilution curves. With the technique, a rapidly responsive thermistor is attached near the end of a Swan-Ganz catheter (see Fig 5-14), and an exact amount of

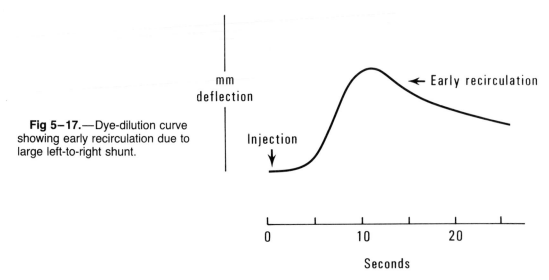

Fig 5–17.—Dye-dilution curve showing early recirculation due to large left-to-right shunt.

a solution of known temperature is injected into the right atrium or superior vena cava; the resultant change in blood temperature between the injection site and the thermistor in the pulmonary artery allows a cooling curve to be recorded. Adequate mixing of blood with the cold injectate occurs during passage of the mixture through two valves and one cardiac chamber. Ten milliliters of 5% glucose is injected. The liquid may be cooled to near 0 C in an ice bath or injected at room temperature (which is still less than body temperature). In either situation, the appropriate correction factor is entered into the cardiac output computer. The decrease in temperature is detected in the pulmonary artery. From the thermodilution curve so obtained, cardiac output can be computed manually or by a thermodilution cardiac output computer.

The technique has the advantage that the substances injected are more physiologic than dye and determinations can be repeated at short intervals (about twice per minute). Duplicate or triplicate sequential determinations of cardiac output are usually done, and a mean is calculated.

TEMPERATURE

The anesthetized patient tends to become poikilothermic because of central depression

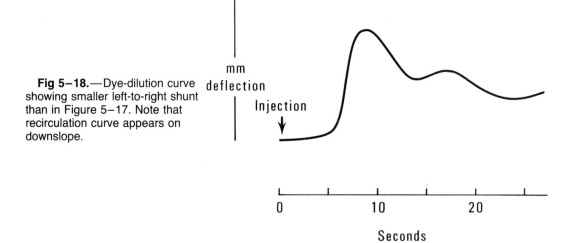

Fig 5–18.—Dye-dilution curve showing smaller left-to-right shunt than in Figure 5–17. Note that recirculation curve appears on downslope.

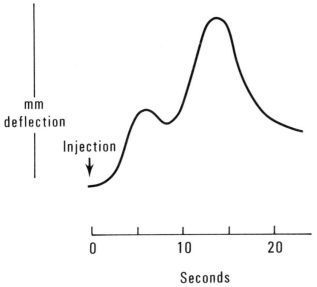

Fig 5-19.—Dye-dilution curve showing large right-to-left shunt. Note early appearance of dye curve after injection.

and loss of vascular control. Hence, the body temperature, being less accurately controlled, tends to drift according to the environmental conditions. A downward drift of body temperature is accelerated if the thorax is open, as during cardiac surgery, so that heat can be lost from the body core by both evaporation and radiation. As a result, body temperature should be monitored continuously during cardiac surgery.

ARTERIAL BLOOD GASES, pH, AND SERUM POTASSIUM

Facilities for measuring Po_2, Pco_2, and pH and for determining electrolyte levels in blood are an indispensable part of the cardiovascular anesthesia practice. Facilities for these measurements should be located near the operating room and should be sufficiently responsive to obviate undue delays in the reporting of results. Samples of arterial blood are sent routinely for Po_2, Pco_2, and pH determinations before, during, and after bypass. Samples should be analyzed at other times when there is a possibility of an acid-base abnormality or inadequate oxygenation. Serum potassium levels are determined whenever low levels of body and serum potassium are suspected or when unexplained arrhythmias appear on the ECG screen.

By placing a three-way stopcock in the intra-arterial pressure line, arterial blood samples can be obtained easily.

URINARY OUTPUT

Patients routinely have an indwelling urinary bladder catheter during surgery. The volume of urine present in the collection container before surgery and during each succeeding hour of anesthesia is recorded. Urinary output of the patients before, during, and after bypass and its significance are discussed in chapter 16.

REFERENCES

1. Allen E.V.: Thromboangiitis obliterans: Methods of diagnosis of chronic occlusive arterial lesions distal to the wrist with illustrative cases. *Am. J. Med. Sci.* 178:237, 1929.
2. Baker J.D. III, Wallace C.T.: Internal jugular central venous pressure monitoring—a panacea? *Anesthesiol. Rev.* 3:15, Mar. 1976.
3. Bedford R.F., Wollman H.: Complications of percutaneous radial-artery cannulation: An objective prospective study in man. *Anesthesiology* 38:228, 1973.
4. Blitt C.D., et al.: Central venous catheterization via the external jugular vein: A technique employing the J-wire. *J.A.M.A.* 229:817, 1974.
5. Branthwaite M.S., Bradley R.D.: Measurement of cardiac output by thermal dilution in man. *J. Appl. Physiol.* 24:434, 1968.
6. Buchbinder N., Ganz, W.: Hemodynamic monitoring: Invasive techniques. *Anesthesiology* 45:146, 1976.
7. Coleman S.S., Anson B.J.: Arterial patterns in

7. the hand based upon a study of 650 specimens. Surg. Gynecol. Obstet. 113:409, 1961.
8. Defalque R.J.: Percutaneous catheterization of the internal jugular vein. Anesth. Analg. 53:116, 1974.
9. Downs J.B., et al.: Hazards of radial-artery catheterization. Anesthesiology 38:283, 1973.
10. English I.C.W., et al.: Percutaneous catheterisation of the internal jugular vein. Anaesthesia 24:521, 1969.
11. Fegler G.: Measurement of cardiac output in anaesthetized animals by a thermo-dilution method. Q.J. Exp. Physiol. 39:153, 1954.
12. Fitzpatrick G.F., Hampson L.G., Burgess J.H.: Bedside determination of left atrial pressure. Can. Med. Assoc. J. 106:1293, 1972.
13. Forrester J.S., et al.: Thermodilution cardiac output determination with a single flow-directed catheter. Am. Heart J. 83:306, 1972.
14. Ganz W., et al.: A new technique for measurement of cardiac output by thermodilution in man. Am. J. Cardiol. 27:392, 1971.
15. Gilston A.: Anaesthesia for cardiac surgery. Br. J. Anaesth. 43:217, 1971.
16. Greenhow D.E.: Incorrect performance of Allen's test—ulnar-artery flow erroneously presumed inadequate. Anesthesiology 37:356, 1972.
17. Jernigan W.R., et al.: Use of the internal jugular vein for placement of central venous catheter. Surg. Gynecol. Obstet. 130:520, 1970.
18. Kamienski R.W., Barnes R.W.: Critique of the Allen test for continuity of the palmar arch assessed by Doppler ultrasound. Surg. Gynecol. Obstet. 142:861, 1976.
19. Kaplan J.A., King S.B. III: The precordial electrocardiographic lead (V_5) in patients who have coronary-artery disease. Anesthesiology 45:570, 1976.
20. Korshin J., et al.: Percutaneous catheterization of the internal jugular vein. Acta Anaesthesiol. Scand. [Suppl.] 67:27, 1978.
21. Miyasaka K., Edmonds J.F., Conn A.W.: Complications of radial artery lines in the paediatric patient. Can. Anaesth. Soc. J. 23:9, 1976.
22. Rao T.L.K., Wong A.Y., Salem M.R.: A new approach to percutaneous catheterization of the internal jugular vein. Anesthesiology 46:362, 1977.
23. Rudolph A.M.: *Congenital Diseases of the Heart: Clinical-Physiologic Considerations in Diagnosis and Management*. Chicago, Year Book Medical Publishers, 1974, p. 49.
24. Seldinger S.I.: Catheter replacement of the needle in percutaneous arteriography: A new technique. Acta Radiol. 39:368, 1953.
25. Swan H.J.C., et al.: Catheterization of the heart in man with use of a flow-directed balloon-tipped catheter. N. Engl. J. Med. 283:447, 1970.
26. Walston A. II, Kendall M.E.: Comparison of pulmonary wedge and left atrial pressure in man. Am. Heart J. 86:159, 1973.
27. Webre D.R., Arens J.F.: Use of cephalic and basilic veins for introduction of central venous catheters. Anesthesiology 38:389, 1973.
28. Wisheart J.D., Hassan M.A., Jackson J.W.: A complication of percutaneous cannulation of the internal jugular vein. Thorax 27:496, 1972.

6 / Anesthesia for Surgical Repair of Congenital Heart Defects in Children

FROUKJE M. BEYNEN

SAIT TARHAN

THE REPORTED incidence of congenital heart defects varies somewhat in different countries. The incidence in the United States is approximately eight per 1,000 live births.[130]

Age is an important determinant in mortality (Table 6–1). Of the children with congenital heart defects who died in the Toronto Hospital for Sick Children between 1950 and 1970, about one third died during the first month of life, another third died between 1 month and 1 year, and another third died after 1 year of age.

Usually, the cause of congenital heart defects is obscure, although teratogens like thalidomide, folic acid antagonists, and maternal rubella infection have been identified (Table 6–2). Also, the incidence of congenital heart defects in the offspring of mothers with diabetes mellitus is increased, which suggests that this metabolic disease also may have some effect.[131] Maternal age and parity are apparently not major determinants; however, 40% to 50% of patients with Down syndrome have congenital heart defects, and Down syndrome occurs more frequently in the offspring of older mothers.[138]

Careful studies have suggested that genetic-environmental interaction ("multifactorial inheritance") accounts for approximately 90% of the cases. In this situation, a hereditary predisposition to cardiovascular maldevelopment interacts with an environmental trigger (virus or drug) at the vulnerable period of cardiogenesis (Table 6–3). The etiologic basis is environmental (for example, rubella) in 1% to 2% and primarily genetic in the remaining 8% to 9%.

The obscure cause makes effective prevention infeasible. Therefore, treatment, which means surgical intervention in most patients, continues to be of major importance. With the remarkable advances in open-heart surgery during the past 20 years, correction of complex congenital heart defects will continue to be attempted in progressively younger age groups. As a result, the anesthesiologist needs to be thoroughly familiar with both the pathophysiology of the congenital heart defects and the pathophysiology of the infant. Valuable information on pediatric cardiac anesthesia can be found in recently published books on pediatric and cardiac anesthesia.[18, 21, 146, 152, 169]

TABLE 6–1.—AGE AT DEATH AMONG 2,870 INFANTS AND CHILDREN WITH CONGENITAL HEART DISEASE*

AGE	DEATHS NO.	%
1st mo of life	980	34.14
1 mo to 1 yr	1,047	36.48
1 to 5 yr	449	15.64
≥5 yr	394	13.72
Total	2,870	100.00

*Represents 27.2% of 10,535 cases of congenital heart disease seen at the Hospital for Sick Children in Toronto between 1950 and 1970. (From Keith J.D.: Prevalence, incidence, and epidemiology, in Keith J.D., Rowe R.D., Vlad P. (eds.): *Heart Disease in Infancy and Childhood*, ed. 3. New York, Macmillan Publishing Co., 1978. Used by permission.)

CLASSIFICATION OF CONGENITAL HEART DEFECTS

Congenital heart defects can be classified in several ways, none of which is entirely satisfactory. The following classification is probably most useful for the anesthesiologist. Patients

TABLE 6-2.—CARDIOVASCULAR TERATOGENS*

TERATOGEN	DRUGS	VIRUSES
Proved	Thalidomide, folic acid antagonists	Rubella
Highly suspected	Dextroamphetamine, anticonvulsants, lithium chloride, alcohol, progestogen-estrogen	Cytomegalovirus, herpes virus hominis B, coxsackievirus B

*From Nora J.J.: Etiologic aspects of congenital heart diseases, in Moss A.J., Adams F.H., Emmanouilides G.C. (eds.): *Heart Disease in Infants, Children, and Adolescents*, ed. 2. Baltimore, Williams & Wilkins Co., 1977. Used by permission.

TABLE 6-3.—PRESUMED VULNERABLE PERIOD FOR TERATOGENIC INFLUENCE ON CARDIOVASCULAR DEVELOPMENT*

ABNORMALITY	EMBRYONIC EVENT COMPLETED, DAYS	LIMITS OF VULNERABLE PERIOD, DAYS	MOST SENSITIVE VULNERABLE PERIOD, DAYS
Truncoconal septation	34	14–34	18–29
Endocardial cushions	38	14–38	18–33
Ventricular septum	38–44	14–44	18–39
Atrial septum secundum	55	14–55	18–50
Semilunar valves	55	14–?	18–50
Ductus arteriosus		14–?	18–60
Coarctation of aorta		14–?	18–60

*From Nora J.J.: Etiologic aspects of congenital heart diseases, in Moss A.J., Adams F.H., Emmanouilides G.C. (eds.): *Heart Disease in Infants, Children, and Adolescents*, ed. 2. Baltimore, Williams & Wilkins Co., 1977. Used by permission.

with congenital heart defects are classified into two groups according to their different behavior during induction of anesthesia: (1) children who have cyanosis and a right-to-left or a bidirectional shunt with dominating right-to-left direction, and (2) children who have acyanotic congenital heart defects. The latter group is further divided into two subgroups: those without a shunt and those with a dominant left-to-right shunt. A classification of congenital heart defects discussed in this chapter is as follows:

Cyanotic
    Pulmonary stenosis and atresia
    Tetralogy of Fallot
    Transposition of the great arteries
    Common ventricle
    Total anomalous pulmonary venous drainage
    Tricuspid atresia
    Ebstein's anomaly
Acyanotic
    Without shunt
        Coarctation of aorta
        Aortic stenosis
        Vascular ring anomalies
    With left-to-right shunt
        Atrial septal defect
        Endocardial cushion defects
        Ventricular septal defect
        Patent ductus arteriosus
        Truncus arteriosus

This is a simplified classification, and the presence of additional anomalies, such as pulmonary stenosis in truncus arteriosus or the absence of right ventricular outflow obstruction in patients with an overriding aorta, may place a particular congenital heart defect into the other group. The necessity for the anesthesiologist to understand the pathologic anatomy and its impact on the circulatory physiology is obvious.

PREOPERATIVE EVALUATION AND PREMEDICATION

The aim of the preoperative visit of the anesthesiologist is to obtain as much information as possible on the condition of the child to decide what anesthetic management is indicated.

A thorough physical examination is done. The history, medications, and records of fluid intake and output, temperature, heart rate, and blood pressure are reviewed, as are the data on the heart catheterization, blood gases, echocardiogram, chest roentgenogram, ECG, hemoglobin, hematocrit, serum electrolytes, and creatinine. In newborns, the levels of blood glucose and calcium should be determined because they may be low. Tests of hemostasis are done when indicated. The planned surgical procedure is discussed with the surgeon, and if there is any doubt whether the patient is in as "optimal" a condition as possible, the opinion and help of the pediatrician, cardiologist, or chest physiotherapist are obtained.

The premedication, induction, and further anesthetic management are planned on the basis of the results of this thorough evaluation. However, the preoperative visit is also valuable in obtaining good rapport with the child and his parents. If the child is of appropriate age, it is helpful to talk about topics in which he is interested (for instance, a pet at home, the hero of his favorite television program, and so forth), because the next morning during preinduction or induction, one may be able to divert the child's attention by talking about his favorite subjects. Also, the routine that will be followed the morning of the operation, including the premedication and transportation to the operating room, and the appearance of the operating room should be explained. When possible, the choice between inhalation induction and intravenous induction is left to the child. Also, the child should be familiarized with the situation that he will find himself in after surgery.

Preoperative Assessment of Abnormal Hemostasis

The importance of being aware of preexisting hemostatic defects in children who are going to have surgery is obvious. If the history is indicative of hereditary bleeding disorders, specific hemostatic tests are ordered and the hematologist will advise the anesthesiologist about the management.[141, 142] Certain medications affect platelet function.[134] Therefore, the parents are asked specifically whether the child may have used any such medication during the ten days before the scheduled day of surgery—for instance, products containing aspirin, antihistamines, furosemide, propranolol, and so forth. If such agents have been used, tests of bleeding time and platelet function are indicated and, if necessary and possible, surgery is postponed.

Cyanotic patients with high hematocrit levels tend to have hemostatic abnormalities.[119] The most frequent hemostatic irregularities in patients with cyanotic congenital heart disease are platelet function abnormalities and prolonged bleeding time, but also reported have been prolonged prothrombin time, prolonged partial thromboplastin time, prolonged thrombin time, decreased plasma activity of factors I, II, V, VII, and VIII, thrombocytopenia, accelerated fibrinolysis, presence of split products of fibrin, and others.[56, 57, 82, 120, 183, 184] Patients with congestive hepatic dysfunction also may have coagulation defects (low activity of factors II, VII, IX, and X).[142] In children with congenital heart disease

TABLE 6-4.—PREMEDICATION*

		INTRAMUSCULAR PREMEDICATION	
WEIGHT, KG	TIME PREOP, HR	ANTICHOLINERGIC	SEDATIVE†
<2	3/4	Atropine (0.05 mg) or glycopyrrolate (0.025 mg)	Not sedated
2–5	3/4–1	Atropine (0.1 mg) or glycopyrrolate (0.05 mg)	If indicated, morphine (0.05 to 0.1 mg/kg)
5–8	3/4–1	Atropine (0.02 mg/kg) or glycopyrrolate (0.01 mg/kg)	If indicated, morphine (0.2 mg/kg)
>8	1–1½	Scopolamine (0.01 mg/kg)	Morphine (0.2 mg/kg), pentobarbital (1 mg/kg)

*Evening before surgery, if child is nervous: pentobarbital (2 mg/kg oral), triclofos elixir (30 mg/kg oral), or valium (0.2 mg/kg oral). In children with tetralogy of Fallot and histories of hypoxic spells, oxygen with anesthesia mask and bag should be present in the room when the intramuscular premedication is given; the same for very ill children. In children in whom intramuscular medication has previously provoked hypoxic spells, oral premedication is given: two hours preoperatively, atropine (0.03 mg/kg to maximal dose of 1 mg) and valium (0.2 to 0.4 mg/kg to maximal dose of 10 mg).
†In severely sick patients, the doses are decreased or the morphine is omitted completely.

TABLE 6-5.—DRUGS AND INTRAVENOUS (IV) DOSAGES IN PEDIATRIC CARDIAC ANESTHESIA*

DRUG	HOW SUPPLIED	USUAL DOSES
Epinephrine	1 mg/ml IV drip 4 mg in 250 ml D_5/W = 16 µg/ml	1–10 µg/kg, repeat as needed; initial 0.1–0.2 µg/kg/min; adjust rate to response
Isoproterenol	0.2 mg/ml IV drip 4 mg in 250 ml D_5/W = 16 µg/ml	Initial 0.02–0.1 µg/kg/min; adjust rate to response
Dopamine	40 mg/ml IV drip 200 mg in 250 ml D_5/W = 800 µg/ml	Usual, 5–10 µg/kg/min
Dobutamine	250 mg powder in vial IV drip 250 mg in 250 ml D_5/W = 1 mg/ml	Usual, 5–15 µg/kg/min
Phenylephrine	1 mg/ml	5–10 µg/kg, repeat as needed
Norepinephrine	1 mg/ml IV drip 4 mg in 250 ml D_5/W = 16 µg/ml	Initial 0.1–1 µg/kg/min; adjust rate to response
Ephedrine	25 mg/ml	0.2–0.5 mg/kg
Calcium chloride	100 mg/ml	10–15 mg/kg
Calcium gluconate	100 mg/ml	50–60 mg/kg
Digoxin†	0.25 mg/ml	Digitalizing dose: 0.75 mg/sq m for newborns and prematures; 0.9 to 1.2 mg/sq m for older infants
Theophylline	25 mg/ml	Slowly max 3 mg/kg over ten minutes; 12 mg/kg/24 hr
Sodium nitroprusside	50 mg powder in vial IV drip 50 mg into 500 ml D_5/W = 100 µg/ml	Start 0.1 µg/kg/min; if needed, up to 5 µg/kg/min; adjust rate to response
Nitroglycerin	To be prepared by hospital pharmacy	Start 0.2–0.6 µg/kg/min; adjust rate to response
Trimethaphan	50 mg/ml IV drip 250 mg in 250 ml D_5/W	Start 5 µg/kg/min; adjust rate to response
Phentolamine	5 mg powder in vial	0.1 mg/kg, repeat as needed
Chlorpromazine	25 mg/ml	0.05–0.1 mg/kg, repeat as needed
Sodium bicarbonate‡	1 mEq/ml	Start 1–2 mEq/kg
Potassium chloride§	2 mEq/ml	Calculated dose at normal pH in mEq KCl = 1/3 kg body wt (desired K − actual serum K)
Propranolol	1 mg/ml	Start 10 µg/kg; in cyanotic spell up to 100–200 µg/kg may be necessary
Edrophonium	10 mg/ml	0.1–0.2 mg/kg
Lidocaine	20 mg/ml IV drip 1,000 mg in 250 ml D_5/W	1 mg/kg 10–30 µg/kg/min
Procainamide	100 mg/ml	2–5 mg/kg
Bretylium	50 mg/ml	5–10 mg/kg
Verapamil	2.5 mg/ml	0.1–0.2 mg/kg
Furosemide	10 mg/ml	0.5–1 mg/kg
Ethacrynic acid	50 mg powder in vial	0.5–1 mg/kg
Mannitol (10%–25%)	100–250 mg/ml	0.5 gm/kg
Glucose (50%)‖	500 mg/ml	250–500 mg/kg
Atropine	0.4 mg/ml	0.01–0.03 mg/kg
Scopolamine	0.33 mg/ml	0.006–0.01 mg/kg
Glycopyrrolate	0.2 mg/ml	0.005–0.01 mg/kg
Neostigmine	1 mg/ml	0.06 mg/kg
Pyridostigmine	5 mg/ml	0.2 mg/kg
Gallamine	20 mg/ml	1.5–2 mg/kg
Metocurine	2 mg/ml	0.10–0.25 mg/kg
Pancuronium	1 mg/ml	0.04–0.1 mg/kg
d-Tubocurarine	3 mg/ml	0.25–0.5 mg/kg
Succinylcholine	20 mg/ml	1–1.5 mg/kg (2–4 mg/kg IM)
Thiopental	25 mg/ml	2–5 mg/kg

(continued)

TABLE 6–5.—Drugs and Intravenous (IV) Dosages in Pediatric Cardiac Anesthesia* *(Cont.)*

DRUG	HOW SUPPLIED	USUAL DOSES
Ketamine	10, 50, and 100 mg/ml	1–2 mg/kg (4–7 mg/kg IM)
Fentanyl	50 µg/ml	Induction 5–40 µg/kg; maintenance 0.5–2 µg/kg as needed, up to about 100 µg/kg
Morphine	8 mg/ml	0.1–0.2 mg/kg; open cardiac surgery, up to about 2 mg/kg
Meperidine	50 mg/ml	0.5–2 mg/kg; open cardiac surgery, up to about 10 mg/kg
Naloxone	0.4 mg/ml	5–10 µg/kg
Diazepam	5 mg/ml	0.2 mg/kg
Diphenhydramine	50 mg/ml	0.5–1.5 mg/kg
Methylprednisolone	125 and 500 mg powder in vial	15–30 mg/kg

*D_5/W indicates 5% dextrose in water; IV, intravenous; IM, intramuscular.
†Give one third to one fourth of digitalizing dose slowly IV in 20 minutes; repeat every six hours until fully digitalized.
‡Dilute and inject slowly, especially in newborns; repeat as needed, according to negative base excess; calculated dose bicarbonate in mEq = 1/3 × kg body weight × negative base excess. Initially, half the calculated dose is given; arterial blood gases are checked before the next dose is given.
§Give diluted one third to one half of calculated dose slowly in 20 to 30 minutes (maximum, 0.5 mEq K^+/kg/30 min).
‖If the blood sugar is below 40 mg/dl, a bolus dose of 250 to 500 mg/kg (dextrose 50% diluted 1:1 with water) should be given, followed by a maintenance dose of approximately 4 to 8 mg/kg/min. Blood sugar should be repeatedly checked and, if indicated, adjustments made.

accompanied by cyanosis and an elevated hematocrit level, screening should be done for hemostasis, such as tests for bleeding time, prothrombin time, activated partial thromboplastin time, thrombin time, platelet count, platelet aggregation, and euglobulin lysis. The hematologist usually decides the advisability of whether, when, and how to treat these abnormalities.

Preoperative hemodilution by removal of the patient's blood, followed by infusion of fresh-frozen plasma,[154] has been beneficial. On rare occasions, ε-aminocaproic acid has been given to patients with cyanotic congenital heart disease before surgery to correct their hemostatic defects.[75] In our institution, however, such preoperative correction usually is not attempted. If treatment is necessary, we wait until after bypass (except for hemodilution in patients with severe polycythemia, the correction usually being performed by the cardiologist during heart catheterization).

Premedication

Effective premedication is important in the anesthetic management of children with congenital heart defects. The arrival of a well-sedated child in the operating room will make the induction of anesthesia, often considered a potentially hazardous time, considerably smoother. Also, since smaller amounts of anesthetic agents during induction will be required, the risk of hypotension during induction is reduced.[160] To minimize the incidence of bradycardia during induction, with its resulting decrease in cardiac output, possibly decreased tissue oxygenation, decreased pH, systemic vasodilation, increased pulmonary vascular resistance, and, in children with a right-to-left shunt, increased shunting, an anticholinergic agent can be routinely added to the premedication.

Especially in premature infants or other infants with histories of bradycardic episodes, it is important to consider premedication with atropine (0.02 mg/kg intramuscularly; minimal dose, 0.05 mg) or glycopyrrolate (0.01 mg/kg intramuscularly; minimal dose, 0.025 mg).

A fairly heavy premedication should be given to children with right-to-left shunts in whom crying and struggling during induction may greatly increase the cyanosis. After the child is premedicated, close bedside observation by an experienced nurse is necessary. The child should not be left alone from the moment that this premedication has been given because of the possibility of respiratory depression. Oxygen and equipment for intubation and ventilation should be available in the room. Children with respiratory decompensation or airway obstruction should not receive narcotics or tranquilizers

TABLE 6-6.—APPROXIMATE SIZE AND LENGTH OF PEDIATRIC ENDOTRACHEAL TUBES (UNCUFFED, CLEAR POLYVINYL CHLORIDE)

AGE OF PATIENT	INTERNAL DIAMETER, MM	LENGTH, CM ORAL	LENGTH, CM NASAL
Premature	2.5-3	9-10	12-13.5
Full-term newborn	3	10-11	13-14
1-3 mo	3-3.5	11-12	14-15
3-12 mo	3.5-4	12-13	15-16
1-2 yr	4-4.5	14	16
4 yr	5	15	17
6 yr	5.5	17	19
8 yr	6	19	21
10 yr	6.5	20	22

preoperatively, unless they are already intubated and mechanically ventilated.

Many different premedication schedules are used. Although none is 100% satisfactory, premedication given according to the schedule of Table 6-4 generally produces a well-sedated child. However, several other schedules also can achieve a similar satisfactory result. The essence of a good preoperative preparation consists of the combination of a correct preoperative evaluation, good rapport with the child, and adequate premedication.

INDUCTION OF ANESTHESIA

Preparation and Induction

Before the child arrives in the operating room, the anesthesia and monitoring equipment are checked. All drugs that may be needed (Table 6-5) are made readily available in a drug cabinet placed within the reach of the anesthesiologist.

For small infants, drugs like atropine and calcium chloride, which may be needed in an emergency, are diluted in advance. For example, for a 2-kg infant, atropine is diluted to 0.04 mg/ml and calcium chloride is diluted to 40 mg/ml, so that the injection of 0.5 to 1 ml will administer the correct dose. For small infants, succinylcholine (1 ml = 20 mg) is used undiluted in a 1-ml syringe, whereas for bigger infants a 3-ml syringe is used.

One endotracheal tube of a size appropriate for age (Table 6-6), another endotracheal tube with a diameter that is 0.5 mm smaller, and a third with a diameter that is 0.5 mm greater are prepared, with oral Magill connectors tightly inserted into the tubes (Fig 6-1). Tapes* are cut at appropriate lengths to secure the endotracheal tube. Figure 6-2 shows an effective way of securing the orotracheal tube to prevent inadvertent extubation.

Two sets of intravenous fluids, 250 ml of 5% dextrose in water and 250 ml of 5% dextrose in 0.2% sodium chloride, with a Buretrol system (for children smaller than 12 kg) and a three-way stopcock in each line, are readied and are checked to be sure that they are free of air bubbles. When the Buretrol system is used, the weight of the child determines the maximal allowable amount of clear fluids (4 ml/kg of body weight) present in the Buretrol to prevent inadvertent overloading of the patient. In children who weigh less than 8 kg, the use of a constant-infusion pump is preferred. The drug line (5% dextrose in water) of this system has a small-volume (<0.5 ml) extension set† connected to the three-way stopcock at the end of the regular intravenous infusion tubing. After the drug is injected by way of the three-way stopcock, approximately 0.5 ml of fluid is used for flushing the medication into the patient. The patient's hand connected to the drug line is positioned in such a way that, during surgery, there is easy access to the three-way stopcock. Before any fluids or drugs are injected, the stopcock is opened to the intravenous fluid bag, and a small amount of fluid is aspirated to clear out any air bubbles. The medication can then be safely injected. A microfilter and blood warmer are used

---

*Microfoam surgical tape (1 inch), No. 1528, Minnesota Mining and Manufacturing Co., St. Paul, Minn.
†Cook disposable connecting tube, DPT 5.2 30 P FM, Cook, Bloomington, Ind.

Induction of Anesthesia

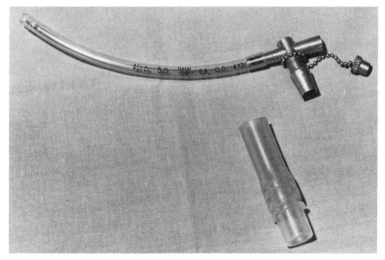

Fig 6–1.—Orotracheal tube and Magill connector.

when blood or fresh-frozen plasma is administered. The setup for arterial and central venous pressure monitoring is the same as for adults (see chap. 5).

The method of induction depends on the condition in which the child arrives in the operating room.

Child Arrives Asleep

If the child arrives asleep or adequately sedated and if inhalation induction is preferred, a prewarmed precordial stethoscope is placed on the child's chest, and after preoxygenation, inhalation induction is performed, with the child still lying on the stretcher on which he arrived in the operating room. The Jackson-Rees modification of the T-piece system is used for the anesthetic induction in all infants. After intubation, the child is connected to a volume ventilator, except for the infant with a lateral thoracotomy, in whom hand ventilation is preferred. Adequate humidification of the anesthetic gases is provided.

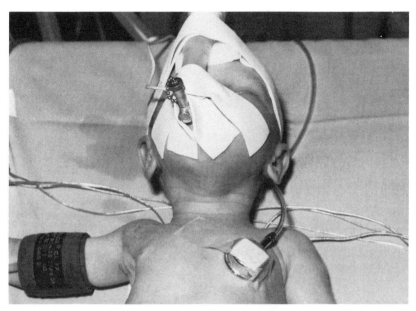

Fig 6–2.—Fixation of orotracheal tube.

When the patient is positioned for lateral thoracotomy, the "precordial" stethoscope is placed and taped at the lateral chest wall of the downward lung, such that after positioning, clear breath sounds of the dependent lung are audible. In this way, the anesthesiologist will immediately detect any decrease in ventilation of the dependent lung (for instance, when secretions are obstructing or when the tip of the endotracheal tube inadvertently advances into the upward bronchus) and can make adjustments before signs of hypoxia develop.

The oxygen and anesthetic gas mixture is initially blown across the face of the child without using a mask, while the hands of the anesthesiologist are gently placed alongside the patient's mandible and chin. In acyanotic children, 70% nitrous oxide with oxygen is used, whereas in cyanotic children, 50% nitrous oxide with oxygen is used. Halothane to between 1.5% and 2% is gradually added.* As soon as tolerated, a mask is placed on the child's face and the halothane concentration is decreased to between 0.5% and 1%. A Doppler blood pressure cuff is positioned, and the blood pressure is checked. A Teflon intravenous cannula is inserted into one of the veins of the dorsal side of the hand and is connected to the drug line, with care being taken that air bubbles are not present. The dangers of air bubbles entering the left side of the circulation and carrying air emboli into the coronary or cerebral vessels are well known. However, this may happen not only in the child with congenital heart defect and a frank right-to-left shunt but also in an infant with a foramen ovale, when a momentary increase in right atrial pressure can create right-to-left shunting.

After the intravenous line is secured, the child is moved gently over onto the operating room table and ECG leads are attached. An ECG strip of leads I, II, III, aV_R, aV_L, aV_F, and V_5 is made. Any arrhythmias that may occur during anesthesia, as well as any changes in the ECG complexes, are recorded. A "complete" seven-lead ECG is repeated after bypass.

The child is intubated after receiving pancuronium, 0.1 mg/kg intravenously, or succinylcholine, 1 to 1.5 mg/kg intravenously (older children are pretreated with d-tubocurarine, 0.1 mg/kg, to decrease fasciculation). At this point, patients who will be undergoing bypass surgery usually receive a narcotic agent—for instance, fentanyl (5–15 μg/kg, or more if indicated).

After injection of the depolarizing relaxant, the use of halothane and nitrous oxide is discontinued, and the patient is ventilated manually with 100% oxygen until muscle relaxation is obtained. After injection of the nondepolarizing relaxant, ventilation is also taken over as soon as indicated, but initially a 50% nitrous oxide and oxygen gas mixture is used. About one minute before intubation, the flow of nitrous oxide is discontinued and the patient is ventilated with 100% oxygen. After intubation, the ventilation of both lungs is checked, the endotracheal tube is securely taped (see Fig 6–2), and the breath sounds are rechecked. A nasogastric tube is inserted; however if there are any difficulties, the gastric tube is inserted through the mouth because trauma to the nasal mucosa may result in brisk nasal bleeding after heparinization. However, a change to a nasogastric tube should be made at the end of the surgery. If the patient is to be left intubated at the end of surgery, the oral endotracheal tube should be removed and a nasotracheal tube should be inserted, because the latter can be better secured and is tolerated well by the child during the postoperative period. An esophageal stethoscope and a nasopharyngeal temperature probe also are inserted.

If a prolonged bypass time or a decreased postoperative cardiac output is expected, a urinary catheter is placed by the surgical assistant. In the meantime, the patient would start receiving 50% nitrous oxide and oxygen and 0.1% to 1% halothane, with frequent checking of the blood pressure and adjusting the halothane concentration when indicated. The radial artery line is inserted percutaneously. A Teflon 20-gauge cannula is used, except in small infants, in whom a 22-gauge cannula is used. If the radial artery cannot be cannulated, either a 20-gauge Teflon cannula is inserted percutaneously in the femoral artery or the surgeon exposes the artery and inserts the cannula under direct vision. In the patient undergoing open-heart surgery, a second intravenous cannula is inserted in the other arm or leg. If a sizable external jugular vein is present, an 18-gauge cannula is placed, and with the use of a J-wire, a longer cannula is

---

*It is unfortunate that in many institutions, ours included, the use of cyclopropane is no longer feasible. We consider inhalation induction with 50% cyclopropane and oxygen to be the technique of choice in acyanotic children.

advanced down into the superior vena cava.[19] If this procedure is not possible or if there is no external jugular vein visible, a 20-gauge cannula* is inserted into the internal jugular vein. We prefer to use the patient's right side because there is no chance to damage the entrance site of the thoracic duct, unless insertion on the left side is indicated, as in patients with a persistent left superior vena cava. Especially in small infants, one has to be careful that the longer intravenous cannula is not advanced too far, since it can easily enter the right atrium or the proximal part of the superior vena cava. This position is undesirable because it makes impossible the detection of malposition of the superior vena caval bypass cannula (which may obstruct the venous flow from the upper part of the body and cause increase of venous pressure). On request, when the child is going on bypass, the surgeon may temporarily occlude the superior vena caval bypass cannula to verify the position of the central venous pressure cannula: an increase in central venous pressure indicates that the cannula is in the right position. However, during bypass, a check should frequently be made for the presence of facial plethora and other signs of obstruction of the venous return from the head, since malfunction or disconnection of the central venous cannula may occur.

If a central venous pressure line cannot be easily inserted into the internal or external jugular vein, the attempts should be discontinued so as not to damage the anatomic structures in the neck, and the surgeon should proceed with preparing and draping of the patient. After the chest is opened, it usually is easy to determine if the heart is adequately filled, and, if indicated, some extra fluid can be infused before the surgeon starts inserting the aortic cannula. Because this maneuver may be accompanied by a relatively considerable loss of blood in small infants, the patient should not be hypovolemic at that moment but should be mildly hypervolemic. At the end of the bypass, the surgeon inserts left and right atrial pressure catheters; the right atrial catheter can be used for intravenous administration of drugs, or, if indicated, another catheter, placed in the right atrium, may be used as a drug line.

---

*Arrow pediatric internal jugular puncture kit, product #AK 04100, Arrow International, Reading, Penn

Child Arrives Awake

If, on arrival in the operating room, the child is awake and prefers an intravenous induction, a Teflon intravenous cannula is inserted after injection of a local anesthetic. The drug line is attached and the ECG leads, blood pressure cuff, and precordial stethoscope are positioned.

Thiopental (2 to 5 mg/kg) is slowly injected intravenously until lid reflex is lost; this is followed by the injection of pancuronium, 0.1 mg/kg, or succinylcholine, 1 to 1.5 mg/kg, while oxygen is administered by mask as soon as the patient is asleep. However, induction with a combination of diazepam (0.1 to 0.3 mg/kg), fentanyl (15 to 40 μg/kg), and pancuronium (0.1 mg/kg) is also frequently performed.

Especially if the child has a low cardiac output or is severely cyanotic, one may not wish to use thiopental for intravenous induction, even though its cardiac depressant effect is mild. Induction with intravenous fentanyl (5 to 15 μg/kg, or more if indicated), slowly titrated, generally will not significantly change the hemodynamics. However, administration of 10 to 15 mg of calcium chloride per kilogram of weight during induction may be useful to lessen the decrease in blood pressure that frequently accompanies induction of anesthesia. If fentanyl is elected for induction, pancuronium (0.1 mg/kg) should be gradually administered as soon as the patient shows signs of heavy sedation during the titration of fentanyl. In this way the patient is asleep before the pancuronium has paralyzed him, and by giving the pancuronium fairly early, a "rigid chest," which may occur if a large dose of fentanyl is given during a short time interval and may endanger the ventilation of the patient during induction, is prevented. If used with fentanyl for induction, succinylcholine may increase the bradycardia that often accompanies the administration of a large dose of fentanyl. If this is undesirable, a small dose of atropine should be given before the succinylcholine.

Child Arrives Uncooperative

If, however, on arrival in the operating room, the child is uncooperative, crying, or struggling, intramuscular ketamine (4 to 7 mg/kg) is preferred instead of a mask induction. As soon as the ketamine takes effect, a Teflon cannula is inserted intravenously, succinylcholine or pancuronium is given intravenously in the usual dose, and the child is ventilated with oxygen and mask until intubation can be performed.

Also successfully used is the combination of intramuscular ketamine (4 to 7 mg/kg) and intramuscular succinylcholine (3 to 4 mg/kg), followed by ventilation by mask with oxygen and intubation, after which the patient is ventilated with 50% N_2O and oxygen; if indicated, halothane is added, with careful monitoring of the blood pressure. This method is especially useful in infants who do not have easily accessible veins and when the intravenous insertion of a cannula is expected to take longer than the duration of the intramuscular ketamine effect.

Small or Very Ill Infants

Newborns and small premature or desperately ill infants are intubated while awake, after preoxygenation.

To decrease the incidence of infection in cardiac surgery, a meticulous sterile technique is used when placing intravenous and arterial lines. Also, prophylactic antibiotics (for instance, cefazolin 25 to 50 mg/kg) are infused slowly after induction and repeated as indicated during surgery and during the postoperative period.

Factors Affecting Induction

Blood-Gas Partition Coefficient

In a healthy child, inhalation induction can be achieved quickly by using a poorly soluble anesthetic inhalation agent (that is, a gas with a low blood-gas partition coefficient, like nitrous oxide or cyclopropane[55]). Because the anesthetic agent is not very soluble in blood, only a small amount of the anesthetic agent is removed from the lungs by the blood. This factor decreases the alveolar partial pressure only slightly, and the inspiratory alveolar and arterial partial pressures will rapidly equilibrate. Furthermore, as the arterial partial pressure increases rapidly, so will the partial pressure of the brain, an organ with a high blood perfusion, and thus induction of anesthesia occurs fairly rapidly.

With a highly soluble anesthetic agent, a large amount of the agent is removed from the alveoli by the blood; thus, the alveolar partial pressure of that agent is considerably lower. Therefore, during the early phase of induction, the arterial partial pressure and consequently the partial pressure in the brain will not increase as fast as it would with a poorly soluble agent.

However, besides the solubility of the inhalation agent, two other factors are important for the rate of induction: the ventilation and the cardiac output.

Ventilation

An increase in ventilation increases the alveolar concentrations of anesthetic agents. The effect is minimal with a poorly soluble agent, as is the effect on the rate of induction. This characteristic is in contrast to the effect of ventilation on the alveolar concentration of a highly soluble anesthetic agent, in which increased ventilation can considerably accelerate the induction.

The increased ventilation refills the alveoli of the lungs so rapidly with a fresh amount of anesthetic agent at inspired partial pressure that, despite the rapid uptake of the highly soluble agent by the blood, the decrease in alveolar partial pressure is not so rapid as during normal ventilation. In addition, as the alveolar partial pressure begins to equal the inspired partial pressure, the arterial partial pressure begins to do so as well, and thus blood with higher anesthetic partial pressure reaches the brain, which results in a faster induction. However, when a poorly soluble agent is used, an increase in ventilation will not make much difference: as occurs with normal ventilation, the alveolar partial pressure rapidly equals the inspired partial pressure.

Cardiac Output

With an increase in cardiac output, more blood passes through the lungs during a specific amount of time and is exposed to a certain amount of anesthetic agent with a certain inspired partial pressure. This action affects anesthetic agents with varying solubilities differently. With a highly soluble agent, an increase in blood flow increases considerably the amount of anesthetic agent removed from the alveoli, and consequently alveolar partial pressure decreases more than with a poorly soluble agent. Therefore, with increased cardiac output, as compared with a normal cardiac output, the induction will be prolonged to a greater degree with a highly soluble anesthetic agent than with a poorly soluble agent, if all other factors are constant.

With a decrease in cardiac output, one may expect for the same reason a substantially increased rate of induction of a highly soluble agent. However, if the reduced cardiac output also decreases the cerebral blood flow, the longer brain time constant balances the effect of the acceleration of increase in the alveolar partial pressure. In this situation, the induction rate for a poorly soluble agent is decreased, compared with the rate when cardiac output is normal.

Induction in Patients With Right-to-Left Shunt

As expected, inhalation induction in a patient with a right-to-left shunt is prolonged because the shunt significantly decreases the anesthetic partial pressure in the blood that reaches the brain, compared with the partial pressure of the blood leaving the lungs, because it is being diluted with mixed venous blood bypassing the lungs and containing a much lower anesthetic concentration. (However, a drug injected intravenously will reach the brain sooner, and the effect of an intravenously injected induction agent will start sooner than in patients without right-to-left shunt.)

As discussed previously, in the normal patient cardiac output and ventilation affect the inhalation induction of a poorly soluble agent and of a highly soluble agent differently. The same is true for the patient with a right-to-left shunt. However, the following requires consideration: the patient with a right-to-left shunt who has a normal $Paco_2$ is, in fact, hyperventilating.

Because carbon dioxide cannot be removed from the nonventilated shunted blood, the blood passing through the lungs has to be hyperventilated to maintain a normal $Paco_2$.

Hyperventilation increases the pulmonary alveolar partial pressure of anesthetic agents. For a highly soluble agent, this may increase the rate of induction enough to overcome the diluting effect of a 50% right-to-left shunt on the arterial partial pressure.[55] As a result, in patients with a right-to-left shunt and a normal $Paco_2$, the rate of induction of a highly soluble agent is about normal, whereas that of a poorly soluble agent is slowed down compared with the normal situation.

So far, the effects of poorly soluble agents (nitrous oxide) and highly soluble agents (ether, methoxyflurane) on inhalation induction in patients with a right-to-left shunt have been discussed. However, a moderately soluble agent (halothane) instead of a highly soluble agent is used during induction. Consequently, its effect on the rate of induction can be expected to be between that of the poorly and highly soluble agents—that is, compared with the induction rate of halothane in a normal child, there will be a slightly prolonged induction in most children with a right-to-left shunt. However, induction with nitrous oxide will be more prolonged (compared with the normal situation).

In cyanotic patients who preoperatively are not receiving oxygen, the induction effect of 50% nitrous oxide should be combined with that of halothane, although the combination may not be as effective as in a normal child. This method makes possible the use of lower concentrations of halothane than if 100% oxygen with halothane were used. If the child is receiving a high oxygen concentration preoperatively and is not already intubated, one can use either an intravenous induction with thiopental or fentanyl and pancuronium or an intramuscular induction with ketamine and succinylcholine while 100% oxygen is being administered by mask.

Generally, patients with right-to-left shunt have to be observed both for peripheral systemic vasodilation (which may increase the shunt) and for a decrease in cardiac output. A decrease in cardiac output in a cyanotic patient increases the cyanosis by decreasing peripheral perfusion and partial pressure of oxygen in the tissues. As a result, metabolic acidosis may develop, which in turn can cause a greater depression of the heart function.

Also, in patients with poor pulmonary perfusion (for instance, pulmonary stenosis or atresia, tricuspid atresia, and severe tetralogy of Fallot) in whom a systemic pulmonary artery shunt is present, acceptable oxygenation depends on an adequate systemic blood pressure. A decrease in systemic blood pressure lessens the flow through the shunt and consequently decreases the pulmonary perfusion. The resulting deterioration of Pao_2, with an increase in acidosis, will increase hypoxic pulmonary vasoconstriction and cause even greater hypoxia.

Peripheral systemic vasodilation may result in a temporary increase in a right-to-left shunt, as

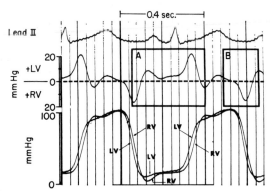

Fig 6–3.—Pressure gradient relationships throughout cardiac cycle in moderate tetralogy of Fallot. Simultaneously recorded ECG, instantaneous pressure gradient, and left *(LV)* and right *(RV)* ventricular pressures are shown. **A,** period favoring left-to-right gradient. During diastole, left ventricular pressure remains slightly higher than right, with accentuation of left-to-right ventricular pressure gradient during isovolemic ventricular contraction. **B,** period favoring right-to-left shunt. During isovolemic ventricular relaxation, pressure in left ventricle decreases faster than right ventricular pressure. Decrease in peripheral systemic resistance may create right-to-left shunting (directed from right ventricle into aorta) in the early ejection phase. (From Levin et al.[104] Used by permission.)

in patients with tetralogy of Fallot, in whom the decrease in systemic resistance may cause blood to be shunted from the right ventricle into the aorta during the early ejection phase[104] (Fig 6–3).

Also, in patients with truncus arteriosus, systemic peripheral vasodilation increases peripheral systemic blood flow, and as a consequence pulmonary blood flow will decrease. Patients with overperfusion of the lungs may benefit from this effect, but in the presence of pulmonary stenosis or banding, hypoperfusion of the lungs may result.

If anesthetic agents with cardiodepressant or vasodilating properties are used in cyanotic patients, one should be aware of these potentially dangerous side effects.

The increased metabolic acidosis accompanied by a decrease in PaO_2, which is occasionally detected when arterial blood gases are checked soon after the start of anesthesia, may be related to the (mild) myocardial depressant action of the anesthetic agent.

In hearts already in failure, prevention of myocardial depression and of reduced cardiac output during the prebypass period are most likely of the same importance for a favorable outcome of surgery as is optimal myocardial preservation by hypothermia and cardioplegic solution during bypass.

The anesthesiologist also should be aware that mechanical ventilation in some patients with decreased pulmonary perfusion may create such extensive ventilation-perfusion maldistribution that the $PaCO_2$ may increase considerably when the patient is ventilated with a normal minute volume.[103] Repeated determinations of the arterial blood gases are necessary in these patients to adjust the ventilation appropriately.

Induction in Patients With Left-to-Right Shunt

The concentration of intravenously injected induction agents will be decreased before they reach the brain because of dilution by the shunted blood. The degree of shunting determines whether this has a measurable effect on induction.

An increased amount of thiopental injected rapidly during induction would overcome this effect. However, the depressant effect of a large dose of thiopental on the cardiac output may be dangerously great. Therefore, thiopental is titrated slowly, often combined with a preinduction dose of meperidine (0.5 to 1.5 mg/kg) or fentanyl (2 to 5 μg/kg), also slowly injected. With this method, an excessive dose of thiopental is not required. An intravenous induction with morphine, between 1 and 3 mg/kg, or with fentanyl, between 15 and 40 μg/kg, in combination with pancuronium is also effective.

The effect on inhalation induction is also influenced by the solubility of the anesthetic agent, the cardiac output, and the ventilation. For instance, in a patient with a left-to-right shunt who has a normal systemic perfusion, an increased pulmonary perfusion, and a normal or decreased $PaCO_2$, the rate of induction is expected to be increased over the rate for a normal person, when a highly soluble anesthetic agent is used. In this situation, the increased pulmonary perfusion diminishes the decrease in alveolar partial pressure because the partial pressure of the anesthetic agent in the blood returning to the lungs is higher than normal as a result of the admixture of the shunted blood returning to the lungs with a high partial pressure. However, inhalation induction of a poorly soluble agent is, as expected, barely influenced by changes in ventilation or cardiac output. As inhalation induction of patients with a left-to-right shunt is accomplished by using both the more rapid-acting, poorly soluble agent nitrous oxide and the slower-acting halothane, the rate of induction is comparable to that in normal patients.

If there is a left-to-right and a right-to-left shunt, the induction rate of intravenous agents, as well as inhalation agents, will be nearer to normal.[55]

ANESTHESIA FOR CLOSED-HEART SURGERY

Patent Ductus Arteriosus

Anatomical closure of a ductus arteriosus occurs within the first nine weeks after birth in 90% of infants.[33] However, the functional closure is usually complete within 15 hours after birth in the full-term infant. Infants with patent ductus arteriosus can be placed into three groups according to their fairly distinct clinical presentation: (1) those without pulmonary disease; (2) those recovering from the respiratory distress syndrome; and (3) those with associated respiratory distress syndrome. The anesthetic management of infants with associated respiratory distress syndrome will be discussed, because these patients generally present the greatest problems.

In premature infants, the ductus may not close in time, and the persistence of an open ductus, especially in combination with the respiratory distress syndrome, can be life-threatening. Heart failure may easily occur in these infants. The left ventricular volume load is increased by the volume shunted left to right through the ductus arteriosus. The resultant increase of pulmonary venous return to the left atrium and left ventricle increases ventricular diastolic volume and results in a high left ventricular end-diastolic pressure with an increase in left atrial pressure, giving the clinical pattern of overt left heart failure with left atrial dilation and pulmonary edema. Secondary to this, right heart failure may develop. The elevated left ventricular end-diastolic pressure may decrease subendocardial perfusion and therefore oxygenation, and this increases the possibility of left heart failure. The tissue oxygenation already may be jeopardized as a result of a combination of (1) decreased blood oxygen content because of the respiratory distress syndrome and the often-present anemia in small infants (which may be due to recurrent blood sampling) and (2) the shift to the left of the fetal hemoglobin saturation curve. The fact that premature infants often have lower-than-normal serum calcium ion concentration also may affect myocardial performance.

In children who are 3 years old or less, the increase in pulmonary blood flow is usually accompanied by only a moderate increase in pulmonary vascular resistance. However, if pulmonary hypertension develops, a right-to-left shunt may become dominant instead of the previously present left-to-right shunt. This late and probably irreversible stage is rare, but, when seen, occurs in older children and surgical closure is usually not advised.[59]

In pulmonary hypertension with still dominant left-to-right shunt, surgery is indicated, but it involves considerable risk.

Generally, in the premature infant with or without the respiratory distress syndrome, surgical repair is not done unless there is severe cardiac failure that is not improved by the usual medical treatment of digoxin, diuretics, and, if indicated, extra oxygen, mechanical ventilation, and intravenous hyperalimentation. Fluids are restricted, the hematocrit level is kept above 45%, and the electrolytes, blood glucose, calcium, and PaO_2 are carefully monitored. Regularly, the eye fundi of the premature infants are checked by an ophthalmologist for retrolental fibroplasia.

The effectiveness of the prostaglandin E_1 synthetase inhibitor indomethacin in closing the patent ductus is currently under investigation.[67,84] If optimal medical treatment fails to control cardiac failure, surgical repair is needed.

One is often confronted with the problem of a premature infant (birth weight < 1,500 gm) in heart failure, sometimes with pulmonary edema, idiopathic respiratory distress syndrome, often mechanically ventilated, with an increased inspiratory oxygen concentration, and the inherent dangers of pulmonary oxygen toxicity and retrolental fibroplasia. The ability for adequate thermoregulation is decreased, metabolic acidosis is likely to develop, and if the infant is not receiving ventilatory assistance, respiratory acidosis is also likely. Blood glucose and calcium levels may be low, and with diuretic and digoxin therapy, the importance of maintaining a normal serum and intracellular potassium concentration is great.

Anemia, resulting from the obtaining of frequent samples for blood gas and electrolyte determinations, has to be prevented. As a result of the diuretic treatment, some hypovolemia may be present, which may create severe hypotension if even a low concentration of halothane is used. In addition to the usual preanesthetic preparation in the operating room, the operating room temperature should be approximately 25.5 to 26.7 C (78 to 80 F) before the baby arrives. When the infant arrives, a heat lamp is placed above the baby and is kept on until the patient is draped. Also, Chemstrip (Bio-Dynamics, Indianapolis, Ind.) is available to measure the baby's blood sugar level during surgery.

If the infant was not receiving ventilatory assistance while in the neonatal intensive care unit, episodes of apnea associated with bradycardia may have occurred during the preoperative period. If this has happened, the child is left intubated after surgery for 12 to 24 hours, if possible breathing spontaneously with a continuous positive airway pressure setup. The eye fundi should be checked[12] to determine the presence or absence of signs of retrolental fibroplasia.

If the child is already intubated and the PaO_2 with the FIO_2 is known, initially the same FIO_2 may be used if the PaO_2 is about 80 mm Hg. However, if the preoperative PaO_2 is approximately 60 mm Hg, anesthesia is started using initially an FIO_2 of 10% to 15% higher than that administered in the intensive care unit. Adjustments are made according to the intraoperative arterial blood gases.

If the child is not intubated, preoxygenation should be done for approximately two minutes and he should be intubated while awake; assisted or controlled ventilation then should be started. Temporarily, a mixture of nitrous oxide and oxygen is administered, with an FIO_2 similar to that given in the neonatal unit. Because this type of patient may be hypovolemic (because of the use of diuretics), halothane should not be given before the intravenous line is secured. A 22-gauge Teflon needle is inserted into a peripheral vein, and a constant-infusion pump is used for the delivery of 5% to 10% dextrose in 0.2% sodium chloride (if indicated, extra dextrose is added according to the result of the Chemstrip test, which is done by an assistant at the time that the intravenous needle is inserted). For relaxation, 0.03 to 0.08 mg/kg of pancuronium is injected intravenously.[11] An esophageal stethoscope is positioned, which also can be used to hear the murmur of the ductus. Between the end of the intravenous administration tubing and the Teflon needle, two three-way stopcocks and a low-volume extension set are placed. One of the stopcocks can be connected to the blood transfusion line and the other to a 10- or 3-ml syringe; these are used for the rapid and accurate administration of blood or drugs. Generally, fluid administration is minimal (1 ml/kg/hour) in the sick infant with heart failure. Because the estimated blood volume of most of these infants is between 100 and 150 ml, blood replacement, if necessary, is adequately accomplished with this system. (However, an older child with pulmonary hypertension and a large, thin-walled, friable pulmonary artery may experience massive blood loss during exposure and transection of the ductus. At least two intravenous lines with adequately sized Teflon cannulas are indicated, as is the presence of a central venous pressure line.)

In the very sick infant, an arterial line is present or will be inserted, usually in the umbilical artery, although the right radial artery is preferred, as its PaO_2 will be equal to that of the blood perfusing the eye fundi; this is helpful both for monitoring the blood pressure (otherwise done by a Doppler blood pressure cuff) and for determining a suitable FIO_2. In the otherwise healthy premature or full-term infant, an attempt to insert percutaneously a radial artery catheter should be made. However, if the attempt is not successful, surgery is performed without an arterial line.

Anesthesia consists usually either of nitrous oxide, halothane, and oxygen or of oxygen, air, and halothane as tolerated. Pancuronium is used for relaxation. In vigorous infants, a small dose of fentanyl, 1 to 2 µg/kg, can be given before the incision is made. This dose does not com-

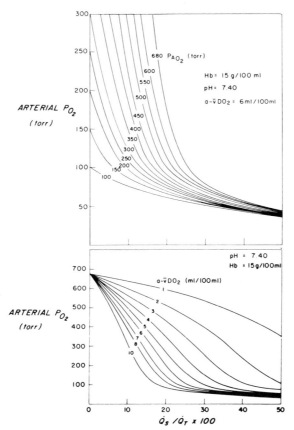

Fig 6–4.—*Top,* relationships between Pa_{O_2} and intrapulmonary right-to-left shunt at different levels of alveolar P_{O_2}, calculated for a specific hemoglobin, pH, and arterial mixed venous oxygen content difference [$C(a-\bar{v})_{O_2}$] (illustration shows arterial mixed venous oxygen content difference as a-$\bar{v}$ DO_2). Note that influence of the PA_{O_2} on the Pa_{O_2} decreases rapidly with increased shunt fraction. *Bottom,* effect of changes in $C(a-\bar{v})_{O_2}$ on Pa_{O_2}. Note that the effect is greatest at moderate levels of right-to-left shunting. An increase in $C(a-\bar{v})_{O_2}$, for instance, by decreasing cardiac output or closure of left-to-right shunt in patient with patent ductus, causes considerable decrease in Pa_{O_2} in the presence of a moderate intrapulmonary right-to-left shunt. (From Pontoppidan H., Laver M.B., Geffin B.: *Adv. Surg.* 4:163, 1970. Used by permission.)

promise the respiration at the end of surgery. In very sick infants, fentanyl (0.5 to 2 μg/kg), air, and oxygen are used.

The muscle relaxant effect is reversed at the end of the surgery by the use of neostigmine (0.06 mg/kg) given slowly with atropine (0.03 mg/kg), unless the child is to be ventilated postoperatively. During the procedure, the nasopharyngeal temperature of the infant should be approximately 36 C and the Pa_{O_2} should be between 60 and 80 mm Hg. Metabolic acidosis, if present, should be gradually corrected by the use of sodium bicarbonate.

In infants with patent ductus arteriosus and pulmonary edema, a considerable ventilation-perfusion maldistribution may be expected. The Pa_{O_2} will be determined by the size of the intrapulmonary right-to-left shunt; in mild-to-moderate shunts, a clinically significant increase in Pa_{O_2} may be accomplished by increasing the FI_{O_2} (Fig 6–4, *top*).

As long as the ductus is patent, relatively oxygen-rich blood will return to the lungs through the ductus and thus increase the oxygen content of the mixed venous blood in the lungs. As a result, the difference between the arterial and mixed venous oxygen content ($C(a-\bar{v})_{O_2}$) will be decreased, and in turn, the Pa_{O_2} will be increased (Fig 6–4, *bottom*). However, after ligation of the ductus, the partial pressure of oxygen in the blood entering the lungs will decrease, as will the Pao$_2$. Therefore, an increase of the F$_{IO_2}$ is usually indicated after closure of the ductus in infants with ventilation-perfusion abnormalities. Also, at this stage halothane should not be used as an anesthetic agent. Because of its depressant action on the cardiac output, halothane may increase the C(a-v̄)O$_2$ and decrease the Pao$_2$ even more.

The surgical procedure is usually straightforward. Exposure is from either a left anterolateral or a posterolateral incision through the third interspace (Fig 6–5). The pleura is incised over the pulmonary artery between and parallel to the vagus and phrenic nerves. If bradycardia occurs when the incision nears the vagal nerve, the surgeon should be notified. If needed, atro-

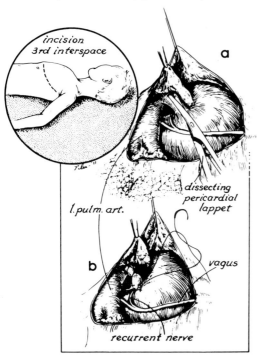

Fig 6–5.—Operative treatment of patent ductus arteriosus by ligation. After exposure of ductus, nonpenetrating pursestring sutures are placed at either end, with perforating mattress suture placed between to obliterate ductus over distance of 8 to 10 mm. (From Bahnson H.T.: Patent ductus arteriosus, in Ravitch M.M., et al. (eds.): *Pediatric Surgery.* Chicago, Year Book Medical Publishers, 1979. Used by permission.)

pine (0.02 mg/kg) can be injected intravenously. The ductus is mobilized and either ligated or transected. Damage to the recurrent nerve may cause unilateral vocal cord paresis. With the ductus ligated, the murmur cannot be heard anymore through the esophageal stethoscope. Usually, the diastolic blood pressure becomes somewhat higher than before.

Before closure of the chest, the lungs are inflated until all atelectatic areas that have developed during surgical manipulation are well expanded. During the remainder of the procedure, ventilation with positive end-expiratory pressure of 2 to 4 cm is used. Manual instead of mechanical ventilation is preferred in all operations requiring lateral thoracotomy.

Coarctation of the Aorta

The coarctation may be opposite, proximal, or distal to the ductus arteriosus. The constriction of the lumen either may be localized or may involve an extensive area, such as the entire isthmus, as is sometimes seen in infants.

Frequently, associated congenital heart anomalies may be present with symptomatic coarctation, such as patent ductus arteriosus, ventricular septal defect, left ventricular outflow obstruction, atrial septal defect, and transposition of the great arteries.

The child born with preductal coarctation of the aorta (Fig 6–6) frequently is initially seen with congestive heart failure within a short time because of the absence of collateral vessels, which would decrease the afterload of the left ventricle. During fetal life, preductal coarctation does not promote the development of collateral vessels because most of the blood that enters the right atrium, which normally would flow via the open foramen ovale to the left side of the heart and through the aorta, instead will flow into the right ventricle because of the increased resistance caused by the coarctation. Via the ductus arteriosus, the blood perfuses the rest of the body. Soon after birth, left ventricular failure may develop, precipitated by the substantially elevated afterload. When the ductus starts to close, the situation will deteriorate rapidly, in contrast to the course of postductal coarctation, in which life in the fetal period would not be possible unless collateral vessels develop and blood through the ductus or the aortic arch can reach the distal part of the peripheral circulation

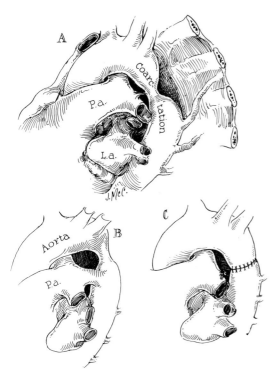

Fig 6–6.—Coarctation of aorta. **A,** postductal coarctation with obliterated ductus arteriosus. Enlarged intercostal arteries participate in collateral circulation. Note pulmonary artery *(P.a.)* and left atrium *(L.a.)*. **B,** preductal coarctation with large patent ductus. **C,** excision of coarctation, followed by end-to-end anastomosis. (From Lewis F.J.: The heart, great vessels and pericardium, in Davis L. (ed.): *Christopher's Textbook of Surgery.* Philadelphia, W.B. Saunders Co., 1964. Used by permission.)

(Fig 6–7). As a consequence, an infant with postductal coarctation is born with already adequate collateral vessels and most often will be asymptomatic.

The patency of the ductus arteriosus is important for the infant with preductal coarctation because right-to-left shunting occurs through it when the increased left ventricular end-diastolic pressure impedes the pulmonary venous drainage into the left side of the heart. Closure increases the pulmonary blood flow and thus produces a diastolic overload of a left ventricle already burdened with an increased afterload. Infusion of prostaglandin E_2 or E_1[102, 162] frequently is used to delay the closure of the ductus while the patient is prepared for surgery.

Also, digoxin and diuretics usually are administered for treatment of left ventricular failure. The stresses that the left ventricle has to endure during surgery are impressive: (1) when the ductus is ligated, more blood is suddenly presented to the pulmonary circulation and the left ventricle, producing a sudden increase in left ventricular preload, and pulmonary edema may develop unless the ventricle can handle this extra load; (2) the cross-clamping of the aorta produces an acute increase in afterload, which may readily induce left ventricular failure.[185]

The combination of additional congenital heart defects and coarctation of the aorta increases the seriousness of the situation even more. For instance, a ventricular septal defect with a left-to-right shunt increases the pulmonary blood flow and may rapidly lead to pulmonary congestion or pulmonary hypertension. More than 60% of these patients are seen initially with congestive heart failure.[137] In patients with coarctation and ventricular septal defect, the coarctation is usually repaired first, followed by measurements of the aortic and pulmonary artery pressures. Previously, if these measurements still indicated a large pulmonary blood flow, pulmonary artery banding was done at the same session, after repair of the coarctation. However, recent policy is for the patient to return for closure of the ventricular septal defect if congestive failure persists, since the situation may gradually improve because of the tendency of the ventricular septal defect to spontaneously decrease in size.

Usually, the child with postductal coarctation is initially asymptomatic; however, complications of the hypertension in the upper part of the body will develop eventually, such as cerebrovascular hemorrhage, aortic dissection or rupture, and chronic congestive heart failure. Also, the incidence of subacute bacterial endocarditis is increased. Therefore, because life expectancy is decreased considerably (approximately 80% die before the age of 50 years), elective surgical correction of uncomplicated coarctation is strongly advised and usually performed when the patient is between 2 and 5 years old (the cross-sectional area of the aorta at that age is already more than 50% of that in the adult, and even if the repaired area does not grow anymore, the diameter still may be wide enough when the child is fully grown so that no significant gradient across the area of repair will

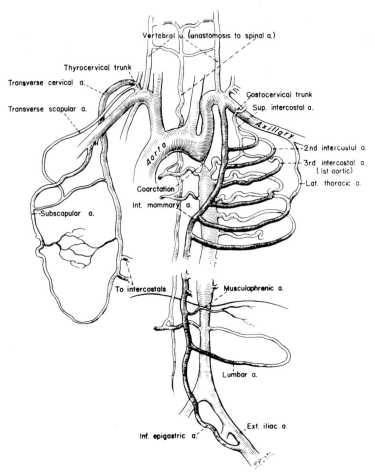

Fig 6–7.—Collateral circulation in coarctation of aorta. Right side of diagram pictures arteries that perfuse thoracic cage, abdominal wall, and lower extremity. Left side shows vessels concerned with circulation around scapula and adjacent tissues. Collateral flow from subclavian arteries (by way of internal mammary, intercostal, transverse cervical, transverse scapular, and subscapular arteries) carries blood from above coarctation to perfuse circulation distal to coarctation. (From Edwards J.E., et al.: The collateral circulation in coarctation of the aorta. *Mayo Clin. Proc.* 23:333, 1948. Used by permission.)

develop). To delay surgical repair until the child is older, therefore, would be of no benefit, whereas the deleterious effects of prolonged hypertension on the cardiovascular system justify early repair.[81]

The most commonly used anesthetic agents are nitrous oxide and halothane (unless left ventricular failure is present). In older children, a small amount of a narcotic drug is added. In patients with left ventricular failure, oxygen and nitrous oxide and narcotics are preferred. Pancuronium is used for relaxation. An arterial line should be inserted into the right radial artery (the left subclavian artery may have to be clamped during surgery), and two venous lines are placed, one of them preferably being an internal jugular line. If there is sudden large loss of blood, which may occur during this operation (a unit of crossmatched blood should be available in the operating room before the start of surgery), the ability to determine the central venous pressure is helpful in assessing the necessary amount of blood for transfusion. In patients with poor collateral circulation or in heart failure, a Swan-Ganz catheter should be placed when possible to monitor the deterioration of the left ventricular function when the aorta is cross-clamped. Also, the catheter is helpful in making the decision whether a vasodilator agent with or without a cardioinotropic drug will be useful or, more rarely, whether a temporary shunt is indicated.

The child is placed in the right lateral position. The incision is made through the fourth intercostal space. If the collateral circulation is well developed, extensive loss of blood may occur during thoracotomy. This loss may have to be replaced because severe hypotension may follow the release of the aortic cross-clamp in a hypovolemic patient. The surgeon isolates the aorta above and below the coarctation and mobilizes the ductus or ligamentum arteriosum. Arterial blood gases are usually determined by this time and are used as a reference value, unless the patient's age or condition (for instance, congestive heart failure or the necessity to keep the PaO_2 within a narrow range to prevent retrolental fibroplasia) dictates that the determination be made earlier.

If the ductus is patent, it is tied off and the aorta is cross-clamped (Fig 6–8). In the presence of adequate collateral circulation, the perfusion of the distal aorta is sufficient most of the time. One is especially concerned about the in-

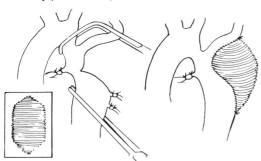

Fig 6–8.—Surgical procedure in patch grafting of coarctation of aorta in small infant. Intercostal arteries close to aorta are tied off, as is ductus arteriosus. Cross-clamp proximal and distal to surgical area is placed. Longitudinal incision is made, extending to left subclavian artery, and Dacron patch is sutured in place, thus enlarging considerably the cross-sectional area of repaired aorta. (From Fleming W.H., et al.: Critical aortic coarctation: Patch aortoplasty in infants less than age 3 months. *Am. J. Cardiol.* 44:687, 1979. Used by permission.)

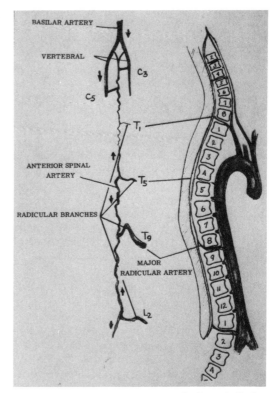

Fig 6–9.—Blood supply to spinal cord. Perfusion of spinal cord is by continuous or interrupted anterior spinal artery, which derives its blood supply from branches (varying from one to three) of intercostal arteries and usually one lumbar radicular artery. Because anterior spinal artery is not always a wide continuous vessel, perfusion of portions of spinal cord may depend on adequate blood flow through radicular arteries. Transection of an intercostal artery from which a radicular branch comes can severely endanger perfusion of a part of the spinal cord in such a patient. Also, hypotension may decrease perfusion of the cord below acceptable levels. Therefore, the surgeon transects as few intercostal arteries as possible while freeing the area of coarctation and takes care that perfusion pressure is adequate in the distal aorta during cross-clamping period. If this is not possible, hypothermia with the use of a bypass will be necessary to help prevent spinal cord damage by hypoperfusion. (From Brewer et al.[23] Used by permission.)

adequate perfusion of the anterior spinal artery (Fig 6–9), because ischemic damage of the spinal cord may occur. The incidence of spinal cord complications is approximately 0.5%.

A mean aortic pressure of 50 mm Hg, measured distal from the aortic cross-clamp, is considered adequate, and the surgeon proceeds with the operation. If there is any doubt about the adequacy of the perfusion of the distal aorta or if a coarctation repair has been previously performed, with the risk that the aorta may be friable where the cross-clamp will have to be applied, the use of hypothermia and left atrial-femoral or femoral-femoral bypass is advised to prevent damage to the spinal cord by hypoperfusion or severe bleeding.[23] When the aorta is cross-clamped, moderate to severe hypertension usually develops in the upper part of the body. Before cross-clamping is done, heparinization is advised[87] because spinal cord complications may result from the formation of clots in the cul-de-sacs above and below the occluding clamps, with resulting distal embolization after release of the clamps. Protamine should be given after the clamps are removed. If halothane (used only in low concentrations in patients with histories of left ventricular failure) is not sufficient to lower the proximal aortic pressure to mild hypertensive values, a nitroprusside drip of 50 mg in 250 ml of 5% dextrose in water is used.[37] No attempt should be made to reach normotension or hypotension because of the danger of a too low perfusion pressure in the distal aorta, with insufficient perfusion of the spinal cord. An infusion pump is used for titrating the necessary doses to reach a mean distal aortic pressure of at least 50 mm Hg and mild hypertension in the proximal aorta. Instead of the short-acting nitroprusside, one may administer the longer-acting trimethaphan (Arfonad) (250 mg in 250 ml of 5% dextrose in water), slowly titrated until the desired blood pressure is reached, or pentolinium tartrate,[10] up to a maximum of 0.5 mg/kg initially, followed by repeated doses of 0.125 to 0.25 mg/kg. Nitroprusside is preferred in our institution because of its fast onset of action and short duration. The fast onset is helpful in rapidly reducing an acutely increased blood pressure after the cross-clamps have been placed. The short duration is convenient because one is able to discontinue the hypotensive action of the drug just before release of the cross-clamps.

Shortly before and after release of the cross-clamps, arterial blood gases are checked and metabolic acidosis, when present, is corrected by the use of sodium bicarbonate. Patients with histories of poor left ventricular function should be tested more frequently for metabolic acidosis during the cross-clamping period, and the acidosis should be corrected vigorously; if necessary, inotropic agents or vasodilators (or both) should be given. Surgical correction is either by direct end-to-end anastomosis after resection of the narrowed area (see Fig 6–6,C) or by a longitudinal incision performed across the coarctation. An internal diaphragm is often present and is excised as much as possible,[158] and a Dacron patch is sutured to create an adequate diameter, which is often necessary in infants (see Fig 6–8).

Before the cross-clamp is released, the anesthesiologist takes care that (1) a normal acid-base status is present, (2) the patient is at least normovolemic or mildly hypervolemic, (3) the use of nitroprusside is discontinued for about four minutes, (4) the use of halothane is discontinued for several minutes, and (5) blood is available if there is a sudden large loss of blood after the release of the cross-clamp. The surgeon then slowly releases the distal aortic cross-clamp first and then the proximal one. Some brisk bleeding is not unusual at this time. Severe hypotension generally reacts well to rapid fluid replacement, but temporary (partial) reclamping of the aorta may be indicated if loss of blood is severe, to give the surgeon time to repair the defects and the anesthesiologist time to treat the hypovolemia.

In some patients, when the condition is stabilized after release of the cross-clamp, hypertension develops either immediately or after two to three days, despite an adequate repair. In these patients, antihypertensive treatment can be started to prevent vasculitis of the small mesenteric arteries and arterioles, with secondary ischemia of the bowel,[40, 65] which may happen in as many as 25% of the patients who have the delayed type of postoperative hypertension. Nitroprusside drip may be continued or the longer-acting chlorpromazine may be titrated slowly intravenously (initial dose 0.1 mg/kg), until an acceptable blood pressure has been reached. During the postoperative period, the treatment is usually continued with orally administered hydralazine or reserpine.

After surgery, the muscle relaxant action is reversed (neostigmine, 0.06 mg/kg; atropine, 0.03 mg/kg). As was mentioned earlier, in older infants (>1 year) the anesthetic usually consists of a combination of halothane with 50% nitrous oxide and oxygen and meperidine (1 to 2 mg/kg) given early during the procedure. This regimen should provide analgesia during the early postoperative period.

Children who are not in cardiac failure before operation and who are without any other cardiac defect are, when breathing well, extubated at the end of the procedure; otherwise, they should be ventilated postoperatively until extubation can be safely performed.

Postoperative analgesia provided by an intercostal block is used by some[40]; however, it is not without hazards, because the greatly enlarged intercostal arteries can be punctured easily.

Complications after repair are infrequent. As mentioned before, bowel ischemia due to mesenteric vasculitis can be prevented by the use of antihypertensive agents. Because of hypoperfusion after cross-clamping of the aorta, spinal cord damage may occur, and the chance of such damage is greatly dependent on the anatomic variations of the anterior spinal artery and the presence of adequate collateral circulation. However, the chance of this complication may be decreased by the use of hypothermia with left heart bypass when the perfusion of the distal aorta is inadequate after cross-clamping. The left recurrent nerve may be damaged, which results in left vocal cord paralysis. In small infants who have end-to-end anastomosis, coarctation may recur.

Vascular Ring Anomalies

Vascular malformations compressing the trachea may cause respiratory distress, especially where the trachea and esophagus are completely encircled by a true vascular ring.[83] Feeding often aggravates the respiratory obstruction. If the obstruction is severe enough, the child prefers to hold his head in a hyperextended position; this position stretches the trachea and lessens the constricting effect of the compressing vessel. The anesthesiologist should observe the position of the head that is preferred by the infant, because less airway problems usually will be encountered if the head is kept in the same position during induction. Frequently, the compressed area is above the carina; however, it also may be located more distally in one of the main bronchi. Anomalies that may be encountered are double aortic arch with small anterior limb (Fig 6–10,A and B) or with small posterior limb (Fig 6–10,C and D), right aortic arch with left-sided ligamentum arteriosum (Fig 6–10,E and F), anomalous innominate artery (Fig 6–10,G and H), and an aberrant right subclavian artery (Fig 6–10,I and J).

Usually, a thoracotomy is made through the left third or fourth intercostal space.[165] Division of the smaller branch of the ring or of the ligamentum arteriosum usually provides the necessary relief. However, if there is an anomalous left pulmonary artery, the left main pulmonary artery must be divided and anastomosed to the pulmonary artery trunk, anterior to the trachea.[127]

Because the airway is usually partially obstructed, an arterial line is important for monitoring the adequacy of ventilation by means of blood gas determinations. Monitoring of arterial blood gases is even more important if there is an anomalous left pulmonary artery, a situation in which perfusion to the left lung is blocked during the suturing of the anastomosis.

Two venous lines are inserted when there is a possibility of sudden extensive bleeding; otherwise one intravenous line is sufficient. In patients with severe stenosis of the airway, inhalation induction is preferred while continuous positive airway pressure is being applied with a modified Ayres T-piece. Until the anesthesiologist is satisfied that adequate ventilation can be performed in this way, intravenous anesthetics and relaxants should not be administered.[152] Usually, halothane, nitrous oxide, and oxygen are used for inhalation induction. However, compression of the airway may have involved the lungs, and repeated pulmonary infections, atelectatic areas, or lobar emphysema may have impaired pulmonary function to such a degree that halothane in 100% oxygen is preferred. This situation is especially true in sick infants in whom bronchoscopy is indicated partly for diagnosis and partly for endobronchial toilet. Usually, the trauma inflicted to the epithelium lining the airway is such with bronchoscopy in small infants that ventilation afterward is even more impaired. Therefore, one should be prepared, after the bronchoscopy is finished and the diagnosis is made, to proceed with the actual surgery during the same session. The situation determines whether the anesthesia is given through the bronchoscope or whether the scope is removed and an endotracheal tube that is long enough to reach the compressed area is inserted. If the airway becomes obstructed dur-

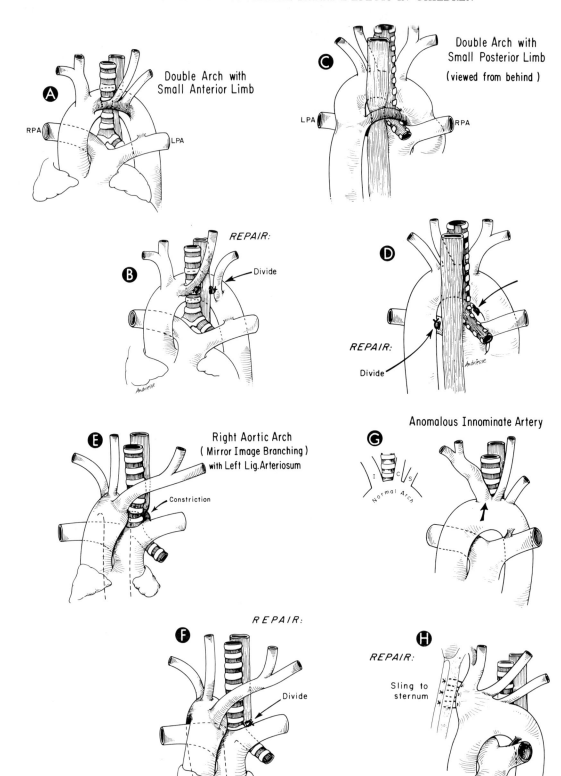

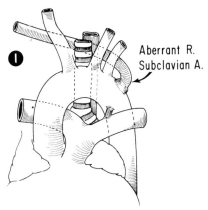 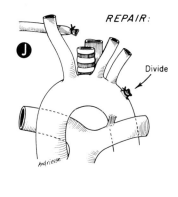

Fig 6–10.—**A** and **B,** the most common variety of vascular ring anomaly. Division of smaller anterior arch corrects the compression. Note right pulmonary artery *(RPA)* and left pulmonary artery *(LPA).* **C** and **D,** meticulous surgical technique is necessary for correction of this defect (division of posterior limb) because if bleeding occurs after division, access to bleeding can be extremely difficult. **E** and **F,** simple division of ligamentum arteriosum is treatment of this anomaly. **G** and **H,** because origin of innominate *(I)* artery is near left common carotid artery *(C),* trachea is caught between these vessels. Suspension of ascending aorta and innominate artery to sternum solves this problem. (*S* indicates left subclavian artery.) **I** and **J,** this anomaly does not often cause symptoms. If so, division may be easily performed. (From Hendren and Kim.[83] Used by permission.)

ing surgery, the tube may need to be advanced beyond the compressed area.

In small infants with severe airway compression, ventilation by bronchoscopy is preferred to ventilation by the usual endotracheal tube because the former affords an opportunity to evaluate, under direct vision, the condition of the tracheal wall when the repair is done, inasmuch as the long-term compression may have weakened the wall and the lumen may collapse after the wall has been dissected free from the compressing vessel and its surroundings. In this situation, an endotracheal tube must be inserted to provide continuous positive airway pressure to keep the airway open as long as necessary during the postoperative period.

Palliative Procedures for Congenital Heart Disease

In conditions in which the pulmonary blood flow is not sufficient and corrective surgery is contraindicated, the creation of a left-to-right shunt will often improve the condition of the patient sufficiently so that corrective surgery may be delayed until a more favorable time.

In infants with transposition, in whom the pulmonary circulation and the systemic circulation are almost completely separated, an acceptable degree of mixing of the blood may be accomplished by the creation or enlargement of an atrial septal defect.

In patients with excessive blood flow through the pulmonary arteries, pulmonary hypertension may develop. To prevent this occurrence, the pulmonary artery is sometimes banded, followed by correction of the defect at a later date.

In cyanotic patients, the anesthetic management is as follows. Induction is with 50% nitrous oxide–oxygen and halothane, with 100% oxygen and halothane, or preferably intravenously with fentanyl. After the chest is opened, 100% oxygen is used in combination with halothane in low concentration, or if not tolerated, doses of fentanyl (1 to 2 µg/kg) are given intermittently as indicated, usually one or two doses during surgery, more if the infant is vigorous. Relaxation is achieved with pancuronium (0.03 to 0.05 mg/kg), if needed, followed by successive doses that are one half to one third of the initial dose. At the end of surgery, muscle relaxation is reversed by neostigmine (0.06 mg/kg) given with atropine (0.03 mg/kg). Usually, the child is extubated at the end of surgery.

During the operation, fluids should be administered generously as tolerated in cyanotic infants with high hematocrit levels to decrease the blood viscosity, improve the flow, and consequently reduce the incidence of intraoperative and postoperative clotting of the shunt. Five percent dextrose in 0.2% normal saline, with or without salt-poor albumin, is preferred to Ringer's solution because, during the procedure, the administration of sodium bicarbonate may be necessary, with the inherent danger of sodium overloading. In patients with a high hematocrit level, blood loss less than 10% to 15% of the estimated blood volume is replaced by this crystalloid solution (the volume given is about three times the volume of estimated blood loss). Of course, a much smaller volume is needed if albumin is also given. In newborns with increased bleeding tendency, the use of fresh-frozen plasma, in addition to vitamin K given intramuscularly before surgery, may be preferred to replace the blood loss. If the hematocrit level is fairly normal for patient age and if the loss of blood is between 10% and 15% or more, blood is transfused, because the cyanotic child will continue to need an elevated hemoglobin level after shunt repair to ensure an adequate blood oxygen-carrying capacity.

Rashkind Procedure (Balloon Atrial Septostomy)

The Rashkind procedure is usually done at the end of catheterization in infants with, for instance, transposition of the great arteries or tricuspid atresia, in whom adequate intercommunication between the pulmonary and the systemic circulation is required for survival. A balloon catheter, introduced into the femoral vein, is passed up into the right atrium and then is manipulated through the foramen ovale. When the position in the left atrium is confirmed, the balloon is inflated by injecting about 2 ml of radiopaque liquid down the catheter. The catheter is then jerked sharply through the atrial septum. This maneuver is repeated several times, with as much as 3 ml of fluid in the balloon, until no further resistance is encountered. The efficacy of the atrial septal defect so created can be immediately determined by repeating the diagnostic studies.

Blalock-Taussig Shunt (Subclavian-Pulmonary Artery Anastomosis)

In the past, the Blalock-Taussig shunt was preferably done on the side opposite the descending aorta, which is the right side in most patients. Ideally, the subclavian branch of the innominate artery is used for the anastomosis[17] because the angle at which the subclavian artery originates from the innominate artery is more favorable and has less of a chance for kinking at its origin than when the subclavian branch of the aorta is used (Fig 6–11,A and B). This consideration is still valid. However, if it seems likely that in the future a Waterston shunt will be necessary, one generally prefers to perform a Blalock-Taussig shunt on the left side. When the right subclavian artery is used for the anastomosis, radial artery cannulation should be performed on the left side; when the left subclavian artery is used, the cannulation should be performed on the right side.

Compression of the lung tissue by the surgeon frequently decreases the PaO_2[133]; therefore, ventilation with 100% oxygen is started as soon as the surgeon opens the chest. Vagal stimulation by the surgeon may occur during freeing of the subclavian artery (Fig 6–12). The surgeon should be notified when this happens, and atropine may be necessary, although discontinuation of the stimulation is generally sufficient.

Another hazardous time is during clamping of the right or left pulmonary artery (Fig 6–13). Any metabolic acidosis should be corrected before the pulmonary artery is cross-clamped. After cross-clamping, the patient is hyperventilated to prevent respiratory acidosis, which may develop because dead space is increased in this situation when only one lung is perfused. Any bradycardia (most often a sign of hypoxia) or hypotension should be aggressively treated during this time, because once the cardiac output is considerably depressed, resuscitation is usually not successful in a patient with hypoxemia, rapidly developing acidosis, and only one lung perfused. Before the start of the anesthesia, atropine, calcium, sodium bicarbonate, and epinephrine are drawn up in syringes in the appropriate dilutions for an infant of this particular weight, so they can be administered immediately when indicated.

Waterston Anastomosis (Ascending Aorta–Right Pulmonary Artery)

The Waterston anastomosis[2] (Fig 6–14) is frequently done in small infants when the diameter of the subclavian artery is too small to ensure a good flow if used for a Blalock-Taussig shunt.

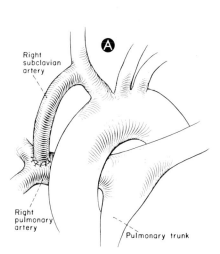
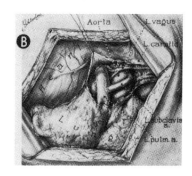

Fig 6–11.—**A,** anastomosis of right subclavian artery and right pulmonary artery. **B,** anastomosis of left subclavian artery as it arises from aorta to left pulmonary artery. Note that angle of left subclavian is less favorable with a left-sided aortic arch. The reverse is true with a right-sided aortic arch. (From Blalock A.: Surgical procedures employed and anatomical variations encountered in the treatment of congenital pulmonic stenosis. *Surg. Gynecol. Obstet.* 87:385, 1948. Used by permission.)

However, if the diameter of the Waterston shunt is made too large, the pulmonary blood flow can increase too much and result in pulmonary edema, and pulmonary hypertension may eventually develop over a long period. Another side effect is kinking or stenosis of the pulmonary artery proximal to the anastomosis, which may create a preferential flow to the right lung, and the left pulmonary artery may become hypoplastic.

A right thoracotomy is performed (the radial artery cannula can be placed on either side), the

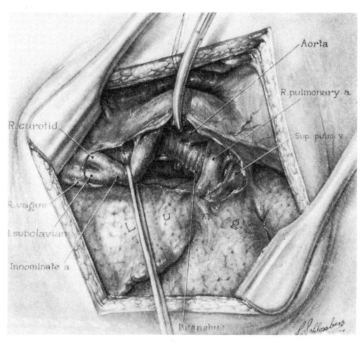

Fig 6–12.—Dissection of right subclavian artery. Note close proximity of vagus nerve. (From Blalock A.: Surgical procedures employed and anatomical variations encountered in the treatment of congenital pulmonic stenosis. *Surg. Gynecol. Obstet.* 87:385, 1948. Used by permission.)

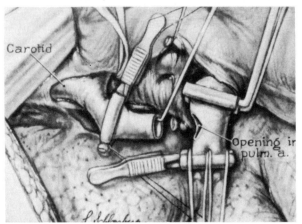

Fig 6–13.—Right subclavian artery is divided and right pulmonary artery is clamped. (From Blalock A.: Surgical procedures employed and anatomical variations encountered in the treatment of congenital pulmonic stenosis. *Surg. Gynecol. Obstet.* 87:385, 1948. Used by permission.)

ascending aorta and right pulmonary artery are dissected free, and a vascular clamp is placed so that one blade is beneath the pulmonary artery and the other is anterior to the ascending aorta (Fig 6–15). An incision is made in the anterior wall of the right pulmonary artery and on the lateral and slightly posterior aspect of the ascending aorta. The diameter of the anastomosis is approximately 4 mm. The anesthetic management is essentially the same as for the Blalock-Taussig shunt.

Both the Blalock-Taussig and the Waterston anastomoses can be taken down relatively easily during bypass surgery when complete repair of the cardiac defect is attempted. The Blalock-Taussig shunt is easily ligated when the bypass is started. The Waterston shunt is kept tightly closed by use of the surgeon's fingers while the patient is rapidly cooled to about 25 C. In this way, excessive pooling of blood in the pulmonary circulation is prevented. The aorta is cross-clamped just distal to the anastomosis, cardioplegic solution is infused, the shunt is transected, and the defect in the ascending aorta is repaired by suturing, while the pulmonary artery is repaired by a Dacron or pericardial patch to prevent this area from later becoming stenotic. Usually, during this time, the flow of the bypass machine is decreased from 2.4 to between 1.5 and 1 L/minute/sq m to reduce the blood reaching the lungs by collateral vessels and interfering with the surgeon's repair of the pulmonary artery defect.

Potts Anastomosis (Descending Aorta to Left Pulmonary Artery)

Potts anastomosis is rarely done anymore, because the late complications are higher than those after the previously discussed shunt operations[157]—that is, the anastomosis may become too large and may result in congestive heart failure or pulmonary hypertension, and a pulmonary artery aneurysm may develop at the site of the anastomosis. In short, the procedure is as follows: A specially designed clamp is positioned around the descending aorta, allowing a small area of the aorta to be isolated while at the same time uninterrupted flow through the aorta continues. A suitable length of the left pulmonary artery is brought side to side with the aorta, ligatures around the pulmonary artery are tightened, and an anastomosis with a diameter of approximately 4 to 5 mm is created (Fig 6–16).

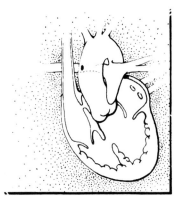

Fig 6–14.—Ascending aorta-to-right pulmonary artery shunt. Anastomosis has a diameter of approximately 4 mm and is situated on posterior side of ascending aorta and anterior wall of right pulmonary artery. (From Cooley D.A., Smith J.M.: Repair of pulmonary arterial stenosis after Waterston-Cooley anastomosis. *J. Thorac. Cardiovasc. Surg.* 77:474, 1979. Used by permission.)

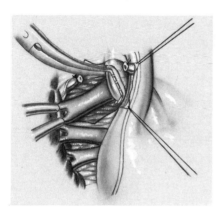

Fig 6–15.—Ascending aorta-to-right pulmonary artery anastomosis. Clamp only partially occludes aorta but totally occludes right pulmonary artery. Snares are tightened around primary branches of pulmonary artery. (Redrawn from Aberdeen.[2] Used by permission.)

Also, closure of the anastomosis during the complete repair is somewhat more complicated than closure of the previous shunts, necessitating a period of circulatory arrest.

After going on bypass, the child is cooled rapidly while the surgeon temporarily compresses the shunt (Fig 6–17,A) with his finger to prevent flow through it from the aorta into the pulmonary circulation. Additional muscle relaxant is administered before circulatory arrest is established, usually at a nasopharyngeal temperature of about 20 C. After cross-clamping of the aorta and the infusion of cold cardioplegic solution, the innominate and left carotid arteries are cross-clamped at their origin to prevent the possibility of air emboli reaching the brain via the aorta when the pulmonary artery is opened for repair of the stoma (Fig 6–17,B).

After repair, the bypass circulation is restarted, while aspiration will remove any air present in the aortic arch; next, the cross-clamps are removed from the carotid and innominate arteries. According to the preference of the surgeon, the temperature either is kept at 20 C or is increased to 25 C while the cardiac defect is repaired.

Blalock-Hanlon Operation (Atrial Septectomy)

When, in infants with transposition of the great arteries, the atrial septal defect created by the Rashkind septostomy is not large enough (usually the Rashkind procedure is adequate for the first 3 months of life), the Blalock-Hanlon operation may be performed,[3] creating a large atrial septal defect. This operation is effective and of relatively low risk in infants. However, some surgeons prefer definitive repair at an early age if septostomy is ineffective.

A right lateral thoracotomy is performed through the fifth interspace,[1] the right pulmonary artery and veins are dissected free, and a silk ligature is passed around each vessel. A partial occlusion clamp is positioned, one jaw behind the right pulmonary veins and one jaw in front, in such a way that, when the clamp is closed, the interatrial groove with a reasonable area of atrial wall is excluded from the rest of the atria (Fig 6–18). To decrease the loss of blood, this operation is frequently performed with inflow occlusion, in which the surgeon tightens snares around the venae cavae just before and during the time septectomy is performed. The anesthetic measures mentioned previously (see under Blalock-Taussig shunt) also apply in this situation. When the patient is

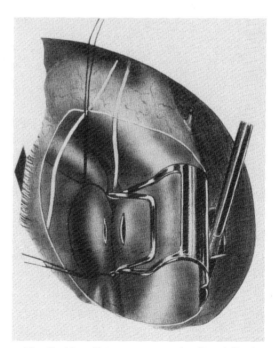

Fig 6–16.—Potts anastomosis. Specially designed clamp is placed around descending aorta. Ligatures are tightened around adjacent part of left pulmonary artery. Incision of about 5 mm is made in each vessel. (From Sellors T.H.: Blalock's and Potts' Operations, in Rob C., Smith R. [eds.]: *Operative Surgery.* London, Butterworth & Co., 1968. Used by permission.)

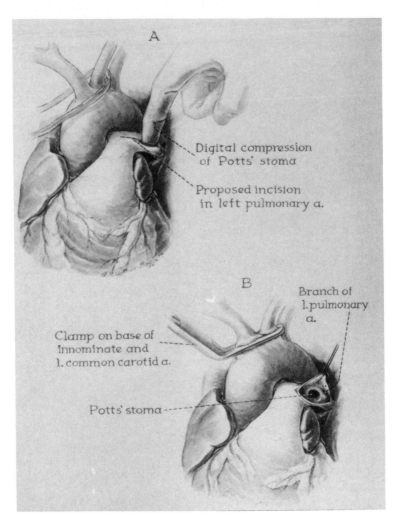

Fig 6–17.—Closure of Potts anastomosis. **A,** during cooling to 20 C, surgeon compresses with his finger Potts shunt. **B,** circulatory arrest is established. Arteries leading toward the head are clamped to prevent air emboli from reaching the brain. Left pulmonary artery is incised, and stoma is visualized. (From Kirklin and Karp.[97] Used by permission.)

ready from the anesthetic standpoint (normal pH, normovolemic, and a normal heart rate), the snare around the right pulmonary artery is closed first, followed after about 15 seconds (to allow for the emptying of the blood from the right lung) by tightening of the snares around the right pulmonary veins, after which the partial occlusion clamp is tightened. If bradycardia occurs, the clamp and snares are released, and another attempt is made after several minutes, usually without any further incident. Otherwise, both bradycardia and hypotension are just as aggressively treated as they are with the previously mentioned shunt operations. An incision close to the interatrial groove is made in the right and the left atrium, the free edge of the atrial septum is grasped with two mosquito forceps, and a part of the atrial septum is excised. (By gently releasing the partial occlusion clamp while at the same time pulling the atrial septum out somewhat farther, a larger atrial septal defect can be created.) A second, smaller partial occlusion clamp is applied so that only the edges of the atrial incision are clamped together (Fig 6–19). The first partial occlusion clamp is released, as are the snares around the right pul-

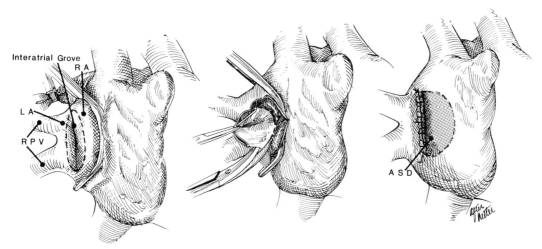

Fig 6–18.—Blalock-Hanlon operation. *Left,* clamp has been applied so as to exclude the interatrial groove and right pulmonary veins. *Center,* clamp has been momentarily loosened to permit interatrial septum to be drawn out and excised. *Right,* large atrial septal defect has thus been created. (Redrawn from Netter F.H.: *The Ciba Collection of Medical Illustrations.* Summit, N.J., Ciba Pharmaceutical Company, 1969. Used by permission.)

monary veins and pulmonary artery. Next, the incision in the atrial wall is sutured. The large atrial septal defect will make adequate bidirectional shunting possible and improve the blood oxygen saturation (Fig 6–20).

Damage to the phrenic nerve, which lies close to the incision of the pericardium, must be avoided. The occurrence of pulmonary congestion may necessitate mechanical ventilation during the early postoperative period.

Brock Procedure (Closed Infundibular Resection With Pulmonary Valvotomy)

The Brock procedure is still considered to be useful in the treatment of patients with tetralogy of Fallot and right ventricular outflow obstruction associated with hypoplasia of the pulmonary artery and annulus.[118] The procedure improves the blood flow through the hypoplastic pulmonary artery, which frequently enlarges considerably after this operation and therefore favors subsequent successful total correction. Also, the procedure may be successful in patients with pulmonary stenosis or atresia. Because loss of blood may be considerable, two adequate intravenous lines are inserted, one preferably a jugular vein line.

A left anterior incision is made in the fourth intercostal space.[174] After insertion of a purse-string suture high in the right ventricle immediately below the infundibular obstruction, a small incision is made in the heart, through which are inserted intermittently a specially designed valvotome, dilators, and an infundibular punch, which widen the stenotic valve and remove obstructing infundibular muscle (Fig 6–21). When the outflow obstruction is relieved, the right ventriculotomy is sutured.

Because the operation is performed in a blind fashion and in a relatively short time (obstruction of the right ventricular outflow tract by the instruments should be as short as possible) and the result therefore is somewhat unpredictable, the open correction of the right ventricular outflow tract is frequently preferred.

Glenn Shunt (Superior Vena Cava–Right Pulmonary Artery Anastomosis)

Because the long-term results of the Glenn shunt may not be favorable and because other options usually exist, this operation is rarely performed anymore, except in a few centers.[157, 175] The advantages of this operation are that (1) only systemic venous blood (from the superior vena cava) is shunted to the lung, (2) left ventricular workload is not increased, as it is in systemic-pulmonary artery shunts, (3) the blood pressure in the pulmonary arteries is not in-

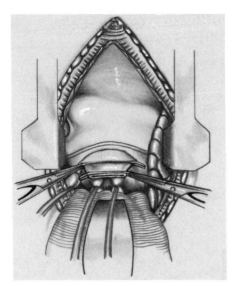

Fig 6–19.—Second, smaller occlusion clamp is now applied so that only edges of atrial incision are clamped together. Next, first clamp, which contained atrial walls and atrial septum, is released, and defect in atrial septum is created. (Redrawn from Aberdeen.[1] Used by permission.)

creased and thus does not lead to pulmonary artery hypertension, as is sometimes seen in systemic–to–pulmonary artery shunts, and (4) the operation is technically easy to perform. However, there are several disadvantages. Shunts made in patients less than 6 months old are associated with a high mortality, probably because of the increased pulmonary resistance in young infants and because the diameter of the right pulmonary artery has to be at least 50% of the diameter of the superior vena cava, a condition that is not often met in young infants. The patients die of cerebral edema caused by a serious superior vena cava syndrome. Incomplete ligation of the caval-atrial junction decreases the incidence of this syndrome; however, such ligation also will decrease its effectiveness.

Even if the initial result of the Glenn shunt is favorable, during the course of several years, function of the shunt frequently deteriorates. The reason for this deterioration is not always clear. In patients with congenital heart defects and pulmonary stenosis, and thus initially with some perfusion of the left lung, infundibular hypertrophy may occur and gradually decrease the pulmonary blood flow. As a consequence of the decrease in Pao_2, the hematocrit level, and thus the blood viscosity, increases, which creates increased resistance to flow through the caval-pulmonary shunt. The pressure in the superior vena cava increases and leads to the development of collateral vessels from the superior vena cava to the inferior vena cava, which decreases the amount of blood available to the right lung for oxygenation.

Also, bronchial collateral vessels may develop, and their blood flow may displace the flow from the superior vena cava in the lung vessels such that the vena cava is perfusing a smaller area of the right lung, which will decrease the effectiveness of the Glenn shunt. Other possible side effects of the placement of a Glenn shunt are chylothorax and hydrocephaly in young infants and the formation of pulmonary arteriovenous pulmonary fistulas. A rare but serious complication is occlusion of the shunt by thrombosis.

The surgical procedure is as follows[70]: A right anterolateral thoracotomy is performed through the fourth interspace. The azygos vein is ligated

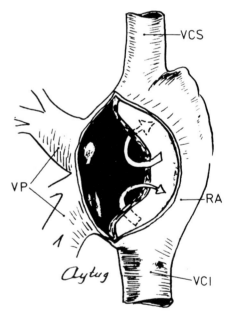

Fig 6–20.—Situation after Blalock-Hanlon septectomy. Part of wall of right atrium is removed in the figure to show septal defect created. Note vena cava superior *(VCS)*, vena pulmonis *(VP)*, right atrium *(RA)*, vena cava inferior *(VCI)*. (From Rohmer J., Geldof W.C.P., Bergmeijer J.H.: Behandeling van transpositie van de grote vaten. *Ned. Tijdschr. Geneeskd.* 118:532, 1974. Used by permission.)

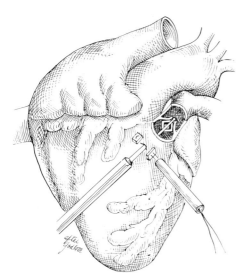

Fig 6–21.—Infundibular valvotome is inserted through small right ventriculotomy. Pursestring suture keeps blood loss under control.

and transected. The superior vena cava is side-clamped (Fig 6–22). The right pulmonary artery is divided near its point of origin (bulldog clamps are placed on the first two branches of the right pulmonary artery to prevent backflow), and an end-to-side anastomosis of the right pulmonary artery to the superior vena cava is performed. The clamps are removed, and the superior vena cava is ligated with two ligatures just below the anastomosis (Fig 6–23). The same anesthetic precautions are taken as with the previous shunt operations.

Venous drainage from the head can be improved by maintaining the patient in a head-up position (about 45 degrees) for at least one year after surgery.

Pulmonary Artery Banding

In some infants with transposition of the great arteries and ventricular septal defect or with univentricular heart, truncus arteriosus, or other complex malformations with increased pulmonary blood flow, pulmonary artery banding is still justifiable as a temporary solution to alleviate the heart failure and pulmonary congestion with which these infants may be seen initially. Because surgery is usually performed only on severely ill infants, the mortality is high, as much as 15% to 25%,[108, 173] depending on the primary defect.

Anesthesia is given with the usual precautions, as in a severely ill infant. Frequently, only oxygen, air, and fentanyl are administered, combined with pancuronium for muscle relaxation. Repeated arterial blood gas determinations are necessary for adequate correction of metabolic acidosis and monitoring of the ventilation. Fluid administration is minimal in cardiac failure, and intravenously administered digoxin (if the patient is not already digitalized) or a dopamine infusion may be necessary. Emergency drugs appropriately diluted (epinephrine, calcium chloride, atropine, sodium bicarbonate) are drawn up into syringes. A small, left anterior thoracotomy is performed in the third or fourth intercostal space, with the patient lying supine. A Silastic or Teflon band of 0.5 to 1 cm width is placed around the main pulmonary artery (Fig 6–24). The degree of tightness of the band is important because (1) if it is too tight, cyanosis and polycythemia will develop since the lungs are insufficiently perfused, and (2) if it is too loose, overperfusion of the lungs and cardiac failure will continue and may lead to pulmonary vascular obstructive disease. Before and after the band is placed, systemic arterial pressure and pulmonary artery pressure distal to the band are measured. After banding of the pulmonary artery, the systemic arterial pressure will generally increase about 10 to 20 mm Hg and be accompanied by slight slowing of heart rate.

The surgeon usually tries to tighten the band until the pulmonary arterial pressure distal to

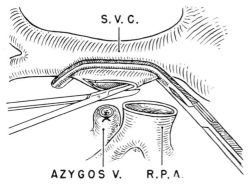

Fig 6–22.—Superior vena cava (S.V.C.) is side-clamped, and incision is made to match diameter of distal end of right pulmonary artery (R.P.A.). (From Glenn.[70] Used by permission.)

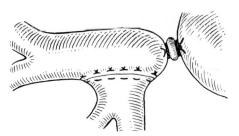

Fig 6–23.—Glenn anastomosis between superior vena cava and right pulmonary artery. Double ligature is placed at distal end of vena cava. (From Glenn.[70] Used by permission.)

the banding is one half to one third of the systemic pressure. However, if the right ventricle cannot overcome the higher resistance, then increased right-to-left shunting occurs, the patient becomes more cyanotic, and his condition deteriorates rapidly. In such a situation, the band tension has to be released slightly.

Because the infant is almost always severely ill, postoperative mechanical ventilation is needed until his condition improves. Pulmonary artery banding may create several problems that may complicate total correction at a later age: for example, fibrosis and scarring of the pulmonary trunk, causing stenosis; right ventricular hypertrophy, leading to infundibular stenosis; and partial or complete obstruction of the pulmonary artery branches at the bifurcation of the pulmonary trunk.

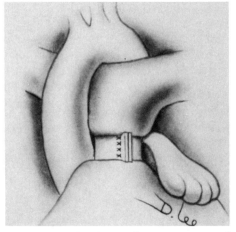

Fig 6–24.—Banded pulmonary artery. Anchoring sutures are placed in adventitia to prevent migration. (From Danielson.[41] Used by permission.)

Summary

Whatever palliative procedure is used, most patients can be extubated after successful systemic–pulmonary artery shunt surgery. However, the endotracheal tube should be left in patients who are in heart failure before surgery or in patients with a doubtful shunt flow, so that their condition can be better controlled and evaluated for several hours postoperatively. In the presence of severely increased pulmonary vascular resistance, a drug with pulmonary vasodilating action, such as prostaglandin E_1, tolazoline, nitroprusside, or, if indicated, isoproterenol, may also be useful during the early postoperative phase.

ANESTHESIA FOR OPEN-HEART SURGERY

Anesthetic Management During Prebypass, Bypass, and Postbypass Periods

Anesthetic Agents

Once the child is intubated and stable, the anesthesiologist has a choice of agents for the maintenance of anesthesia. A thorough knowledge of the pharmacology of drugs and especially of their effects on the patient's hemodynamics is essential. For instance, an agent with a vasodilating effect is contraindicated in a hypovolemic patient or in a patient with left ventricular outflow obstruction, unless adequate amounts of fluids have been administered first.

Nitrous oxide (50%) with oxygen is used as the basic anesthetic in nearly all patients, except in cyanotic patients with hypoxic pulmonary vasoconstriction, in whom the administration of 100% oxygen may reduce the pulmonary vascular hypertension. Also, in severely ill patients, 100% oxygen in combination with an intravenous agent is preferred because the cardiodepressant action of nitrous oxide may be too great for these patients. In addition to nitrous oxide, the following agents can be used: halothane, enflurane, meperidine, morphine, and fentanyl. Halothane is usually administered in a concentration of 0.1% to 0.8%. In patients with severe cyanosis, it is used only in a low concentration to prevent a decrease in cardiac output, which may increase the cyanosis. Meperidine can be slowly injected up to a total dose of between 2 and 10 mg/kg of body weight, or more if indicated. Often meperidine is used with halothane in low concentrations. Though morphine is not a cardiodepressant, it too should be administered very slowly because vasodilation may decrease blood pressure. If indicated, infusion of intravenous fluids to correct the decreased preload should accompany its administration. The total dose is usually between 0.5 and 2 mg/kg. Enflurane is less desirable for inhalation induction because it is more irritating than halothane and frequently causes an increased excitation phase. However, if the child agrees to an intravenous induction, enflurane in concentrations up to 1% may be used for the maintenance of anesthesia, often in combination with low doses of meperidine or morphine. Because halothane tends to sensitize the myocardium to epinephrine, enflurane is preferred to halothane in patients with a potential for arrhythmias,[16] especially if epinephrine drip is expected to be needed when the patient comes off bypass. Fentanyl in doses of between 30 and 100 µg/kg, or more if indicated, can be used for maintenance of anesthesia. For muscle relaxation, pancuronium in an initial dose of 0.1 mg/kg can be used, followed by 0.05 mg/kg when the patient goes on bypass.

Fluid Management

Dextrose, 5% in 0.2% normal saline, can be used in a maintenance dose of 3 to 4 ml/kg/hour. Correction for fluid deprivation during the preoperative fasting time is made when the child's urinary output is less than 1 ml/kg/hour or when the history (use of diuretics or nothing by mouth for longer than four hours) or clinical impression (low central venous pressure, considerable blood pressure decrease with the use of halothane) is suggestive of hypovolemia.

Generally, a small infant should be kept slightly hypervolemic before insertion of the aortic cannula because considerable (for the infant's size) loss of blood may occur during this procedure. If the loss is severe during the insertion of the venous cannulas, the pump technician should transfuse blood as needed via the aortic cannula.

During dissection around the heart, hypotension or arrhythmias may occur easily. The anesthesiologist closely watches the blood pressure and ECG and notifies the surgeon of any changes. Discontinuation of the stimulation is usually sufficient to solve the problem. Obviously, the discontinuation of all anesthetic agents and the administration of 100% oxygen are indicated if severe hypotension occurs.

Surface Cooling

In small infants, the use of conventional cardiopulmonary bypass was earlier accompanied by high mortality and morbidity. However, during the last decade, the results have been improving considerably since the use of profound hypothermia, cardioplegic solution, and total circulatory arrest for as long as 60 minutes. The advantages are as follows: optimal surgical exposure of an exsanguinated relaxed heart when the venous cannulas are removed and shortened time for repair of the cardiac defect, combined with adequate myocardial protection by hypothermia and cardioplegic solution.

For shortening the bypass time and providing more uniform cooling of the body, surface cooling has been used in infants who weigh less than 10 kg. The patient is cooled first to between 28 and 29 C with surface cooling, which is followed by bypass cooling, until the nasopharyngeal temperature reaches about 16 to 18 C. Disadvantages of this method are the prolonged anesthesia time, the potential cold injury to the skin, and sometimes the increased irritability of the heart, with the resulting supraventricular and ventricular arrhythmias. Induction and maintenance of anesthesia are as previously described. The vasodilating action of halothane is helpful in the cooling process, and pancuronium is useful as a relaxant to prevent shivering during the cooling. The infant is placed on a cooling blanket, and plastic bags with melting crushed ice in ice water are placed on top of and around the child, especially where the great vessels are close under the skin, as in the groins, axillae, and neck. Also, ice bags are placed around the head and on the abdomen and right side of the chest. Ice bags should not be placed on the left precordial region because the heart may cool too rapidly and arrhythmias may ensue. The ice bags, which are wrapped in gauze, are frequently repositioned to prevent skin damage by cold injury. No ice is placed on the hands or feet.

If halothane is not tolerated during surface

cooling, narcotics are added to the 50% nitrous oxide in oxygen. Also during cooling, up to 5% carbon dioxide is added to the inspired gases to maintain a high-normal (temperature corrected) $PaCO_2$ because the $PaCO_2$ will otherwise decrease with the decrease in the rate of metabolism during cooling. A normal $PaCO_2$ is necessary to prevent peripheral and cerebral vasoconstriction.

Prevention of respiratory alkalosis in this period is also helpful in decreasing the chance of cardiac arrhythmias[88, 170] and in preventing an even further shift to the left of the hemoglobin-oxygen saturation curve, resulting in reduced tissue oxygenation (Fig 6–25).

The viscosity of the blood is highly dependent on the hematocrit. As the viscosity increases during surface cooling (decreasing from 37 to 25 C increases the viscosity by about 50%),[72] patients are given 5% albumin or 5% dextrose in 0.2% saline, which may total between 10% and 20% of the estimated blood volume of the child.

Arterial samples are frequently taken to determine PaO_2, $PaCO_2$, and hematocrit and potassium levels. If the potassium level decreases during cooling, diluted potassium chloride is given intravenously (see Table 6–5) slowly over a 20-minute period. The plasma potassium level is determined after each dose. A plasma potassium level of at least 4 mmole/L is preferred, because hypokalemia may precipitate cardiac arrhythmias. Moderate-to-severe metabolic acidosis should be corrected by the use of sodium bicarbonate. When a nasopharyngeal temperature of 29 to 30 C is reached, the surface cooling is discontinued, and the temperature usually decreases another 1 or 2 C before cannulation of the aorta and right atrium is completed. At this temperature, the blood pressure and heart rate are decreased but a normal sinus rhythm is present. In a desperately ill infant or in the presence of ventricular irritability, the femoral vessels should be cannulated before sternotomy is performed, because the sternotomy may easily precipitate ventricular tachycardia and fibrillation. Although a temperature of approximately 29 C provides some protection against the effects of ventricular fibrillation, the situation is considerably less stressful if the patient can be placed immediately on femoral-femoral bypass and the surgeon can continue the procedure in the chest without haste. If the usual procedure is followed (sternotomy and cannulation of the aorta and right atrium), heparin (300 units/kg) is administered shortly before the sternotomy, and the bypass lines are filled and ready for cannulation so that, if cardiac arrest occurs, the blood is already heparinized and time is not wasted.

The chance for ventricular fibrillation increases at temperatures below 30 C. Most often this happens suddenly without any prior arrhythmia, during either sternotomy or exposure of the heart. Recent digitalis therapy, combined with a low or low-normal serum potassium level, may precipitate ventricular fibrillation. If indicated, lidocaine (1 mg/kg) is administered shortly before sternotomy. During surface cooling, no changes have been found in the serum levels of sodium, magnesium, or ionic calcium. However, blood sugar levels increase significantly, probably because of the reduction in cellular uptake and metabolism of glucose.[88, 170]

Anticoagulation and Its Reversal

The administration of an adequate dose of heparin is necessary to keep the patient safely anticoagulated while attached to the bypass machine.[28, 92] However, the sensitivity of a patient to heparin and the half-life of heparin are not predictable and may differ considerably among patients. Thus, for the heparinization, the method of Bull et al.[29] is used, with some modification. After the determination of the baseline

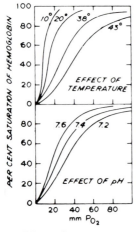

Fig 6–25.—Effect of temperature and pH on hemoglobin-oxygen saturation curve. (From Comroe J.H. Jr.: *Physiology of Respiration: An Introductory Text.* Chicago, Year Book Medical Publishers, 1965. Used by permission.)

activated clotting time,* on a sample taken from the arterial line, a dose of 300 units of heparin per kilogram is given. Before the aspiration of 3 ml of blood for the determination of activated clotting time, 10 ml of blood is aspirated to clear the arterial line of heparin present in the flush solution. The initial activated clotting time is usually between 100 and 130 seconds. After five minutes, the activated clotting time is measured again. Both values are plotted on a graph (Fig 6–26). If, after 300 units of heparin per kilogram, the activated clotting time is below 450 seconds, a line is extrapolated through both activated clotting time values to intersect with the 450-second line, and the calculated amount of heparin is added. When the bypass is started, the heparin that has been added to the perfusate in the bypass machine usually will increase the activated clotting time far above the 450 seconds for the duration of the bypass. The activated clotting time is checked 5 minutes after the start of bypass. At the same time, circulating heparin levels are analyzed by the Hepcon† heparin analyzer system.[84a, 144a] We prefer to keep the heparin concentration during bypass at 300 U/kg. Usually the heparin level is checked every 2 hours at body temperatures below 25 C, every hour when the body temperature is between 25 and 30 C, and every 30 minutes at temperatures above 30 C.

After the patient comes off bypass, both activated clotting time and heparin levels are checked again. Protamine sulfate is usually given slowly during a 5-minute period. The vasodilating effect of protamine may necessitate an increased rate of transfusion during this time. The amount of protamine needed for reversal of heparin is calculated with the Hepcon analyzer system, which computes the estimated blood volume from the body weight, height, and sex of the patient. However, because we generally transfuse using left atrial pressures up to 12 to 20 mm Hg while the patient is coming off bypass, we assume that the patient's blood volume after bypass is increased, compared with that before bypass. Therefore, the protamine reversal dose (as calculated by the Hepcon analyzer) is increased by at least 10%.

*The activated clotting time is determined in the operating room, using a Hemochron 400, International Technidyne Corp., Metuchen, N.J.
†Hepcon Cyotom A-10, Hemotech, Inc., Englewood, Colo.

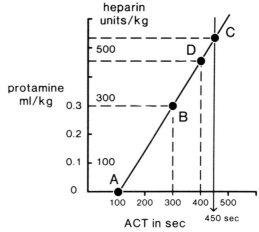

Fig 6–26.—Initial activated clotting time *(ACT)* (point *A*) is determined. Heparin, 300 units/kg (1,000 units = 1 ml) is administered. After five minutes, ACT is repeated (point *B*). If ACT is considerably below 450 seconds, line drawn through A and B, intersecting with 450-second line (point *C*) provides information about additional dose of heparin necessary to obtain ACT of 450 seconds (in this example, about 230 units/kg = 0.23 ml/kg). ACT measured after coming off bypass (for instance, 400 seconds) is plotted (point *D*), and necessary neutralizing dose of protamine (here, 0.46 ml/kg) is given for reversal of circulating heparin. However, lately the Hepcon heparin analyzer system is being used for calculating the neutralizing dose of protamine (see text).

About 10 minutes after administration of protamine, the adequacy of the heparin reversal is checked by the activated clotting time and the Hepcon analyzer system, and additional protamine is given if necessary.

If both determinations suggest that adequate reversal took place, another 10% of the initial protamine dose is slowly infused during the next 2 to 4 hours, in order to decrease the incidence and severity of postoperative heparin rebound.[24, 144a] The use of both activated clotting time and a heparin analyzing system has several advantages. The adequacy of the initial heparin dose in providing effective anticoagulation should be confirmed by a clotting test instead of by measuring the blood heparin level. Although the latter may be 300 U/kg of body weight, this does not guarantee adequate anticoagulation, as for instance in the patient with low antithrombin III.[87a, 152a] Therefore, if additional (above the calculated 300 U/kg) heparin is necessary before bypass in order to obtain an activated clotting time of 450 seconds,[4] the blood heparin level is measured with the Hepcon analyzer, and this increased level, which ensures an adequate anticoagulation, will be maintained during bypass.

The results obtained by the activated clotting time fluctuate during bypass much more than heparin levels as measured by the Hepcon analyzer. Monitoring of heparin levels during bypass, therefore, is preferable.

If increased bleeding occurs after bypass, more information may be obtained when both the heparin level and the activated clotting time are measured. For instance, if the activated clotting time is increased and the Hepcon analyzer shows the presence of residual heparin, the treatment will consist of the administration of protamine. However, if no heparin is detected by the Hepcon analyzer and the activated clotting time is either prolonged or normal, the clotting mechanism probably is, respectively, severely or moderately disturbed. In this situation, blood is sent for clotting studies; and the bleeding will be treated with the administration of clotting factors. This obviates the need to add additional protamine "just in case."

Cardiopulmonary Bypass

During surgical repair of the heart, adequate oxygenation and perfusion of the body is provided by the bypass machine. Its task is facilitated by the use of hypothermia, which decreases considerably the body oxygen consumption.

However, several problems are associated with hypothermia and the use of the bypass machine: (1) the blood viscosity is increased during hypothermia, (2) additional protection of the myocardium is necessary, (3) protection of the brain must be adequate, and (4) anomalies of hemostasis may be present after bypass.

The general principles of cardiopulmonary bypass are discussed in chapter 9. However, several details of importance for pediatric patients should be mentioned. The size of the aortic cannula depends on the highest flow rate that will be used to perfuse the body. A gradient of less than 100 mm Hg across the cannula (at the highest flow to be used) is preferred to minimize the turbulence as blood leaves the cannula's tip. Furthermore, the arterial line pressure (measured by the arterial line manometer on the pump oxygenator) should be less than 250 mm Hg because the metal or plastic connectors located in the bypass circuit may become disconnected from the bypass tubing if the pressure in the line is too high. For instance, in a child with a surface area of 0.5 sq m, the maximal flow rate will be 1.2 L/minute (maximal perfusion flow rate is 2.4 L/minute/sq m), and, therefore, a 14 F cannula is the smallest that can be used (Table 6–7). Also, the size of the venous cannula depends on the maximal perfusion flow rate to be used for that patient (Table 6–8). This is to assure as low a venous pressure as possible during bypass.

Intracardiac Suction

Suction lines are required to aspirate blood from the opened heart and return it to the pump oxygenator as part of the venous return and to decompress the heart (especially the left side) when needed. Therefore, as a routine just after establishing cardiopulmonary bypass, a small suction catheter is inserted in the left ventricle via the left atrium or superior pulmonary vein near the left atrium. At the end of bypass, air may be evacuated by using this catheter or by direct needle aspiration of the left ventricle.

An aortic vent in the ascending aorta is used for evacuation of air before the release of the aortic cross-clamp. The intracardiac suction system is more traumatic to blood than any other part of the bypass system. Also, blood returning via the suction lines usually contains more debris than that returning through the venous lines. Therefore, a filter is interposed between the suction line and the oxygenator. Another suction line is connected to the wall suction for the removal, from the pericardial space, of blood and iced saline that is used for surface cooling of the heart and, if indicated, for the removal of cardioplegic solution that returns to the right atrium after perfusion of the coronary arteries.

Perfusion Flow and Temperature

Experimental studies at 37 C show that total-body oxygen consumption is directly related to the perfusion flow rate, up to a flow of approximately 2.5 L/minute/sq m, after which oxygen consumption does not increase.[100] Presumably,

TABLE 6–7.—PRESSURE GRADIENTS (MM HG) BY FLOWS ACCORDING TO SIZE OF ARTERIAL CANNULAS*

SIZE (FRENCH)	FLOW, L/MIN							
	0.5	1.0	1.5	2.0	2.5	3.0	3.5	4.0
10	60	175	350					
12	40	100	225	325				
14	25	60	140	240	350			
16		25	50	90	150	200	260	
18		20	40	60	80	120	150	200
20			25	40	60	80	100	120
22			25	40	50	60	75	90
24				40	50	60	70	80

*From Kirklin et al.[100] Used by permission.

TABLE 6–8.—VENOUS CANNULAS CHART*

TOTAL FLOW, L/MIN	SINGLE TYGON CANNULA, IN.	TWO TYGON CANNULAS, IN.	DOUBLE RYGG CANNULAS, MM
<0.7	...	...	4
0.7–0.9	3/16	...	4
0.91–1.75	4/16	3/16	5
1.76–2.2	4/16	4/16	6
2.21–2.8	5/16	4/16	6
2.81–3.2	5/16	5/16	6
3.21–3.7	6/16	5/16	7
>3.7	7/16	6/16	7

*From Kirklin et al.[100] Used by permission.

at these flows most of the microcirculation is perfused. At lower flows only a part is perfused, and consequently oxygen consumption is reduced. Therefore, under the usual conditions of mild-to-moderate hypothermia, a flow rate of 2.2 L/minute/sq m at a mean systemic pressure of 50 to 70 mm Hg should be adequate to assure satisfactory oxygenation of the patient. With profound hypothermia (less than 28 C), a flow rate of about 1.6 L/minute/sq m is adequate for up to two hours. A low flow rate (0.5 L/minute/sq m) is considered acceptable for 30 minutes at 26 C and for 45 minutes at 22 C.[6, 100]

Perfusion at low flow is preferred to total circulatory arrest.[103] However, in small infants removal of the venous cannulas may be necessary for adequate surgical exposure. During the phases of cooling and rewarming, high flow rates are used to shorten these phases. The temperature difference between the body and the perfusate should never be more than 10 or 12 C during cooling, to prevent cold injury of the tissues, or during rewarming, to prevent the formation of gas bubbles in the blood (with increasing temperature the solubility of gas decreases). The temperatures of the water bath and perfusate are kept below 42 and 38 C, respectively.

Blood is equilibrated in the oxygenator with a mixture of oxygen and 2% to 5% carbon dioxide. A continuous P_{aO_2} and $P_{\bar{v}O_2}$ monitoring device connected, respectively, to the arterial and venous pump line enables the P_{aO_2} to be maintained between 100 and 200 mm Hg and the $P_{\bar{v}O_2}$ to be maintained above 40 mm Hg. The temperature-corrected P_{aCO_2} is approximately between 30 and 40 mm Hg, as measured by blood gas analysis.

Perfusate

Because the blood viscosity increases both with the hematocrit value and with increased hypothermia, there has been concern about the cyanotic child with a high hematocrit reading having bypass while under deep hypothermia, especially if total circulatory arrest is planned.[72, 73, 103] However, too much hemodilution will cause problems with adequate oxygenation of the tissues when the patient is rewarmed, and also the colloid osmolar pressure should not decrease too much, to prevent excessive fluid moving into the extravascular compartment. A hematocrit reading of 25% seems to be an acceptable compromise.

With the bypass solutions used in our institution, as mentioned in chapter 9, the hematocrit value of the patient during bypass will usually decrease to about 30%. However, for deep hypothermia, we recently started to use less blood prime to obtain a hematocrit reading of 25%. With the following equation, the necessary amount of blood and clear prime that will provide a hematocrit (Hct) value of 25% during bypass can be calculated:

$$25\% \; Hct = (BV \times Hct + BP \times Hct)/TF$$

where BV is the estimated blood volume of the patient in liters, BP is the blood prime in liters, and TF is the total amount of fluids in liters (total fluids equals the child's blood volume plus blood prime plus clear prime). Suppose, for instance, in the following situation, the priming volume of oxygenator and pump lines is 1 liter, the blood volume of a 3-kg infant (hematocrit, 60%) is 270 ml, and the hematocrit of the blood prime is 30%: thus,

$$Hct \; (25\%) = (0.270 \times 60 + X \times 30)/1{,}270$$

in which the denominator (1,270 ml) is obtained from 270 ml child's blood volume plus X ml of blood prime plus $(1{,}000 - X)$ ml of clear prime. One unit of blood (actually 518 ml) is required in this situation.

The urine production during bypass usually tends to increase the hematocrit. However, if during rewarming the hematocrit is too low, furosemide or mannitol, if necessary combined with packed RBCs, may be given during rewarming or early in the postbypass period. When the patient is coming off bypass, a hematocrit value of between 35% and 45% is the goal, because the oxygen delivery is maximal in this range.

Myocardial Protection

Preservation of cardiac function by protection from ischemia before, during, and after bypass forms an important part of the successful outcome of surgery (see chap. 14). Subendocardial myocardial necrosis, most likely caused by a discrepancy between energy supply and demand,[26] is the most frequent cause of morbidity and death after technically successful cardiac operations. Its manifestations are a low cardiac output state (from mild to so severe that the patient is unable to come off bypass) and arrhythmias. The left ventricular subendocardial myocardium is most susceptible to ischemia. When the heart is beating, this area receives its blood supply only during diastole. Recent animal studies[85] suggest that subendocardial ischemia may occur when the ratio of the diastolic pressure time index and tension time index is near 0.4 in a normal heart with normal blood oxygen content. In cyanotic heart diseases or severe left ventricular hypertrophy, a higher ratio is likely to be necessary to decrease the chance of myocardial ischemia. Unfortunately, anesthesia frequently has a negative inotropic effect on the myocardium and may actually reduce the diastolic pressure time index in patients already in cardiac failure by increasing the left ventricular end-diastolic pressure. However, in hyperactive hearts, decrease of the tension time index, as occurs with decrease in the left ventricular systolic pressure, and decrease of the heart rate have a beneficial effect on the myocardial oxygen consumption.

The protection of the myocardium against ischemia during bypass is also a matter of great concern. Recently, promising results have been reached by use of a combination of hypothermia (which decreases myocardial oxygen requirements) and rapid cardiac arrest by cardioplegia,[96] thus allowing the small amount of energy produced by anaerobic metabolism during the aortic cross-clamping to be used for the maintenance of cellular structure and of the energy-dependent cell membrane pumps necessary in preserving the transcellular gradients of sodium, potassium, calcium, and magnesium, instead of allowing the energy to be wasted on useless electromechanical activity (beating or fibrillation). However, because of noncoronary collateral blood flow, the cold cardioplegic solution is washed away fairly rapidly. Consequently, both the energy-sparing low myocardial temperature (perfusion of cold cardioplegic solution brings the myocardial temperature down, usually to between 11 and 14 C) and the beneficial action of the cold cardioplegic solution will be of short duration. Therefore, repeated doses of cold cardioplegic solution (approximately every 20 minutes or whenever the myocardial temperature reaches about 20 C or if the electromechanical activity of the heart reappears) are necessary for protection against myocardial damage.

The use of whole-body hypothermia and repeated infusions of cold cardioplegic solution allows the following to be accomplished:[27] (1) production of immediate cardiac arrest after cross-clamping of the aorta to avoid the energy depletion by ischemic electromechanical work; (2) further reduction of energy demands and prevention of recurrence of electromechanical activity; (3) provision of substrate for continued anaerobic or aerobic (or both) energy production during aortic clamping; (4) buffering to counteract anaerobic acidosis and maintain a pH optimal for continued metabolism; (5) hyperosmolarity to reduce edema; and (6) membrane stabilization, either by the addition of procaine or steroids or by the repeated administration of cardioplegic solution.

There are different opinions about the proper composition of cardioplegic solutions. At our institution, two different solutions are in use (see chap. 14).

Administration of Cardioplegic Solution (Practical Aspects)

A plastic bag with cardioplegic solution is kept in the operating room at a temperature of about 4 C (submerged in a container filled with melting ice). The cardioplegic solution is infused in the aortic root via the aortic vent needle (before infusing the cardioplegic solution, the infusion line is thoroughly flushed to remove air bubbles). Later, this needle functions as a vent to aspirate air that may have entered the left side of the heart during surgical repair. The patient is cooled to the "desired temperature"* and the aorta is cross-clamped, followed immediately (and preferably before fibrillation occurs) by the infusion by a roller pump of the cold cardioplegic solution, until a myocardial temperature (measured by a thermistor needle in the myocardium) of between 11 and 14 C is reached. The amount of cardioplegic solution necessary is usually between 10 and 25 ml/kg. The necessity of removing the cardioplegic solution by suction (connected to a wall suction bottle) from the right atrium to prevent a dangerous increase in potassium level depends more on the urine output during bypass and the number of times that perfusion with the solution is performed than on the size of the patient. For instance, if a child of 3 kg receives 60 ml of cardioplegic solution once or twice, this will add each time (if a cardioplegic solution containing 30 mEq of KCl per liter is used) about 2 mEq of potassium chloride to the fluid pool formed by the bypass priming fluid and the blood volume of the child, which amounts to at least about 1,000 ml and therefore is of no concern. However, in older children with complicated congenital heart defects who will need multiple myocardial perfusions of cardioplegic solutions, one may wish to prevent the cardioplegic solution from mixing with the pump perfusate, especially if the urine output is low. Generally, in uncomplicated heart defects, the mixing of cardioplegic solution with the pump perfusate is of some benefit, because it decreases the incidence of hypokalemia, which frequently develops during bypass.

During aortic cross-clamping, the goal is for a mean perfusion pressure of between 50 (30 to 40 in newborns) and 80 mm Hg. Sometimes immediately after the start of bypass or near the end after release of the aortic cross-clamp, the mean perfusion pressure decreases to an "unacceptably" low level of about 20 to 30 mm Hg. As the body temperature is nearly normal in these situations, one is concerned about possibly inadequate perfusion not only of organs like the brain and kidneys but also of the myocardium. Especially if the patient has a history of heart failure or left ventricular hypertrophy or another condition in which adequate coronary perfusion pressure is essential to prevent (further) myocardial damage, the perfusion pressure may have to be increased to an acceptable level by the administration of small amounts (5 to 10 µg) of an α-adrenergic drug like phenylephrine, which may be repeated until the desired result has been reached. However, especially near the end of bypass, phenylephrine may not be the correct choice. Because its action is somewhat prolonged, its vasoconstricting effect, which also affects the pulmonary vessels, may extend into the immediate postbypass period. This effect may be undesirable, especially for patients with

---

*Depending on the preference of the surgical team, the desired temperature is usually 20 to 25 C. If fibrillation occurs before this temperature is reached, the aorta is cross-clamped and cold cardioplegic solution is infused while patient cooling continues until the desired temperature has been reached.

a modified Fontan repair or with a right ventriculotomy when an increased pulmonary resistance is not easily tolerated. The other method of increasing the systemic blood pressure in this situation is asking the pump technician to decrease the venous return slightly while the left atrial pressure is closely monitored.

In the presence of profuse systemic-pulmonary artery collateral circulation, the perfusion pressure will decrease considerably as soon as the patient is placed on bypass, because the perfusion of the systemic circulation is less than usual inasmuch as part of the perfusate will flow via the collateral vessels, the pulmonary circulation, left ventricle, and left ventricular suction line back into the pump and thus will bypass the systemic circulation. The administration of an α-adrenergic drug is not effective in this situation and may even result in more volume displacement from the systemic into the pulmonary circulation. Rapid cooling is indicated to provide adequate protection. An additional advantage of such a low temperature is that the perfusion flow can be brought down to between 1.5 and 0.5 L/minute/sq m, or to circulatory arrest if necessary, to provide a dry surgical field, because frequently too much blood flows via the collateral vessels into the pulmonary circulation and the left side of the heart and interferes with adequate visualization. Unfortunately, as just mentioned, the systemic circulation receives a smaller volume of cooled perfusate per time unit from the pump, with the result that the rate of cooling in patients with systemic-pulmonary artery collaterals is slower than normal. Because the adequacy of tissue perfusion and oxygen supply to the brain (and probably of other organs too) is questionable during this period of low perfusion pressure and only slowly decreasing body temperature, 5 mg of thiopental per kilogram is administered just before bypass is started in the hope of providing some protection for the brain. The use of a short-acting vasodilating agent to increase the rate of cooling may be indicated.

An increase in mean aortic pressure above 80 mm Hg is a sign of peripheral vasoconstriction and is an undesirable situation, because it decreases peripheral tissue perfusion. Adequate vasodilation may be provided by halothane administered by a vaporizer inserted in-line in the tubing that delivers oxygen and carbon dioxide to the bubble oxygenator in a concentration of, at most, 1% during mild hypothermia or 0.5% during moderate hypothermia. However, the administration of a vasodilating agent that does not have a cardiodepressant side effect is generally preferred. Therefore, chlorpromazine (between 2.5 and 5 mg) or a nitroprusside drip (50 mg in 250 ml of 5% dextrose in water) is frequently used to obtain adequate vasodilation during bypass.

Emergence From Bypass

After completion of the repair, the patient is rewarmed. At a nasopharyngeal temperature of between 29 and 31 C, the aortic cross-clamp is removed. If ventricular fibrillation results, the heart is defibrillated. An adequate coronary perfusion pressure is important for the perfusion and oxygenation of the myocardium in this last part of the bypass period in which the heart is beating and the temperature is increasing to reach 37 C. If the mean perfusion pressure after removal of the aortic cross-clamp is considered to be too low for adequate perfusion of the coronary arteries, increase in perfusion pressure can be obtained either by administration of a short-acting α-adrenergic drug or by slightly decreasing the venous blood return from the patient to the pump when the patient is on partial bypass (the ties that kept both venae cavae tightly closed around the venous return cannulas are released when the right atrium wall is closed). An increase of several millimeters of mercury in the right and left atrial pressures (pressure lines have been inserted by the surgeon) is usually sufficient to provide a mean aortic pressure of about 70 mm Hg. If halothane is used during bypass, its use is discontinued when rewarming is started,[156] to provide enough time for its washout and to minimize its cardiodepressant effects when the patient comes off bypass.

When the patient is rewarmed (nasopharyngeal temperature of 36.5 to 37 C) and the left atrial pressure line is inserted, manual ventilation with 100% oxygen is started, initially with continuous positive airway pressure, which is helpful for getting all areas of the lung reexpanded. The lungs are not kept inflated with air or oxygen as was done previously during bypass. Since the establishment of this practice, there has not been an increase in postoperative pulmonary complications.

During anesthesia, the urine output should be adequate (at least 1 ml/kg/hour, except during periods of low perfusion flow or total circulatory arrest). If the urinary production is low, furosemide, 0.5 to 1 mg/kg, is given. (If the potassium level is low, potassium chloride is given as needed, as soon as urinary production starts.)

Arterial blood gases and electrolytes are checked as indicated—for instance, when pump time is prolonged, after total circulatory arrest, and before the patient comes off bypass. In infants, the blood sugar level is checked with a Chemstrip after rewarming.

Total Circulatory Arrest

As mentioned before, in small infants, not only the space in the heart occupied by the venous return bypass tubing but also the collateral blood flow that shunts into the pulmonary circulation and the left side of the heart may create problems for the surgeon. Total circulatory arrest, which allows the cannulation tubing to be removed from the operating field and eliminates collateral flow, solves these problems. Small infants less than 10 kg sometimes are surface cooled to a nasopharyngeal temperature of about 28 C before being connected to the bypass machine.

The hematocrit reading of the perfusate probably should be less than 25% to decrease the impact of the low temperature on the viscosity and consequently on tissue perfusion. Aggregation of RBCs and other particles within the microvasculature may require high pressures to reinstitute flow after circulatory arrest. During the cooling of the patient to between 16 and 18 C, a full paralyzing dose of pancuronium is given to prevent the child from starting to breathe after circulatory arrest has been established. Also, the heparin level is determined with the Hepcon analyzer system and, if indicated, an additional dose of heparin is given.

When a nasopharyngeal temperature of about 17 C is reached, the aorta is cross-clamped and 10 to 20 ml of cardioplegic solution per kilogram is administered until a myocardial temperature of about 11 or 12 C is reached. Next, the arterial bypass cannula is clamped, blood is drained via the right atrial or vena cava cannulas into the bypass pump, the pump is stopped, and the venous cannulas are clamped and removed from the right atrium. During total circulatory arrest, the cardioplegic solution is removed from the opened right atrium by wall suction.

The bypass is reestablished by inserting the venous cannulas into the right atrium and removing the clamp from the aortic cannula. Pump perfusion is started at low flows while the clamps from the venous cannulas are slowly released, and air from the aortic root and heart is aspirated. Rewarming occurs at flows between 2.2 and 2.4 L/minute/sq m.

Adequacy of Cerebral Protection

Hypothermia protects the brain from irreversible damage during circulatory arrest, or when using low perfusion flows, in several ways. First, the normal metabolic rate is reduced. Second, the quantity of oxygen in the tissues is increased owing to the enhanced solubility of oxygen at low temperatures. Third, when the available oxygen is used, anaerobic metabolism provides enough energy to maintain cellular integrity.

However, several factors may threaten an adequate perfusion, and therefore the oxygen and substrate supply of the brain, and may cause obvious and not-so-obvious neurologic dysfunction after open-heart surgery.[176, 186] The incidence is considerably decreased, compared with that during the early years of cardiopulmonary bypass, because of the following factors:

1. Filters are used in the pump lines; this factor has decreased and hopefully virtually eliminated damage by microemboli[22] (air, aggregated formed elements of the blood, fat emboli).

2. Cerebral air emboli originating from the left side of the heart are prevented during repair because air is meticulously removed by the surgeon before the aortic cross-clamp is opened.

3. A certain minimal perfusion pressure is necessary at mild and moderate hypothermia to provide adequate survival conditions to the brain. A pressure of 50 mm Hg (30 to 40 mm Hg in newborns and young infants) probably is a safe minimal mean perfusion pressure[171]; this value probably is high, considering the young age and the absence of arteriosclerotic brain vessels.

4. A high blood-tissue temperature gradient is prevented.[32] Such a gradient may cause gas bubbles during rewarming when the perfusate is more than 12 to 15 C warmer than the body temperature of the child.

5. Electrolyte imbalance, hyperglycemia

(which may happen if dextrose solutions are administered during hypothermia, probably because insulin secretion is decreased at lower temperatures[25]), and hypoglycemia during rewarming, which also may cause neurologic damage,[159] are prevented.

6. The use of perfusate with lower hematocrit levels[72, 73, 103] (approximately 25%) may be beneficial for the brain tissue perfusion and may decrease the phenomenon of impaired cerebral perfusion at the microvascular level after circulatory arrest.[25]

7. The prevention of hypotension or low cardiac output after bypass is also probably important because it may avoid or minimize ischemic damage suffered during bypass.

The Presence of Hemostatic Anomalies After Bypass

Many different explanations have been suggested[14, 15, 66, 71, 89, 155, 179] for the excessive bleeding that may occur after cardiopulmonary bypass: insufficient surgical hemostasis, inadequate heparin neutralization, inadequate dosage of heparin during bypass, protamine excess, heparin rebound, thrombocytopenia, abnormal platelet function, hypofibrinogenemia, primary fibrinolysis, disseminated intravascular coagulation, coagulation factor deficiencies or the presence of inhibitors of coagulation factors, transfusion reactions, hypocalcemia, use of prosthetic materials, renal or hepatic failure, preoperative medication, prolonged cardiopulmonary bypass, and low cardiac output with poor tissue perfusion.

Insufficient surgical hemostasis, inadequate heparin neutralization (heparin rebound), and abnormal platelet function are among the most frequent causes of excessive bleeding after bypass.

Frequently occurring hemostatic anomalies, their treatment, and the value of certain survey tests in the diagnosis of these anomalies are listed in Table 6–9[20, 46, 47] and shown in Figure 6–27. These tests are routinely ordered when excessive bleeding after bypass occurs, both to prevent unnecessary surgical reexploration and to enable specific treatment of the bleeding disorder.

PLATELET DYSFUNCTION AND THROMBOCYTOPENIA.—Usually after prolonged bypass, serious platelet dysfunction and thrombocytopenia are present. The latter occurs also when a large prosthetic graft (Dacron conduit, for instance) is used for repair of the cardiac defect. Transfusion of platelets, therefore, is indicated in these situations. However, the consumption of platelets and the incidence of bleeding through the conduit can be decreased considerably by preclotting of the conduit with unheparinized blood of the patient.

HEPARIN EXCESS.—The Hepcon analyzing system and the activated clotting time[150] are used to determine the presence of free heparin. Although the activated clotting time is a test of the intrinsic and common coagulation system (see Fig 6–27), the result of this test is abnormal only when a severe deficiency of (one of) those factors exists. Therefore, the activated clotting time is useful after uncomplicated routine cardiac bypass, where a prolonged activated clotting time, easily determined in the operating room with a Hemochron 400, usually implies the presence of free heparin in the blood. However, especially in the presence of coagulation abnormalities, a more reliable method to detect the presence of heparin is the use of the protamine-heparin neutralizing principle of the Hepcon analyzer. This guarantees an adequate heparin level during bypass, where the activated clotting time frequently remains prolonged despite decreasing blood heparin levels. Diffuse intravascular coagulation caused by insufficient heparin concentration during bypass (followed by diffuse bleeding after bypass as a result of consumption of the clotting factors) thus can be prevented.

PRIMARY HYPERFIBRINOLYSIS AND DISSEMINATED INTRAVASCULAR COAGULATION.—Clinically significant primary hyperfibrinolysis without the presence of disseminated intravascular coagulation[20] is extremely rare after bypass. Laboratory tests are helpful in making the diagnosis: for instance, disseminated intravascular coagulation differs from primary hyperfibrinolysis by the presence of thrombocytopenia and a positive protamine gel test. The protamine gel test measures the presence of fibrin monomers of fibrin split products but not of fibrinogen split products. Fibrin monomers are the breakdown products of fibrin, which is obviously present in large amounts in disseminated intravascular coagulation but not in primary hyperfibrinolysis, in which fibrinogen is broken down by plasmin into fibrinogen split products, which are not de-

TABLE 6-9.—LABORATORY DIAGNOSIS AND TREATMENT OF FREQUENTLY OCCURRING HEMOSTATIC ANOMALIES DURING POSTBYPASS PERIOD*

ANOMALY	ACT	aPTT	PT	TT	FSP	PROTAMINE GEL TEST	FIBRINOGEN	PLATELETS	TREATMENT
Platelet dysfunction	N	N	N	N	—	—	N	N	Platelets
Thrombocytopenia	N	N	N	N	—	—	N	N→	Platelets
Heparin excess	←	←	←	←	—	—	N	N	Protamine
Primary hyperfibrinolysis	←	←	←	←	←	—	N→	N	ε-Aminocaproic acid
Presence of inhibitors to:									
Intrinsic system	←	←	N	N	—	—	N	N	FFP
Extrinsic system	N	N	←	N	—	—	N	N→	FFP
Disseminated intravascular coagulation	←	←	←	←	←	+	←	←	(1) Volume replacement, treatment of hypotension and acidosis; (2) use of vasodilating agents; (3) replacement of consumed factors (FFP, platelets, cryoprecipitate [VIII, I]); (4) corticosteroids to "cement the capillaries"; (5) if no success, heparin (?)

*This table shows the changes in laboratory tests caused by such hemostasis defects as are usually present after bypass. However, in extreme cases, the test results may be different (for instance, usually the degree of thrombocytopenia that occurs after bypass does not affect the clotting tests. However, the clotting times can be prolonged in the presence of severe thrombocytopenia). Abbreviations are as follows: ACT, activated clotting time; aPTT, activated partial thromboplastin time; PT, prothrombin time; TT, thrombin time; FSP, fibrin (fibrinogen) split products; FFP, fresh-frozen plasma.

tected by the protamine gel test. However, frequently the diagnosis is not that easy[54] when the patient has profuse bleeding after bypass, and one is tempted, when transfusions with fresh-frozen plasma and platelets are not successful, to stop the bleeding by giving ε-aminocaproic acid. ε-Aminocaproic acid, which prevents fibrinogenolysis by plasmin (fibrinogen → fibrin split products), may be useful to stop the profuse bleeding present in primary hyperfibrinolysis. However, administration of ε-aminocaproic acid in disseminated intravascular coagulation prevents fibrinolysis and therefore may result in generalized diffuse obstruction of the microvasculature with fibrin clots, because, in disseminated intravascular coagulation, fibrinolysis is necessary to dissolve the fibrin deposits that resulted from the massive diffuse intravascular

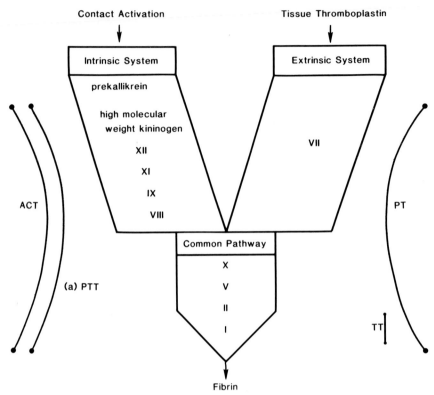

Fig 6-27.—Interpretation of common screening tests of blood coagulation. Activated clotting time *(ACT)* is insensitive test in which time is prolonged only when factors of intrinsic common system are severely decreased. Activated partial thromboplastin time *[(a)PPT]* is a more sensitive test in which time becomes prolonged when level of coagulation factors of intrinsic common system decreases to between 10% and 40% of normal level. Prothrombin time *(PT)* detects low levels (up to approximately 10% of their normal value) of factors of extrinsic common system. Thrombin time *(TT)* is prolonged in the presence of low (abnormal) fibrinogen. In all of the above-mentioned tests, the times are also prolonged in the presence of heparin, fibrin (fibrinogen) split products *(FSP)*, and other inhibitors of the coagulation factors measured by these tests.

coagulation. Because the differential diagnosis between disseminated intravascular coagulation and primary hyperfibrinolysis after bypass is not always straightforward, it is recommended that a hematologist be consulted before ε-aminocaproic acid is given to a patient who has an assumed primary hyperfibrinolysis. Administration of heparin, followed by that of ε-aminocaproic acid in massive diffuse bleeding not reacting to the usual treatment of disseminated intravascular coagulation, has been advised when there is considerable doubt as to the presence of disseminated intravascular coagulation or primary hyperfibrinolysis.

The fibrin(ogen) split products, which are produced in significant amounts in disseminated intravascular coagulation and hyperfibrinolysis, cause a widespread disturbance of hemostasis because they interfere with activated coagulation factors, fibrin polymerization, and platelet aggregation. However, the mild elevation of fibrin split products, which is commonly seen after bypass, will not interfere with hemostasis.

INHIBITORS TO FACTORS OF THE INTRINSIC OR EXTRINSIC (OR BOTH) SYSTEMS.—Prolongation of clotting tests may result not only from too low a level of coagulation factors but also from circulating inhibitors, like heparin, fibrin split products, and protein after extracorporeal circulation[36] (which is an inhibitor of the extrinsic coagulation system). In vitro, the addition of a small amount of fresh normal plasma to the test solution is sufficient to give a normal clotting test result if a low level of a coagulation factor was the cause of the prolonged test; however, the addition of even an equal quantity of fresh plasma is not sufficient to correct the anomaly in the presence of a significant amount of circulating inhibitors. As a consequence, in the postbypass period, the latter situation may require transfusion of considerably more fresh-frozen plasma. Although inhibitors to the coagulation factors are frequently present after bypass, they usually do not occur in great enough concentration to interfere with the hemostasis.

The Postbypass Period

Several factors, such as the presence or absence of cardiac failure before operation, whether complete anatomic correction of the defect has been accomplished and whether adequate protection of the myocardium was provided during surgery, are important in deciding the need for pharmaceutical support when coming off bypass.

A slightly increased preload (left atrial pressure between 12 and 18 mm Hg) is usually necessary and frequently sufficient in establishing an adequate cardiac output, which is temporarily depressed because of the surgical trauma. However, if the arterial blood pressure remains too low, administration of a single dose of calcium chloride (10 to 15 mg/kg) may be indicated to increase the cardiac output adequately and is frequently the only support needed when the patient comes off bypass. After repair of complex congenital defects, however, inotropic support for a more prolonged time is sometimes indicated, and either an infusion of dopamine, isoproterenol, or dobutamine (the latter two are preferred when a decrease in the pulmonary vascular resistance is important, for instance, after a modified Fontan repair) or an infusion of epinephrine is started.

Patients who were previously in cardiac failure and patients with increased systemic resistance may benefit considerably from reduction of the afterload (by an infusion of nitroprusside).

Sinus rhythm at an adequate rate is an important factor in providing sufficient cardiac output. Sinus bradycardia usually responds well to the use of atropine. If its administration is not beneficial, an isoproterenol infusion or atrial or sequential pacing may be indicated. Severe supraventricular tachycardia can be terminated by carotid massage or the administration of edrophonium, propranolol, or verapamil. However, such tachycardia frequently is responsive to cardioversion, using 5 to 10 W-second, with the defibrillation paddles applied to the atria.

Disturbing ventricular arrhythmias are treated with lidocaine, procainamide, bretylium, or verapamil, while abnormal arterial blood gas levels and the presence of hypokalemia should be excluded as possible causes.

Heparin is neutralized, as described before. For an extensive review of the use of blood components, see chapter 20. However, an additional consideration about the use of blood components in the small infant after bypass should be emphasized. Owing to the extensive dilution of its clotting factors and platelets by the priming fluid of the bypass pump (usually packed RBCs and clear prime), the administration of fresh-frozen plasma and platelets is indicated.

Complete Repair of Specific Congenital Heart Defects

Atrial Septal Defect—Secundum Type

PATHOPHYSIOLOGY.—The atrial septal defect is usually large, and the shunt depends on the respective filling resistances in the right and left ventricles. The pressures in the atria, and thus the direction of the shunted blood, are determined by the relative compliances of their ventricles in diastole. Because the right ventricle is thin-walled and more easily distensible, the dominant shunt is normally from left to right (Fig 6–28).

During the first several weeks of life, the thicknesses of the walls of the two ventricles are nearly equal, with similar filling characteristics, and thus minimal shunting results. With increasing age, the initially elevated pulmonary vascular resistance decreases and the thickness of the right ventricular wall decreases, resulting in an increasing left-to-right shunt. However, at the onset of ventricular contraction and also at the time of rapid filling of the ventricles as the atrioventricular valves open, the right atrial pressure may briefly exceed the left, and small amounts of blood may shunt from right to left.[105]

The pulmonary blood flow is increased, with the ratio of pulmonary blood flow to systemic

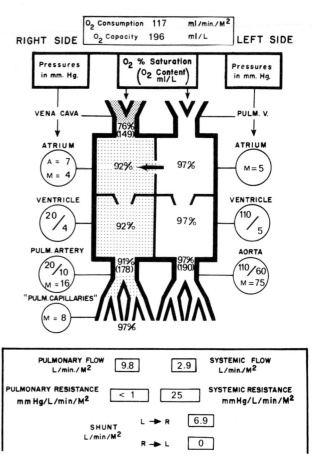

Fig 6-28.—Catheterization findings in patient with secundum atrial septal defect. (From Nadas and Fyler.[136] Used by permission.)

blood flow ($\dot{Q}p/\dot{Q}s$) ranging between 1.2 and 6[35]; however, until early adult life, the pulmonary arterial resistance is almost always normal or only slightly elevated.

The systemic blood flow is usually slightly below normal and is associated with a below-normal left ventricular end-diastolic pressure; therefore, the decreased systemic blood flow seems to be mainly due to impaired delivery of blood to the left ventricle, secondary to the left-to-right shunt, and does not relate to an intrinsic abnormality of left ventricular function.[62]

CLINICAL IMPLICATIONS.—A small atrial septal defect is tolerated without any difficulty and is compatible with normal life expectancy, except for an increased incidence of bacterial endocarditis. Therefore, surgical treatment is not considered in uncomplicated cases. Also, spontaneous closure of atrial septal defect occurs occasionally. Most patients with moderate left-to-right shunt ($\dot{Q}p/\dot{Q}s = 1.5$) and normal pulmonary arterial pressure are asymptomatic. However, the incidence of fatigue and dyspnea increases in patients with a larger left-to-right shunt ($\dot{Q}p/\dot{Q}s>3$), and cardiac failure may occur, occasionally even in infancy. The pulmonary artery resistance, which usually remains normal until the patient reaches the early teens, tends to become elevated (though generally only mildly to moderately) in adult patients.

If pulmonary vascular disease develops, its course is progressive and is accompanied by severe exertional dyspnea, diminution of the left-to-right shunt, shunt reversal, and cyanosis. Cardiac failure, caused by the large diastolic overloading, increases in frequency during the second and third decades of life.

Precipitating causes of death occurring from the fourth decade on are pulmonary vascular disease, cardiac failure, coronary artery disease, and atrial arrhythmias.

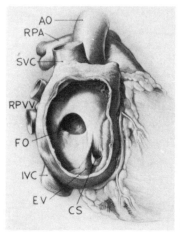 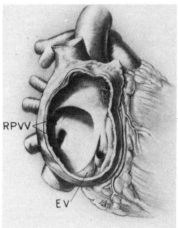 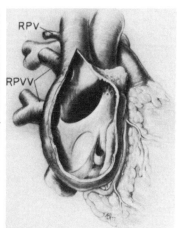

Fig 6–29.—Patent foramen ovale. Sizable foramen is seen in central portion of atrial septum. Aorta *(AO)*; right pulmonary artery *(RPA)*; superior vena cava *(SVC)*; right pulmonary veins *(RPVV)*; foramen ovale *(FO)*; inferior vena cava *(IVC)*; eustachian valve *(EV)*; coronary sinus *(CS)*. (From Lindesmith.[106] Used by permission.)

Fig 6–30.—Ostium secundum type of atrial septal defect. Openings of right pulmonary veins *(RPVV)* are near margin of defect. Eustachian valve *(EV)*. (From Lindesmith.[106] Used by permission.)

Fig 6–31.—Sinus venosus defect in characteristic superior portion of atrial septum. Right pulmonary veins *(RPVV)* enter into superior vena cava. Right pulmonary vein *(RPV)*. (From Lindesmith.[106] Used by permission.)

Surgery is usually recommended after cardiac catheterization has demonstrated a significant increase in pulmonary blood flow ($\dot{Q}p/\dot{Q}s > 1.5$) without the presence of severe pulmonary vascular obstructive disease (ratio between pulmonary vascular resistance and systemic resistance is less than 0.7). Although most children have few or no symptoms, it is usually advised that surgery be done before the age of 5 or 6 years because of the complications of uncorrected atrial septal defect in later life.

PATHOLOGIC ANATOMY, CLASSIFICATION, AND INTRAOPERATIVE MANAGEMENT.—Defects of the septum secundum can be divided into three categories[106]: (1) patent foramen ovale (Fig 6–29), which is often associated with other intracardiac defects; (2) ostium secundum defect (Fig 6–30), which is most frequently encountered as an isolated lesion (the area of the septum involved most frequently includes that of the foramen ovale and the septal tissue lateral and inferior to it); and (3) sinus venosus defect. This last type is regularly accompanied by anatomic drainage of a portion of the right pulmonary veins into either the right atrium or the superior vena cava (Fig 6–31). The anomalous location of the right pulmonary veins has to be corrected at surgery, because significant left-to-right shunting may occur through them. Surgery usually is conducted through a median sternotomy; sometimes, however, a right thoracotomy is performed. Cardiopulmonary bypass and moderate hypothermia are used. Before insertion of the atrial cannulas into the right atrium, the pump technician is asked to transfuse a small amount of pump prime by way of the aortic cannula until a central venous pressure of 8 to 10 mm Hg is reached. This decreases the chance of air being sucked into the right atrium and, via the atrial septal defect, into the left atrium.

After a temperature of 20 to 25 C is reached or after the heart fibrillates, the aorta is cross-clamped and about 10 to 20 ml of cardioplegic solution per kilogram are infused, until a myocardial temperature of 11 to 14 C has been reached.

A longitudinal atriotomy is made in the right atrium, exposing the atrial septum. The intracardiac suction should not enter the left atrium, because evacuation of blood may introduce air into the left atrium. For the same reason, usually no venting of the left side of the heart is used. The repair is either by direct suturing of the small defect or by the use of a patch (Fig 6–32). At the end of the repair, blood must completely fill and spurt from the left atrium through the remaining opening before the suture line is tightened to ensure that no air is left in the left atrium. If necessary, needle aspiration of air is performed.

Atrial septal defect repair is also sometimes performed while the heart is beating in sinus rhythm. On partial bypass, the patient is cooled to 30 C. An aortic vent is inserted, the aorta is cross-clamped, and the venae cavae ties are tightened as in the previous operation. The right atrium is opened, and the defect is closed while the heart is beating. Immediately before the repair is finished, the lungs are gently inflated by the anesthesiologist to remove any air that may have entered the pulmonary circulation. By this maneuver, blood and any air present are squeezed through the pulmonary vessel bed into the left atrium, from where the air is removed by needle aspiration. The aortic vent removes any air that accumulates in the aortic root.

Sutures placed too close to the coronary sinus or atrioventricular node may cause conduction disturbances. If repair is done with the heart beating in sinus rhythm, such disturbances are detected at once and immediate removal of the offending suture frequently solves the problem.

If possible, anomalous right pulmonary veins draining into the superior vena cava should be drained into the left atrium. If the anomalous veins are near the caval-atrial junction, the inferior portion of the superior vena cava may be divided by a pericardial patch, such that the blood from the anomalous veins drains beneath the patch through the atrial septal defect into the left atrium (Fig 6–33).

POSTOPERATIVE COMPLICATIONS.—During the postoperative period, supraventricular arrhythmias can occur, although they are not frequent after repair of secundum atrial septal defects in children. The incidence of postoperative arrhythmias increases with increasing patient age. During the early postoperative period, arrhythmias occur in more than 30% of the patients.[35] Supraventricular arrhythmias, of which atrial flutter, atrial fibrillation, and nodal rhythm are the most frequent, constitute the usual arrhythmia. Children rarely experience atrial fibrillation. Third-degree conduction defects are of major importance because of their association with asystole and death. The reported incidence of first- and second-degree heart block has generally not exceeded 5%. Disorders of sinus node function can occur.[34] In patients with increased pulmonary vascular resistance, postoperative complications are more common, including low cardiac output, arrhythmias, and respiratory insufficiency.

Endocardial Cushion Defects (Atrioventricular Canal Defects)

Abnormalities in the development of the endocardial cushions[42] produce defects of the atrial septum, ventricular septum, and atrioventricular valves. These defects may occur together or singly. They are divided into two groups: partial atrioventricular canal and complete atrioventricular canal. In partial atrioventricular canal or septum primum defect, the posterobasal part of the ventricular septum, as well as the caudal portion of the atrial septum, is absent, but there is no interventricular communication because the atrioventricular valves are fused to the crest of the underlying ventricular septum (Fig 6–34). Complete atrioventricular canal also has a centrally situated septal defect; however, the leaflets of the valves are connected to the ventricular septum only by chordae or are free-floating above the crest of the septum. Thus, there is both an interatrial and an interventricular communication present. Abnormalities in the formation of the mitral and tricuspid valves are always part of the defect in complete atrioventricular canal and often in partial atrioventricular canal, in which the ostium primum defect usually is associated with a cleft in the mitral leaflet.

PARTIAL ATRIOVENTRICULAR CANAL.—The left-to-right shunt is usually large, as in the secundum-type atrial septal defect, and produces a volume overload of the right ventricle, with an increased pulmonary blood flow. There is also a variable degree of mitral insufficiency, resulting in volume overload of the left ventricle. The jet through the insufficient mitral valve may be directed back into the left atrium, but often the regurgitant stream passes directly through the atrial septal defect into the right atrium. The calculated left-to-right shunt usually exceeds 50%. Most patients have insignificant right-to-

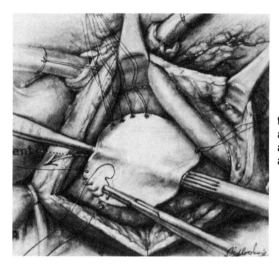

Fig 6-32.—Patch repair of ostium secundum-type atrial septal defect. Before the last sutures are drawn tight, great care is taken to evacuate any air present from left atrium. (From Cohn et al.[35] Used by permission.)

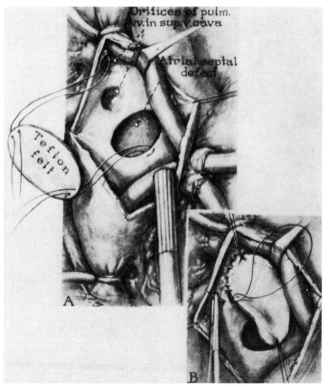

Fig 6-33.—Repair of sinus venosus type of atrial septal defect. High-lying interatrial defect and orifices of right pulmonary veins are exposed. Patch is sutured such that blood draining from right pulmonary veins will flow into left atrium. Currently, atriotomy is performed slightly differently from that shown in this figure, where incision cuts through area of sinus node. (From Cohn et al.[35] Used by permission.)

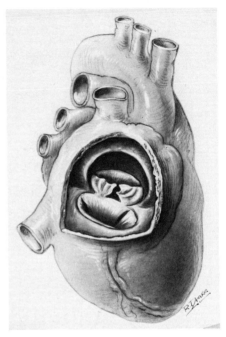

Fig 6–34.—Partial atrioventricular canal. Cleft in anterior leaflet of mitral valve can be seen through atrial septal defect, which is located in inferior portion of atrial septum. (Modified from McGoon D.C., DuShane J.W., and Kirklin J.W.: The surgical treatment of endocardial cushion defects. *Surgery* 46:185, 1959. Used by permission.)

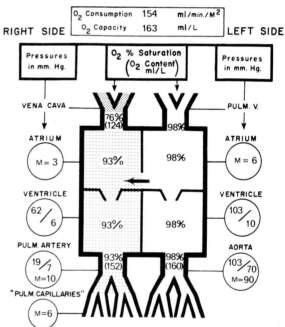

Fig 6–35.—Catheterization findings in partial atrioventricular canal. (From Nadas and Fyler.[136] Used by permission.)

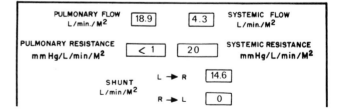

left shunting; the right ventricular pressure is usually considerably lower than the systemic pressure; significant elevation of pulmonary vascular resistance is unusual (Fig 6–35).

Volume overload of both the right and the left ventricles may create symptoms of congestive heart failure. The incidence is highest in childhood, but such overload may not manifest itself until the fourth or fifth decade.

Dysrhythmias such as atrial fibrillation, nodal bradycardia, paroxysmal ventricular tachycardia, and complete heart block occur in approximately 20% of patients.[166] There may be recurrent respiratory infections and growth failure. The severity of symptoms frequently depends on the degree of insufficiency of the atrioventricular valve. Repair is indicated at any age if cardiac failure that is not easily manageable by medical treatment is present, and repair is performed electively when the child is about 5 years old.[109]

The main problem of the surgical repair relates to the mitral deformity. Usually, accurate alignment of the anterior and posterior portions of the anterior (aortic) mitral leaflet reduces the mitral regurgitation sufficiently. If deficient leaflet tissue or gross deformity of the valve precludes a successful repair, mitral valve replacement can be performed at the initial operation in older children. Double-sampling dye curves, performed by injecting indocyanine green into the left ventricle and sampling simultaneously from the left atrium and ascending aorta, are indicated after the patient comes off bypass to assess the mitral regurgitation.[124] If there is any doubt about the location of the conduction system, the heart may be allowed to beat while the atrial septal patch is being sutured into position (Fig 6–36).

Residual or increasing (or both) mitral regurgitation necessitated subsequent mitral valve surgery in 4% of 210 patients after surgery for partial atrioventricular canal.[129] Heart block, congestive heart failure, and arrhythmias also may occur after repair.

COMPLETE ATRIOVENTRICULAR CANAL.— Three types of complete atrioventricular canal are identified[147]: In type A, the most common, the anterior leaflet is divided and the medial

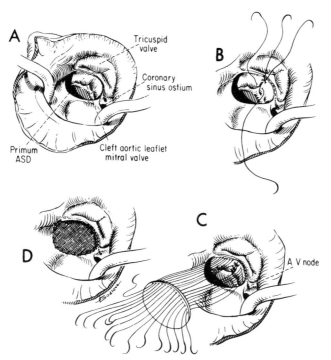

Fig 6–36.—Partial atrioventricular canal repair. **A** and **B,** cleft in anterior leaflet of mitral valve is approximated with interrupted sutures. Next, interrupted sutures are placed in anterior leaflet 1 mm from annulus, staying to left of conduction bundle. **C,** sutures are placed through patch, which is lowered into place and tied. **D,** continuous suture laterally and superiorly completes closure. Atrial septal defect (ASD). (From Danielson.[42] Used by permission.)

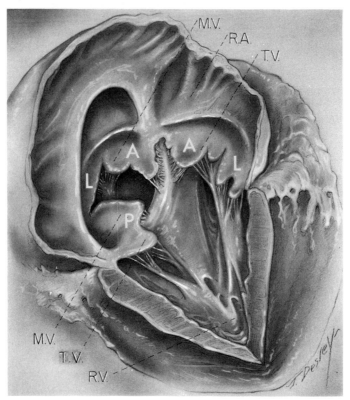

Fig 6–37.—Type A complete atrioventricular canal. This is most common type. Anterior leaflet *(A)* of common atrioventricular valve is divided and both portions are attached by chordae to ventricular septum. Mitral and tricuspid portions of anterior and posterior leaflets *(M.V. and T.V.)*, right atrium and right ventricle *(R.A. and R.V.)*, posterior common leaflet *(P)*, lateral leaflet *(L)*. (From Rastelli et al.[147] Used by permission.)

chordae are inserted into the crest of the muscular ventricular septum (Fig 6–37). In type B, the anterior common leaflet is divided and the medial chordae are inserted into an abnormal papillary muscle in the right ventricle (Fig 6–38). In type C, there often are other major defects, such as pulmonary stenosis, transposition of the great arteries, and common ventricle. The anterior common leaflet is a single structure, undivided and free-floating, without insertion of chordae into the ventricular septum (Fig 6–39). In all three types, the posterior leaflet has a variable attachment to the underlying ventricular septum and a variable division between its tricuspid and mitral portions.

In complete atrioventricular canal, the four heart chambers communicate and both ventricles function at systemic pressures. If no pulmonary stenosis is present, there will be pulmonary hypertension with high pulmonary blood flow. As pulmonary vascular hypertension develops, the left-to-right shunt may decrease while the right-to-left shunt increases. Usually, surgery should be done before the patient is 2 years of age to prevent severe pulmonary vascular disease.

The operative approach[42, 128, 182] is the same as for partial atrioventricular canal.

The components of the mitral valve are approximated with interrupted sutures (Fig 6–40,A). The anterior common leaflet is, if necessary, incised to the annulus at the junction of the mitral and the tricuspid portions. If needed, a similar incision of the posterior common leaflet is done in patients with an interventricular communication beneath this leaflet. The lower portion of a Teflon patch with an oval size equal to the overall ventricular and atrial septal defect is

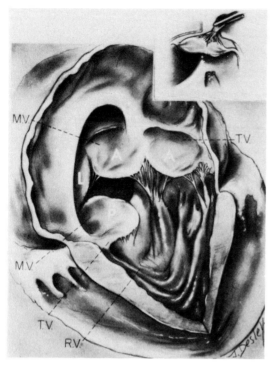

Fig 6-38.—Type B complete atrioventricular canal. Common anterior leaflet *(A)* is divided; both portions are attached by chordae to a papillary muscle in right ventricle. Abbreviations as in Figure 6-37. (From Rastelli et al.[147] Used by permission.)

sutured to the right side of the ventricular septum (Fig 6-40,B). Sometimes, the sutures in the region of the conduction bundle are placed and tied while the heart is beating to immediately detect any damage to this area. The mitral margins of the naturally divided anterior common leaflet (types A and B) (Fig 6-40,C) or the mitral and tricuspid margins of the surgically incised leaflet (type C) are sutured to the patch at a level corresponding to the plane of the normal mitral and tricuspid annuli. The incised or naturally divided posterior common leaflet is attached to the patch in a similar manner. Next, the atrial portion of the Teflon septum is sutured in place (Fig 6-40,D).

Damage to the conduction bundle by sutures placed near the coronary sinus, where the sinus is crossed by the Teflon patch, is of concern. In older patients with severe mitral or tricuspid valve incompetence, prosthetic valve(s) attached to the septal patch may be inserted. Mild-to-moderate valvular incompetence is well tolerated by most patients. Postoperative ventilation with positive end-expiratory pressure, followed by continuous positive airway pressure, may be indicated in some of these patients. Supraventricular arrhythmias may also occur during the early postoperative period. Usually, these arrhythmias are hemodynamically benign. A low cardiac output may require the use of inotropic drugs for several days. The use of digoxin is usually continued after surgery.

Ventricular Septal Defect

PATHOPHYSIOLOGY AND CLASSIFICATION OF VENTRICULAR SEPTAL DEFECT.—The magnitude and direction of the shunt across a ventricular septal defect depend on the size of the defect and the pressure gradient across it during the various phases of the cardiac cycle (Table 6-10).

Small defect.—The small defect has a small left-to-right shunt because the ventricular septal defect offers considerable resistance to flow, and its small size preserves the large systolic pressure difference between the left and the right ventricle. Thus, there is little or no tendency for an increase in pulmonary vascular resistance, and the interventricular pressure relationships are near normal (Fig 6-41).

Moderate defect.—The moderate defect with mild increase of pulmonary vascular resistance

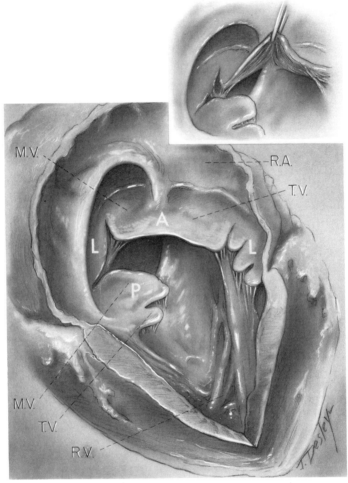

Fig 6–39.—Type C complete atrioventricular canal. Anterior common leaflet is undivided and is unattached to ventricular septum. Abbreviations are as in Figure 6–37. (From Rastelli et al.[147] Used by permission.)

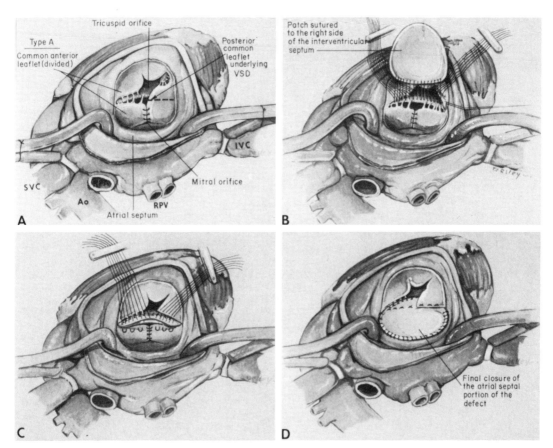

Fig 6–40.—Surgical repair of complete atrioventricular canal, type A. **A,** anterior and posterior components of anterior leaflet of mitral valve are approximated by interrupted sutures. Posterior common leaflet will be incised (broken line) because interventricular communication is present underneath. Inferior vena cava *(IVC)*; superior vena cava *(SVC)*; aorta *(Ao)*; right pulmonary vein *(RPV)*. **B,** septal patch is sutured to right side of interventricular septum, thus avoiding bundle of His. **C,** mitral margin of divided anterior common leaflet is sutured to patch at level corresponding to normal plane of mitral valve. Similarly, mitral and tricuspid edges of incised posterior common leaflet are attached to patch. **D,** complete repair, as seen from right atrium. (From McMullan et al.[128] Used by permission.)

TABLE 6-10.—CLASSIFICATION OF VENTRICULAR SEPTAL DEFECTS*

SIZE OF DEFECT	PULMONARY ARTERIAL HYPERTENSION		PULMONARY BLOOD FLOW (MAGNITUDE OF INCREASE)	Qp/Qs‡	PULMONARY VASCULAR DISEASE	
	DEGREE	Pp/Ps†			SEVERITY	RPU§
Small	None	<0.25	Mild	<1.4	None	<5
Moderate	Mild	0.25–0.45	Moderate	1.4–2	None	<5
Large	Mild	0.25–0.45	Large	>2	Mild	<5
	Moderate	0.45–0.75	Large	>2	Mild	5–7
	Severe	>0.75	Large	>2	Mild	5–7
			Moderate	1.4–2	Moderate	8–10
			Small	<1.4	Severe	>10

*From Kirklin J.W., Karp R.B., Bargeron L.M. Jr.: Surgical treatment of ventricular septal defect, in Sabiston D.C. Jr., Spencer F.C. (eds.): *Gibbon's Surgery of the Chest*, ed. 3. Philadelphia, W.B. Saunders Co., 1976. Used by permission.
†Pp/Ps is the ratio between peak pressure in pulmonary artery and that in a systemic artery. (ratio between mean pressures may be used, and is similar).
‡Qp/Qs is the ratio between pulmonary and systemic blood flow.
§RPU is pulmonary resistance units (units sq m).

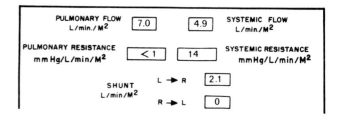

Fig 6-41.—Catheterization findings in patient with small ventricular septal defect. (From Nadas and Fyler.[136] Used by permission.)

is large enough to permit a moderate shunt, yet small enough to offer some resistance to flow. Although the difference in pressure between both ventricles is decreased in this group during ventricular ejection, the systolic pressure difference from the left to the right ventricle continues to be at least 15 mm Hg.[74] In this group, large elevations of pulmonary vascular resistance are rare.

Large defect with mild-to-moderate elevations of pulmonary vascular resistance.—This type of large defect does not restrict flow, and as a result, the pulmonary circulation is subjected to the common ejectile force of both ventricles during most of the period of ventricular ejection. A large left-to-right shunt ensues, with systemic pressure in both ventricles (Fig 6–42). Frequently, there is a small right-to-left shunt into the systemic circulation. This factor is explained as follows: With the onset of systole, the left ventricular pressure increases more rapidly than the right ventricular pressure. This gradient is maintained until the later part of ventricular ejection, when the right ventricular pressure equals or exceeds the left. As the cycle continues into the initial portion of isovolemic relaxation, the earlier and more rapid decrease in left ventricular pressure accentuates the right-to-left gradient, with resulting right-to-left shunting (Fig 6–43). The anesthesiologist who places an intravenous line or injects a drug intravenously should be aware of this phenomenon. An air bubble entering the body via an intravenous line and arriving in the right ventricle at this moment of the cardiac cycle may pass into the left side of the circulation, with the danger of air embolization of the coronary and cerebral vessels.

The greatly increased pulmonary blood flow results in an increased pulmonary arterial pressure, and muscular contraction of the pulmonary arterioles may eventually cause a permanent increase in pulmonary vascular resistance. The pa-

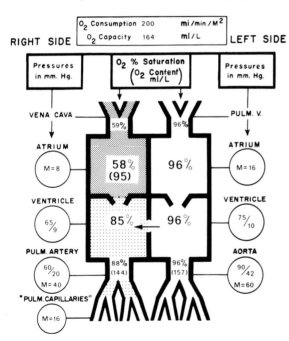

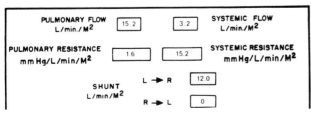

Fig 6–42.—Catheterization findings in patient with large ventricular septal defect, high pulmonary blood flow, and low pulmonary resistance. (From Nadas and Fyler.[136] Used by permission.)

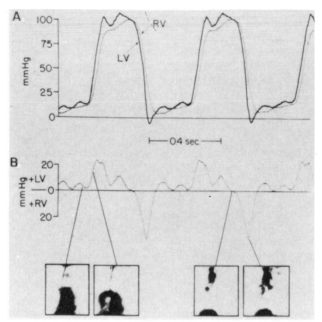

Fig 6–43.—Interventricular pressure relationships and their influence on flow across large defects. **A,** simultaneous right *(RV)* and left *(LV)* ventricular pressures. **B,** continuous pressure difference across the defect throughout the cardiac cycle. Note that during diastole the pressure gradient is predominantly left to right. During this interval diastolic shunting from left ventricle to right ventricle occurs, with augmentation of shunt during atrial contraction. With onset of isovolemic contraction, there is augmentation of the pressure gradient, with an increased left-to-right shunt during this interval prior to opening of the aortic valve. Although right ventricle has a "systemic" pressure, during early ejection instantaneous pressure of left ventricle is greater than that of right ventricle. During later part of ventricular ejection, right ventricular pressure exceeds that of the left. Period of "isovolemic" relaxation is characterized by more rapid decrease in left ventricular pressure, with prominent right-to-left gradient that results in right-to-left flow across defect into left ventricle. Cineangiocardiographic pictures demonstrate effect on flow of pressure difference across defect. (From Graham et al.[74] Used by permission.)

tient who has the hyperdynamic type of pulmonary hypertension with a large ventricular septal defect, large pulmonary blood flow ($\dot{Q}p/\dot{Q}s > 2$), and a mild elevation of pulmonary resistance (<8 units sq m) will be in danger of progressing into the next stage.

Large defect with marked elevation of pulmonary vascular resistance.—This type of large defect is characterized by decreased pulmonary blood flow. When pulmonary vascular resistance finally exceeds that of the systemic circulation, the flow across the ventricular septal defect becomes predominantly right to left—the so-called Eisenmenger complex.

CLINICAL IMPLICATIONS.—Small ventricular septal defects usually produce no detrimental effects on the circulation, and there are no data that suggest a decreased life expectancy for these patients in the absence of infectious endocarditis. Also, there is a 50% to 80% chance that the defect will close spontaneously.[5, 86] Because the long-term prognosis is excellent, surgery is not indicated.

In the infant with a moderate to large defect with large left-to-right shunt, as soon as the physiologic high fetal pulmonary arterial resistance decreases (usually between 7 and 14 days after delivery in a term infant), the effects of severe left ventricular volume overload will develop. These effects include increased left atrial pressure, elevated pulmonary venous pressure with mild-to-moderate pulmonary edema, decreased lung compliance, frequent respiratory tract infections, and, because the infant tires easily with feeding, no or minimal gain in weight. Initial therapy is with digoxin and a diuretic. Cardiac catheterization is usually recommended within the first 6 months of life to determine, among other variables, the degree of pulmonary artery resistance. If the initial catheterization in the young infant discloses an elevated pulmonary artery pressure, usually medical therapy is started, and, within a few months, recatheterization is done. If there is no improvement, surgery is recommended. The development of pulmonary vascular disease usually occurs only in patients with a large ventricular septal defect and is rarely irreversibly advanced in patients less than 2 years old.[38] Because of high operative risk and poor late results, surgery is generally not recommended for patients with a pulmonary resistance of more than 10 units sq m and a Qp/Qs of less than 1.4. However, an exception to this rule is made in patients who are younger than 2 years of age. In one study,[49] partial or complete reversal of the severe pulmonary arterial hypertension occurred in all 18 patients (less than 2 years old). In a group of patients older than 2 years with severe increased pulmonary resistance, the severe pulmonary hypertension continued five years or more after repair in more than 50% of patients and decreased only to moderate hypertension in another 20%.

The results of primary repair of the ventricular septal defect, even in small infants, compared with results of initial banding of the pulmonary artery followed by repair of ventricular septal defect at a later age, favor the first procedure.[38] However, in small infants with multiple muscular ventricular septal defects of the "Swiss-cheese" type or with the combination ventricular septal defect and coarctation of the aorta, initial banding of the pulmonary artery may still be preferred.[76]

PATHOLOGIC ANATOMY AND SURGICAL MANAGEMENT.—The pathologic anatomy is depicted schematically in Figure 6–44. The membranous or infracristal defect is the most frequent (approximately 80% of ventricular septal defects). The defect lies in the outflow tract of the left ventricle, immediately beneath the aortic valve. The bundle of His lies in a subendocardial position as it courses along the posteroinferior margin of the defect. The surgeon should prevent damage to this area, which can produce complete heart block. In muscular ventricular septal defect and supracristal defects,

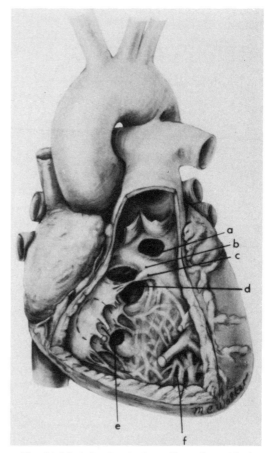

Fig 6–44.—Anatomical position of ventricular septal defects as seen from right side with right ventricular wall removed. Supracristal defect *(a)*; crista supraventricularis *(b)*; papillary muscle of conus *(c)*; membranous defect *(d)*; isolated defect of atrioventricular canal type *(e)*; muscular defect *(f)*—often multiple. (From Graham et al.[74] Used by permission.)

there is little danger of heart block because the conduction tissue is far removed from the defect. Right bundle-branch block occurs frequently after surgery for ventricular septal defects, supposedly caused either by the right ventriculotomy with disruption of a distal branch of the right bundle or by damage to the right bundle itself, which can course along the posteroinferior margin of infracristal defects.[74]

Most ventricular septal defects can be repaired from the right atrial approach (Fig 6–45). Supracristal defects nearly always require right ventriculotomy (Fig 6–46). With multiple ventricular septal defects of the muscular type or a

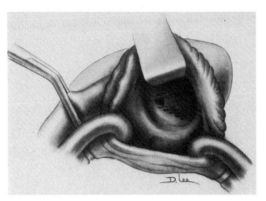

Fig 6-45.—Approach from right atrium allows good exposure for most high ventricular septal defects and defects of atrioventricular canal type. (From Cartmill T.B., et al.: Results of repair of ventricular septal defect. *J. Thorac. Cardiovasc. Surg.* 52:486, 1966. Used by permission.)

low-placed (near apex) muscular-type ventricular septal defect, a left ventriculotomy is sometimes necessary.

Cardiopulmonary bypass with moderate-to-profound hypothermia and cardioplegia (and, if needed, circulatory arrest in young infants) is

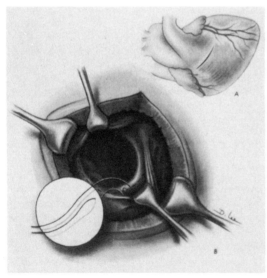

Fig 6-46.—Repair of supracristal ventricular septal defect by transverse right ventriculotomy. *A*, site of ventriculotomy. *B*, exposure of septal defect. (From Cartmill T.B., et al.: Results of repair of ventricular septal defect. *J. Thorac. Cardiovasc. Surg.* 52:486, 1966. Used by permission.)

established as previously discussed. When the desired temperature (20 to 25 C) is reached, the blood flow can be reduced to 0.5 L/minute/sq m and intracardiac repair is started. This low flow at a body temperature of about 22 C may be maintained as long as 45 minutes, if necessary. (If with this low flow the exposure is difficult because of intracardiac return, the patient is cooled further, until a nasopharyngeal temperature of about 18 C is reached, after which total circulatory arrest is established.) The right atrium is opened, and the foramen ovale is inspected and closed if necessary. Also, the accessibility of the ventricular septal defect through the tricuspid valve is determined (see Fig 6-45), and if indicated, a right (see Fig 6-46) or a left ventriculotomy is done. Large defects are repaired by suturing a patch of Teflon into place. Small defects may be repaired by direct suturing, though the incidence of recurrent ventricular septal defect after suture closure is higher.[139] When the defect is repaired, full perfusion flow is reestablished and rewarming is begun. After termination of bypass, a left atrial pressure of between 15 and 18 mm Hg is the goal.

COMPLICATIONS AFTER SURGERY FOR VENTRICULAR SEPTAL DEFECT.—Residual defects with persistent left-to-right shunting and trauma to the conduction system are the most common complications.[139, 149] Less frequently, ventricular dysfunction, tricuspid regurgitation, hemolysis, and ventricular septal aneurysm occur.

Residual shunt is caused either by disruption of the patch suture line or by the failure to detect one or more multiple ventricular septal defects. Fortunately, most of those residual defects are not hemodynamically significant and may not need surgical reexploration. A transient heart block may be related to trauma from suction catheters placed in the coronary sinus or to edema or a tissue reaction involving suture material near the conduction tissue. Infrequently, permanent heart block occurs by actual damage to the conduction bundle.

Damage to the sinoatrial node or the internodal tracts, causing intermittent periods of supraventricular tachycardia and bradycardia, is uncommon. Ventriculotomies may cause ventricular dysfunction during the early postoperative phase, necessitating the use of inotropic agents and digitalization. Tricuspid regurgitation may follow direct injury (for instance, incorporation of valve leaflets or chordae tendineae in the sutures used for closing the septal defect) or may be secondary to right ventricular failure.

Mild hemolysis is a common complication of cardiopulmonary bypass. However, after patch repair, RBCs may be damaged by the bloodstream's forceful striking of the patch surface (usually in the presence of mitral or aortic insufficiency). Mannitol to produce diuresis and sodium bicarbonate to alkalinize the urine are used to decrease renal tubular damage from excreted hemoglobin.

A ventricular septal aneurysm may develop when pericardium is used for closure of large ventricular septal defects. It can obstruct the right ventricular outflow tract or rupture and cause a recurrence of the left-to-right shunt.

Truncus Arteriosus

In this rare heart defect, only one main arterial trunk leaves the base of the heart, supplying branches to the coronary, pulmonary, and systemic circulations. Four major types can be recognized according to Collett and Edwards' classification[111, 181] (Fig 6–47).

In type I, a single arterial trunk gives rise to the aorta and main pulmonary artery. In type II, the right and left pulmonary arteries arise close together from the dorsal wall of the truncus arteriosus. In type III, the right and left pulmonary arteries arise independently from either side of the truncus arteriosus. In type IV, pulmonary arteries are absent. The arterial circulation to the lungs is by way of bronchial arteries. This type is no longer classified under truncus arteriosus but is classified as pulmonary atresia with ventricular septal defect and absence of pulmonary arteries.[111, 112]

Another classification by van Praagh divides the lesions into two major groups (Fig 6–48): type A, with a ventricular septal defect; type B, without a ventricular septal defect. Type B is extremely rare. The two groups are further subdivided. In subtype 1, the main pulmonary artery separates from the truncus (Collett and Edwards' type I). In subtype 2, the pulmonary arteries arise directly from the common trunk (Collett and Edwards' types II and III). In subtype 3, either the right or the left pulmonary artery is absent, the lung being supplied by collateral vessels. In subtype 4, there is hypoplasia, coarctation, or atresia of the aortic isthmus. This subtype is associated with a large ductus arteriosus.

In almost all patients, a ventricular septal defect is present. Generally, the truncus straddles the ventricular septum or arises entirely from the right ventricle. About one third of the patients have mild truncal valve incompetence. A patent ductus arteriosus, persistent left superior vena cava, or atrial septal defect is present in about 20% of the patients.

Because the pulmonary vascular bed is submitted to high perfusion pressures, pulmonary resistance increases and pulmonary vascular obstructive disease eventually develops that reduces pulmonary blood flow and thus decreases arterial saturation. There seems to be a relationship between pulmonary vascular resistance and arterial saturation. In the absence of other anatomical abnormalities, patients with an arterial saturation of less than 85% have advanced pulmonary vascular obstructive disease.[112]

During the first few weeks of life, symptoms are usually minimal because of the normally increased pulmonary vascular resistance in the newborn. Soon, however, the pulmonary blood flow increases and precipitates congestive heart failure. Unless pulmonary artery stenosis or significant pulmonary vascular disease is present, the resting arterial saturation is usually above 85%, and except during crying or exercise, the child is acyanotic.

As expected in children with a dominant left-

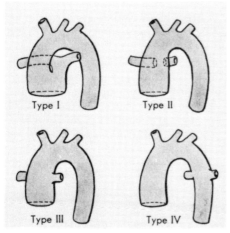

Fig 6–47.—Anatomical types of truncus arteriosus, Collett and Edwards' classification. (From Keith J.D., Rowe R.D., Vlad P.: *Heart Disease in Infancy and Childhood.* New York, Macmillan Publishing Co., 1958. Used by permission.)

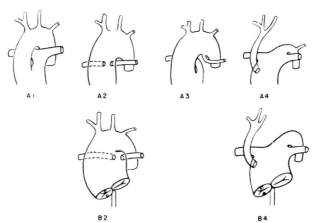

Fig 6–48.—Van Praagh's anatomical classification of truncus arteriosus. (From Van Praagh R., Van Praagh S.: The anatomy of common aorticopulmonary trunk (truncus arteriosus communis) and its embryologic implications: A study of 57 necropsy cases. *Am. J. Cardiol.* 16:406, 1965. Used by permission.)

to-right shunt, inhalation induction of anesthesia should occur as fast as in normal children. Systemic vasodilatation increases the right-to-left shunt and may cause cyanosis. However, systemic vasodilatation may be beneficial in the patient with pulmonary hyperperfusion.

The young infant in cardiac failure is intubated while awake, after preoxygenation. In the older infant with cardiac failure and greatly increased pulmonary blood flow, an intravenous induction is preferred; however, if halothane is chosen for induction, it should be used only in low concentrations because of its cardiodepressant effect. As soon as can be tolerated, an intravenous route should be established and pancuronium should be administered with fentanyl (5 to 10 μg/kg), while the use of halothane is discontinued or the concentration is decreased to between 0.1% and 0.2%, if tolerated, while blood pressure is closely monitored. Careful administration of nitroprusside may increase the ratio between systemic and pulmonary blood flow.[69]

In small infants with increased pulmonary artery flow, pulmonary artery banding may be indicated for treating the congestive heart failure and for delaying the progression of pulmonary vascular obstructive disease; however, this procedure has a high mortality. (In the rare case of truncus arteriosus, with a severely decreased pulmonary blood flow due to stenosis of the pulmonary arteries, a systemic pulmonary artery shunt is indicated.) Complete correction of the defect is probably preferable, even in infancy. Because of the size of the conduit and the future growth of the patient, complete repair is usually delayed until the child is at least 2 years old. Recently, promising results of repair at a younger age have been published.[50]

If pulmonary artery banding has been done successfully, one prefers to wait for definitive repair until the child is several years older, because the pulmonary band decreases the danger of the development of pulmonary vascular disease. Complete surgical correction is done by establishing the continuity between the right ventricle and the pulmonary artery by use of a Dacron conduit containing a porcine semilunar valve. After the origin of the pulmonary arteries is excised from the truncus (Fig 6–49), the defect in the truncus (aorta) is closed. An incision is made in the right ventricle, and the ventricular septal defect is closed with a Teflon patch. Next, the distal end of the conduit is sutured to the pulmonary arteries, after which the proximal end is anastomosed to the right ventricle.

If severe truncal valve incompetence is present, either valve repair or valve replacement is necessary; moderate or mild incompetence is tolerated well by the patient. Low cardiac output is treated with the usual inotropic agents, frequently in combination with vasodilators. The use of digoxin is generally started during the early postoperative period. Arrhythmia, re-

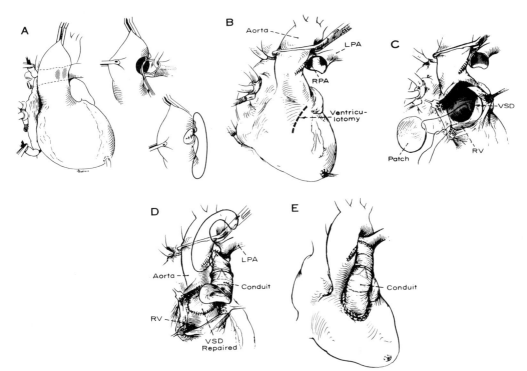

Fig 6–49.—Repair of truncus arteriosus. *A,* origin of the pulmonary arteries is excised from truncus. Defect in truncus is sutured. (From McGoon D.C., Rastelli G.C., Ongley P.A.: An operation for the correction of truncus arteriosus. *J.A.M.A.* 205:69, 1968. Used by permission of the American Medical Association.) *B,* right ventriculotomy is done. Left pulmonary artery *(LPA);* right pulmonary artery *(RPA). C,* ventricular septal defect *(VSD)* is closed with Teflon patch. Right ventricle *(RV). D,* distal end of Hancock conduit is sutured to pulmonary arteries. *E,* proximal end of conduit is anastomosed to right ventricle. (From Wallace.[181] Used by permission.)

spiratory insufficiency (requiring mechanical ventilation for 72 hours or more), and bleeding are among the postoperative complications.[116] Fresh-frozen plasma and platelets are routinely used to decrease postoperative bleeding, part of which is inherent to the use of the Dacron conduit. Exposing the conduit to fresh blood drawn from the patient before the administration of heparin can be helpful in decreasing this bleeding.[161]

Congenital Aortic Stenosis

Valvular aortic stenosis is most frequent, followed in frequency by subvalvular (either by a fibrous diaphragm or by diffuse muscular hypertrophy involving primarily the ventricular septum) and supravalvular stenosis.[80, 185] Severe aortic stenosis can result in heart failure early in infancy. Syncope, angina, and sudden death may occur at a later age.

If the child is symptomatic or has a gradient of 60 mm Hg or more, or if progressive left ventricular hypertrophy is present, surgical treatment is recommended. Repair is done using cardiopulmonary bypass.[41]

If surgical repair is expected to require a short time, mild hypothermia may be sufficient; however, when repair is expected to take longer than 20 minutes or when the left ventricle is severely hypertrophied, moderate hypothermia combined with a cold cardioplegic solution is preferred.

SUPRAVALVULAR AORTIC STENOSIS.—After aortic cross-clamping, a vertical incision is made in the right anterolateral aspect of the aorta, beginning above the constricted area and extending across into the noncoronary sinus of Valsalva. If the stenosis is sharply localized, the protruding narrow ridge may be excised, or excision of the narrowed segment and primary anastomosis may be done. To widen the previously constricted area, an elliptical Dacron patch is sutured into the incision in the ascending aorta (Fig 6–50).

VALVULAR STENOSIS.—In valvular stenosis (Fig 6–51), the valve is usually bicuspid. After incision of the aorta, valvotomy is performed by incision of the fused commissures to a distance of 1 to 2 mm short of the annulus to avoid unhinging the leaflets and thus producing aortic insufficiency. In older patients, excision and replacement of the valve with a prosthesis may be indicated.

SUBVALVULAR STENOSIS.—If subvalvular stenosis is due to a fibrous membrane (Fig 6–52), a transverse or oblique incision is made in the proximal ascending aorta, the aortic valve leaflets are gently retracted, and the membrane is excised. Trauma to the conduction bundle, aortic cusps, and mitral valve should be prevented (Fig 6–52). A less common variety of subvalvular aortic stenosis is idiopathic hypertrophic subaortic stenosis (Fig 6–53). The hypertrophic process primarily involves the ventricular septum. Repair is done preferably via an incision in the aorta (right or left ventriculotomy has also been performed) after which about two thirds of the thickness of the ventricular septum is excised. In patients who are in heart failure preoperatively, inotropic agents or systemic vasodilation (or both) may temporarily be necessary while coming off bypass and during the early postoperative period. Aortic valve insufficiency and heart block may complicate repair of subaortic stenosis.

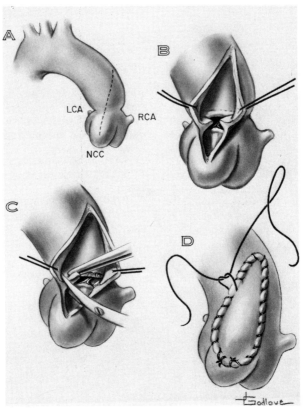

Fig 6–50.—Supravalvular aortic stenosis. *A* and *B*, vertical incision is made across constricted area extending to noncoronary sinus of Valsalva. *C*, well-localized constriction is excised. *D*, aortotomy is enlarged with pericardial or Dacron patch both in diffuse and in localized stenosis. Left coronary artery *(LCA);* right coronary artery *(RCA);* noncoronary cusp *(NCC).* (From Danielson.[41] Used by permission.)

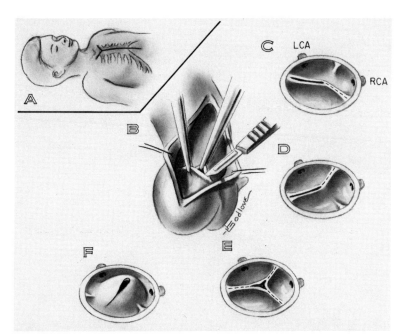

Fig 6–51.—Valvular aortic stenosis. After median sternotomy (A), aorta is incised (B) and well-developed commissures are divided. Most common types (C and D) are incised along interrupted lines and result in functional bicuspid valves. Variety E is rare. Type F needs replacement by prosthesis, as incision of valve will produce unacceptable aortic insufficiency. Left coronary artery (LCA); right coronary artery (RCA). (From Danielson.[41] Used by permission.)

ANESTHETIC MANAGEMENT.—Light anesthesia resulting in tachycardia and increased cardiac contractility should be prevented, as this increases myocardial oxygen consumption. At the same time, it decreases the ratio between the diastolic pressure time index and the tension time index and therefore decreases the oxygen delivery to the hypertrophied myocardium. In idiopathic hypertrophic subaortic stenosis (IHSS), light anesthesia is even more undesirable because it may increase considerably the functional left ventricular outlet stenosis. Anesthesia consisting of a combination of a narcotic—for instance, fentanyl—and a carefully administered cardiodepressant agent like enflurane or halothane is frequently beneficial in patients with IHSS. Also, administration of propranolol (given in increments of 0.05 mg/kg) or verapamil (0.1 mg/kg), slowly injected, may be indicated and may improve the ratio of myocardial oxygen supply and demand. During bypass, and especially during aortic cross-clamping, effective myocardial protection from ischemia is important, as the hypertrophied myocardium is easily insulted and may react with increased irritability. Consequently, sometimes the ventricular fibrillation that follows release of the aortic cross-clamp may be difficult to convert into sinus rhythm. Therefore, lidocaine (1 to 2 mg/kg) is given before the aorta is cross-clamped and again just before release of the aortic cross-clamp. Administration of verapamil (0.1 to 0.2 mg/kg) is probably even more effective.

Besides light anesthesia, vasodilatation or hypovolemia, which may cause hypotension, should also be prevented because the heart with severe aortic stenosis does not compensate as efficiently for hypotension as does a normal heart. Hypotension—either by hypovolemia or cardiodepression—should be treated vigorously because the hypertrophied myocardium will not tolerate inadequate perfusion of the coronary arteries, and arrhythmias combined with further decrease in cardiac output will result. In the acute situation where hypotension is caused by sudden severe loss of blood, temporary infusion of phenylephrine (10 mg in 50 ml of 5% dextrose in water, with a drip rate as indicated) may in-

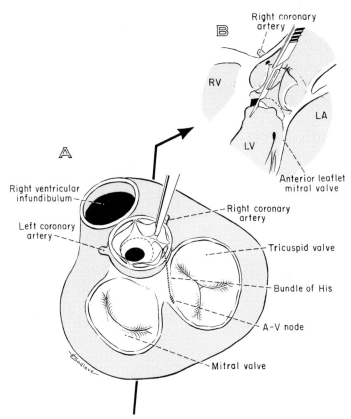

Fig 6–52.—Subvalvular stenosis. Most common form is caused by localized ring of fibrous tissue. During excision, injury to aortic cusps, mitral valve, and conduction bundle should be avoided. Right ventricle *(RV)*; left ventricle *(LV)*; left atrium *(LA)*; atrioventricular *(A-V)*. (From Danielson.[41] Used by permission.)

crease the peripheral resistance rapidly and therefore increase the diastolic blood pressure and coronary perfusion. Another side effect is the decrease in heart rate, which is also beneficial for the myocardial perfusion. In the meantime, replacement of the blood loss is continued while the phenylephrine drip is gradually decreased.

Management of anesthesia in the failing heart with severely increased left ventricular end-diastolic pressure may involve the use of a peripheral vasodilator to decrease the left ventricular end-diastolic pressure and improve subendocardial perfusion of the left ventricle. In this situation, nitroglycerin by infusion is the treatment of choice, if indicated, combined with an inotropic agent. Preferably, induction of anesthesia in patients with aortic stenosis is done intravenously with fentanyl (25 to 50 μg/kg), diazepam (0.1 to 0.2 mg/kg), and pancuronium (0.08 mg/kg) (or a combination of dimethyl tubocurarine [0.1 mg/kg] and pancuronium [0.04 mg/kg] in the presence of tachycardia). This provides a stable blood pressure and heart rate. However, if inhalation induction is preferred by the patient and the anesthesiologist, induction with nitrous oxide, oxygen, and 0.5 to 1% halothane, followed by intravenously administered narcotics (fentanyl 10 to 40 μg/kg) and a relaxant, enables a smooth intubation in a deeply analgesic patient. Maintenance of anesthesia is with narcotics, diazepam, and, if indicated, enflurane or halothane. Again, prevention of ischemia and damage of the hypertrophied myocardium is of great concern in these patients. During bypass, protection of the myocardium may be obtained by the use of hypothermia and cardioplegia and by maintaining a high-normal (70 to 80 mm Hg) mean perfusion pressure during the time that the aorta is not cross-clamped and oxygenation

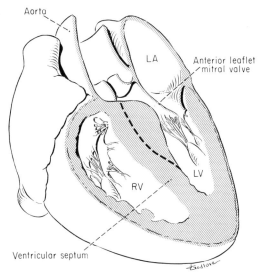

Fig 6–53.—Idiopathic hypertrophic subaortic stenosis. Left ventricular outflow tract obstruction is caused by hypertrophied septum that encroaches on anterior leaflet of mitral valve. Repair is accomplished by excision of septal hypertrophy through transaortic or transcardiac incision. Left atrium *(LA)*; left ventricle *(LV)*; right ventricle *(RV)*. (From Danielson.[41] Used by permission.)

of the myocardium is dependent on the adequacy of the coronary perfusion. Therefore, the administration of an α-adrenergic drug may be indicated in these time intervals.

Pulmonary Atresia With Intact Ventricular Septum

In more than 90% of patients, pulmonary atresia involves the pulmonary valve, the cusps of which are fused and form a diaphragm-like membrane. Also, the pulmonary valve ring and main pulmonary trunk may be hypoplastic.[60, 125] Usually, the right ventricle is small, but in about 20% of patients, the ventricle is normal or enlarged (the latter is accompanied by tricuspid insufficiency). The right atrium is always dilated.

The venous blood returning into the right atrium cannot enter the pulmonary artery because of the atretic pulmonary valve (Fig 6–54). Instead, the blood flows through a defect in the atrial septum (which has to be present to make life possible) into the left atrium, where it mixes with the pulmonary venous return. Next, it passes through the left ventricle, and part of the blood flows through the ductus arteriosus to the lungs, where it is oxygenated, while the other part follows the normal pathway of the systemic circulation.

Both the defect in the atrial system and the presence of an open ductus arteriosus are essential for life in an infant with pulmonary atresia and an intact ventricular septum. The diameter of the ductus is of great importance. If the ductus is narrow or tends to close, the pulmonary circulation becomes insufficient, less and less blood flows through the lungs to be oxygenated, and the child becomes increasingly cyanotic and acidotic. Therefore, infusion with prostaglandin E_1 is started to try to slow down the closure of the ductus during the time that preparations for emergency surgery are being made.

However, if the ductus is large, a substantial blood flow will go through the lungs and enter the left atrium, where it will impede the blood flow coming from the right atrium. As a result, a higher right atrial pressure is needed to maintain the flow of systemic venous return into the left atrium. The first situation, with decreased pulmonary blood flow because of a narrow ductus, is more frequent. Besides an adequate ductus arteriosus, the defect of the atrial septum has to be large enough to enable flow to be adequate. When indicated, balloon septostomy is performed at the end of catheterization, or, if necessary, a Blalock-Hanlon septectomy is done.

Surgical treatment depends on the anatomical findings. In patients with a normal-sized right ventricle and pulmonary valve atresia, valvotomy according to the method of Brock or while on cardiopulmonary bypass under direct vision gives excellent results if there is normal ventricular function and no significant tricuspid insufficiency.

In patients with a hypoplastic right ventricle and hypoplastic or atretic infundibulum, a systemic-pulmonary artery shunt (either a Waterston or a Blalock-Taussig) is preferred. However, there are some patients in whom valvotomy is not successful but is still desirable for improvement of the size and the function of the right ventricle and the pulmonary artery.[51, 132] In these patients, both valvotomy and systemic-pulmonary artery shunting are performed. When in due time cardiac catheterization shows that the size of the right ventricle and that the pulmonary valve and artery are adequate, the

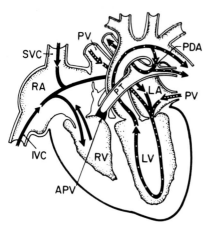

Fig 6–54.—Pulmonary atresia with intact ventricular septum. Systemic venous blood enters left atrium through patent foramen ovale or atrial septal defect. After mixing with oxygenated pulmonary blood coming via pulmonary veins, blood flows through left ventricle and enters aorta, where part of blood will perfuse systemic circulation and part will perfuse pulmonary circulation through ductus arteriosus. Superior vena cava *(SVC)*; inferior vena cava *(IVC)*; right ventricle *(RV)*; left ventricle *(LV)*; atretic pulmonary valve *(APV)*; pulmonary vein *(PV)*; patent ductus arteriosus *(PDA)*; pulmonary trunk *(PT)*; right atrium *(RA)*; left atrium *(LA)*. (From Emmanouilides.[60] Used by permission.)

systemic-pulmonary artery shunt may be discontinued and, if necessary, the atrial septal defect may be closed. In a hypoplastic infundibulum but with adequate right ventricular function, one may consider correcting the defect when the patient is about 5 or 6 years old by discontinuing the systemic-pulmonary artery shunt, closing the atrial septal defect, and inserting a valved conduit between the right ventricle and the pulmonary artery. If the right ventricle is too small, a connection between the right atrium and the pulmonary artery may be performed (see "Tricuspid Atresia"). The essentials of anesthetic management of the cyanotic infant with a decreased pulmonary flow, narrow ductus arteriosus, and acidosis have been discussed previously in the section on palliative procedures. Important factors are infusion of prostaglandin E_1, the correction of the acidosis, an attempt to obtain a PaO_2 of near 40 mm Hg, and the prevention of peripheral systemic vasodilatation, cardiodepression, or hypovolemia to avoid a decrease of blood flow through the ductus. Also, ventilation with low (but adequate) inspiratory pressures is advisable because high inspiratory pressures may worsen the already insufficient perfusion of the lungs.

Pulmonary Valvular Stenosis With Intact Ventricular Septum

Clinically, the patients with pulmonary valvular stenosis with intact ventricular septum[60] can be grouped into two categories: (1) patients with severe-to-moderate pulmonary stenosis (Fig 6–55) and (2) asymptomatic patients with moderate or mild pulmonary valvular stenosis. Besides a regular follow-up for evaluation of pos-

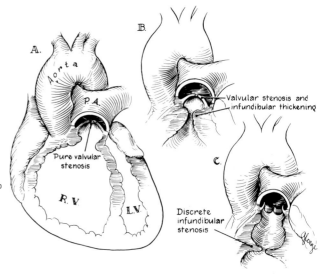

Fig 6–55.—Diagrammatic portrayal of pulmonary valvular stenosis with intact ventricular septum *(A)*, valvular stenosis with secondary infundibular thickening *(B)*, and primary infundibular stenosis with discrete narrowing in proximal portion of infundibulum *(C)*. Pulmonary artery *(P.A.)*; right ventricle *(R.V.)*; left ventricle *(L.V.)*. (From Emmanouilides.[60] Used by permission.)

sible progression and prophylaxis against bacterial endocarditis, patients belonging to this group usually do not need medical or surgical attention. Conversely, patients with moderate-to-severe pulmonary stenosis and right ventricular pressures equal to or greater than left ventricular pressures essentially have the same problems as do patients with pulmonary atresia. However, because there is some flow from the right ventricle into the pulmonary artery, closure of the ductus arteriosus does not have that immediate disastrous impact on the patient's life that closure in pulmonary atresia has.

If the stenosis of the pulmonary valve is so severe that the elevated end-diastolic pressure of the right ventricle is high enough to cause a right-to-left shunt through the foramen ovale (or atrial septal defect) and the child becomes cyanotic, large bronchial collateral vessels may develop.[123] This also will happen in patients with pulmonary atresia, unless early closure of the ductus occurs and the condition deteriorates too fast. Tricuspid insufficiency may develop if the right ventricle dilates, thus increasing the load of the right atrium and consequently the right-to-left shunt.

The size of the right ventricular cavity may be decreased, but usually this decrease occurs because of hypertrophy of the wall, and in moderate-to-severe stenosis the right ventricular pressures are often higher than those of the left ventricle. Hypertrophy of the wall of the right ventricle is common, which may necessitate resection of the hypertrophied infundibular muscle during repair. In severe obstruction, a large increase in heart rate should be prevented, because the shortening of the diastolic filling time may result in a decreased cardiac output from the greater impedance to filling of the stiff, hypertrophied muscle mass of the right ventricle.

Because surgical repair of pulmonary stenosis is usually not done at such a young age as is repair of pulmonary atresia and, more important, because the anatomy of both the right ventricle and the pulmonary artery is fairly normal, primary correction is the treatment of choice. When present, the bronchial collateral vessels are tied off before the patient goes on bypass. A defect in the atrial septum is repaired. The pulmonary artery is incised, and valvotomy is done. In the presence of infundibular obstruction, a right ventriculotomy may be necessary for excision of the hypertrophied infundibular muscle.

If the annulus of the pulmonary valve is narrow, widening of the annulus and proximal pulmonary artery is done by insertion of a pericardial graft or Dacron patch. Any resulting pulmonary valvular insufficiency is better tolerated than is a persistent obstruction. When the patient is coming off bypass, the difference in pressure between the right ventricle and the pulmonary artery is measured. A gradient of 20 to 40 mm Hg is acceptable. If the pressure is greater, bypass is reestablished, and further correction (most often infundibular resection) is performed.

Tetralogy of Fallot

Tetralogy of Fallot anatomically (Fig 6–56) comprises the following: (1) ventricular septal defect; (2) right ventricular outflow obstruction involving one or more of the following locations: infundibulum, pulmonic valve or annulus, and the pulmonary artery (in some patients—the so-called pink Fallots—the right ventricular outflow obstruction is minimal, resulting in a predominant shunt from left to right); (3) dextroposition of the aorta; and (4) hypertrophy of the right ventricle. The basic physiologic disturbance is a reduced pulmonary blood flow because of the right ventricular outflow obstruction, with direct shunting of blood from the right ventricle to the systemic circulation. The pulmonary blood flow is determined by the fixed anatomical right ventricular outflow obstruction, the relatively fixed right ventricular pressure, and the variable systemic resistance (Fig 6–57).

The anesthesiologist who is aware of this characteristic will take great care to prevent a decrease in systemic blood pressure by peripheral systemic vasodilatation because it will increase the right-to-left shunt and decrease the tissue oxygenation. As a result, metabolic acidosis may develop, which increases pulmonary vascular resistance and increases systemic vasodilation. This process gives more shunting from right to left, and a vicious circle is created. When halothane is used, it should be administered with the utmost care. Hypovolemia should be prevented or treated immediately if it occurs. If blood pressure decreases suddenly, accompanied by a deterioration of Pao_2, the administration of phenylephrine (5 to 10 μg/kg body weight) is sometimes indicated and helpful in breaking this vicious circle. The use of this

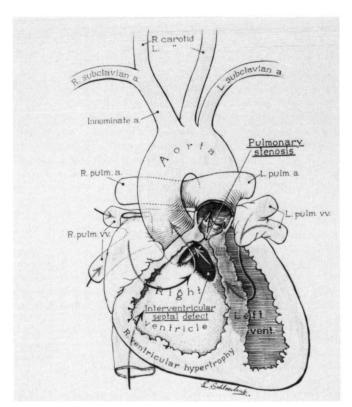

Fig 6–56.—Tetralogy of Fallot. Diagram shows pulmonary stenosis, ventricular septal defect with overriding aorta, and right ventricular hypertrophy. (From Blalock A.: Surgical procedures employed and anatomical variations encountered in the treatment of congenital pulmonic stenosis. Surg. Gynecol. Obstet. 87:385, 1948. Used by permission.)

agent will temporarily increase the peripheral resistance, more than the pulmonary resistance, and therefore will decrease the right-to-left shunt. In addition to this, the increased right ventricular pressure leads to elevated pulmonary blood flow and higher PaO_2[172] (Fig 6–58).

In a patient with tetralogy of Fallot, the total resistance to flow across the pulmonic circuit exceeds the systemic vascular resistance, sometimes three to four times, which may decrease pulmonary blood flow to between one third and one fourth the systemic blood flow. The right-to-left shunt will compensate for the decreased left atrial preload but not for the hypoxia that results from the low pulmonary blood flow. The patient compensates for the hypoxia by the development of collateral circulation to the lungs (which usually takes several years) and polycythemia. There is a correlation between the increased incidence of thrombosis and the elevated viscosity present at high levels of hematocrit (>60%). Also, polycythemia appears to have a role in the bleeding tendency that can cause problems during the postoperative period. Another hazard the anesthesiologist may encounter is the so-called hypoxic spell, of which the cause still is unknown.[77] The incidence seems to be greatest in patients 2 to 4 months old, but these spells may occur at any age. Usually, apprehension or pain causes the child to cry, which increases the right-to-left shunt and eventually results in hypoxemia, acidosis, and increased pulmonary vasoconstriction.[90]

The treatment of a cyanotic spell during induction is as follows: Oxygen is administered by mask while halothane is gradually added (as necessary up to 1.5%)—its negative inotropic effect supposedly decreases the pulmonary outflow obstruction. A muscle relaxant is given either intramuscularly or intravenously to abolish the straining and crying and the concomitant increase in oxygen consumption and cyanosis. If

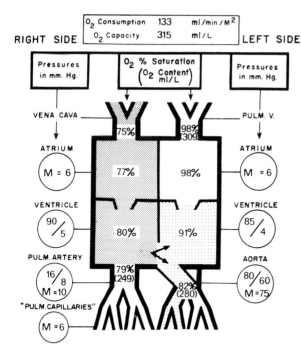

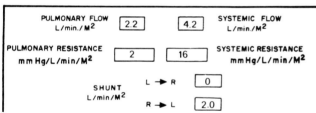

Fig 6–57.—Catheterization findings in tetralogy of Fallot. Pressure in right ventricle is slightly higher than on left side because of stenosis in pulmonary outflow tract. Degree of resulting right-to-left shunt determines amount of cyanosis with which patient is seen initially. (From Nadas and Fyler.[136] Used by permission.)

metabolic acidosis is present or suspected to be present, sodium bicarbonate is administered and arterial blood samples are repeatedly taken to enable adequate treatment of the acid-base disturbance. As soon as an intravenous line is established, fentanyl (2 to 15 μg/kg) or morphine (0.1 to 0.2 mg/kg) is given.

Most useful in the treatment of a severe cyanotic spell is propranolol. It is given slowly intravenously, if necessary up to 0.2 mg/kg, though usually a smaller dose (0.05 to 0.1 mg/kg) is sufficient. Its negative inotropic effect may necessitate the use of inotropic agents later when coming off bypass.

Generally, there is a reluctance to continue the oral propranolol treatment (1 mg/kg four times daily, which is given for prevention of hypoxic spells) until the morning of surgery because of the frequent occurrence of postoperative low cardiac output. However, in children with histories of severe spells, oral propranolol should be continued up to six hours before surgery. As mentioned previously, effective premedication that provides adequate preoperative sedation is essential in these patients.

SURGICAL TREATMENT.—Palliative surgery by creation of various shunts in symptomatic patients has been discussed previously. Complete repair may be performed successfully in infants who are only a few weeks old and is becoming the operation of choice for symptomatic infants who do not respond to medical treatment unless the anatomy is unfavorable (hypoplasia of the distal pulmonary arteries and anomalies of the right coronary arterial system which preclude outflow patching). In such patients, a palliative operation is performed first, followed later by complete repair. Early primary repair has the advantage of preventing the development of

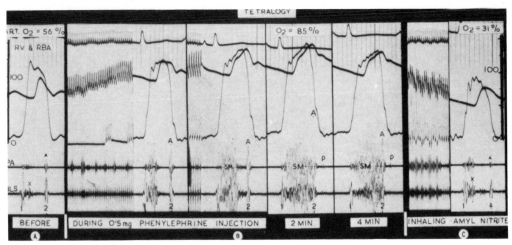

Fig 6-58.—Effects of increasing and decreasing systemic resistance on right ventricular *(RV)* and systemic (right brachial artery, *RBA*) pressures and arterial oxygen saturation in tetralogy of Fallot. From top to bottom are depicted ECG, RV, and systemic pressure curves, and two recordings of a phonocardiogram. *A,* before phenylephrine injection; arterial oxygen saturation 56%, RV pressure 125/5 mm Hg, systemic pressure 100/70 mm Hg. Phonocardiogram record shows low pulmonary blood flow. *B,* during and after injection of phenylephrine, arterial oxygen saturation and both systemic and RV systolic pressures increase. Increase in RV pressure causes progressive increase in pulmonary blood flow (compare recordings of phonocardiogram during and two and four minutes after). *C,* reduction of systemic resistance by inhalation of amyl nitrite. Both RV and systemic pressures decrease rapidly, respectively, to 95/2 and 80/52 mm Hg. As decrease in systemic pressure is greater than that of systolic pressure in right ventricle, increase in right-to-left shunt will occur and pulmonary perfusion will deteriorate. Phonocardiogram is consistent with large decrease in pulmonary blood flow. Arterial oxygen saturation decreased to 31%. (From Vogelpoel L., et al.: The use of phenylephrine in the differentiation of Fallot's tetralogy from pulmonary stenosis with intact ventricular septum. *Am. Heart J.* 59:489, 1960. Used by permission.)

progressive infundibular obstruction, with decreasing pulmonary blood flow, decreasing left ventricular stroke volume and capacity, and increasing polycythemia with thrombosis and bleeding tendency. However, in patients with mild cyanosis, mild polycythemia, and mild disability, the operation can be safely deferred until the age of about 4 years, when it can be performed with a low mortality risk.[97]

The surgical repair of the defects is as follows: If large bronchial collateral vessels or surgical shunts are present, they have to be ligated before bypass is begun, to prevent blood shunting into the pulmonary circulation during cardiopulmonary bypass. After insertion of the arterial and venous cannulas, bypass is started and the patient is cooled to between 20 and 25 C. During cooling, the right atrium is opened and, if present, the foramen ovale is closed, followed by closure of the right atrium. When the nasopharyngeal temperature reaches 25 C, or as soon as ventricular fibrillation starts, the aorta is cross-clamped and a cold cardioplegic solution is given. Small infants who are to undergo surgical repair under circulatory arrest are cooled to a nasopharyngeal temperature of about 18 C. In infants of about 3 months and older, total circulatory arrest is usually not necessary. If working conditions require, the flow can be reduced to between 0.5 and 1 L/minute/sq m for about 30 to 45 minutes at a temperature of 20 C, followed by a flow of 1.6 L/minute/sq m for as long as required.[98] The right ventricle is incised. The choice of direction for the ventriculotomy depends on the anatomy.[122] Dependent on the necessity for a pulmonary outflow patch, a vertical incision in the infundibulum of the right ventricle may have to be extended across the pulmonary valve ring (Fig 6-59). Before surgery, the possibility of an anomalous coronary artery run-

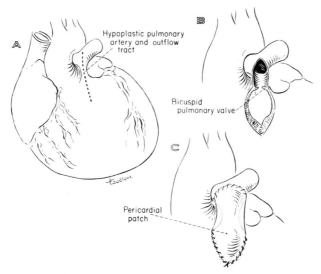

Fig 6–59.—Repair of hypoplastic pulmonary artery and pulmonary valve ring. *A* and *B,* vertical incision of infundibulum extends upward into hypoplastic pulmonary artery trunk. *C,* outflow tract is enlarged with pericardial patch. (From McGoon D.C.: Technics of open heart surgery for congenital heart disease. *Curr. Probl. Surg.,* April 1968, p. 1. Used by permission.)

ning deep under the myocardium of the right ventricular outflow tract has to be excluded by coronary arteriography to prevent a catastrophe if the artery is inadvertently incised.

If stenotic, the pulmonary valve is opened as much as possible by direct incision of its commissures. Infundibular muscle and parietal muscle bands are resected as necessary to provide an adequate outlet from the right ventricle, followed by repair of the ventricular septal defect with a patch. There is a risk of complete atrioventricular block due to injury of the conducting tissue that lies close to the posteroinferior border of the ventricular septal defect where the bundle of His perforates the fibrous ring. Next, the decision has to be made whether enlargement by a patch graft of the outflow tract should be done. Measurement of the diameter of the pulmonary valve with Hegar's dilators is helpful in making this decision.[98] However, if a patch graft is not placed and, after termination of bypass, if the ratio of the peak pressure in the right ventricle to that in the left is greater than 0.6, bypass usually needs to be reestablished and a patch graft enlargement across the pulmonary valve ring should be performed.

POSTOPERATIVE PERIOD.—The cardiac output in patients with tetralogy of Fallot tends to be depressed during the early postoperative period.[97] Cardiac performance may be affected by several factors. First, right ventriculotomy may depress right ventricular performance; both contractility and compliance (because of edema near the incision) are depressed. As a result, both right ventricular end-diastolic and right atrial pressures increase and the right ventricular stroke volume decreases, as do the left ventricular end-diastolic pressure, left atrial pressure, and cardiac output. A transverse ventriculotomy decreases right ventricular performance less than does a vertical ventriculotomy. Second, residual right ventricular hypertension from incomplete relief of pulmonary stenosis increases the afterload of the right ventricle, again increasing right atrial pressure and right ventricular end-diastolic pressure, while decreasing these values on the left side and decreasing the cardiac output. Another cause of increased right ventricular afterload is pulmonary arterial hypertension—for instance, in patients with prior Potts shunt, residual ventricular septal defect, or multiple diffuse pulmonary arteriolar thrombosis.[95] Third, a patch across the pulmonary valve ring results in pulmonary valvular incompetence. Fourth, the relatively small left ventricle in patients with a severe (75%) overriding of the aorta decreases its functional reserve, causing higher left ventricular end-diastolic and atrial pressures.[77]

In the management of decreased postoperative cardiac output, adequate ventricular filling pressures are indicated—the higher of the two atrial pressures is kept between 10 and 15 mm Hg. However, overloading has to be prevented, especially when the left ventricle is the restricting ventricle, because pulmonary edema may develop relatively easily. Usually, an inotropic drug is needed, and digitalization is started immediately after surgery (digitalization dose of digoxin is 0.9 mg/sq m of body surface area); usually, one third to one fourth of the digitalization dose is given, followed as indicated by additional doses, depending on the renal function and potassium level. The incidence of digitalis toxicity is greatly increased during the postbypass period.

During the postoperative period, ventilation with positive end-expiratory pressure (4 to 8 mm Hg) is frequently beneficial. The patient usually can be weaned from mechanical ventilation on the second postoperative day (see chap. 24). Frequently, a diuretic is needed during the postoperative period to ensure a good urinary output and to decrease the excessive fluid retention that easily develops in these patients. Con-

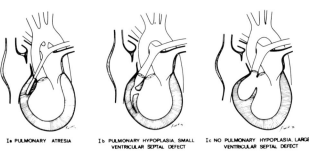

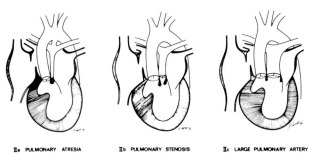

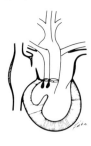

Fig 6–60.—Classification of tricuspid atresia according to associated lesions. (From Sade and Castaneda.[157] Used by permission.)

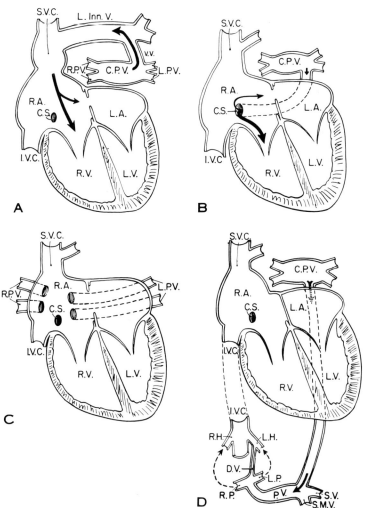

Fig 6–80.—Common forms of total anomalous pulmonary venous connection. **A,** supracardiac type. **B** and **C,** cardiac type. (In **B,** pulmonary veins join and from their confluence a common pulmonary vein connects to coronary sinus. In **C,** right and left pulmonary veins enter right atrium separately.) **D,** infracardiac type. From confluence of pulmonary veins, a venous channel arises, which connects to portal vein. Common pulmonary vein *(C.P.V.)*; vertical vein *(V.V.)*; left innominate vein *(L.Inn.V.)*; superior vena cava *(S.V.C.)*; right, left atrium *(R.A., L.A.)*; coronary sinus *(C.S.)*; inferior vena cava *(I.V.C.)*; right, left ventricle *(R.V., L.V.)*; right, left pulmonary vein *(R.P.V., L.P.V.)*; splenic vein *(S.V.)*; superior mesenteric vein *(S.M.V.)*; portal vein *(P.V.)*; right, left portal vein *(R.P., L.P.)*; ductus venosus *(D.V.)*; right, left hepatic vein *(R.H., L.H.)*. (From Lucas and Schmidt.[107] Used by permission.)

lar resistance decreases, newborns with TAPVC without pulmonary venous obstruction will show improved oxygen saturation. The pulmonary blood flow may be as much as three to five times the systemic blood flow.[107] Systemic blood flow is usually normal. Because the mixed venous pool in the right atrium receives three to five parts of fully saturated blood for each part of desaturated systemic venous blood, the oxygen saturation in the right atrium may be 90% or higher.[53] Because of the mixing of oxygenated and deoxygenated blood in the right atrium, the oxygen saturations in the right ventricle, pulmonary artery, left atrium, left ventricle, and aorta are approximately equal to those in the right atrium.

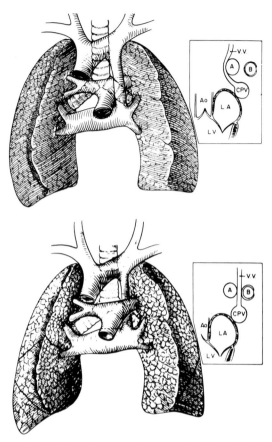

Fig 6–81.—Supracardiac type. Relationship of vertical vein to thoracic structures. **Top,** usually, vertical vein passes anterior to left pulmonary artery. **Bottom,** if vertical vein, coming from confluence of pulmonary veins *(CPV)*, ascends between left pulmonary artery *(A)* and left mainstem bronchus *(B)* to join left innominate vein, pulmonary venous obstruction may result because of extrinsic compression. Aorta *(Ao)*; left atrium *(LA)*; left ventricle *(LV)*; vertical vein *(v.v.)*. (From Elliott L.P., Edwards J.E.: The problem of pulmonary venous obstruction in total anomalous pulmonary venous connection to the left innominate vein, editorial. *Circulation* 25:913, 1962. Used by permission of the American Heart Association.)

Dilatation and hypertrophy of the right ventricle and dilatation of the pulmonary artery occur. In time, the increase in pulmonary artery pressure results in pulmonary vascular disease. Right heart failure is commonly seen. Except when these complications occur, cyanosis may be clinically inapparent.

Infants with TAPVC and pulmonary venous obstruction are seen initially with pulmonary hypertension, edema, and severe cyanosis. Reflex pulmonary arteriolar constriction worsens the condition by decreasing pulmonary blood flow, which increases pulmonary artery hypertension and right ventricular hypertrophy and eventually causes right heart failure.

These infants become severely cyanotic and acidotic and may deteriorate rapidly. Ventilation with positive end-expiratory pressure may improve the pulmonary edema and therefore the pulmonary hypoxic vasoconstriction. Mechanical ventilation also decreases the oxygen consumption by taking over the work of breathing. If necessary, the use of pancuronium for relaxation may be helpful in improving the preoperative condition of the infant. Acidosis is corrected by the use of bicarbonate.

In patients with pulmonary venous obstruction because of a narrow interatrial defect, balloon septostomy[39, 107] may improve the condition sufficiently to decrease the risk of operation. Other palliative treatment is not possible.

The anesthetic management is the same as for a very sick infant: awake intubation after preoxygenation and insertion of two venous lines, one arterial line, and preferably an external or internal jugular vein line. In the infant weighing less than 10 kg, surface cooling is performed and arterial blood gas and serum potassium levels are determined frequently. The $PaCO_2$ is maintained between 45 and 50 mm Hg while 2% to 5% carbon dioxide is added to the anesthetic gases (low-concentration halothane, and nitrous oxide and oxygen in a ratio dependent on the PaO_2). If necessary, diluted potassium is slowly injected intravenously to keep the serum level around 4 mEq/L, especially in infants receiving digoxin. When the temperature reaches between 28 and 30 C, the patient is placed on bypass and is further cooled to between 18 and 20 C. A present ductus arteriosus is ligated, the aorta is cross-clamped, and a cardioplegic solution is infused. Pancuronium (0.05 mg/kg) is given. Next, the aortic cannula is clamped, venous blood is drained into the bypass machine, the superior and inferior venae cavae are occluded, and the venous cannula is removed from the right atrium. Under total circulatory arrest, repair is performed. In the supracardiac type, the apex of the heart is lifted upward to expose the common venous trunk, which lies behind the left atrium.

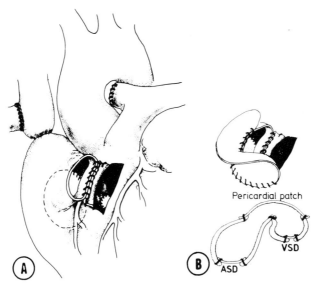

Fig 6-65.—**A,** anastomosis of right atrium to right ventricular outlet chamber. First, atrial septal defect *(ASD)* and ventricular septal defect *(VSD)* are repaired. Next, posterior wall of right atrial appendage is sutured to right ventricular incision, after which pericardial patch is used to complete the anastomosis **(B).** (Note: In this patient, a Glenn operation was previously performed, with end-to-side anastomosis of distal part of right pulmonary artery and superior vena cava. Proximal end of right pulmonary artery is closed.) (From Björk V.O., et al.: Right atrial right ventricular anastomosis for correction of tricuspid atresia. *J. Thorac. Cardiovasc. Surg.* 77:452, 1979. Used by permission.)

the great arteries (aorta located anterior or lateral to the pulmonary artery instead of posterior), other malalignments may be present in the heart defects classified in this group: inverted position of the atria, discordant atrioventricular connection, inverted ventricles, and discordant ventricular–great arterial connection. The wide variety of anatomic anomalies present in this group made a subclassification necessary. Unfortunately, a confusing variety of descriptions and terminology resulted.[94, 136, 144, 167, 178]

Classification based on the anatomical position of the atria, ventricles, and great arteries, as well as on their relative position, is currently preferred. Occasionally, the direction of the anatomical axis of the heart is abnormal, and this should also be described. The heart defects of the malposition group are classified according to their (1) atrial position, (2) ventricular position, (3) position of the great arteries, and (4) axis of the heart.

ATRIAL POSITION.—The position of the atria and that of the abdominal organs are related, and, therefore, if there is doubt at which sides the morphologic left and right atria are located, the position of the abdominal organs will provide the answer. Three possibilities exist: (1) the atria and abdominal organs are in their usual position, situs solitus (S); (2) the abdominal organs are a mirror image of the normal, and thus the atria are also reversed in position (morphologic right atrium on the left and left atrium on the right side), situs inversus (I); and (3) situs ambiguus (A), in which there is doubt about the visceral position. The bronchial anatomy may be the most reliable guide to the atrial and visceral situs.[143] Asplenia or polysplenia frequently is present in type A.

VENTRICULAR POSITION.—During fetal development, the cardiac loop formation takes place either in the normal direction (D-loop formation, resulting in the morphologic right ventricle on the right and the morphologic left ventricle on the left side [D]) or toward the left (L-loop formation, resulting in inverted ventricles [L]).

Regarding the atrial-ventricular relationship, in concordant connection, the morphologic right atrium connects to the morphologic right ventricle and the left atrium connects to the left ventricle. If the atria are connected to the opposite ventricles, discordant connection exists.

POSITION OF THE GREAT ARTERIES.—The great arteries are positioned as follows: (1) In solitus normally related great arteries (S), the aorta arises posterior and to the right of the pulmonary artery. (2) In inverted normally related great arteries (I), the aorta arises posterior and to the left of the pulmonary artery. (3) In D-malposition (D), the aorta is anterior or lateral and to the right of the pulmonary artery. (4) In L-malposition (L), the aorta arises anterior or lateral and to the left of the pulmonary artery.

Regarding the ventricular–great arterial relationship, in concordant connection, the aorta arises from the morphologic left ventricle and the pulmonary artery from the right. In discordant connection, the aorta arises from the morphologic right ventricle and the pulmonary artery from the left.

AXIS OF THE HEART.—If the apex of the heart is directed to the right and the heart located in the right side of the chest, the condition is called "isolated dextrocardia." For the patient, this position of the heart is of no consequence; however, dextrocardia is frequently associated with transposition and other congenital heart defects or bronchiectasis. Normally, the heart is positioned in the left side of the chest, with the axis directed to the left. However, usually the term "levocardia" is not used to describe this normal condition. The term "isolated levocardia" is used to delineate the condition in which the heart is in the normal position but the atria and viscera are either in situs inversus or ambiguus. In the latter group, which is almost invariably associated with asplenia or polysplenia and absence of the inferior vena cava, the venous atrium and superior vena cava remain on the right side.

Anomalies of the systemic venous return,

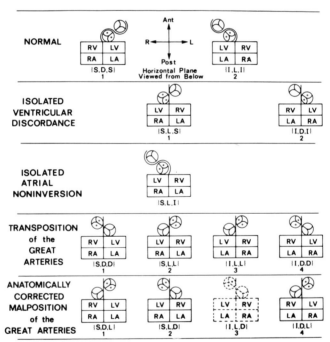

Fig 6–66.—A few of many atrioventricular and ventriculoarterial connections that are possible in the human heart. *Broken lines* indicate anomaly that has not yet been documented. Heart diagrams are viewed from below. Notations under heart diagrams describe first visceroatrial situs, followed by ventricular loop and relationship of conotruncus. For instance, in S.D.L., S indicates situs solitus of viscera and atria (both in normal position), D indicates fetal development of cardiac loop took place in normal direction. Thus, morphologic right ventricle is on right and morphologic left ventricle is on left. L indicates levotransposition (malposition) of conotruncal part, such that aorta is positioned on left of and anterior to pulmonary artery. (From van Praagh et al.[178] Used by permission.)

transposition, or other congenital heart defects frequently occur in patients with isolated levocardia.

Symbolic notation is frequently used in describing various cardiac malpositions (Fig 6–66).

With the above descriptive classification, the anatomy of any particular heart defect belonging to this group of malposition of the great arteries is easier to understand. For instance, complete transposition of the great arteries is described as follows: atria in situs solitus, D-loop formation of ventricles, and D-malposition, or SDD. Of course, information about the presence of other defects, such as atrial or ventricular septal defect, will have to be added as indicated. From this classification, an even simpler way of describing a particular heart defect evolved: After having described the position of the atria and if necessary of the axis of the heart, one follows with the description of the atrioventricular and ventricular–great arterial connections. This method makes understanding the anatomy much easier: atria in situs solitus, concordant atrioventricular connection, and discordant ventricular-arterial connection indicate to a noncardiologist more about the situation than just the diagnosis D-transposition.

In addition to complete or D-transposition, which is the most frequent type and which will be discussed more thoroughly, two other types are sometimes mentioned and can be confusing because of their terminology.

In congenitally corrected transposition, there is atrioventricular and ventricular-arterial discordance. As a result, unsaturated systemic venous blood reaches the pulmonary artery via the right atrium and left ventricle, while saturated pulmonary venous blood reaches the aorta via the left atrium and right ventricle. Thus, functionally the circulation is normal or "corrected" (Fig 6–67). However, frequently a ventricular septal defect with or without an atrial septal defect is present that may need surgical repair. The abnormal position of the conduction tissue, which is common in atrioventricular discordance, may give the surgeon some difficulties.[48, 99]

In anatomically corrected transposition (the preferred terminology is now "anatomically corrected malposition of the great arteries"), the aorta arises from the left ventricle but anterior to and frequently to the left of the pulmonary artery. In this rare anomaly, atrioventricular discordance, ventricular septal defect, and pulmonary stenosis may be present.

In complete transposition of the great arteries, the pulmonary and systemic circulations are completely separate and independent. Adequate communication between these circulations is necessary for survival. The pulmonary circuit, with a low resistance and a powerful pump (left ventricle), has a rapid rate of circulation; the systemic circulation, with a higher resistance, is slower. Output on the pulmonary side is usually considerably greater than on the systemic side, except in severe pulmonary stenosis or increased pulmonary vascular resistance (Fig 6–68).

Communication between both circulations is generally at the atrial level; other possibilities are a ventricular septal defect, open ductus, bronchopulmonary collateral vessels, and iatrogenic systemic–pulmonary artery shunts. The systemic arterial oxygen saturation is greatly de-

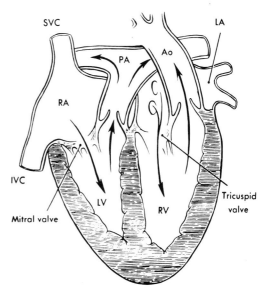

Fig 6–67.—Congenitally corrected transposition (malposition) of great arteries. Unless ventricular septal defect or atrial septal defect is present, surgery is not indicated in this condition. Superior vena cava *(SVC)*; inferior vena cava *(IVC)*; right atrium *(RA)*; pulmonary artery *(PA)*; aorta *(Ao)*; left ventricle *(LV)*; left atrium *(LA)*; right ventricle *(RV)*. (From Kidd B.S.L.: Congenitally corrected transposition of the great arteries, in Keith J.D., Rowe R.D., Vlad P. [eds.]: *Heart Disease in Infancy and Childhood.* New York, Macmillan Publishing Co., 1978. Used by permission.)

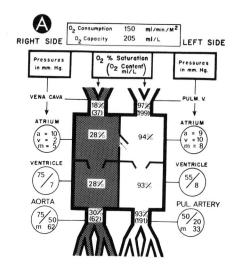
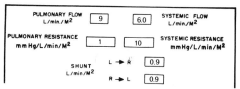
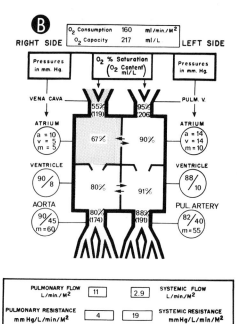
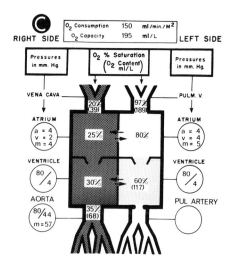
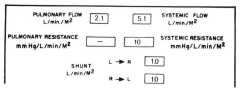

Fig 6–68.—Catheterization data. **A,** in complete transposition of great arteries and atrial septal defect. Note, right-to-left and left-to-right shunts have to be equal in the two parallel circulations. **B,** in complete transposition with atrial septal defect and ventricular septal defect, both increased pulmonary-to-systemic-flow ratio and increased communication between both separated circulations improve oxygenation of blood perfusing systemic circulation. **C,** in complete transposition, atrial septal defect, ventricular septal defect, and subpulmonic stenosis, the reduction in pulmonary blood flow greatly affects oxygenation of systemic circulation, as increased resistance in pulmonary circuit prevents adequate pulmonary blood flow and therefore decreases effective pulmonary and systemic blood flow despite adequate-sized shunting sites. (From Nadas and Fyler.[136] Used by permission.)

pendent on the anatomical left-to-right shunt (Fig 6–69) (which is the effective systemic blood flow because it carries oxygenated pulmonary venous return to the systemic circulation). The anatomical right-to-left shunt (representing the effective pulmonary blood flow) is equal to the effective systemic blood flow. With adequate mixing between both circulations, the level of arterial oxygen saturation is determined primarily by the pulmonary-to-systemic blood flow ratio; a high pulmonary blood flow will result in a relatively high arterial oxygen saturation,[110] as long as the left ventricle can maintain the high-output state. Pulmonary stenosis or increased pulmonary vascular resistance can decrease pulmonary blood flow and lower systemic oxygen saturation, despite adequate-sized anatomical shunting sites between both circulations (see Fig 6–68,C).

In transposition of the great arteries with an adequate ventricular septal defect but without elevated pulmonary vascular resistance, the blood flow in the pulmonary circulation may be increased, resulting in a high arterial oxygen saturation, unless heart failure and pulmonary edema intervene.

More than 30% of infants less than 2 years of age with transposition of the great arteries have bronchopulmonary collateral vessels that enter the pulmonary vascular bed proximal to the pulmonary capillary bed. The widespread and accelerated occurrence of pulmonary vascular disease found in patients with transposition of the great arteries is probably related to this anomaly, because the flow of low saturated systemic blood may induce hypoxemic pulmonary vasoconstriction in regions of the lungs perfused by these collateral vessels.[9]

In about 50% of patients with D-transposition, blood flow to the right lung is considerably greater than to the left, probably because the main pulmonary artery has an abnormal right-

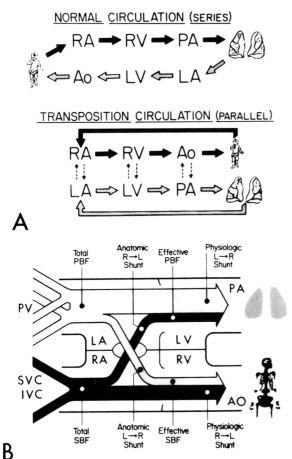

Fig 6–69.—Circulation pathways in complete transposition. **A,** normally, systemic and pulmonary circulatory pathways are in series. In patients with complete transposition, circulations are parallel. **B,** circulation schema of complete transposition with intact ventricular septum. Desaturated blood from inferior and superior venae cavae *(IVC, SVC)* flows through right atrium, where anatomical shunt from left to right through atrial septal defect adds oxygenated blood. At same time, equal amount of desaturated blood will shunt from right to left (the anatomical right-to-left shunt), which is actually effective pulmonary blood flow *(PBF)* (desaturated blood perfusing lungs). Previously mentioned anatomical left-to-right shunt provides oxygenated blood to systemic circulation and therefore represents effective systemic blood flow *(SBF)*. In addition to this oxygenated blood, systemic circulation will be perfused by that part of desaturated blood flow from systemic circulation that did not shunt to pulmonary circulation and that actually represents physiologic right-to-left shunt. (From Paul.[144] Used by permission.)

ward inclination.[135] However, the clinical implications usually are of no great significance.

The clinical findings in an infant with transposition of the great arteries vary considerably. If an adequate connection between both circulations exists, mild-to-moderate cyanosis may be present. With a large ventricular septal defect and sufficient pulmonary blood flow, the cyanosis is only mild because of the adequate mixing, but soon heart failure and pulmonary vascular disease will develop. If the connection between both circulations is inadequate, the cyanosis may be severe. The systemic hypoxemia lowers the peripheral systemic resistance, increases the systemic blood flow and the physiologic right-to-left shunt (Fig 6-69), and will thus further increase systemic hypoxemia, because the inadequate anatomic shunting sites make increase in effective pulmonary or systemic flow impossible.[114]

1. Infants with inadequate communication between the two circulations (either intact ventricular septum or small ventricular septal defect) are seen initially with hypoxia (Pao_2 about 25 mm Hg), acidosis (pH 7.0 to 6.8), and often hypoglycemia, and will develop congestive failure unless surgical treatment creates an adequate communication between both circulations.

2. In infants with transposition of the great arteries and a large ventricular septal defect, cyanosis and acidosis are less (Pao_2 between 30 and 40 mm Hg, pH about 7.3), but congestive heart failure with pulmonary edema and increasing cyanosis will develop between 2 and 6 weeks.

3. In infants with left ventricular outflow tract obstruction and ventricular septal defect, the symptoms usually will be seen later. Heart failure is late and cyanosis is mild. However, if the subvalvular pulmonary stenosis is severe, severe cyanosis and acidosis will soon develop. Closure of the ductus arteriosus may precipitate sudden deterioration.

Infants with transposition of the great arteries, especially with a large ventricular septal defect, suffer pulmonary vascular disease at an early age, with secondary cyanosis and increased polycythemia. Other complications of transposition of the great arteries are thrombocytopenia and impaired blood coagulation mechanisms[180, 183] (which may develop in infants 6 months of age or older), and an increased incidence of thrombotic lesions, spontaneous cerebrovascular accidents, and brain abscesses.

OPERATIVE TREATMENT.—In newborns and infants up to approximately 8 weeks of age who have inadequate mixing in the two circulations, balloon septostomy according to the method of Rashkind will usually enlarge the defect in the atrial septum sufficiently for a period of several months.

Atrial septectomy (Blalock-Hanlon operation) may give excellent improvement. Preferably, the procedure is performed in infants who are older than 3 months of age, when the shunting by the Rashkind balloon septostomy is no longer adequate, but the Blalock-Hanlon also can be performed in patients who are younger. Definitive repair, even in infancy, is preferred over septectomy by most groups.

In infants with severe pulmonary stenosis, a systemic–pulmonary artery shunt (preferably a Blalock-Taussig shunt, a Waterston shunt, or a Gore-Tex [5- to 6-mm diameter] prosthetic graft anastomosed end-to-side between the subclavian and the pulmonary artery) is still a useful palliative procedure.[144]

In infants with a large ventricular septal defect, pulmonary artery banding is advisable before the age of 4 months because of the early development of pulmonary vascular obstructive changes. Frequently atrial septectomy is done at the same session to ensure adequate mixing between both circulations.

For corrective surgery with the Mustard operation, an age of 8 to 12 months is considered optimal. However, in patients in whom balloon septostomy (or atrial septectomy) provides inadequate palliation, the Mustard operation can be performed at an earlier age.

In patients with a large ventricular septal defect or ductus arteriosus in whom pulmonary banding has not been performed, early (before the age of 6 months) repair by the Mustard operation may be indicated. The Mustard operation[167] is performed with cardiopulmonary bypass, moderate hypothermia, and the use of a cold cardioplegic solution, which enables the surgeon to use periods of low flow rate or, after cooling the child further to a nasopharyngeal temperature of about 20 C, short periods of circulatory arrest if pulmonary venous return is interfering with the surgical repair. Surface cooling, circulatory arrest at a nasopharyngeal temperature of 16 to 18 C, and cold cardioplegic solution are used in infants who are less than 6 months of age. The pericardium between the phrenic nerves is excised and is used for the atrial patch (Fig 6–70).

After insertion of the cannula into the aorta, the inferior vena cava is cannulated at its junction with the right atrium. The superior vena cava is cannulated at least 1.5 cm above its junction with the right atrium, preventing damage to the sinoatrial node and sinus node artery. A right ventricular vent is placed.

The right atrium is opened, and the atrial septum is excised. A ventricular septal defect (if present) is repaired through the tricuspid orifice if possible; otherwise, a left or right ventriculotomy may be necessary. The pericardial patch is now sutured in place so that blood from the inferior and superior venae cavae will flow through the mitral valve and the left ventricle into the pulmonary artery to be oxygenated in the lungs (Fig 6–71). Saturated pulmonary venous blood will flow around the patch through the tricuspid valve and right ventricle into the aorta. Frequently, a Dacron patch sutured into the initial atrial incision is necessary to expand the pulmonary venous atrium.

An infant previously in cardiac failure or severely hypoxemic will frequently need inotropic support when coming off bypass. The left atrial pressure (pulmonary venous return) is preferably kept below 15 mm Hg to prevent pulmonary congestion and edema. High systemic vascular resistance may have to be lowered by the use of chlorpromazine or a nitroprusside drip.

The following complications of the Mustard operation have been reported[167]: obstruction of the inferior or superior vena cava, chylothorax, obstruction to the pulmonary venous return, damage to the phrenic nerves, dysrhythmias (atrial flutter, complete atrioventricular dissociation, junctional rhythm, transient supraventricular tachycardia), tricuspid valve regurgitation, interatrial shunts, and decreased right ventricular function.

In patients with severe pulmonary vascular obstructive disease, the so-called palliative Mustard repair provides excellent symptomatic improvement.[30, 114] In this operation, an intra-atrial baffle, according to the method described by Mustard, is placed, but the ventricular septal defect is not closed. This procedure will allow unsaturated blood to shunt from the pulmonary (left) ventricle into the systemic ventricle when the pulmonary resistance is too high. However, as the increase in "effective" flow[114] (oxygenated blood reaching the systemic circulation) by this operation will also increase the systemic mixed venous saturation significantly, the systemic arterial oxygen saturation improves considerably. Before surgery, these patients will have a systemic arterial oxygen saturation of (considerably) less than 75%; after palliation they have an arterial saturation of more than 80% and, not infrequently, more than 90%.

The reduction in polycythemia that accompanies this improvement in the oxygen saturation decreases the risk of bleeding tendencies and thromboembolic complications. Although the immediate results of the Mustard repair are encouraging, long-term follow-up[78, 113] shows a relatively high incidence of late death and morbidity secondary to serious dysrhythmias, caval or pulmonary venous obstruction, and tricuspid insufficiency. Also, the postoperative decrease in right ventricular function supports efforts to surgically correct the transposition of the great arteries with the use of the left ventricle as the systemic ventricle.[113] Options to the Mustard operation are the Senning operation[79, 145, 163] and the switching of the great vessels with or without transplanting the coronary arteries. With the Senning operation, or a modification of it,[140, 164] repair is by intra-atrial correction (Fig 6–72).

Although arrhythmias and venous obstruction apparently seem to occur less frequently with the Senning repair than with the Mustard operation, the work load of the systemic circulation is still supplied by the right ventricle.

In transposition of the great arteries with pulmonary stenosis and ventricular septal defect, repair according to the method of Mustard usually gives poor results, partly because of the inability to adequately relieve the pulmonary stenosis. The Rastelli operation[148, 167] is the operation of choice in these patients. Because the results are better in older children, one usually prefers to wait at least until the patient is 2 to 3 years old, or preferably 4 to 5 years old. (If the child requires surgery before that age, a systemic–pulmonary artery shunt is used to increase the pulmonary blood flow.) Hypothermia

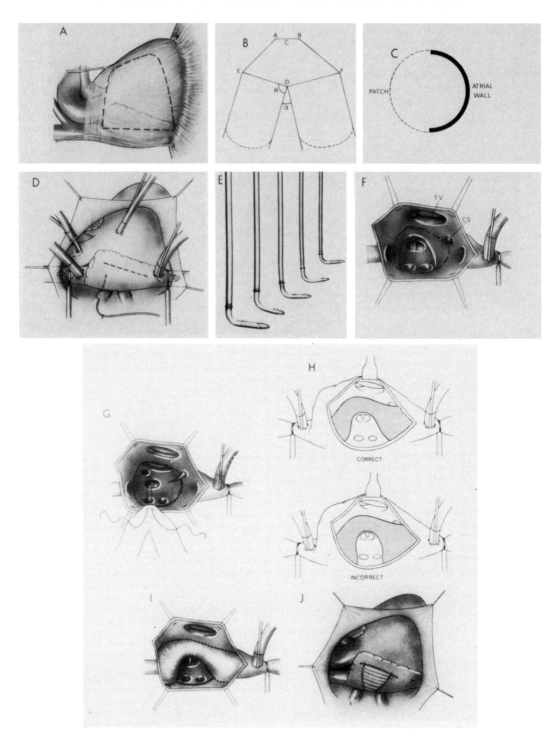

Fig 6–70.—**A** and **B**, after pericardium is excised, it is cut into a kind of trouser shape. Note that excision of pericardial patch has to be done carefully to prevent damage to phrenic nerves. **C**, the newly formed pathway comprises at least 50% of circumference of atrial wall. **D**, arterial and venous cannulas are placed, as are a right ventricular vent and left atrial pressure line. **E**,

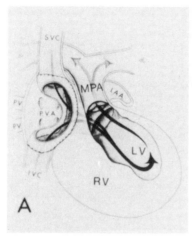 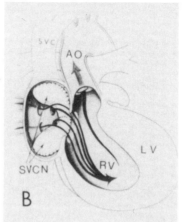

Fig 6–71.—Circulation pathways of systemic (**A**) and pulmonary venous return (**B**) after intra-atrial patch repair. Pulmonary veins *(PV)*; pulmonary venous atrium *(PVA)*; right/left ventricle *(R/LV)*; main pulmonary artery *(MPA)*; inferior/superior vena cava *(I/SVC)*; systemic venous baffle conduit *(SVCN)*; aorta *(AO)*; left atrial appendage *(LAA)*. (From Paul.[144] Used by permission.)

to between 20 and 25 C and a cold cardioplegic solution are used. The right atrium is opened (Fig 6–73,A) so that the atrial septum can be inspected and an atrial septal defect or a patent foramen ovale can be closed. The position of the ventricular septal defect and papillary muscles is checked to determine whether the anatomy is suitable for the Rastelli repair. A right ventriculotomy is done. If necessary, the ventricular septal defect is enlarged to ensure a wide outflow from the left ventricle to the aorta (Fig 6–73,B). The pulmonary valve is sutured closed, and the pulmonary artery is doubly ligated above the valve (Fig 6–73,C). A large patch of Teflon is sutured around the ventricular septal defect to connect the left ventricle to the aorta (Fig 6–73,D). Next, the pulmonary artery is opened widely at the bifurcation, so that a large anastomosis with the valved conduit can be performed (Fig 6–73,E). Finally, the proximal end of the conduit is sutured to the right ventricle (Fig 6–73,F).

Postoperative complications include bleeding from the porous Dacron conduit, which can be decreased by preclotting the conduit. Residual defects of the ventricular septum have been frequent. Aneurysm of the right ventricle, compression or obstruction of the conduit, and obstruction of the newly constructed left ventricular outflow tract have been described. Usually, the left ventricular wall is well developed and postoperative cardiac output is adequate.

As mentioned previously, intra-atrial correction of transposition of the great arteries is accompanied by problems. Therefore, the logical solution to correction of transposition of the great arteries is by switching the great arteries, and this technique has been used by a few centers for several years.[8, 13, 45, 93, 187]

A modification[8] of the switching of the great vessels described by Jatene is performed at our institution. The pulmonary artery and aorta are transected, the latter distal to the ostia of the coronary arteries, and an aortopulmonary win-

---

different sizes of Rygg cannulas are used for venous cannulation. **F,** interrupted line is line of excision of interatrial septum. Tricuspid valve *(TV)*; coronary sinus *(CS)*. **G,** patch is sutured in place. **H,** correct and incorrect placement of interatrial patch. Lower and upper suture lines should diverge to avoid obstruction of pulmonary venous return. **I,** completed patch. Caval and coronary sinus returns enter the left atrium, while the pulmonary veins drain in the right atrium. **J,** Dacron patch is frequently necessary for enlargement of pulmonary venous (right) atrium. (From Stark J.: Mustard's operation for transposition of the great arteries, in Jackson J.W. [ed.]: *Operative Surgery: Cardiothoracic Surgery.* London, Butterworth & Co., 1978. Used by permission.)

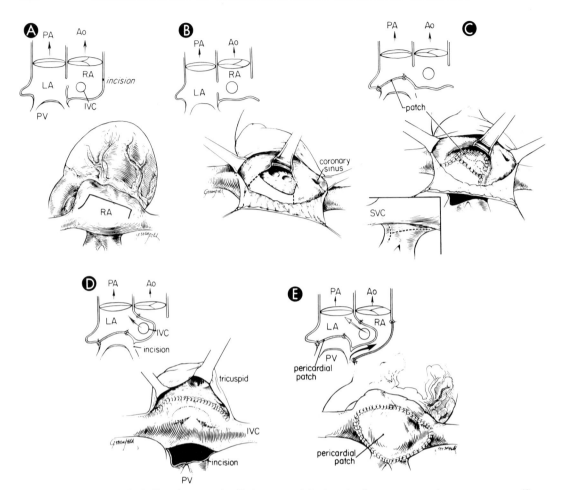

Fig 6–72.—Modified Senning repair. Pulmonary artery *(PA)*; aorta *(Ao)*; left atrium *(LA)*; right atrium *(RA)*; pulmonary vein *(PV)*; inferior and superior venae cavae *(IVC and SVC)*. **A,** right atrium is incised. **B,** atrial septum (often supplemented with Gore-Tex patch or pericardial patch—modified Senning—because atrial septum is often deficient by previous balloon atrial septostomy or Blalock-Hanlon) is sewn between left pulmonary vein orifices and the mitral valve. **C,** to increase mobility of septal flap, left atrium is first incised posterior to interatrial groove. Later on, right atrial wall will be sutured in here, thus connecting newly created pulmonary venous outflow area with right atrium. **D,** next, right atrial wall flap is sutured at its superior angle from crista terminalis, over superior vena cava orifice, via remnant of distal part of intra-atrial septum to free edge of the eustachian valve, thus creating pathway from venae cavae through mitral valve and left ventricle into pulmonary artery reaching lungs. Coronary sinus is left to drain with oxygenated pulmonary venous blood. **E,** remnant of atrial wall, in small infants often enlarged by insertion of pericardial patch, is sutured to incision site previously made posterior to interatrial groove (see **C**). Blood coming from pulmonary veins will now flow through this newly created space underneath the enlarged right atrial wall, through tricuspid valve and right ventricle into aorta. (From Otero Coto et al.[140] Used by permission.)

dow is created. Next, a pericardial patch is sutured to the posterior wall of the artery coming from the right ventricle (previously the aorta), such that a tunnel is made connecting the aortopulmonary window with both coronary artery ostia. Consequently, the coronary arteries will receive well-oxygenated blood from the left ventricle by way of the aortopulmonary window and pericardial tunnel. The next step is the switching of the great arteries. To enable end-to-end

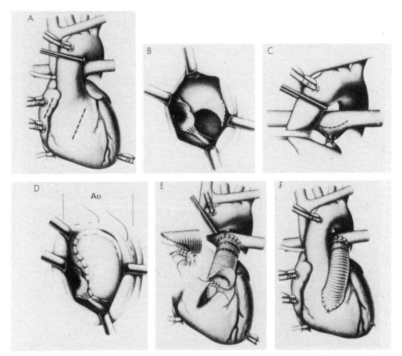

Fig 6–73.—Rastelli operation (see text for details). (From Stark J.: The Rastelli operation, in *Operative Surgery: Cardiothoracic Surgery*. London, Butterworth & Co., 1978. Used by permission.)

anastomosis of the proximal end of the aorta with the pulmonary artery, incorporation of a pericardial patch is necessary in order to increase the circumference of the new pulmonary trunk. Another method of switching the great arteries without relocation of coronary arteries is also performed (Fig 6–74). The pulmonary artery is transected, and the proximal end is anastomosed to the posterior aspect of the aorta. A valved conduit is placed between the distal pulmonary arteriotomy site and the right ventricle. Systemic venous blood will reach the lungs via the right atrium, right ventricle, the valved conduit, and the pulmonary arteries. Oxygenated blood from the lungs passes through the left atrium and left ventricle and will reach the aorta via the proximal part of the pulmonary artery. A competent aortic valve (positioned between the right ventricle and the aorta) will prevent backflow from the aorta into the right ventricle, because the greater systemic aortic pressure will keep this valve closed.

Apparently, after a short period of depressed function, the left ventricle can function normally after correction of transposition by switching of the great arteries, but long-term results are not yet available. However, when performed in one session, correction of transposition of the great arteries with an intact interventricular septum is not possible by this method because rapid decrease in left ventricular mass occurs shortly after birth, and the left ventricle soon becomes incapable of supporting the systemic circulation. Therefore, the left ventricle will first have to be redeveloped by the use of pulmonary artery banding, usually performed after a balloon atrial septostomy or an atrial septectomy (Blalock-Hanlon) and infrequently accompanied by a systemic pulmonary artery shunt if the pulmonary perfusion is decreased too much by the banding. In time, surgical correction at the arterial level with or without coronary relocation will be performed in these patients.

In patients with transposition of the great arteries accompanied by other defects that cause a high left ventricular systolic pressure, such as a large ventricular septal defect or subpulmonary stenosis, the left ventricle develops normally and the problem of decreased left ventricular mass, as just mentioned in transposition of

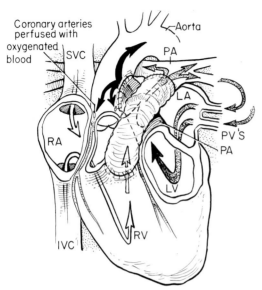

Fig 6–74.—Correction of transposition by switching of great arteries without relocation of coronary arteries. Diagrammatic representation of blood flow after correction. Inferior vena cava *(IVC)*; left atrium *(LA)*; left ventricle *(LV)*; pulmonary artery *(PA)*; pulmonary veins *(PV's)*; right atrium *(RA)*; right ventricle *(RV)*; superior vena cava *(SVC)*. (From Kaye.[93] Used by permission.)

the great arteries with intact ventricular septum, does not develop.

ANESTHETIC MANAGEMENT.—As expected, inhalation induction of anesthesia will be extremely slow because the effective systemic blood flow (blood passing through the lungs that reaches the systemic circulation, see Fig 6–69) is relatively low. The induction time may be decreased by the use of a high concentration of halothane. However, such an attempt is dangerous; when the necessary anesthetic induction concentration is reached in the systemic circulation, the level of anesthesia will deepen further for some time because the concentration of the anesthetic agent in the lungs is high and will continue to slowly increase the systemic level. Although discontinuation of halothane decreases the high concentration of halothane in the pulmonary circulation fairly rapidly, the washout from the systemic circulation will be extremely slow because of the relatively small effective pulmonary blood flow. Because these patients are often severely hypoxemic and frequently acidotic, the heart rate is easily depressed by concentrations of halothane in the systemic circulation, which may be harmless in normal patients and in most other patients with congenital heart disease. The result of this "rapid" inhalation induction is thus a prolonged decrease in cardiac output. With a decrease in cardiac output, the hypoxemia and acidosis increase, followed by a greater decrease in cardiac output, and so forth. If such a situation develops, one should hyperventilate with oxygen (to counteract the metabolic acidosis and to try to wash out the halothane as fast as possible), rapidly insert an intravenous cannula, and administer 2 to 3 mEq/kg bicarbonate diluted in water. Calcium chloride, 10 to 15 mg/kg, may be beneficial and, if necessary, repeated within several minutes, especially in neonates in whom the calcium level may be low. If there is relative hypovolemia secondary to peripheral vasodilatation caused by the acidosis, about 4 ml/kg of 5% dextrose in 2% normal saline should be rapidly infused, followed, if needed, by another 2 to 4 ml/kg.

Determination of arterial blood gases to evaluate the necessity for further administration of bicarbonate is essential. Usually, the fastest way to obtain a sample in this situation is from the femoral artery.

Our method of induction and maintenance of anesthesia in transposition of the great arteries is the following. Neonates are intubated awake after preoxygenation. In severe cyanosis, 100% oxygen is continued with intravenous pancuronium (0.1 mg/kg) and fentanyl slowly (0.5 to 1.0 µg/kg); this regimen can be repeated if necessary. If an intravenous line is not rapidly available for the administration of pancuronium and fentanyl, an intramuscular injection of ketamine (4 to 5 mg/kg) and succinylcholine (2 to 3 mg/kg) can be given to relax the infant temporarily while intravenous and arterial lines are inserted. Halothane may be used for maintenance, but only in low concentration.

In older infants, in whom an intravenous line may be difficult to insert, intramuscular ketamine (4 to 7 mg/kg) is preferred as an induction agent, accompanied by either 50% nitrous oxide or, again, in severely cyanotic children, by 100% oxygen in an attempt to decrease the hypoxic pulmonary vasoconstriction and so maybe slightly improve the oxygenation.

After insertion of an intravenous line, pancuronium (0.1 mg/kg) is administered, accompanied by fentanyl (3 to 5 μg/kg, or more in vigorous children), but this additional medication is rarely necessary after the intramuscular dose of ketamine. The blood pressure is monitored continuously. The child is intubated, an arterial line is inserted, and a second intravenous line and a central venous line are inserted. Anesthesia is maintained by narcotics with 50% nitrous oxide or 100% oxygen. If necessary, halothane in low concentration (0.1% to 0.5%) is added slowly while the blood pressure and pH are closely observed.

Arterial blood gases are checked as soon as possible in all patients with transposition of the great arteries and cyanosis, because metabolic acidosis not only may be already present but also may frequently worsen, despite attempts to give anesthetic agents that have minimal cardiodepressant action. Metabolic acidosis is completely corrected in patients in whom palliative surgery is being performed and also if the negative base excess is more than 5 mEq/L in patients with bypass surgery.

In older children and in infants in whom intravenous lines can be inserted easily, intravenous induction with fentanyl (5 to 25 μg/kg or more) is preferred. The induction is rapid because the pulmonary circulation is nearly completely bypassed by the drugs. Maintenance is as described previously.

Bradycardia is a serious dysrhythmia in the cyanotic infant with transposition of the great arteries and should be treated aggressively. Administration of anesthetic agents is discontinued, and 100% oxygen is given.

Usually, mild bradycardia will react favorably to atropine (0.02 mg/kg), but severe bradycardia, often based on hypoxemia and accompanied by a considerable decrease in cardiac output, may necessitate the administration of epinephrine in doses of 1 to 3 μg/kg (repeated if improvement does not rapidly occur, for which sodium bicarbonate, 1 to 2 mEq/kg, should be given intravenously because metabolic acidosis will develop rapidly and will decrease the efficacy of epinephrine).

Univentricular Heart

Univentricular heart is a congenital defect characterized by one ventricular chamber that receives both the tricuspid and the mitral valves or that has a common atrioventricular valve, with or without an outlet chamber.[43, 52] The entity can be divided into four types according to van Praagh's classification (Fig 6–75).

Type A is the classic single ventricle with a rudimentary outlet chamber. The single ventricle is composed of left ventricular myocardium, whereas the outflow chamber is composed of right ventricular myocardium. In type B, the ventricle is formed entirely of right ventricular myocardium. In type C, the common ventricular chamber is composed of approximately equal portions of right and left myocardia, with a rudimentary ventricular septum at the apex of the heart. No outlet chamber is present. In type D, the ventricle is formed completely from underdeveloped ventricular myocardium.

Subclassification is according to the relationship of the great arteries: I, normal relationship; II, regular transposition (aorta anterior); and III, L-transposition, with the aorta anterior and to the left, originating from a leftward outlet chamber.

Associated anomalies are common, such as transposition of the great arteries, aortic or pulmonary stenosis or atresia, dextrocardia,

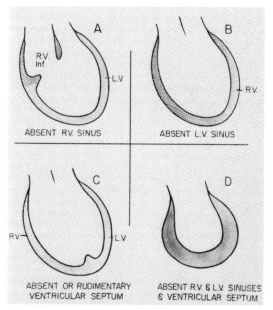

Fig 6–75.—Van Praagh classification of single ventricle. *Crosshatched portions* represent right ventricular *(RV)* myocardium, while *smooth print* represents left ventricular *(LV)* myocardium. (From Edie R.N., et al.: Surgical repair of single ventricle. *J. Thorac. Cardiovasc. Surg.* 66:350, 1973. Used by permission.)

asplenia, atrioventricular canal, atrial septal defect, and coarctation of the aorta.

Patients seen initially without obstruction to pulmonary blood flow have features of a large left-to-right shunt,[58] an elevated pulmonary blood flow, usually an enlarged left atrium, and symptoms of heart failure. There is no or minimal cyanosis; however, when pulmonary vascular obstructive disease develops, cyanosis becomes evident. In pulmonary obstruction, the amount of pulmonary blood flow determines the degree of cyanosis. Usually, no heart failure is present. Bronchial collateral flow may develop.

The infant with a single ventricle and severely reduced pulmonary blood flow will need a systemic–pulmonary artery anastomosis, while infants with excessive pulmonary blood flow and heart failure may need intensive medical treatment and pulmonary artery banding. Total correction should be delayed until significant disability develops because of the generally poor or undefined result of operation. However, waiting too long may increase the risk or create secondary, irreversible changes in the pulmonary vasculature.

The anesthetic management is as usual for the patient with a (potential) right-to-left shunt. Prevention of systemic vasodilation and cardiac depression is important. Because of the unpredictable position of the conduction system and the danger of damaging this system when the ventricular septum is sutured, intracardiac mapping is valuable in preventing postoperative arrhythmias or complete heart block.

A systemic pulmonary artery shunt is clamped before bypass is started. Initially, the temperature is lowered to 30 C during bypass to enable the surgeon to locate the intraventricular conduction system while the heart is beating in sinus rhythm.[115]

Next, the child is cooled to between 20 and 25 C. The aorta is cross-clamped, and a cold cardioplegic solution is injected. The injection of solution is repeated approximately every 20 minutes, or sooner if electrical myocardial activity returns.

One method of surgical repair is by septation of the ventricle. This procedure is basically as follows[126]: A longitudinal ventriculotomy is made in the anticipated plane of the ventricular septal patch, avoiding large coronary arteries. The prosthetic septum (intracardiac knitted Teflon) is then sutured in place. In the absence of pulmonary stenosis, the septum is placed between the semilunar valves, with care being taken not to injure the bundle of His (Fig 6–76,A). If pulmonary stenosis is present, resection and reconstruction of the pulmonary outflow tract usually are contraindicated because of the location of the proximal conduction bundle and of a major coronary artery. Repair is accomplished by suturing the prosthetic septum to the right of both semilunar valves, combined with transection of the pulmonary artery, closure of the proximal part of the pulmonary artery, and insertion of a valved conduit between the right-sided chamber and the distal part of the pulmonary artery (Fig 6–76,B).

In addition to this septation type of repair of a univentricular heart with two atrioventricular valves, associated defects should be corrected when indicated, such as replacement of abnormal atrioventricular valves, atrioventricular annuloplasty, repair of atrial septal defect, and so forth.

In a univentricular heart with a common atrioventricular valve, the interatrial septum is corrected in such a way that there remains no open connection between the right atrium and the ventricle. The pulmonary artery is transected, the proximal side is closed, and the distal part is connected via a (valved) conduit with the appendix of the right atrium (a modified Fontan procedure[68]). This approach is currently preferred also for any patient with univentricular heart and pulmonary stenosis in whom the pulmonary vascular resistance is not significantly elevated.

Inadequate cardiac performance frequently necessitates the use of inotropic agents while the patient is coming off bypass and for several days after operation. Postoperative bleeding is frequently increased as a result of the considerable amount of prosthetic material used. Fresh-frozen plasma and platelets are administered routinely to these patients. Residual ventricular shunt or atrioventricular regurgitation may necessitate reoperation for congestive heart failure. Heart block requires permanent pacing.

Ebstein's Anomaly

In Ebstein's anomaly (Fig 6–77), the frequently hypoplastic septal and posterior leaflets of the tricuspid valve are displaced downward, while the anterior leaflet forms a deep curtain-

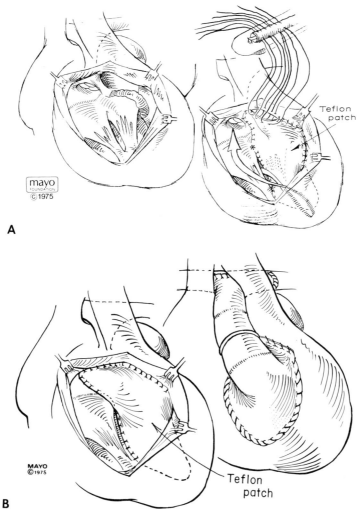

Fig 6–76.—**A,** type AIII univentricular heart (right ventricular outlet chamber and levotransposition). Superior edge of septation patch is sutured between semilunar valves and thus separates pulmonary and systemic flow pathways. **B,** in presence of pulmonary stenosis, septation patch is placed to right of both semilunar valves, creating double-outlet left ventricle. Next, main pulmonary artery is divided, and proximal part is oversewn, followed by placement of valved conduit between right ventriculotomy and distal part of main pulmonary artery.

like structure extending from the annulus fibrosus to the papillary muscle of the right ventricle.[7, 68, 188] Sometimes, however, this leaflet is also partially adherent to the wall. This downward displacement of the tricuspid valve partitions the right ventricle into a proximal, thin-walled atrialized portion and a small distal chamber. The malformed and, in a kind of spiral line, inferiorly displaced leaflets may result in variable obstruction and insufficiency. The right atrium and the atrialized portion of the right ventricle may become enlarged as a result. Both the obstruction and the insufficiency of the abnormal valve may increase right atrial pressure, resulting in a right-to-left shunt if an open foramen ovale or atrial septal defect is present. The neonate, with an increased pulmonary vascular pressure, may be intensely cyanotic; the cyanosis decreases spontaneously during the subsequent weeks of life.

Other lesions associated with Ebstein's anomaly are ostium primum defect, ventricular septal

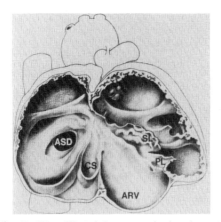

Fig 6–77.—Ebstein's anomaly is characterized by abnormal, displaced tricuspid valve in which posterior and often medial leaflet are not attached in normal way to annulus fibrosus but rather to ventricular wall near apex. Anterior leaflet, which originates at annulus, either may be seen as a loose, curtain-like structure inserting at papillary muscle of right ventricle or—as occurs in most cases—may be attached to ventricular wall to greater or lesser degree (see Fig 6–78). As a result, upper part of right ventricle is incorporated into right atrium. Annulus fibrosus divides original atrium from atrialized ventricle part, the wall of which is often as thin as that of the atrium. Consequently, right ventricular cavity is small and comprises only apical portion and outflow tract. Frequently, considerable regurgitation is present through tricuspid valve; stenosis is rare. In about 75% of patients, either open foramen ovale or atrial septal defect is present. Septal leaflet *(SL)*; posterior leaflet *(PL)*; atrial septal defect *(ASD)*; coronary sinus *(CS)*; and atrialized right ventricle *(ARV)*. (From Netter F.H.: *The Ciba Collection of Medical Illustrations.* Vol. 5: *Heart.* Edited by Yonkman F. F. Summit, N.J., Ciba Pharmaceutical Co., 1969. Used by permission.)

defect, pulmonary atresia, pulmonary stenosis, patent ductus arteriosus, and hypoplastic aorta.

The variability of the tricuspid valve anomaly and the involvement of the right ventricle determine the severity of the right-sided heart failure and the right-to-left shunt if an atrial septal defect is present.

The degree of impairment of right ventricular function depends considerably on the extent to which the right ventricular inflow portion is atrialized and whether the wall in that area has become extremely thin or has remained almost normal, except for the redundant valve leaflets, which are superficially adherent to the trabeculae carneae (Fig 6–78).

Most patients with Ebstein's anomaly can be managed medically. However, surgical intervention is indicated in patients with moderate-to-severe cyanosis, paradoxical emboli, and right ventricular outflow obstruction and in patients in functional classes III and IV.

Atrial and ventricular dysrhythmias are common in Ebstein's malformation and are frequently difficult to manage medically.[31, 44] Sudden death may result from ventricular fibrillation. The Wolff-Parkinson-White syndrome, which is often associated with Ebstein's anomaly, can be treated surgically.

Surgical treatment of Ebstein's anomaly[44, 121, 151] depends largely on the anatomy of the abnormal valve, which may vary greatly among patients, and the surgeon has to decide at operation which repair is indicated for that specific patient.

In the presence of an adequate-sized anterior leaflet, plication of the free wall of the atrialized portion of the right ventricle, posterior tricuspid annuloplasty, reduction of the size of the right atrium, and patch graft of the atrial septal defect has given good results (Fig 6–79). If this procedure is not possible, replacement of the tricuspid valve or repair by a modified Fontan procedure is the other option. In patients with this anomaly, the anesthesiologist must be aware of the propensity to arrhythmias and the potentially lethal outcome. In patients with histories of ventricular arrhythmias, a lidocaine drip should be started before induction and should

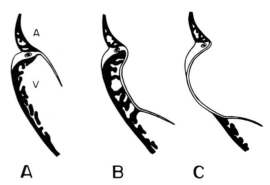

Fig 6–78.—Section through right atrioventricular junction. **A**, normal heart (*A*, right atrium; *V*, right ventricle). **B**, mild Ebstein's anomaly. **C**, severe Ebstein's anomaly. (From van Mierop et al.[177] Used by permission.)

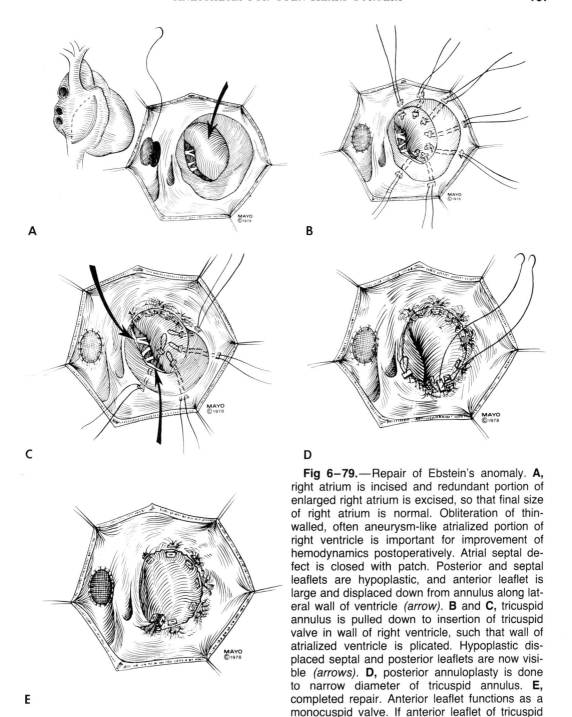

Fig 6–79.—Repair of Ebstein's anomaly. **A,** right atrium is incised and redundant portion of enlarged right atrium is excised, so that final size of right atrium is normal. Obliteration of thin-walled, often aneurysm-like atrialized portion of right ventricle is important for improvement of hemodynamics postoperatively. Atrial septal defect is closed with patch. Posterior and septal leaflets are hypoplastic, and anterior leaflet is large and displaced down from annulus along lateral wall of ventricle *(arrow)*. **B** and **C,** tricuspid annulus is pulled down to insertion of tricuspid valve in wall of right ventricle, such that wall of atrialized ventricle is plicated. Hypoplastic displaced septal and posterior leaflets are now visible *(arrows)*. **D,** posterior annuloplasty is done to narrow diameter of tricuspid annulus. **E,** completed repair. Anterior leaflet functions as a monocuspid valve. If anterior leaflet of tricuspid valve is too small or abnormal, valve replacement may be necessary, although the success rate has not been encouraging.

be continued during and after surgery, while the use of any agent that may sensitize the myocardium to catecholamines is avoided.

Tachycardia, which enhances tricuspid insufficiency[177] and increases the right-to-left shunt, should be prevented. Atropine should not be used for premedication, especially in patients with the Wolff-Parkinson-White syndrome. After cardiopulmonary bypass is started, in patients with Wolff-Parkinson-White syndrome, electrophysiologic mapping is performed. The perfusate temperature is temporarily maintained at 30 C to keep the heart beating while the specialized conduction tissue is mapped. When the anomalous accessory bundle of Kent is detected and cut, the perfusate temperature is reduced. When the nasopharyngeal temperature is 20 to 25 C, the aorta is cross-clamped and a cardioplegic solution is infused. The infusion of the cardioplegic solution is repeated if necessary during surgery. At the end of the repair, the atrium is closed and epicardial electrodes are routinely inserted.

If surgical repair has been successful, the patient usually comes off bypass without the help of inotropic drugs, though dopamine may be beneficial. Because life-threatening arrhythmias usually occur suddenly and without warning, prophylactic antiarrhythmic drugs should be administered in adequate amounts. In our institution, lidocaine is given intravenously on a routine basis for at least 48 hours after surgery, after which treatment is continued with oral procainamide.

Total Anomalous Pulmonary Venous Connections

In total anomalous pulmonary venous connections (TAPVCs), the blood coming from the lungs enters the right atrium, where it mixes with the venous blood from the peripheral circulation.[53, 107] Some of this mixture will shunt to the left atrium through a defect in the atrial septum, which has to be present in this condition to make life possible. The blood then passes through the left ventricle and enters the peripheral circulation, where the partially saturated blood produces cyanosis. The rest of the blood from the right atrium will follow the normal pathway to the lungs. Usually, the aorta, left atrium, and ventricle are smaller (but adequate) than the dilated pulmonary artery and hypertrophied and dilated right atrium and ventricle. There are four different types of TAPVC, based on the location of the entrance of the pulmonary veins into the systemic veins or right atrium:

In the supracardiac type (Fig 6–80,A), or type I, which is the most frequent type, the common pulmonary venous trunk drains into the left innominate vein through an anomalous vertical vein. Less frequently, the pulmonary veins drain straight into the superior vena cava.

In the cardiac type (Fig 6–80,B and C), or type II, the site of connection is usually located in the posteroinferior portion of the right atrium, where the pulmonary veins, draining separately, enter the right atrium (Fig 6–80,C). Another variation is the pulmonary veins joining a common trunk, which connects to the coronary sinus and follows its normal course to the right atrium (Fig 6–80,B).

In the infracardiac type (Fig 6–80,D), or type III, the pulmonary veins from both lungs join immediately behind the left atrium. A common trunk originates from the confluence, descends immediately anterior to the esophagus, penetrates the diaphragm through the esophageal hiatus, and joins the portal vein. Less often, the anomalous trunk connects to the ductus venosus, the hepatic vein, or the inferior vena cava.

In type IV, anomalous connections are present at two or more of the above-described locations.

The presence of associated cardiac anomalies or of obstruction to pulmonary venous drainage may worsen the hemodynamic situation. External obstruction in type III, where the anomalous vein traverses the diaphragm, is frequent. Also, if this vessel joins the ductus venosus, which normally undergoes constriction, pulmonary venous obstruction results. Obstruction of the pulmonary venous flow also may occur in type I, if the vertical vein ascends (Fig 6–81) between (and is compressed by) the left main pulmonary artery and the left main-stem bronchus. A narrow atrial septal defect also will obstruct the blood flowing from the pulmonary veins via the right atrium into the left atrium. Associated cardiac anomalies, which are present in about one third of patients with TAPVC, are single ventricle, truncus arteriosus, transposition of the great arteries, pulmonary atresia, and coarctation of the aorta.

Soon after birth, when the pulmonary vascu-

The vertical vein is ligated, and anastomosis is performed after an incision is made in the long axis of the retrocardiac vein and in the left atrium (Fig 6–82). A right atriotomy is done, and the defect in the atrial septum is closed. At times, the anastomosis is performed via the right and left atria from an anterior approach.

Repair of the cardiac type depends on whether the venous return is directly in the right atrium (for which the atrial septum is excised and a prosthetic septum is sutured in such a way that the pulmonary return is located on the left side of the atrial septum) or whether the pulmonary venous return is via the coronary sinus (Fig 6–83). In the latter condition, after incision of the right atrium, the septum between the coronary sinus and the defect in the atrial septum is excised, and a tunnel is created; a Dacron patch is used such that blood coming from the anomalous pulmonary vein remains on the left side of the atrial septum. Usually, the patch can be placed so that the coronary vein still enters the right atrium; however, if this is not possible, the impact of this desaturated blood on the systemic saturation is not of any importance.

For the repair of the infracardiac type, the apex of the heart is elevated to expose the retrocardiac vein, which runs in a vertical direction (Fig 6–84). The descending vertical vein is ligated at the diaphragm and transected if necessary. A transverse incision is made in the posterior left atrium, and an anastomosis is

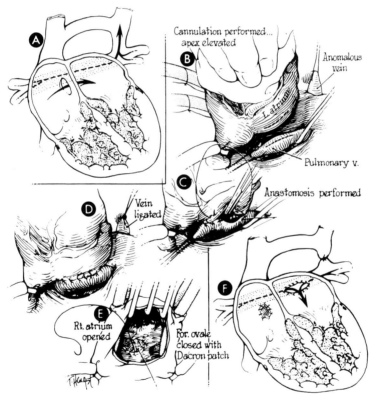

Fig 6–82.—Repair of supracardiac type of total anomalous pulmonary venous connections. **A,** anatomy before repair. In **B,** patient is on bypass and the heart is gently retracted anteriorly. Total circulatory arrest is preferred in small infants, while in older children, great care has to be taken not to obstruct pulmonary venous return during this procedure. In **C,** anastomosis is made between retrocardiac transverse pulmonary venous trunk and left atrium. In **D,** the vertical vein, connecting pulmonary venous circulation with systemic venous circulation, is ligated. In **E,** foramen ovale or atrial septal defect is closed via incision in right atrium. **F** depicts anatomy after repair. (From Cooley and Wukasch.[39] Used by permission.)

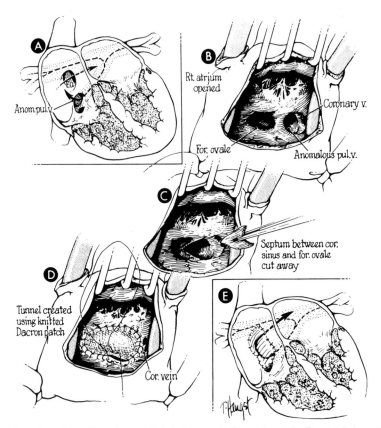

Fig 6–83.—Repair of cardiac type of total anomalous pulmonary venous connections. **A** shows anatomy before repair. In **B**, right atrium is opened and position of coronary sinus and anomalous pulmonary vein is visualized. In **C**, septum between coronary sinus and foramen ovale is excised. In **D**, patch is sutured such that blood from anomalous pulmonary vein is directed into left atrium. Frequently, entrance of coronary vein into right atrium is preserved. **E** shows anatomy after repair. (From Cooley and Wukasch.[39] Used by permission.)

performed between the retrocardiac trunk and the left atrium.

After repair, the usual intra-atrial pressure monitor lines and pacemaker wires are inserted. Frequently, depending on the preoperative condition, these patients need inotropic drugs when coming off bypass.

Postoperatively, mechanical ventilation with positive end-expiratory pressure, followed by spontaneous respiration with continuous positive airway pressure for several days, usually helps improve the lung function in infants with TAPVC and pulmonary edema. Fluid administration is initially kept low (atrial pressures approximately 10 mm Hg) while an adequate urinary output and cardiac output are being maintained. To improve cardiac output,[61] inotropic agents are preferred instead of increasing the ventricular filling pressures.

The results of surgical correction of TAPVC, with an early mortality of at least 30%, are not as favorable as one wishes, although recent results have shown some improvement.[53,91,117] The causes of death include low cardiac output, pulmonary edema, persistent pulmonary venous obstruction with severe postoperative pulmonary hypertension, sudden cardiac arrest, heart block, and respiratory insufficiency. The relatively small size of the left atrium has been blamed for the decreased cardiac output, although this is controversial, because the repair frequently involves an increase in size of the left atrium.[91,117]

duction disturbances such as atrioventricular dissociation, right bundle-branch block (sometimes associated with a left anterior hemiblock), and trifascicular block occur frequently and may develop even years after surgery. Patients with right bundle-branch block and premature ventricular contractions or with trifascicular block are especially at an increased risk for sudden death.[146, 168]

Tricuspid Atresia

Besides the absence of a direct communication between the right atrium and the right ventricle caused by the agenesis of the tricuspid valve, other defects are present in tricuspid atresia[157]: an interatrial defect, a communication between the systemic and the pulmonary artery circulations—usually a ventricular septal defect—and hypoplasia of the right ventricle.

The associated lesions determine the classification (Fig 6-60) of tricuspid atresia (Table 6-11).

An adequate atrial septal defect is necessary because the entire venous return must pass through the atrial septum. If the atrial septal defect is small, the systemic venous pressure is high and imitates the clinical pattern of right heart failure.

The amount of pulmonary blood flow determines whether the patient is seen initially with cyanosis or with heart failure. Patients with tricuspid atresia and diminished or normal pulmonary blood flow (types IA and B, IIA and B, III) are cyanotic and develop polycythemia and its consequences. Hypoxic spells are frequent. Hypoxic spells usually occur in children who are less than 6 months old and who have diminished pulmonary blood flow.[153] These spells are similar to the hypoxic spells seen in infants with tetralogy of Fallot—a warning indicating critically low pulmonary flow and an urgent need for surgery. Because of the relatively low pulmonary blood flow in types IA and IB, IIA and IIB, and III, only a small volume of oxygenated blood is present in the left atrium to mix with the venous return coming from the right atrium. Therefore, the systemic saturation is decreased (may range between 60% and 80%), and the patients are cyanotic. Since complete mixing is achieved in the left atrium, the saturations of the left atrium, right and left ventricles, pulmonary artery, and systemic artery are essentially identical. The degree of hypoxemia is dependent on the pulmonary-to-systemic artery flow ratio. If hypoxemia is severe, metabolic acidosis is present.

The infant born with tricuspid atresia and diminished pulmonary blood flow may need emergency surgery soon after birth. If the atrial septal defect is not sufficient, a balloon septostomy according to the method of Rashkind is done after catheterization. The threatening closure of the patent ductus makes surgery urgent. An infusion with prostaglandin E_1 (about 0.1 µg/kg/minute) may delay closure of the ductus temporarily, while preparations are made for surgery. Correction of the metabolic acidosis and increase of the inspired oxygen concentration—aiming for a PaO_2 of about 40 mm Hg—may decrease hypoxic pulmonary vasoconstriction without the risk that a higher PaO_2 may hasten the closure of the ductus and therefore endanger the child.

In infants less than 3 months of age, the creation of a systemic-to-pulmonary artery shunt (Waterston or an end-to-side anastomosis with a Gore-Tex shunt between the subclavian and a pulmonary artery may be indicated because at that age the diameter of a Blalock-Taussig shunt may not be sufficient to keep the shunt open) is

TABLE 6-11.—CLASSIFICATION OF TRICUSPID ATRESIA

I. Normally related great arteries
  A. Intact ventricular septum with pulmonary atresia and ductus arteriosus.
  B. Small ventricular septal defect, pulmonary stenosis. This is the most common type. The pulmonary artery is hypoplastic and the right ventricle small.
  C. Medium-large ventricular septal defect, normal pulmonary valve and pulmonary artery.
II. D-transposition of the great arteries
  A. Large ventricular septal defect, pulmonary atresia. The aorta arises from the right ventricle, which has a ventricular wall thicker than in type I. The ductus arteriosus is patent.
  B. Large ventricular septal defect, pulmonary stenosis, and overriding aorta.
  C. Usually large ventricular septal defect, large pulmonary artery. The right ventricular infundibular stenosis frequently reduces the systemic blood flow, which also may be reduced by aortic coarctation or hypoplasia, which are commonly associated with this type.
III. Tricuspid atresia with L-transposition. This type is very rare and has been described in association with subpulmonary and subaortic stenosis.

usually performed to improve the critically low pulmonary blood flow. The major disadvantage of the Waterston shunt is that it often tends to become too large. Excessive pulmonary blood flow may result, with the eventual development of pulmonary vascular hypertension, which makes a future surgical correction by creating a right atrial–right ventricular or atrial-pulmonary artery connection impossible.

In an infant between 3 months and 1 year of age, the Blalock-Taussig shunt is preferred. From 1 year to about 4 years, either a Blalock-Taussig or a Glenn shunt is performed, and from about 4 years on definitive repair with a modified Fontan correction is the operation of choice.[64] Recently, the latter approach also has been performed successfully in infants.

In contrast to patients with decreased pulmonary blood flow, patients belonging to types IC and IIC—those with excessive pulmonary blood flow—develop heart failure and later develop pulmonary arterial hypertension and pulmonary vascular disease. Pulmonary artery banding is frequently necessary for patients with type IIC, while the ventricular septal defect of the patients with type IC tends to decrease in size. Therefore, this type may convert spontaneously to type IB, with a decreased instead of an excessive pulmonary blood flow. Requirements for a definitive (Fontan) repair are as follows: (1) a normal pulmonary vascular resistance and a mean pulmonary artery pressure less than 20 mm Hg; (2) adequate-sized main and branch pulmonary arteries; (3) normal left heart with good left ventricular function (left ventricular end-diastolic pressure less than 10 mm Hg); and (4) preferably a normal sinus rhythm.

In the absence of pulmonary vascular obstructive disease, a successful result depends greatly on an adequate gradient between the right and the left atrium. This gradient is the driving pressure for pulmonary flow. With normal or low left atrial pressure, the right atrial pressure may not be greatly elevated postoperatively.

In the presence of pulmonary vascular obstructive disease or left ventricular dysfunction, the Fontan operation is contraindicated because the pressure that the right atrium would have to overcome would be too high. The presence of sinus rhythm, creating an "atrial kick" (thus lowering the left atrial pressure and producing a pulsatile pulmonary flow) is also important for a good outcome of this operation.

The original procedure performed by Fontan[63] is as follows: The superior vena cava is anastomosed to the distal end of the right pulmonary artery, according to the Glenn procedure, with a side-to-end anastomosis. Then, an end-to-end anastomosis is done from the right atrial appendage to the proximal end of the right pulmonary artery by means of an aortic valve homograft. Next, the patient is placed on bypass, the right atrium is incised, and the atrial septal defect is closed. A pulmonary valve homograft is inserted where the inferior vena cava enters the right atrium (Fig 6–61). The right atrium is closed. At the end of the bypass, the cannulas are removed, the superior vena cava is transected at its entry into the right atrium, and both ends are sutured. Also, the main pulmonary artery is ligated (Fig 6–62). In this way, the blood flow from the superior vena cava is led to the right lung and the blood from the inferior vena cava, via an interposed valve in the vena cava (atrial

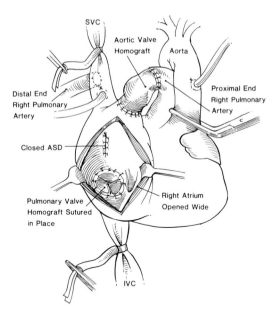

Fig 6–61.—Fontan operation as originally done. Right pulmonary artery is transected, and distal end is connected to superior vena cava *(SVC)*. Proximal end of right pulmonary artery is anastomosed to right atrial appendage by aortic valve homograft. Atrial septal defect *(ASD)* is closed under cardiopulmonary bypass, and pulmonary valve homograft is placed into right atrium at entrance of inferior vena cava *(IVC)*. (Modified from Fontan and Baudet.[63] Used by permission.)

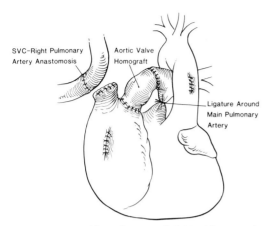

Fig 6–62.—After closure of right atrium, main pulmonary artery is ligated or transected and bypass is discontinued. Next, superior vena cava (SVC) is transected at entry site in right atrium. Blood from superior vena cava will now perfuse right lung, while blood from inferior vena cava will supply left lung. (Modified from Fontan and Baudet.[63] Used by permission.)

junction and another valve between the atrium and the pulmonary artery), will reach the left lung. The valve between the inferior vena cava and the right atrium has proved to be unnecessary, and the need for a valve between the atrium and the pulmonary artery also may be questionable.

Modifications of the Fontan operation are performed instead of the original repair: Evolving from Kreutzer's[101] variation (who connected the right atrium with the pulmonary artery by a valved homograft of the pulmonary artery while omitting the anastomosis between the superior vena cava and the right pulmonary artery, as well as the inferior vena cava allograft), repair is now performed by using a valved conduit that connects the appendage of the right atrium directly to the pulmonary artery (Fig 6–63).

Another variation is the placement of a nonvalved conduit between the right atrial appendage and the right ventricular outlet chamber, if of adequate size (Fig 6–64). In this procedure, the ventricular septal defect has to be closed.

Another modification is to connect the atrial appendage directly to the right ventricular outflow tract, if necessary with the help of a pericardial patch sutured to the right atrium and right ventricle to complete the anastomosis (Fig 6–65). If a Glenn procedure has not been performed (contrary to the anatomy depicted in Fig 6–65), the situation will be as follows: From the inferior and superior venae cavae, blood will flow through the right atrium (atrial septal defect is closed) via the newly formed anastomosis into the right ventricular outflow tract (ventricular septal defect is closed). From there, the blood follows the usual pathway through the pulmonary valve into the main pulmonary artery and perfuses both lungs.

A previously performed Glenn anastomosis is left in place (as in Fig 6–65). However, previously performed systemic–pulmonary artery shunts have to be discontinued because they are no longer helpful and the right atrial pressure would be increased by the increased flow in the pulmonary circulation caused by such a shunt. It is important to remember that the right atrium may serve to some extent as the pumping chamber. Therefore, trauma to the right atrium has to be prevented. Direct vena caval cannulations are performed above and below the right atrium, and no atriotomy or conduit anastomosis to the wall of the right atrium is performed (instead, the appendage is used) so as

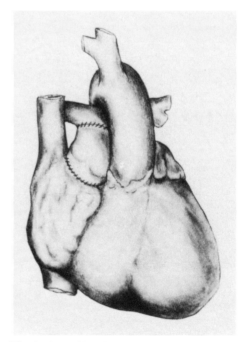

Fig 6–63.—Modification of Fontan operation. Connection of right atrium and distal part of pulmonary artery by a valved conduit. (From Fontan et al.[64] Used by permission.)

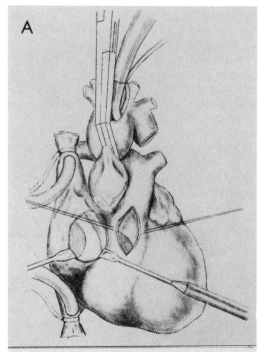

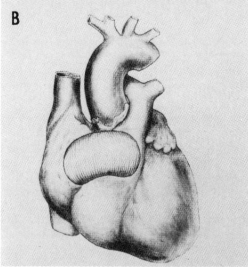

Fig 6-64.—**A** and **B,** connection of right atrium and right ventricular outlet chamber by nonvalved conduit. (From Fontan et al.[64] Used by permission.)

not to interfere with the performance of the atrial muscles or to injure arteries supplying those muscles.

The right atrium needs a generous filling pressure for an adequate performance; therefore, the mean right atrial pressure after operation usually is between 15 and 20 mm Hg, or sometimes higher,[101, 153] while before operation it may have been 5 to 7 mm Hg. Because of this factor, a mild-to-moderate superior vena cava syndrome and hepatomegaly, sometimes accompanied by decreased renal function, tend to develop. Head-up position of the patient is helpful in decreasing the severity of a superior vena cava syndrome.

Inotropic drugs (dopamine, dobutamine, isoproterenol, or epinephrine) are frequently needed postoperatively. Isoproterenol or dobutamine is probably indicated in this situation, because the pulmonary vasodilating effect of these drugs may decrease the right atrial afterload. If arrhythmias are present, great effort has to be made to reestablish a sinus rhythm because it will improve cardiac output considerably. If a pacemaker is necessary, an atrial or a sequential pacemaker is preferred.

After surgery is complete, either spontaneous or intermittent mandatory ventilation is started as soon as possible because positive-pressure ventilation intermittently may increase the resistance to pulmonary blood flow.

D-transposition of the Great Arteries

D-transposition or complete transposition is classified together with several other congenital heart defects under malposition (transposition*) of the great arteries. Besides the malposition of

---

*Instead of transposition, the term "malposition" is preferred because (though infrequently) despite malposition of the great arteries (aorta anterior to the pulmonary artery), the anatomical configuration of the heart is such that the aorta arises from the left ventricle and the pulmonary artery arises from the right. Therefore, the term "transposition" should not be used unless malposition of the great arteries actually occurs together with discordant ventricular–great artery connection, and consequently the aorta arises from the right ventricle and the pulmonary artery from the left ventricle (which is the situation in the great majority of patients with this anomaly). Originally, transposition was used to describe the situation in which the aorta arises from the right ventricle and the pulmonary artery arises from the left ventricle. Because the aorta is anterior to the pulmonary artery in these patients, the term "transposition" became associated with this particular position of the great arteries. However, the situation became confused when patients had concordant ventricular–great artery relationship and the aorta located anterior to the pulmonary artery. Initially, "transposition" continued to be used for these defects. However, the more logical term, "malposition," is now preferred.

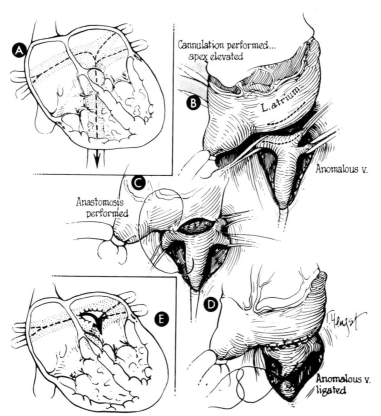

Fig 6–84.—Repair of infracardiac type of total anomalous pulmonary venous connections. **A** shows anatomy before repair. In **B**, the heart is elevated, with same precautions to prevent pulmonary venous obstruction if total circulatory arrest is not used. In **C**, transverse incision is made in anomalous vein behind left atrium and also in left atrium, after which anastomosis is made. **D**, next, anomalous vein distal to anastomosis is ligated. **E** shows anatomy after repair. (From Cooley and Wukasch.[39] Used by permission.)

REFERENCES

1. Aberdeen E.: Blalock-Hanlon operation and Rashkind procedure, in Rob C., Smith R. (eds.): *Operative Surgery*. Vol. 2: *Thorax*, ed. 2. London, Butterworth & Co., 1968, p. 193.
2. Aberdeen E.: The Waterston operation: Ascending aorta–right pulmonary artery anastomosis, in Rob C., Smith R. (eds.): *Operative Surgery*. Vol. 2: *Thorax*, ed. 2. London, Butterworth & Co., 1968, p. 234.
3. Aberdeen E.: Transposition of the great arteries, in Sabiston D.C. Jr., Spencer F.C. (eds.): *Gibbon's Surgery of the Chest*, ed. 3. Philadelphia, W.B. Saunders Co., 1976, p. 1092.
4. Akl B.F., et al.: Clinical experience with the activated clotting time for the control of heparin and protamine therapy during cardiopulmonary bypass. *J. Thorac. Cardiovasc. Surg.* 79:97, 1980.
5. Alpert B.S., et al.: Spontaneous closure of small ventricular septal defects: Ten-year follow-up. *Pediatrics* 63:204, 1979.
6. Andersen M.N., Senning Å.: Studies in oxygen consumption during extracorporeal circulation with a pump-oxygenator. *Ann. Surg.* 148:59, 1958.
7. Anderson K.R., et al.: Morphologic spectrum of Ebstein's anomaly of the heart: A review. *Mayo Clin. Proc.* 54:174, 1979.
8. Aubert J., et al.: Transposition of the great arteries: New technique for anatomical correction. *Br. Heart J.* 40:204, 1978.
9. Aziz K.U., Paul M.H., Rowe R.D.: Bronchopulmonary circulation in D-transposition of the great arteries: Possible role in genesis of accelerated pulmonary vascular disease. *Am. J. Cardiol.* 39:432, 1977.

10. Bennett E.J., Dalal F.Y.: Hypotensive anaesthesia for coarctation: A method of prevention of post-operative hypertension. *Anaesthesia* 29:269, 1974.
11. Bennett E.J., et al.: Pancuronium and the neonate. *Br. J. Anaesth.* 47:75, 1975.
12. Betts E.K., et al.: Retrolental fibroplasia and oxygen administration during general anesthesia. *Anesthesiology* 47:518, 1977.
13. Bex J.P., et al.: Anatomical correction of transposition of the great arteries. *Ann. Thorac. Surg.* 29:86, 1980.
14. Bick R.L., Schmalhorst W.R., Arbegast N.R.: Alterations of hemostasis associated with cardiopulmonary bypass. *Thromb. Res.* 8:285, 1976.
15. Bick R.L., et al.: Hemostatic defects induced by cardiopulmonary bypass. *Vasc. Surg.* 9:228, 1975.
16. Black G.W.: Enflurane. *Br. J. Anaesth.* 51:627, 1979.
17. Blalock A., Taussig H.B.: The surgical treatment of malformations of the heart: In which there is pulmonary stenosis or pulmonary atresia. *J.A.M.A.* 128:189, 1945.
18. Bland J.W. Jr., Williams W.H.: Anesthesia for treatment of congenital heart defects, in Kaplan J.A. (ed.): *Cardiac Anesthesia.* New York, Grune & Stratton, 1979, p. 281.
19. Blitt C.D.: Monitoring the circulation in the operating room: Catheterization techniques. 29th Annual Refresher Course Lectures, American Society of Anesthesiologists Annual Meeting, Chicago, October 21 to 25, 1978, 204A/p. 1.
20. Bowie E.J.W., Owen C.A. Jr.: Hemostatic failure in clinical medicine. *Semin. Hematol.* 14:341, 1977.
21. Branthwaite M.A.: *Anaesthesia for Cardiac Surgery and Allied Procedures.* Oxford, England, Blackwell Scientific Publications, 1977, p. 155.
22. Brennan R.W., Patterson R.H. Jr., Kessler J.: Cerebral blood flow and metabolism during cardiopulmonary bypass: Evidence of microemboli encephalopathy. *Neurology* 21:665, 1971.
23. Brewer L.A. III, et al.: Spinal cord complications following surgery for coarctation of the aorta: A study of 66 cases. *J. Thorac. Cardiovasc. Surg.* 64:368, 1972.
24. Brögli H.: Der Mechanismus des sogenannten 'Heparin-Rebound' nach extrakorporellem Kreislauf. *Thromb. Diath. Haemorrh.* 13:401, 1965.
25. Brunberg J.A., Reilly E.L., Doty D.B.: Central nervous system consequences in infants of cardiac surgery using deep hypothermia and circulatory arrest. *Circulation* 50 (suppl. 2):60, 1974.
26. Buckberg G.D.: Left ventricular subendocardial necrosis. *Ann. Thorac. Surg.* 24:379, 1977.
27. Buckberg G.D.: A proposed 'solution' to the cardioplegic controversy, editorial. *J. Thorac. Cardiovasc. Surg.* 77:803, 1979.
28. Bull B.S., et al.: Heparin therapy during extracorporeal circulation: I. Problems inherent in existing heparin protocols. *J. Thorac. Cardiovasc. Surg.* 69:674, 1975.
29. Bull B.S., et al.: Heparin therapy during extracorporeal circulation: II. The use of a dose-response curve to individualize heparin and protamine dosage. *J. Thorac. Cardiovasc. Surg.* 69:685, 1975.
30. Byrne J., et al.: Treatment of patients with transposition of great arteries and pulmonary vascular obstructive disease. *Br. Heart J.* 40:221, 1978.
31. Castaneda A.R., Norwood G.A.: Tricuspid atresia and Ebstein's anomaly, in Ravitch M.M., et al. (eds.): *Pediatric Surgery,* ed. 3. Chicago, Year Book Medical Publishers, 1979, vol. 1, p. 741.
32. Castaneda A.R., et al.: Open-heart surgery during the first three months of life. *J. Thorac. Cardiovasc. Surg.* 68:719, 1974.
33. Christie A.: Normal closing time of the foramen ovale and the ductus arteriosus: An anatomic and statistical study, *Am. J. Dis. Child.* 40:323, 1930.
34. Clark E.B., et al.: Should the sinus venosus type ASD be closed? A review of the atrial conduction defects and surgical results in twenty eight children, abstracted. *Am. J. Cardiol.* 35:127, 1975.
35. Cohn L.H., Morrow A.G., Braunwald E.: Operative treatment of atrial septal defect: Clinical and haemodynamic assessments in 175 patients. *Br. Heart J.* 29:725, 1967.
36. Cole E.R., et al.: The hemostatic mechanism after open-heart surgery: III. Correlation between the appearance of an abnormal protein demonstrated by gel electrophoresis and of an inhibitor of the extrinsic coagulation system (PEC). *Thromb. Haemost.* 39:474, 1978.
37. Cole P.: The safe use of sodium nitroprusside. *Anaesthesia* 33:473, 1978.
38. Collins G., et al.: Ventricular septal defect: Clinical and hemodynamic changes in the first five years of life. *Am. Heart J.* 84:695, 1972.
39. Cooley D.A., Wukasch D.C.: Anomalous pulmonary venous return, in Ravitch M.M., et al. (eds.): *Pediatric Surgery,* ed. 3. Chi-

cago, Year Book Medical Publishers, 1979, vol. 1, p. 659.
40. Dalal F.Y., et al.: Anaesthesia for coarctation: A new classification for rational anaesthetic management. *Anaesthesia* 29:704, 1974.
41. Danielson G.K.: Surgical considerations in congenital heart disease, in Conn H.L. Jr., Horwitz O. (eds.): *Cardiac and Vascular Diseases*. Philadelphia, Lea & Febiger, 1971, vol. 1, p. 686.
42. Danielson G.K.: Endocardial cushion defects, in Ravitch M.M., et al. (eds.): *Pediatric Surgery*, ed. 3. Chicago, Year Book Medical Publishers, 1979, vol. 1, p. 720.
43. Danielson G.K., Giuliani E.R., Ritter D.G.: Successful repair of common ventricle associated with complete atrioventricular canal. *J. Thorac. Cardiovasc. Surg.* 67:152, 1974.
44. Danielson G.K., Maloney J.D., Devloo R.A.E.: Surgical repair of Ebstein's anomaly. *Mayo Clin. Proc.* 54:185, 1979.
45. Danielson G.K., et al.: Great-vessel switch operation without coronary relocation for transposition of great arteries. *Mayo Clin. Proc.* 53:675, 1978.
46. Davey F.R.: Platelets and platelet disorders, in Henry J.B. (ed.): *Clinical Diagnosis and Management by Laboratory Methods*. Philadelphia, W.B. Saunders Co., 1979, p. 1109.
47. Davey F.R.: Blood coagulation and its disorders, in Henry J.B. (ed.): *Clinical Diagnosis and Management by Laboratory Methods*. Philadelphia, W.B. Saunders Co., 1979, p. 1131.
48. De Leval M.R., et al.: Surgical technique to reduce the risks of heart block following closure of ventricular septal defect in atrioventricular discordance. *J. Thorac. Cardiovasc. Surg.* 78:515, 1979.
49. DuShane J.W., Kirklin J.W.: Late results of the repair of ventricular septal defect on pulmonary vascular disease, in Kirklin J.W. (ed.): *Advances in Cardiovascular Surgery*. New York, Grune & Stratton, 1973, p. 9.
50. Ebert P.A., et al.: Pulmonary artery conduits in infants younger than six months of age. *J. Thorac. Cardiovasc. Surg.* 72:351, 1976.
51. Edie R.N., Malm J.R.: Pulmonary atresia with intact ventricular septum, in Sabiston D.C. Jr., Spencer F.C. (eds.): *Gibbon's Surgery of the Chest*, ed. 3. Philadelphia, W.B. Saunders Co., 1976, p. 1138.
52. Edie R.N., Malm J.R.: Single ventricle, in Sabiston D.C. Jr., Spencer F.C. (eds.): *Gibbon's Surgery of the Chest*, ed. 3. Philadelphia, W.B. Saunders Co., 1976, p. 1142.
53. Edmunds L.H. Jr.: Total anomaly of venous return, in Sabiston D.C. Jr., Spencer F.C. (eds.): *Gibbon's Surgery of the Chest*, ed. 3. Philadelphia, W.B. Saunders Co., 1976, p. 1000.
54. Egan E.L., et al.: Effect of surgical operations on certain tests used to diagnose intravascular coagulation and fibrinolysis. *Mayo Clin. Proc.* 49:658, 1974.
55. Eger E.I. II: *Anesthetic Uptake and Action*. Baltimore, Williams & Wilkins Co., 1974, p. 77.
56. Ekert H., Sheers M.: Preoperative and postoperative platelet function in cyanotic congenital heart disease. *J. Thorac. Cardiovasc. Surg.* 67:184, 1974.
57. Ekert H., et al.: Hemostasis in cyanotic congenital heart disease. *J. Pediatr.* 76:221, 1970.
58. Elliott L.P., Bream P.R., Gessner I.H.: Single and common ventricle, in Moss A.J., Adams F.H., Emmanouilides G.C. (eds.): *Heart Disease in Infants, Children, and Adolescents*, ed. 2. Baltimore, Williams & Wilkins Co., 1977, p. 381.
59. Ellis F.H. Jr., et al.: Patent ductus arteriosus with pulmonary hypertension: An analysis of cases treated surgically. *J. Thorac. Surg.* 31:268, 1956.
60. Emmanouilides G.C.: Obstructive lesions of the right ventricle and the pulmonary arterial tree, in Moss A.J., Adams F.H., Emmanouilides G.C. (eds.): *Heart Disease in Infants, Children, and Adolescents*, ed. 2. Baltimore, Williams & Wilkins Co., 1977, p. 226.
61. Fiser B., et al.: Infradiaphragmatic total anomalous pulmonary venous drainage. *J. Cardiovasc. Surg.* 20:69, 1979.
62. Flamm M.D., Cohn K.E., Hancock E.W.: Ventricular function in atrial septal defect. *Am. J. Med.* 48:286, 1970.
63. Fontan F., Baudet E.: Surgical repair of tricuspid atresia. *Thorax* 26:240, 1971.
64. Fontan F., et al.: Repair of tricuspid atresia—Surgical considerations and results, in Anderson R.H., Shinebourne E.A. (eds.): *Paediatric Cardiology 1977*. Edinburgh, Churchill Livingstone, 1978, p. 567.
65. Fox S., Pierce W.S., Waldhausen J.A.: Pathogenesis of paradoxical hypertension after coarctation repair. *Ann. Thorac. Surg.* 29:135, 1980.
66. Friedenberg W.R., et al.: Platelet dysfunction associated with cardiopulmonary bypass. *Ann. Thorac. Surg.* 25:298, 1978.
67. Friedman W.F., et al.: Pharmacologic closure of patent ductus arteriosus in the premature infant. *N. Engl. J. Med.* 295:526, 1976.
68. Gale A.W., et al.: Modified Fontan operation

for univentricular heart and complicated congenital lesions. *J. Thorac. Cardiovasc. Surg.* 78:831, 1979.
69. Glass D.D.: Sodium nitroprusside, in Hershey S.G. (ed.): *Refresher Courses in Anesthesiology 5*. Philadelphia, J.B. Lippincott Co., 1977, p. 87.
70. Glenn W.W.L.: The Glenn operation: Superior vena cava–pulmonary artery anastomosis, in Rob C., Smith R. (eds.): *Operative Surgery*. Vol. 2: *Thorax*, ed. 2. London, Butterworth & Co., 1968, p. 240.
71. Gomes M.M.R., McGoon D.C.: Bleeding patterns after open-heart surgery. *J. Thorac. Cardiovasc. Surg.* 60:87, 1970.
72. Gordon R.J., Ravin M.B., Daicoff G.R.: *Cardiovascular Physiology for Anesthesiologists*. Springfield, Ill., Charles C Thomas, Publisher, 1979, p. 27.
73. Gordon R.J., Ravin M.B., Daicoff G.R.: *Cardiovascular Physiology for Anesthesiologists*. Springfield, Ill., Charles C Thomas, Publisher, 1979, p. 179.
74. Graham T.P. Jr., Bender H.W., Spach M.S.: Defects of the ventricular septum, in Moss A.J., Adams F.H., Emmanouilides G.C. (eds.): *Heart Disease in Infants, Children, and Adolescents*, ed. 2. Baltimore, Williams & Wilkins Co., 1977, p. 140.
75. Gralnick H.R.: ε-Aminocaproic acid in preoperative correction of haemostatic defect in cyanotic congenital heart-disease. *Lancet* 1:1204, 1970.
76. Griepp E., et al.: Is pulmonary artery banding for ventricular septal defects obsolete? *Circulation* 50(suppl. 2):14, 1974.
77. Guntheroth W.G., Kawabori I.: 'Tetrad of Fallot,' in Moss A.J., Adams F.H., Emmanouilides G.C. (eds.): *Heart Disease in Infants, Children, and Adolescents*, ed. 2. Baltimore, Williams & Wilkins Co., 1977, p. 276.
78. Hagler D.J., et al.: Clinical, angiographic, and hemodynamic assessment of late results after Mustard operation. *Circulation* 57:1214, 1978.
79. Hagler D.J., et al.: Right and left ventricular function after the Mustard procedure in transposition of the great arteries. *Am. J. Cardiol.* 44:276, 1979.
80. Hallman G.L., Cooley D.A.: Congenital aortic stenosis, in Sabiston D.C. Jr., Spencer F.C. (eds.): *Gibbon's Surgery of the Chest*, ed. 3. Philadelphia, W.B. Saunders Co., 1976, p. 1076.
81. Hartmann A.F. Jr., et al.: Coarctation of the aorta, in Moss A.J., Adams F.H., Emmanouilides G.C. (eds.): *Heart Disease in Infants, Children, and Adolescents*, ed. 2. Baltimore, Williams & Wilkins Co., 1977, p. 199.
82. Hastreiter A.R., van der Horst R.L.: Hemodynamics of neonatal cyanotic heart disease. *Crit. Care Med.* 5:23, 1977.
83. Hendren W.H., Kim S.H.: Pediatric thoracic surgery, in Scarpelli E.M., Auld P.A.M., Goldman H.S. (eds.): *Pulmonary Disease of the Fetus, Newborn and Child*. Philadelphia, Lea & Febiger, 1978, p. 166.
84. Heymann M.A., Rudolph A.M., Silverman N.H.: Closure of the ductus arteriosus in premature infants by inhibition of prostaglandin synthesis. *N. Engl. J. Med.* 295:530, 1976.
84a. Hill A.G., Lefrak E.A.: Monitoring heparin and protamine therapy during cardiopulmonary bypass procedures. *Proc. Am. Soc. Extracorporeal Technology* 6:10, 1978.
85. Hoffman J.I.E.: Determinants and prediction of transmural myocardial perfusion. *Circulation* 58:381, 1978.
86. Hoffman J.I.: Ventricular septal defect: Indications for therapy in infants. *Pediatr. Clin. North Am.* 18:1091, 1971.
87. Hughes R.: Discussion. *J. Thorac. Cardiovasc. Surg.* 64:379, 1972.
87a. Jaques L.B.: Heparins—anionic polyelectrolyte drugs. *Pharm. Rev.* 31:99, 1979.
88. Johnston A.E., et al.: Acid-base and electrolyte changes in infants undergoing profound hypothermia for surgical correction of congenital heart defects. *Can. Anaesth. Soc. J.* 21:23, 1974.
89. Kalter R.D., et al.: Cardiopulmonary bypass: Associated hemostatic abnormalities. *J. Thorac. Cardiovasc. Surg.* 77:427, 1979.
90. Kam C.A.: Infundibular spasm in Fallot's tetralogy—An account and its management in anaesthesia. *Anaesth. Intensive Care* 6:138, 1978.
91. Katz N.M., Kirklin J.W., Pacifico A.D.: Concepts and practices in surgery for total anomalous pulmonary venous connection. *Ann. Thorac. Surg.* 25:479, 1978.
92. Kaul T.K., et al.: Heparin administration during extracorporeal circulation: Heparin rebound and postoperative bleeding. *J. Thorac. Cardiovasc. Surg.* 78:95, 1979.
93. Kaye M.P.: Anatomic correction of transposition of great arteries. *Mayo Clin. Proc.* 50:638, 1975.
94. Kidd B.S.L.: Complete transposition of the great arteries, in Keith J.D., Rowe R.D., Vlad P. (eds.): *Heart Disease in Infancy and Childhood*, ed. 3. New York, Macmillan Publishing Co., 1978, p. 590.
95. Kinsley R.H., et al.: Pulmonary arterial hy-

pertension after repair of tetralogy of Fallot. *J. Thorac. Cardiovasc. Surg.* 67:110, 1974.
96. Kirklin J.W., Conti V.R., Blackstone E.H.: Prevention of myocardial damage during cardiac operations. *N. Engl. J. Med.* 301:135, 1979.
97. Kirklin J.W., Karp R.B.: *The Tetralogy of Fallot: From a Surgical Viewpoint.* Philadelphia, W.B. Saunders Co., 1970.
98. Kirklin J.W., Pacifico A.D.: Tetralogy of Fallot, in Ravitch M.M., et al. (eds.): *Pediatric Surgery,* ed. 3. Chicago, Year Book Medical Publishers, 1979, vol. 1, p. 706.
99. Kirklin J.W., et al.: Cardiac repair in anatomically corrected malposition of the great arteries. *Circulation* 48:153, 1973.
100. Kirklin J.W., et al.: Cardiopulmonary bypass for cardiac surgery, in Sabiston D.C. Jr., Spencer F.C. (eds.): *Gibbon's Surgery of the Chest,* ed. 3. Philadelphia, W.B. Saunders Co., 1976, p. 846.
101. Kreutzer G., et al.: An operation for the correction of tricuspid atresia. *J. Thorac. Cardiovasc. Surg.* 66:613, 1973.
102. Lang P., et al.: Use of prostaglandin E_1 in infants with D-transposition of the great arteries and intact ventricular septum. *Am. J. Cardiol.* 44:76, 1979.
103. Laver M.B., Bland J.H.L.: Anesthetic management of the pediatric patient during open-heart surgery. *Int. Anesthesiol. Clin.* 13:149, fall 1975.
104. Levin A.R., et al.: Ventricular pressure-flow dynamics in tetralogy of Fallot. *Circulation* 34:4, 1966.
105. Levin A.R., et al.: Atrial pressure-flow dynamics in atrial septal defects (secundum type). *Circulation* 37:476, 1968.
106. Lindesmith G.G.: Secundum type atrial septal defects, in Ravitch M.M., et al. (eds.): *Pediatric Surgery,* ed. 3. Chicago, Year Book Medical Publishers, 1979, p. 714.
107. Lucas R.V. Jr., Schmidt R.E.: Anomalous venous connections, pulmonary and systemic, in Moss A.J., Adams F.H., Emmanouilides G.C. (eds.): *Heart Disease in Infants, Children, and Adolescents,* ed. 2. Baltimore, Williams & Wilkins Co., 1977, p. 437.
108. Mahle S., et al.: Pulmonary artery banding: Long-term results in 63 patients. *Ann. Thorac. Surg.* 27:216, 1979.
109. Mair D.D., McGoon D.C.: Surgical correction of atrioventricular canal during the first year of life. *Am. J. Cardiol.* 40:66, 1977.
110. Mair D.D., Ritter D.G.: Factors influencing intercirculatory mixing in patients with complete transposition of the great arteries. *Am. J. Cardiol.* 30:653, 1972.
111. Mair D.D., Ritter D.G.: Truncus arteriosus, in Moss A.J., Adams F.H., Emmanouilides G.C. (eds.): *Heart Disease in Infants, Children, and Adolescents,* ed. 2. Baltimore, Williams & Wilkins Co., 1977, p. 417.
112. Mair D.D., et al.: Selection of patients with truncus arteriosus for surgical correction: Anatomic and hemodynamic considerations. *Circulation* 49:144, 1974.
113. Mair D.D., et al.: Long-term follow-up of Mustard operation survivors. *Circulation* 50(suppl. 2):46, 1974.
114. Mair D.D., et al.: The palliative Mustard operation: Rationale and results. *Am. J. Cardiol.* 37:762, 1976.
115. Maloney J.D., et al.: Identification of the conduction system in corrected transposition and common ventricle at operation. *Mayo Clin. Proc.* 50:387, 1975.
116. Marcelletti C., et al.: Early and late results of surgical repair of truncus arteriosus. *Circulation* 55:636, 1977.
117. Mathew R., et al.: Cardiac function in total anomalous pulmonary venous return before and after surgery. *Circulation* 55:361, 1977.
118. Matthews H.R., Belsey R.H.R.: Indications for the Brock operation in current treatment of tetralogy of Fallot. *Thorax* 28:1, 1973.
119. Maurer H.M.: Hematologic effects of cardiac disease. *Pediatr. Clin. North Am.* 19:1083, 1972.
120. Maurer H.M., et al.: Impairment in platelet aggregation in congenital heart disease. *Blood* 40:207, 1972.
121. McFaul R.C., et al.: Ebstein's malformation: Surgical experience at the Mayo Clinic. *J. Thorac. Cardiovasc. Surg.* 72:910, 1976.
122. McGoon D.C.: Intracardiac repair of tetralogy of Fallot, in Kidd B.S.L., Keith J.D. (eds.): *The Natural History and Progress in Treatment of Congenital Heart Defects.* Springfield, Ill., Charles C Thomas, Publisher, 1971, p. 96.
123. McGoon D.C., Baird D.K., Davis G.D.: Surgical management of large bronchial collateral arteries with pulmonary stenosis or atresia. *Circulation* 52:109, 1975.
124. McGoon D.C., et al.: Correction of complete atrioventricular canal in infants. *Mayo Clin. Proc.* 48:769, 1973.
125. McGoon D.C., et al.: Late results of surgical treatment of pulmonary atresia: Preliminary report, in Kidd B.S.L., Rowe R.D. (eds.): *The Child With Congenital Heart Disease After Surgery.* Mount Kisco, N.Y., Futura Publishing Co., 1976, p. 135.
126. McGoon D.C., et al.: Correction of the univentricular heart having two atrioventricular

127. McLeskey C.H., Martin W.E.: Anesthesia for repair of a pulmonary-artery sling in an infant with severe tracheal stenosis. *Anesthesiology* 46:368, 1977.
128. McMullan M.H., et al.: Surgical treatment of complete atrioventricular canal. *Surgery* 72:905, 1972.
129. McMullan M.H., et al.: Surgical treatment of partial atrioventricular canal. *Arch. Surg.* 107:705, 1973.
130. Mitchell S.C., Korones S.B., Berendes H.W.: Congenital heart disease in 56,109 births: Incidence and natural history. *Circulation* 43:323, 1971.
131. Mitchell S.C., et al.: Etiologic correlates in a study of congenital heart disease in 56,109 births. *Am. J. Cardiol.* 28:653, 1971.
132. Moulton A.L., et al.: Pulmonary atresia with intact ventricular septum: Sixteen-year experience. *J. Thorac. Cardiovasc. Surg.* 78:527, 1979.
133. Murphy D.A., et al.: Effect of unilateral pulmonary artery occlusion on the arterial oxygen pressure of children undergoing pulmonary systemic artery shunt procedures. *Can. J. Surg.* 20:107, 1977.
134. Mustard J.F., Packham M.A.: Factors influencing platelet function: Adhesion, release, and aggregation. *Pharmacol. Rev.* 22:97, 1970.
135. Muster A.J., et al.: Abnormal distribution of the pulmonary blood flow between the two lungs in transposition of the great arteries, in Kidd B.S.L., Rowe R.D. (eds.): *The Child With Congenital Heart Disease After Surgery.* Mount Kisco, N.Y., Futura Publishing Co., 1976, p. 165.
136. Nadas A.S., Fyler D.C.: *Pediatric Cardiology,* ed. 3. Philadelphia, W.B. Saunders Co., 1972, p. 608.
137. Neches W.H., et al.: Coarctation of the aorta with ventricular septal defect. *Circulation* 55:189, 1977.
138. Noonan J.A.: Association of congenital heart disease with syndromes or other defects. *Pediatr. Clin. North Am.* 25:797, 1978.
139. Norwood W.I., Castaneda A.R.: Complications of the surgical repair of defects in the ventricular septum, in Cordell A.R., Ellison R.G. (eds.): *Complications of Intrathoracic Surgery.* Boston, Little, Brown & Co., 1979, p. 117.
140. Otero Coto E., et al.: Modified Senning operation for treatment of transposition of the great arteries. *J. Thorac. Cardiovasc. Surg.* 78:721, 1979.
141. Owen C.A. Jr., Bowie E.J.W.: Surgical hemostasis. *J. Neurosurg.* 51:137, 1979.
142. Owen C.A. Jr., Bowie E.J.W., Thompson J.H. Jr.: *The Diagnosis of Bleeding Disorders,* ed. 2. Boston, Little, Brown & Co., 1975.
143. Partridge J.B., et al.: Visualization and measurement of the main bronchi by tomography as an objective indicator of thoracic situs in congenital heart disease. *Circulation* 51:188, 1975.
144. Paul M.H.: D-transposition of the great arteries, in Moss A.J., Adams F.H., Emmanouilides G.C. (eds.): *Heart Disease in Infants, Children, and Adolescents,* ed. 2. Baltimore, Williams & Wilkins Co., 1977, p. 301.
144a. Pifarré R., et al.: Management of rebound following cardiopulmonary bypass. *J. Thorac. Cardiovasc. Surg.* 81:378, 1981.
145. Quaegebeur J.M., et al.: Revival of the Senning operation in the treatment of transposition of the great arteries: Preliminary report on recent experience. *Thorax* 32:517, 1977.
146. Rodnay P.A., Nagashimo H.: Anesthetic considerations for pediatric cardiac surgery. *Int. Anesthesiol. Clin.,* vol. 18, No. 1, 1980.
147. Rastelli G.C., Kirklin J.W., Titus J.L.: Anatomic observations on complete form of persistent common atrioventricular canal with special reference to atrioventricular valves. *Mayo Clin. Proc.* 41:296, 1966.
148. Rastelli G.C., McGoon D.C., Wallace R.B.: Anatomic correction of transposition of the great arteries with ventricular septal defect and subpulmonary stenosis. *J. Thorac. Cardiovasc. Surg.* 58:545, 1969.
149. Roberts N.K., Yabek S.: Arrhythmias following atrial and ventricular surgery, in Roberts N.K., Gelband H. (eds.): *Cardiac Arrhythmias in the Neonate, Infant, and Child.* New York, Appleton-Century-Crofts, 1977, p. 405.
150. Rodvien R., Salzman E.W.: Thrombotic and hemorrhagic problems in surgery. *Thromb. Haemost.* 39:254, 1978.
151. Roe B.B.: Ebstein's anomaly, in Sabiston D.C. Jr., Spencer F.C. (eds.): *Gibbon's Surgery of the Chest,* ed. 3. Philadelphia, W.B. Saunders Co., 1976, p. 1170.
152. Rogers M.C., Smith R.M.: Anesthesia for intrathoracic and cardiac surgery, in Smith R.M. (ed.): *Anesthesia for Infants and Children,* ed. 4. St. Louis, C. V. Mosby Co., 1980, p. 336.
152a. Rosenberg R. D.,: Actions and interactions of antithrombin and heparin. *New Engl. J. Med.* 292:146, 1975.
153. Rosenthal A.: Tricuspid atresia, in Moss A.J., Adams F.H., Emmanouilides G.C. (eds.):

Heart Disease in Infants, Children, and Adolescents, ed. 2. Baltimore, Williams & Wilkins Co., 1977, p. 289.
154. Rosenthal A., et al.: Acute hemodynamic effects of red cell volume reduction in polycythemia of cyanotic congenital heart disease. *Circulation* 42:297, 1970.
155. Roth J.A., Cukingnan R.A., Scott C.R.: Use of activated coagulation time to monitor heparin during cardiac surgery. *Ann. Thorac. Surg.* 28:69, 1979.
156. Sada T., Maguire H.T., Aldrete J.A.: Halothane solubility in blood during cardiopulmonary bypass: The effect of haemodilution and hypothermia. *Can. Anaesth. Soc. J.* 26:164, 1979.
157. Sade R.M., Castaneda A.R.: Tricuspid atresia, in Sabiston D.C. Jr., Spencer F.C. (eds.): *Gibbon's Surgery of the Chest*, ed. 3. Philadelphia, W. B. Saunders Co., 1976, p. 1152.
158. Sade R.M., Taylor A.B., Chariker E.P.: Aortoplasty compared with resection for coarctation of the aorta in young children. *Ann. Thorac. Surg.* 28:346, 1979.
159. Sade R.M., Williams R.G., Castaneda A.R.: Corrective surgery for congenital cardiovascular defects in early infancy. *Am. Heart J.* 90:656, 1975.
160. Saidman L.J., Eger E.I. II: Effect of nitrous oxide and of narcotic premedication on the alveolar concentration of halothane required for anesthesia. *Anesthesiology* 25:302, 1964.
161. Samuels P.B., Ironside P.A., Kartchner M.M.: A new method of preclotting fabric prostheses: A preliminary report. *Am. J. Surg.* 138:283, 1979.
162. Schumacher G., et al.: Hämodynamische und angiokardiographische Befunde bei Neugeborenen mit zyanotischen Hertzfehlern und verminderter Lungendurchblutung unter der Therapie mit Prostaglandin E_1. *Klin. Paediatr.* 190:465, 1978.
163. Senning Å.: Surgical correction of transposition of the great vessels. *Surgery* 45:966, 1959.
164. Senning Å.: Correction of the transposition of the great arteries. *Ann. Surg.* 182:287, 1975.
165. Sissman N.J.: Anomalies of the aortic arch complex, in Moss A.J., Adams F.H., Emmanouilides G.C. (eds.): *Heart Disease in Infants, Children, and Adolescents*, ed. 2. Baltimore, Williams & Wilkins Co., 1977, p. 210.
166. Somerville J.: Ostium primum defect: Factors causing deterioration in the natural history. *Br. Heart J.* 27:413, 1965.
167. Stark J., Aberdeen E.: Transposition of the great arteries (ventriculo-arterial discordance), in Ravitch M.M., et al. (eds.): *Pediatric Surgery*, ed. 3. Chicago, Year Book Medical Publishers, 1979, vol 1., p. 672.
168. Steeg C.N., et al.: Postoperative left anterior hemiblock and right bundle branch block following repair of tetralogy of Fallot: Clinical and etiologic considerations. *Circulation* 51:1026, 1975.
169. Steward D.J.: *Manual of Pediatric Anesthesia*. New York, Churchill Livingstone, 1979, p. 161.
170. Steward D.J., Sloan I.A., Johnston A.E.: Anaesthetic management of infants undergoing profound hypothermia for surgical correction of congenital heart defects. *Can. Anaesth. Soc. J.* 21:15, 1974.
171. Stockard J.J., et al.: Hypotension-induced changes in cerebral function during cardiac surgery. *Stroke* 5:730, 1974.
172. Strong M.J., Keats A.S., Cooley D.A.: Arterial gas tensions under anaesthesia in tetralogy of Fallot. *Br. J. Anaesth.* 39:472, 1967.
173. Takahashi M., et al.: Clinical and hemodynamic effects of pulmonary artery banding. *Am. J. Cardiol.* 21:174, 1968.
174. Taylor D.G.: The Brock procedure, in Rob C., Smith R. (eds.): *Operative Surgery.* Vol. 2: *Thorax*, ed. 2. London, Butterworth & Co., 1968, p. 247.
175. Trusler G.A., Williams W.G.: Long-term results of the Glenn procedure for tricuspid atresia, in Kidd B.S.L., and Rowe R.D. (eds.): *The Child With Congenital Heart Disease After Surgery*. Mount Kisco, N.Y., Futura Publishing Co., 1976, p. 79.
176. Tufo H.M., Ostfeld A.M., Shekelle R.: Central nervous system dysfunction following open-heart surgery. *J.A.M.A.* 212:1333, 1970.
177. Van Mierop L.H.S., Schiebler G.L., Victorica B.E.: Anomalies of the tricuspid valve resulting in stenosis or incompetence, in Moss A.J., Adams F.H., Emmanouilides G.C. (eds.): *Heart Disease in Infants, Children, and Adolescents*, ed. 2. Baltimore, Williams & Wilkins Co., 1977, p. 262.
178. Van Praagh R., Weinberg P.M., Van Praagh S.: Malposition of the heart, in Moss A.J., Adams F.H., Emmanouilides G.C. (eds.): *Heart Disease in Infants, Children, and Adolescents*, ed. 2. Baltimore, Williams & Wilkins Co., 1977, p. 394.
179. Verska J.J., Lonser E.R., Brewer L.A. III: Predisposing factors and management of hemorrhage following open heart surgery. *J. Cardiovasc. Surg.* 13:361, 1972.
180. Waldman J.D., et al.: Shortened platelet survival in cyanotic heart disease. *J. Pediatr.* 87:77, 1975.

181. Wallace R.B.: Truncus arteriosus, in Sabiston D.C. Jr., Spencer F.C. (eds.): *Gibbon's Surgery of the Chest*, ed. 3. Philadelphia, W. B. Saunders Co., 1976, p. 1066.
182. Wallace R.B., McGoon D.C., Danielson G.K.: Complete atrioventricular canal. *Adv. Cardiol.* 11:26, 1974.
183. Wedemeyer A.L., Edson J.R., Krivit W.: Coagulation in cyanotic congenital heart disease. *Am. J. Dis. Child.* 124:656, 1972.
184. Wedemeyer A.L., et al.: Serial coagulation studies in patients undergoing Mustard procedure. *Ann. Thorac. Surg.* 15:120, 1973.
185. Weldon C.S.: Congenital obstruction to left ventricular outflow, including coarctation of the aorta, in Ravitch M.M., et al. (eds.): *Pediatric Surgery*, ed. 3. Chicago, Year Book Medical Publishers, 1979, vol. 1, p. 633.
186. Wright J.S., Hicks R.G., Newman D.C.: Deep hypothermic arrest: Observations on later development in children. *J. Thorac. Cardiovasc. Surg.* 77:466, 1979.
187. Yacoub M.H.: The case for anatomic correction of transposition of the great arteries. *J. Thorac. Cardiovasc. Surg.* 78:3, 1979.
188. Zuberbuhler J.R., Allwork S.P., Anderson R.H.: The spectrum of Ebstein's anomaly of the tricuspid valve. *J. Thorac. Cardiovasc. Surg.* 77:202, 1979.

7 / Valvular Heart Disease, Cardiovascular Performance, and Anesthesia

JOHN CHRISTOPHER SILL
ROGER D. WHITE

CARDIAC SURGERY has undergone rapid evolution during the last two decades and now offers many patients with congenital and acquired heart disease treatment that ameliorates suffering and prolongs life. Valvular heart disease has become a less frequently encountered complication of group A β-hemolytic streptococcal infection but has by no means disappeared. Valvular heart disease has multiple causes, and while the incidence and severity of rheumatic fever have declined, degenerative heart disease, which may also damage the heart valves, has become more widespread.

Anesthesia for cardiac surgery is necessarily complex and demanding and has undergone evolution as a result of accumulated experience, expanded understanding of hemodynamic principles, and improved ability to monitor and manipulate the circulation. The anesthesiologist's contribution to successful surgery is especially important because patients with valvular heart disease maintain compensatory changes to preserve circulatory homeostasis and thus are vulnerable to any further challenge to hemodynamic integrity.

While valve replacement is effective therapy for valvular heart disease, there are many hazards to its successful outcome. Many of these hazards can be lessened by vigilant anesthetic management. To provide circulatory stability, the anesthesiologist must be familiar with (1) compensatory hemodynamic changes brought about by valvular disease, (2) events that depress cardiac performance, and (3) manipulations that can be introduced to maintain or improve function.

The anesthesiologist's aim is to precisely control the cardiovascular system to provide optimal function while introducing sedation, analgesia, or hypnosis and simultaneous protection of the vital organs.

Valvular heart disease, like most diseases, follows a predictable path, with characteristic alterations in function. The disease may induce a volume or a pressure overload on one or both ventricles and bring about changes in the peripheral and pulmonary circulations. The ventricle responds to the overload by dilatation or hypertrophy or both, but its compensatory mechanisms are limited and may also be accompanied by some decline in performance. While this new equilibrium may be physiologically acceptable to the patient at rest, further stress brought about by surgical stimulation may bring about a precipitous deterioration in function. The anesthesiologist's role can be outlined: either he must prevent such stress from altering homeostasis or he must alter the circulation so that it can adjust to the new demands. Anesthesia becomes a means of maintaining function while valve replacement is being performed.

Surgical stimulation results in the activation of the adrenergic sympathetic axis and the secretion of numerous humoral factors that constitute the evolutionary "fight or flight" response to threat. For the patient with valvular heart disease, such a response may provoke profound and adverse hemodynamic changes. The anesthesiologist must isolate the cardiovascular system from inappropriate stress and, at the same time, pharmacologically manipulate the circulation to an optimal state of function.

VALVE REPLACEMENT

Approximately 18,000 heart valves are replaced annually in the United States, and this number is increasing each year.[74] There are several types of prostheses[18, 74]: ball, caged-disk, tilting disk, and various tissue valves.

Ball Valves

The Starr-Edwards ball-valve prosthesis was introduced in 1960, and the basic design has changed little since then (Fig 7–1,A). One modification has been the use of a cloth covering that permits endothelialization and thus reduces the incidence of thromboembolism. This arrangement may reduce the orifice area and may result in wearing of the cloth that covers the struts, but this has been overcome by the introduction of stellite strips on the inside of each cloth-covered strut in the "track-valve" design. A second modification was the replacement in 1967 of the Silastic ball (which showed considerable early wear) with a stellite ball.

The Silastic poppet of the Braunwald-Cutter ball valve (Fig 7–1,B) has demonstrated accelerated wear with a predicted 12% escape at 5 years. At our institution, patients with the

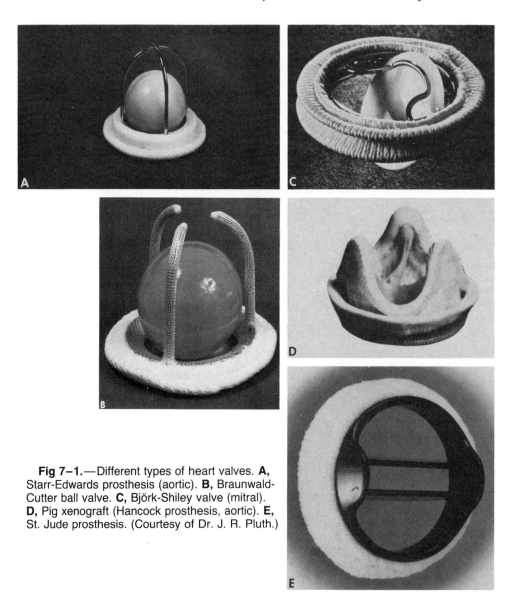

Fig 7–1.—Different types of heart valves. **A,** Starr-Edwards prosthesis (aortic). **B,** Braunwald-Cutter ball valve. **C,** Björk-Shiley valve (mitral). **D,** Pig xenograft (Hancock prosthesis, aortic). **E,** St. Jude prosthesis. (Courtesy of Dr. J. R. Pluth.)

Braunwald-Cutter prosthesis in the aortic position received replacement valves 4½ to 5 years after insertion.

Disk Valves

The Beall prosthesis is a caged disk that was introduced for use in the mitral position because its low profile does not obstruct the ventricular outflow tract. It is not frequently used, because current ball valves have a sufficiently low profile and may wear less rapidly.

The Björk-Shiley valve, introduced in 1969, is an example of a caged-disk valve and has a high internal-to-external diameter ratio, thus permitting a low valvular gradient (Fig 7–1,C). The tilting disk opens 60 degrees, permitting central laminar flow.

Tissue Valves

Tissue valves are associated with less tendency to thromboembolization and may provide better hemodynamic characteristics, but their long-term durability is not as certain when compared with that of synthetic prostheses. A glutaraldehyde-preserved, flexible, strut-mounted pig xenograft (Hancock prosthesis) is popular (Fig 7–1,D). Unfortunately, porcine xenograft valve degeneration is now being encountered and is related to the duration of the implant. Degeneration is especially prevalent in patients less than 25 years of age. Porcine xenograft valves inserted in the aortic position are more likely to degenerate than those implanted in the mitral position. It has become apparent that decreased platelet survival and thromboembolism are more common than previously reported, with a prevalency that may be similar to that incurred after insertion of mechanical prostheses.

The St. Jude prosthesis, a recently introduced bileaflet, low-profile valve of pyrolytic carbon, may provide good durability and a low incidence of thromboembolism (Fig 7–1,E).

DETERMINANTS OF CARDIAC PERFORMANCE

Studies of isolated heart muscle have demonstrated four determinants of cardiac mechanical performance (Fig 7–2). These four factors regulate the performance of the heart in health, maintain the function of the damaged heart in valvular heart disease, and can be used by the anesthesiologist in the operating room to rapidly alter the state of the circulation. The four determinants of performance—preload, afterload, contractile state, and heart rate—govern pump output and are also the major determinants of oxygen consumption. In the healthy person, cardiac output is increased principally by an increase in heart rate, but the patient with a diseased heart relies for the long term on the recruitment of all four mechanisms. Unfortunately, the response of the diseased heart to these determinants of performance may be blunted and even refractory. As valvular heart disease progresses, the role of these factors becomes more important. The deterioration in circulatory performance is frequently prevented, but at the expense of the appearance of symptoms and signs of heart failure—for example, pulmonary congestion as a result of increased preload and angina as a consequence of increased oxygen demand. These determinants of cardiac performance are the basic currency of the cardiac anesthesiologist.

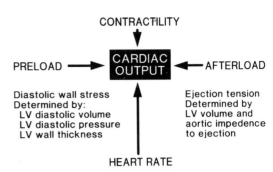

Fig 7–2.—Determinants of cardiac mechanical performance.

Preload

Preload in the isolated papillary muscle is the force that stretches the unloaded muscle. In the intact ventricle, it is the force that distends the ventricular chamber during diastole; it is the end-diastolic wall stress, which in clinical situations is equated with the end-diastolic pressure. The stroke volume increases in proportion to the degree of diastolic stress, that is, the diastolic stretch of the heart muscle fibers (Fig 7–3). Starling's law of the heart states, "The mechanical energy set free on passage from resting to the contracted state is a function of the initial

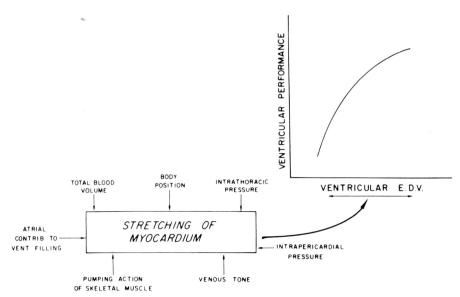

Fig 7–3.—Curve *(top right)* is ventricular function or Starling curve, relating preload, represented by left ventricular end-diastolic volume (E.D.V.), to ventricular performance. Diagram *(lower left)* indicates factors that contribute to distention of heart during diastole. (From Braunwald et al.[16] Used by permission.)

length of the muscle fibre."[16, 77] Cardiac muscle behaves in a way that is dissimilar to skeletal muscle—a critical relationship exists between the diastolic stretch of the muscle fibers and the amount of tension generated during contraction. The sliding-filament mechanism is the microscopic structural model of contraction, although recently this model has undergone some criticism.[75] The greatest force is developed when the sarcomeres of muscle fibrils are stretched during diastole to a length of 2.2 μm.[106]

The force generated decreases at lesser or greater lengths because the number of chemical cross-linkages in the sarcomere between the contractile protein filaments (actin and myosin) is decreased.

The operation of the preload mechanism can be interpreted using different models. If the sarcomere is considered, increased diastolic stress (preload) lengthens the sarcomeres toward the optimal 2.2 μm, a length that corresponds clinically to a left ventricular end-diastolic pressure (LVEDP) of 15 mm Hg or a right ventricular end-diastolic pressure of 10 mm Hg. Unfortunately, these two pressures are a poor approximation of preload and do not accurately represent diastolic stress. Calculation of end-diastolic wall stress is derived not only from the end-diastolic pressure but also from the end-diastolic chamber volume and ventricular wall thickness. If the Laplace equation is considered in a simplified form, then:

$$\text{Wall stress} = \frac{\text{chamber pressure} \times \text{chamber radius}}{\text{wall thickness}}$$

Wall stress is expressed as force per cross-sectional area of the ventricular myocardium. Stress is proportional not only to the pressure but also to the cube root of the chamber volume and is inversely proportional to wall thickness.

If preload and the hypertrophied left ventricle in aortic stenosis are considered, then because the ventricular wall has an increased thickness, to generate a diastolic wall stress (preload) equal to that in a nonhypertrophied ventricle, a higher LVEDP is needed. Because of ventricular hypertrophy and increased wall thickness, if the Laplace equation is applied, diastolic wall stress (preload) is normal despite an elevated LVEDP.

The preload mechanism can be better interpreted using values for left ventricular end-diastolic volume (LVEDV) rather than LVEDP. An increase in end-diastolic volume with muscle fiber stretch permits a more forceful contraction, and the greater ventricular size permits the ejection of a larger stroke volume with less shortening of the ventricle's circumferential muscle fibers.[65] Ventricular dilatation is evidence of the operation of the preload mechanism.

If the sarcomere is again considered, then chronic ventricular failure with increased muscle fiber stretch does not lead to disengagement of the actin-myosin cross-linkages.[65] The sarcomere length remains optimal at 2.2 μm during chronic heart failure.[16] Increased diastolic stress results in slippage among myofibrils rather than in sarcomere stretch beyond 2.2 μm. Along with myofibrillar slippage, there is muscle hypertrophy, resulting in longer myofibrils with more sarcomeres in series. Chronic preload increase results in greater end-diastolic volume and a multiplication of sarcomeres. Further acute preload increase is frequently still possible because not all sarcomeres have reached an optimal length of 2.2 μm; that is, some preload reserve remains.[65]

The heart damaged by valvular disease can recruit the preload mechanism to maintain performance, but there are associated disadvantages. Pulmonary or systemic congestion may accompany increased preload. As myofibrillar slippage occurs, ventricular muscle contractile state is impaired, necessitating greater increases in preload to sustain cardiac performance; that is, the ventricular function curve is depressed. This function curve departs from its steep linear relationship at low filling pressure and becomes flattened, little improvement in performance now occurring despite increased preload (Fig 7–4).

A further disadvantage of increases in preload is the detrimental influence on the myocardial oxygen supply-and-demand relationship. Wall stress is a major determinant of myocardial oxygen needs, and as the diastolic wall stress increases, so does the oxygen requirement. The subendocardial layers of the heart receive coronary blood flow that is easily jeopardized by reduction in coronary perfusion pressure. The pressure gradient between the aorta and the ventricular cavity governs coronary flow, and this gradient during diastole is diminished by an increase in LVEDP.

Atrial Contribution to Preload

The brief atrial contraction that occurs just before conclusion of ventricular diastole is an

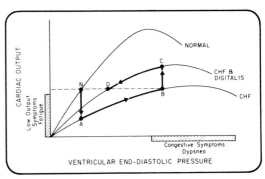

Fig 7–4.—Illustration of Starling mechanism maintaining cardiac output during congestive heart failure (CHF). Top curve represents normal ventricular function curve; bottom curve, CHF curve; middle curve, curve after treatment with digitalis. Decrease in performance leading to decompensation (NA), Starling mechanism restores cardiac output but at the expense of higher filling pressure and congestive symptoms (AB), increased contractility by administration of digitalis, resulting in a new Starling curve (BC), digitalis action permits return to a more normal left ventricular end-diastolic pressure while maintaining cardiac output (CD). (From Mason.[65] Used by permission.)

important mechanism for increasing ventricular preload without exposing the pulmonary vasculature to the adverse effects of increased left atrial pressure.[41, 44, 92] Left ventricular end-diastolic pressure is now greater than mean left atrial pressure because the brief atrial systole contributes little to mean left atrial pressure and is rapidly followed by mitral valve closure. The thick-walled, noncompliant ventricle of aortic stenosis becomes particularly dependent on atrial contraction to maintain even a small increase in diastolic wall stress (preload)[44, 55, 114] (Fig 7–5). The narrowed orifice of mitral stenosis poses a considerable obstruction to left ventricular filling and development of preload and, in the absence of effective atrial systolic flow into the ventricle, is further reduced.[114] This situation is manifested clinically by the deterioration in function seen with the onset of atrial fibrillation in the patient with mitral stenosis.

Descending Limb of the Starling Curve

At high levels of ventricular diastolic wall stress, sarcomeres may be stretched beyond 2.2 μm, resulting in a downward slope of the

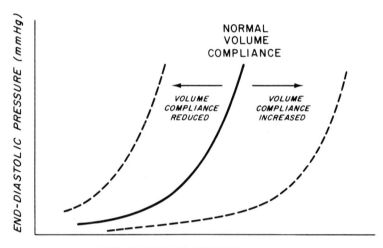

Fig 7–5.—Passive pressure-volume curve of ventricle. Compliance of ventricular wall is determined by relationship of pressure to volume in ventricle. Compliance is decreased by concentric hypertrophy and is increased by ventricular dilatation. Aortic stenosis results in loss of compliance, while mitral insufficiency and aortic insufficiency are usually associated with increased compliance. (From Johnson R.A.: Heart failure, in Johnson R.A., Haber E., Austen W.G. [eds.]: *The Practice of Cardiology.* Boston, Little, Brown & Co., 1980. Used by permission.)

ventricular function curve.[16] Alternatively, this event can be explained in terms of increased afterload. Under these conditions, the ventricle dilates, and according to the principles of the Laplace law, systolic wall tension and stress increase. Systolic wall stress is "afterload," and increased afterload reduces cardiac performance.[16, 91]

Contractility

It is difficult to define contractility because no single measurement can be used in its description. Contractile state of the isolated papillary muscle can be defined as a condition of muscle in which the force of contraction can be altered by stimulation despite a constant preload and afterload. Contractility refers to the intrinsic fiber-shortening property of heart muscle.[16] In clinical practice, cardiac radiologists examine the force, velocity, and length relationships and express these quantities in terms of dp/dt, the rate of increase in ventricular pressure, an isovolumetric index, and V_{CF}, mean rate of circumferential fiber shortening, an ejection index.[65] Increase in ventricular pressure is generated by shortening of the contractile units of the myocardial fibers, exerting a force on the blood contained in the ventricle at the end of diastole. During the isovolumetric phase of ventricular contraction, the rate of increase of ventricular pressure is directly related to the velocity of shortening of the myofibers and is used as a means of assessing muscle performance, independent of the overall pumping function of the heart.[65] The slope of the ventricular function curve, that is, the increase in stroke volume at constant preload, offers some approximation of the contractile state, but the information obtained reflects changes in afterload as much as contractile state.[16, 22] The force-velocity relationship best describes contraction, and the position of this curve reflects contractility (Fig 7–6).

Valvular heart disease frequently leads to ventricular hypertrophy and dilatation. If muscle from such hearts is isolated and examined and the results are expressed in terms of force-velocity relationships, then the performance of this muscle is impaired.[14, 16, 65, 108] The maximal velocity of unloaded shortening, V_{max}, is reduced; and the maximal isometric tension decreases[16, 108] (see Fig 7–6). There is a decrease in dp/dt. Muscle from the failing heart also shows such evidence of depressed contractility but to a more severe degree.[16, 108] A reduced myocardial contractile state is the hallmark of hypertrophied or failing cardiac muscle seen with long-standing valvular heart disease.[65]

In the normal heart, norepinephrine released from nerve endings in the heart is the direct stimulus that regulates the contractile state. Failing heart muscle shows a defect in norepinephrine turnover, with depletion of cardiac norepinephrine. Sympathetic stimulation of the contractile state becomes dependent on circulating catecholamines secreted by the adrenal medulla and other extracardiac adrenergic ganglia, probably within the peripheral vasculature.[16, 54, 65]

Contractility is a major determinant of myocardial oxygen needs. Enhanced contractility results in an elevation of the heart's oxygen consumption.

Afterload

Afterload is the force that resists the shortening of myocardial muscle fibers. It is the stress within the ventricular wall that has to be developed to open the aortic valve and eject blood.[22] Stress is defined as the force per cross-sectional area of the ventricular wall and is determined by ventricular pressure, cavity size, and wall thickness.[94] These quantities can be related, using the principles of the Laplace equation for tension in the wall of a sphere:

$$\text{Wall stress} = \frac{\text{chamber pressure} \times \text{chamber radius}}{\text{wall thickness}}$$

It is important to consider afterload in terms of wall stress rather than wall tension (tension = pressure × radius), because the ventricular wall has thickness.[82] A feature of valvular heart disease is ventricular hypertrophy, with an increase in wall thickness. Although wall tension may not be reduced by this means, wall stress is returned toward more normal values.[81]

Wall stress is expressed as force per cross-sectional area of the ventricular myocardium. In clinical practice, chamber volume is more readily obtained than chamber radius. The radius can be taken as the cube root of ventricular volume. Changes in ventricular wall stress are directly proportional to changes in chamber pressure and the cube root of ventricular volume but are inversely proportional to wall thickness. Afterload is proportional to left ventricular pressure times the cube root of the LVEDV divided by the left ventricular wall thickness. Systolic wall stress or afterload at the time of aortic valve opening can be calculated in the cardiac catheterization laboratory from simultaneous measurements of arterial blood pressure and left ventricular chamber size and wall thickness.

Some difficulty arises in defining afterload, because the term is frequently used loosely. Clinically, afterload has been equated to the ar-

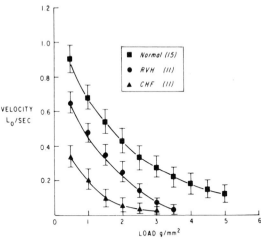

Fig 7–6.—Force-velocity relationships of three groups of cat papillary muscles. Numbers within parentheses represent number of cats. For a given load, velocity of contraction decreases when normal, hypertrophied, and failing muscles are examined. This change implies decrease in contractility. Right ventricular hypertrophy *(RVH),* congestive heart failure *(CHF).* (From Spann.[108] Used by permission of the American Heart Association.)

terial systolic blood pressure, but maximal systolic wall stress (afterload) develops shortly after the opening of the aortic valve and so is determined by LVEDV and diastolic aortic pressure.[82] Wall stress declines after valve opening because ejection of blood reduces end-diastolic volume, and as ventricular contraction occurs, wall thickness increases. From the equation, it can be seen that afterload decreases because ejection of the stroke volume permits a decline in end-diastolic volume and an increase in wall thickness. After aortic valve opening, the pressure generated by the ventricle becomes a function of myocardial fiber shortening and of impedance to the blood as it is ejected.[22] The arterial bed exerts an influence on cardiac performance by the impedance it offers to ventricular ejection. This impedance to flow is governed largely by the compliance of the great arteries and the total systemic vascular resistance. These factors become important determinants of the rate of increase of aortic pressure, ejection velocity, ejection duration, the size and shape of the chamber during ejection, the ejection fraction, and the stroke volume (Fig 7–7). Thus, impedance to ejection is a major de-

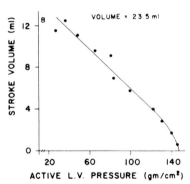

Fig 7–8.—In dogs, if left ventricular end-diastolic volume is held constant, then an inverse relationship between stroke volume and active left ventricular (L.V.) pressure can be seen during isotonic contraction; that is, stroke volume decreases as systolic pressure is increased. (From Burns J.W., Covell J.W., Ross J. Jr.: Mechanics of isotonic left ventricular contractions. *Am. J. Physiol.* 224:725, 1973. Used by permission.)

terminant of cardiac output.[22, 23] At normal or less-than-normal impedance to ejection, stroke volume is a function of preload, but if impedance is increased, then preload has less effect on stroke volume.[16] There is an inverse relationship between stroke volume and afterload (Fig 7–8). The left ventricle functions most efficiently at normal or low afterload. Patients whose hearts are hypertrophied or are failing because of valvular heart disease demonstrate two important characteristics[20, 23]: (1) cardiac output is easily depressed by increases in afterload (Fig 7–9), and (2) systemic vascular resistance is frequently elevated. Thus, a vasodilator (for example, sodium nitroprusside), by reducing systemic vascular resistance, can improve performance[20, 22, 23, 42, 67, 70] (see Figs 7–7 and 7–10).

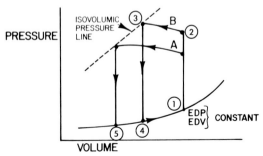

Fig 7–7.—Ventricular pressure-volume relationship. Beat B, 1 2 3 4, begins to contract at point 1, develops pressure until aortic valve opens at point 2, ejects until point 3 is reached—line of maximal pressure that left ventricle can generate at a given end-diastolic volume *(EDV)* if it does not eject blood—and then relaxes to point 4 on the passive pressure-volume curve. Beat A is performed at same level of contractility (isovolumetric pressure line) and EDV (point 1) but with decrease in arterial pressure. As arterial pressure is decreased from beat B to beat A, there is an increase in the stroke volume of beat A. Increase in stroke volume is represented by point 4–5. This beat A can be achieved by vasodilator therapy. *EDP,* end-diastolic pressure. (From Chatterjee and Parmley.[20] Used by permission.)

Of considerable importance is the influence of impedance to ejection on myocardial oxygen consumption.[20] Oxygen requirements of the left ventricle are far more dependent on pressure generated than on volume ejected, because oxygen consumption is partly determined by wall tension. Fiber shortening during ejection of stroke volume consumes little oxygen when compared with the oxygen needed for isovolumetric pressure generation.[16] Thus, in this energy requirement effect, increases in stroke work associated with increases in stroke volume require little extra oxygen, whereas increases in stroke work associated with increases in intra-

buildup of volume and pressure behind the mitral valve and extending through the pulmonary vasculature to the right side of the heart and even to the systemic venous system. Ahead of the obstruction is the ventricle, which suffers a reduction in the volume of blood entering the chamber. Decreased filling and, hence, decreased preload are the hemodynamic impositions on the left ventricle. A pressure difference during diastole between the left atrium and the left ventricle is the circulatory characteristic of mitral stenosis. This pressure difference, the mitral valve gradient, is determined by the area of the mitral orifice and the volume of blood flowing through it. The normal valve area in health is between 4 and 6 sq cm. Serious hemodynamic consequences do not become manifest until this area is decreased by disease to between 1 and 2 sq cm. A valve area of 2.0 to 2.5 sq cm leads to occasional symptoms, and when the area is diminished to between 1.5 and 2.0 sq cm, symptoms are present during exertion. Symptoms occur at rest when the valve area is 1.5 sq cm or less, and an area of 0.3 to 0.4 sq cm seems to be the minimal area compatible with life.[97]

When stenosis is mild, left atrial pressure is usually normal, the valve area being adequate to permit flow without offering significant obstruction. During exercise, left atrial pressure increases, as does the mitral gradient, and greater flow is possible through the stenosis, permitting better filling of the ventricle and an increase in cardiac output. Mitral valve area (*MVA*, square centimeters) can be calculated using the Gorlin modification of standard hydraulic formulas[38]:

$$MVA = BF/(K \times 44.5 \times \sqrt{P_1 - P_2})$$

in which *BF* is blood flow in milliliters per second; *K* is a correction factor for several variables; 44.5 is the value of $\sqrt{2g}$, in which *g* equals the acceleration factor; and P_1 and P_2 represent the mean pressure (millimeters mercury) during the period of flow in the chambers on each side of the valve. Normal cardiac output is associated with a left atrial pressure of about 6 to 10 mm Hg. The orifice area at rest is 1.0 sq cm. When the left atrial pressure reaches 25 mm Hg, transudation of fluid from capillaries to alveoli occurs. Despite further reduction in initial valve area, the left atrial pressure does not seem to increase. Pulmonary vascular changes (for example, hypertrophic arteriolar narrowing and vasoconstriction) reduce output from the right ventricle by presenting adverse afterloading conditions. Now the altered pulmonary vasculature constitutes a second point of obstruction and, in a sense, "protects" the lungs from further increases in left atrial pressure. Increased cardiac output is achieved at the expense of increased left atrial pressure, with a parallel increase of pressure in the pulmonary vasculature. If the stenosis is mild, the gradient may be present only during periods of high mitral flow, which occur in early diastole and at the end of diastole when atrial contraction occurs. When the stenosis is severe, the gradient is present throughout diastole. Eventually, with progression of the disease, at a certain amount of valve narrowing, the left atrial pressure needed to maintain a sufficient gradient to achieve adequate left ventricular filling is also the pressure at which pulmonary edema develops. Such patients live on the borderline of pulmonary edema, and left atrial pressure may be chronically 25 mm Hg or more. Exertion or excitement or anxiety, such as that immediately before surgery, may be sufficient to upset this precarious state and cause acute pulmonary edema.

Aspects of Mitral Stenosis

PULMONARY CHANGES. — Shortness of breath is a frequently encountered symptom of mitral stenosis and is caused by elevated pulmonary venous and capillary pressures and by changes in the structure of the lungs as a consequence of long-standing elevation of these pressures. If left atrial, pulmonary venous, and pulmonary capillary pressures increase rapidly to 30 mm Hg, then hydrostatic pressure exceeds plasma oncotic pressure and fluid passes from the lung vascular compartment, resulting in alveolar flooding or pulmonary edema. If left atrial pressure increases slowly, then the lungs show a remarkable ability to adapt to the higher pulmonary vascular pressures. Lung parenchymal and vascular changes occur, offering some protection against higher hydrostatic pressure, and the lymphatic clearance of pulmonary water is enhanced. When left atrial pressure increases slowly, fluid transudes into the alveolar wall and a physical barrier eventually develops between the capillaries and the alveoli. This barrier consists of thickened capillary basement membrane, collagen deposition, and fibrosis.[27]

The gross pathologic features in the lungs include stiff parenchymal tissue as a result of fibrosis. Also, calcification may occur. The intralobular septa are thickened and edematous. Microscopically, organization of chronic interstitial and alveolar pulmonary edema results in fibrosis. The lymphatic vessels are tortuous and dilated. The entire pulmonary vascular bed undergoes change, with dilatation of the larger arteries and thickening, hypertrophy, and fibrosis of the arterioles and venules. The lungs are stiffer than normal, total lung water is increased, and the resultant decrease in compliance greatly increases the work of breathing.[27]

Interstitial edema may compress pulmonary vessels and so reduce perfusion of lower dependent lung regions, with redistribution of perfusion to upper nondependent areas of lung. Regional ventilation also may be reduced owing to peribronchial edema, which causes narrowing of small airways and progressive shift of ventilation to nondependent areas. Overall ventilation-perfusion relationships in such lungs are imbalanced. Pulmonary hypertension ensues from medial hypertrophy and intimal proliferation in the small muscular arteries, but a further contributing element is hypoxemic vasoconstriction of pulmonary arterioles and small pulmonary arteries. The elevated pulmonary vascular resistance frequently decreases after mitral valve replacement, but if the high resistance is long-standing, the vascular changes may be permanent.

The thin-walled right ventricle is subjected to pressure overload because pulmonary hypertension increases the impedance to ventricular emptying. The anesthesiologist is now confronted with the problems of a right ventricle that is pressure-overloaded and hypertrophied and that may be experiencing a significant decline in performance and a left ventricle that is volume-underloaded. The two ventricles may be separated by a congested pulmonary system.

LEFT VENTRICLE.—Mitral stenosis causes backward pulmonary congestion and forward left ventricular underloading. In a sense, the left ventricle is "protected" by volume underloading, and its function is frequently normal.

The LVEDV and LVEDP are normal in about 85% of patients and low in 15%.[30, 53] Increased LVEDV or LVEDP indicates an element of left ventricular failure or coexistent mitral and aortic regurgitation. Stroke volume is normal or lower than normal and, with severe stenosis, is low even at rest. Usually, the ejection fraction remains normal as LVEDV and left ventricular end-systolic volume (LVESV) are reduced proportionately.[30, 53] The ejection fraction is calculated as follows:

$$EF = \frac{LVEDV - LVESV}{LVEDV} = \frac{SV}{LVEDV}$$

Some patients have low ejection fractions, and this observation probably indicates decreased myocardial contractile state. Left ventricular muscle mass is usually normal, but left ventricular atrophy sometimes occurs, perhaps as a consequence of chronic low preload.

MYOCARDIAL FACTORS.—Because the left ventricle is not subjected to abnormal loads, it would be expected that its contractile state would be unchanged, but some decrease in performance has been noted.[1, 28, 45] This depressed function has been attributed to (1) myocardial damage from the original episodes of rheumatic fever, (2) atrophy as a consequence of long-standing volume underloading, or (3) scarring of the ventricular wall by the same process that involves the valve.

Cineangiography may demonstrate poor contraction of the posterobasal and the anterolateral walls.[28] The valvular scarring process probably converts the valve to a rigid cylinder that acts like an internal cast, immobilizing the posterior wall of the ventricle. Atrophy may follow immobilization.[45]

Right ventricular hypertrophy and dilatation may disturb left ventricular function because of their close anatomical relationship and because some myocardial fibers are common to both ventricles.

TACHYCARDIA.—Left ventricular filling is governed by two factors: gradient and filling period. If the diastolic period is increased, then more time is permitted for flow across the narrowed valve. The reverse is also true. Tachycardia reduces diastolic time, resulting in a decrease in stroke volume. The left ventricle operates at a lower position on the Starling function curve, and at the same time left atrial pressure increases. Pulmonary edema may develop in the presence of an empty left ventricle. From Gorlin's formula:

$$\text{Gradient} = \left(\frac{\text{cardiac output}}{K \times \text{area} \times \text{diastolic filling time}}\right)^2$$

An increase in cardiac output or a decrease in diastolic filling time results in an exponential increase in gradient. Also, if diastolic filling time shortens but the gradient is not increased, then cardiac output decreases. Patients with mitral stenosis are particularly adversely affected by tachycardia, and it must be avoided[2, 116] (Fig 7–12).

LEFT ATRIAL FUNCTION.—The contribution of left atrial contraction to ventricular performance increases as stenosis worsens. The left atrium has three major roles[116] (Fig 7–13): (1) as a conduit for passage of blood from the pulmonary veins to the left ventricle during diastole, (2) as a reservoir for the storage of pulmonary venous blood during systole, and (3) as a booster pump to augment left ventricular filling before systole. Left atrial volume is about 40 ml/sq m, and this volume is maximal at end-systole just before the mitral valve opens. Left atrial contraction maintains flow across the mitral valve during the late phases of ventricular diastole when the left atrial pressure-to-LVEDP gradient is decreasing and when the diastolic compliance curve of the filling ventricle has steepened.[30]

Normally, at rest, left atrial contraction increases LVEDV by about 20%, but in the presence of mitral stenosis, LVEDV may be increased by as much as 33%.[116]

As heart rate increases, the importance of atrial contraction increases, and as stenosis worsens, atrial contraction contributes more significantly to left ventricular filling. The presence of atrial contraction maintains cardiac output at lower levels of mean left atrial pressure (atrial systole does not significantly increase mean left atrial pressure) than would be present under comparable conditions if atrial systole were absent (for example, during atrial fibrillation).[2]

ATRIAL FIBRILLATION.—The onset of atrial fibrillation frequently worsens the symptoms of mitral stenosis.[2, 37] There are three reasons why atrial fibrillation is detrimental: (1) rapid ventricular rate results from atrial fibrillation, and this tachycardia decreases diastolic filling time; (2) active atrial transport provided by atrial systole

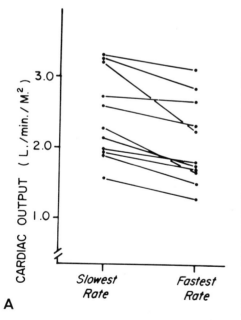
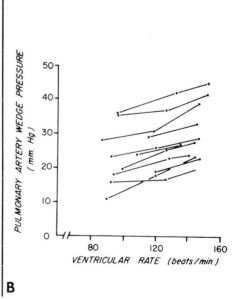
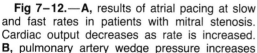

Fig 7–12.—**A,** results of atrial pacing at slow and fast rates in patients with mitral stenosis. Cardiac output decreases as rate is increased. **B,** pulmonary artery wedge pressure increases when heart rate in patient with mitral stenosis is increased by atrial pacing. (From Arani and Carleton.[2] Used by permission of the American Heart Association.)

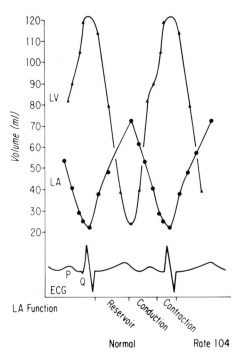

Fig 7–13.—Normal left atrium and ventricle. Volume is plotted against time. Reservoir, conduction, and atrial contraction phases with their effect on left atrial *(LA)* and left ventricular *(LV)* volume are shown. (From Murray J.A., Kennedy J.W., Figley M.M.: Quantitative angiocardiography. II. The normal left atrial volume in man. *Circulation* 37:800, 1968. Used by permission of the American Heart Association.)

is lost; and (3) changing the cycle length adversely affects the above two factors and also directly impairs contractility.

AFTERLOAD.—Generally, diminished performance further deteriorates when impedance to ventricular ejection is increased.[20, 23] The left ventricle in mitral stenosis responds similarly, but afterload reduction may not be of much benefit, because the major feature that disturbs performance is decreased preload caused by obstruction to filling.[8]

Mitral Regurgitation

Etiology

The mitral valve requires the coordinated functioning of a number of cardiac structures to achieve competence[49, 93, 105] (Fig 7–14). Failure of any of these factors results in regurgitation.[51, 78, 87] Because so many structures are involved, there are multiple causes of mitral insufficiency.[83] Rheumatic endocarditis may result in mitral regurgitation, usually associated with mitral stenosis. Infective endocarditis may produce destruction or perforation of the cusps or rupture of the chordae tendineae. Widespread incidence of ischemic heart disease has brought about a high frequency of mitral regurgitation resulting from papillary muscle infarction. The papillary muscles are the most distal structures of the heart to receive arterial perfusion and so are the most vulnerable regions of cardiac muscle.

Left ventricular dilatation from any cause, for example, ischemia, infarction, aortic valve disease, or hypertension, may lead to dilatation of the valve ring. The ensuing regurgitation leads to further left ventricular dilatation and more mitral regurgitation. Of considerable importance when therapeutic measures are considered is the improvement in mitral regurgitation when left ventricular dilatation is reduced.[11]

Acute rupture of the chordae tendineae is a particularly dangerous condition because the left atrium has little time available to dilate, to become more compliant, and to act as a buffer between the lungs and the left ventricle.[49, 97]

In the absence of left atrial dilatation, the pressure wave during left ventricular systole is transmitted without damping through the left atrium and into the pulmonary vasculature, where elevated pressure results in fluid transudation from the vascular compartment into the alveoli. If mitral regurgitation evolves more slowly, then left atrial dilatation absorbs some of the pressure transmitted from the ventricle and limits adverse effects on the lungs and the pulmonary circulation. Pulmonary vascular changes are ameliorated by the buffer effect of increased left atrial compliance, and in the absence of severe pulmonary changes, little afterload stress is placed on the right ventricle. The greater the volume and compliance of the left atrium, the less is the congestion in the pulmonary vasculature and thus the lower is the pressure overload imposed on the right ventricle.[86] Left atrial dilatation sometimes results in a giant left atrium, with a volume of as much as 300 ml or even 400 ml.[30] Because compliance is increased, left atrial pressure does not increase significantly.

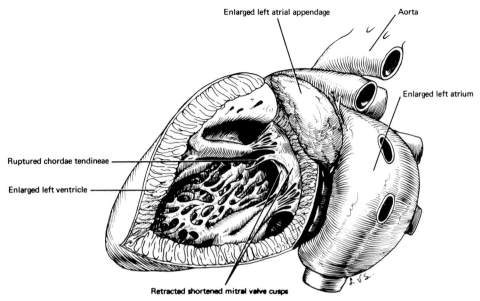

Fig 7-14.—Anatomical features of mitral regurgitation. (From Sokolow and McIlroy.[105] Used by permission.)

Symptoms

Although patients with chronic mitral regurgitation eventually experience dyspnea, they may remain symptom-free for a longer period than those with mitral stenosis, because the large compliant left atrium protects the lungs from pressure-induced changes.

Signs

There is a holosystolic murmur that is maximal at the apex. This murmur is diminished when forward aortic flow is increased by reduction of afterload. Wide splitting of the second heart sound occurs as the aortic valve closes early, owing to rapid ventricular emptying into the left atrium as well as into the aorta.

Investigations

The ECG often shows the altered P wave of left atrial hypertrophy, as well as evidence of left ventricular hypertrophy. The roentgenogram of the chest demonstrates a giant left atrium and left ventricular enlargement, and the lung fields often reveal increased vascularity and even congestion.

Hemodynamics

Dilatation and eccentric hypertrophy are the principal changes that occur in the heart with volume overload.[106] An incompetent mitral valve permits regurgitation of part of the left ventricular stroke volume into the left atrium. The left atrium dilates and delivers a larger than normal volume to the ventricle during diastole, imposing a volume overload. Left ventricular dilatation occurs, and because cavity volume is increased, the wall tension and stress are likewise increased. Eccentric hypertrophy thickens the ventricular wall in proportion to the increased ventricular volume, therefore returning wall stress to a more normal value, that is:

$$\text{Wall stress} = \frac{\text{LV pressure} \times \text{LV volume}}{\text{LV wall thickness}}$$

Both dilatation and hypertrophy occur. Left ventricular volume may be increased by a factor of four or five, but LVEDP is usually normal, owing to an increase in compliance. Eccentric hypertrophy is not associated with an elevated LVEDP unless failure occurs.[30, 80]

Stroke volume is made up of two components: forward stroke volume that enters the aorta and regurgitant stroke volume that is ejected into the left atrium. Together they constitute the "total stroke volume." The incompetent mitral valve enables the left ventricle to empty during systole down a low resistance pathway into the left atrium. Impedance to ejection presented by the partially patent valve and left atrium is lower than that offered by the aorta. This reduced ejection impedance permits greater ventricular emptying, with an enhanced total stroke volume and an increase in the velocity of fiber shortening.[12] The extra volume work is accomplished with little increase in oxygen requirement. The low resistance pathway enables the ventricular volume and thus the wall tension to decrease rapidly. Because tension declines rapidly, oxygen consumption is little increased, despite the ejection of a larger than normal stroke volume.[12]

The left ventricle is obliged to maintain high volume work to provide a normal forward cardiac output. Because an increased volume movement in the presence of low ejection impedance can be accomplished without much extra pressure generation, the extra work involved does not require a great increase in oxygen demand. (The heart uses more oxygen in performing a given amount of work in generating pressure than in achieving flow.[16]) Overall oxygen demand is greater because eccentric hypertrophy results in increased muscle mass.[106]

Mitral regurgitation produces changes in a number of angiographically determined quantities. The LVEDV is almost always increased, and LVEDV per square meter may be as much as 300 ml (normal 70 ml).[30] Stroke volume is also increased.[100] Ejection fraction remains within normal range as stroke volume and LVEDV increase in proportion, but because afterload is reduced by the low resistance pathway into the left atrium, the ejection fraction would be expected to increase. Depressed ejection fraction in the presence of this advantageous afterloading condition implies a significant deterioration in myocardial contractile state.[31]

Chronic volume overload, left ventricular dilatation, and eccentric hypertrophy eventually lead to an overall decline in cardiac function because of a decrease in myocardial contractile state. Hypertrophied heart muscle does not perform as well as normal muscle,[108] and ventricular dilatation may result in a permanent and irreversible slippage between ventricular wall myofibrils.[80] The LVEDV and LVEDP increase, but ejection fraction decreases. The LVEDV now increases without an increase in stroke volume.[93] Further eccentric hypertrophy is unable to ameliorate this deterioration in performance, and forward stroke volume and cardiac output decrease. Increasing the LVEDP leads to pulmonary congestion and increases the already present overload on the right ventricle. Mitral regurgitation has now damaged the left ventricle, induced pulmonary hypertension, impaired pulmonary function, and pressure-overloaded the right ventricle.

Acute Mitral Regurgitation

In acute mitral regurgitation, which is an extremely dangerous condition, there is an acute volume overload placed on the left ventricle, which rapidly dilates, and despite this extensive use of the Starling preload mechanism, forward cardiac output decreases. Wall stress is high because, during the acute hemodynamic disturbance, significant eccentric wall hypertrophy is not possible. The brevity of the illness frequently prevents left atrial dilatation,[5] thus exposing the pulmonary vasculature to the full force of left ventricular systole. The consequences of acute mitral regurgitation are decreasing forward cardiac output and pulmonary congestion.

Aspects of Mitral Regurgitation

OXYGEN CONSUMPTION.—Ventricular wall tension is a major determinant of myocardial oxygen consumption. Because wall tension decreases rapidly when ejection occurs partly into the left atrium, the extra volume work is accomplished with no great increase in oxygen demand.[12, 31] The low expenditure of energy per unit work used for shortening, as opposed to that used for tension development, allows the large stroke volume to be maintained at only a small increase in oxygen consumption by the ventricle. Eccentric hypertrophy increases muscle mass, and, therefore, overall oxygen requirement is increased and angina may be a symptom of mitral regurgitation.[30]

REGURGITATION.—Regurgitation[49] is proportional to (1) the area of the valve orifice during ventricular systole (this area is variable and is significantly increased by left ventricular dilatation), (2) the systolic pressure gradient between the left ventricle and the left atrium, and (3) the duration of systole. Although systolic pressure influences regurgitation, its effect is proportional to the square root of the gradient. From this relationship, it can be appreciated that a large increase in left ventricular systolic pressure and gradient produces a smaller than expected effect on regurgitant flow.

Of considerable importance is the influence of left ventricular dilatation on regurgitation. Factors that increase LVEDV increase both the subvalvular mitral area and the diameter of the mitral ring, thus worsening the degree of regurgitation.[11] This aspect of the hemodynamic properties of an incompetent valve lends itself to therapeutic manipulation; that is, increased ventricular emptying and reduced ventricular volume lessen regurgitation.[11]

REDUCED SYSTEMIC VASCULAR RESISTANCE.—Nitroprusside reduces the impedance to forward flow, permitting greater forward ejection.[21,43] There is more complete emptying of the ventricle and a decline in LVEDV and therefore a reduction in subvalvular area, with lessening of regurgitation.[11] At the same time, the left ventricular systolic-to-left atrial gradient diminishes.

INCREASED SYSTEMIC VASCULAR RESISTANCE.—Systemic vascular resistance dramatically influences the function of the incompetent valve. As resistance increases, regurgitation worsens by two mechanisms: the left ventricular systolic-to-left atrial gradient increases and the hypertrophied, dilated ventricle is particularly sensitive to elevated afterload and responds by decreased ejection fraction and stroke volume.[20,23] Thus, LVEDV is greater, causing further valvular incompetence, with elevated regurgitant fraction.

Diminution of forward stroke volume and increased regurgitant volume are seen during infusion of vasoconstrictors.[11] Of more importance to the anesthesiologist is the elevation of systemic vascular resistance induced by surgical stimulation. Even though arterial blood pressure may change little, this stimulation-induced increased impedance to forward flow reduces cardiac output and increases the regurgitant fraction.[113]

CONTRACTILITY.—Enhanced contractile state improves left ventricular emptying and reduces LVEDV and subvalvular area.[11] Regurgitation is therefore diminished. Likewise, depressants of contractile state (for example, inhalational anesthetic agents) may increase LVEDV and regurgitation.

RATE.—Tachycardia decreases systolic time and the tendency to regurgitation and may lower LVEDP and LVEDV. Bradycardia appears to have a hemodynamically deleterious effect: ventricular volume and regurgitant fraction increase while forward cardiac output decreases.

VOLUME INFUSION.—Volume expansion may worsen conditions for the volume-overloaded ventricle,[11] and although no great increase in filling pressure may be observed, chamber volume may increase substantially. This hemodynamic situation is an example of the unreliability of filling pressure as a guide to preload, because the dilated ventricle may demonstrate an altered relationship between pressure and volume, that is, changed wall compliance (see Fig 7–5).

VENTRICULAR SHAPE.—When the contractile state is augmented and LVEDV reduced, the ventricle becomes more eccentrically shaped, while during afterload increase or volume infusion with elevated LVEDV, the shape is more spherical. Ventricular shape influences the subvalvular mitral region and the degree of regurgitation.[11]

In summary, factors that increase LVEDV (for example, negative inotropic drugs) or that decrease compliance of the arterial bed (for example, vasoconstrictors) worsen mitral regurgitation. The adverse pulmonary effects of regurgitation are limited by the distensibility of the left atrium and the pulmonary veins. Increased left atrial compliance blunts the transmission of the ventricular systolic V wave to the pulmonary circulation. Although this V wave may be substantial, mean left atrial pressure may not be greatly increased. Failure is a result of a decline in myocardial contractile state and is manifest as an increase in regurgitant flow and a decrease in forward cardiac output. Now the lungs become subject to a greater venous pressure and deteriorate in a way similar to that seen in mitral stenosis. Pulmonary hypertension may lead to right ventricular hypertrophy and even failure. The anesthesiologist now must be concerned with a

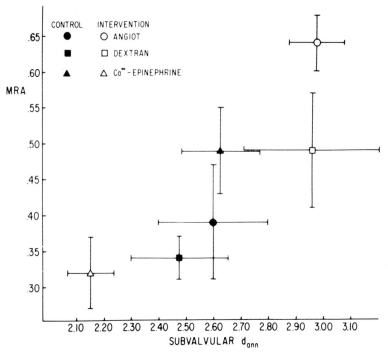

Fig 7-15.—Relationship between calculated area of mitral regurgitation *(MRA)* and observed subvalvular mitral orifice size (d_{ann}) seen on angiography. Increased systemic vascular resistance induced by angiotensin *(ANGIOT)* and volume expansion by dextran increase observed orifice size, while inotropic stimulation from epinephrine decreases diameter of subvalvular mitral orifice. (From Borgenhagen et al.[11] Used by permission of the American Heart Association.)

volume-overloaded left ventricle and a pressure-overloaded right ventricle, separated by a congested pulmonary system. Effects of volume, increased systemic vascular resistance, and inotropic stimulation on the subvalvular mitral area are demonstrated in Figure 7-15.

AORTIC VALVE DISEASE

The aortic valve has three cusps attached to a fibrous valve ring. Immediately above the insertion of the valve cusps are the sinuses of Valsalva. From two of these sinuses arise the left main and the right coronary arteries.

Valvular stenosis produces a pressure overload, and insufficiency results in volume overload. Both forms of overload induce muscle hypertrophy and may eventually lead to failure. Aortic stenosis is distinguished from other valvular lesions by its tendency to cause sudden death. Aortic insufficiency is particularly difficult to manage because the volume overload is not ameliorated by a low-resistance outflow path, as in mitral insufficiency. The total stroke volume must be ejected against the normal impedance of the aorta. This overload eventually diminishes contractile performance. Unfortunately, the jeopardized ventricle is burdened by an additional problem. Aortic insufficiency induces hypertrophy, with increased oxygen needs, but the result is a rapid decline in aortic diastolic pressure. Vital coronary artery perfusion pressure is thus reduced at a time when the myocardial oxygen needs are increased.

Aortic Stenosis

Aortic stenosis may be congenital, rheumatic, or sclerotic in origin. Rheumatic aortic stenosis is usually accompanied by mitral valve damage, while anatomically isolated aortic stenosis results from accelerated degeneration of a congenitally bicuspid or even unicuspid aortic valve (Fig 7-16).

Symptoms

Symptoms are often absent until the late stages of the disease, when angina, dyspnea, and syncope may appear.[17, 76, 85, 86] The freedom from symptoms during much of the disease may represent the ability of the circulation to compensate for aortic stenosis without generating symptoms. Once the disease becomes manifest to the patient, there is a 50% chance of death within four years after the onset of angina or dyspnea. After the onset of congestive heart failure or syncope, there is a 50% chance of death in two years.

Syncope occurs with exercise and results from the inability of the heart to increase cardiac output during exercise-induced peripheral vasodilatation. Syncope also may be associated with rhythm disturbance. Dysrhythmias include intermittent intra-His or infra-His block due to calcification of the valve and septum, with injury to the conducting system.

Signs

A systolic crescendo-decrescendo murmur, radiating into the neck, can be heard over the aortic outflow tract. The second heart sound is diminished in proportion to the stiffness of the calcified valve. Stenosis limits stroke volume, and unless systemic vascular resistance is elevated, blood pressure tends to be low.

Investigations

The ECG demonstrates left ventricular hypertrophy, and if ischemia or calcification has been severe, the ventricular conducting system may have been damaged, resulting in conduction abnormalities. The chest roentgenogram shows left ventricular hypertrophy. Pulmonary congestion is not present unless failure has ensued.

Hemodynamics

Stenosis of the aortic valve necessitates the generation of a high systolic pressure to accomplish ejection, thus subjecting the ventricle to a severe pressure overload. Concentric hypertrophy is the compensatory mechanism introduced to maintain performance, and an extremely thick ventricular wall results.[65, 81]

Normal aortic valve size is 2.5 to 3.0 sq cm,[49, 97] which is smaller than the mitral area. The orifice area at which symptoms appear is also less than in mitral disease, because the hypertrophied ventricle can generate a high systolic pressure and gradient. Symptoms may not appear until the area has diminished to 0.8 sq cm or less.[39]

As the valve area decreases, left ventricular systolic pressure increases in order to increase the gradient and maintain stroke volume. This pressure load increases wall tension and stress. Tension stimulates hypertrophy, and wall thickness increases, thus returning the wall stress to a more normal value[81]:

$$\text{Wall stress} = \frac{\text{pressure} \times \text{volume}}{\text{wall thickness}}$$

Increase in wall thickness is proportional to the increase in intraventricular pressure. The LVEDV tends to remain normal, but left ventricular mass increases so that the ratio of LVEDV to left ventricular muscle mass is elevated from the normal of 1.2:1 to about 2.0:1.[80] The LVEDP increases, but this implies reduced wall compliance rather than ventricular dilatation and "heart failure." The LVEDP may be substantially elevated despite normal cardiac performance, and this factor illustrates the inaccuracy of using LVEDP as an indicator of left ventricular failure and indicates a need for caution in the interpretation of filling pressure (see Fig 7–5). The ejection fraction during this phase of compensated aortic stenosis is normal and may be greater than normal. If the pressure-volume loop (Fig 7–17) is considered during well-compensated stenosis, the most pronounced abnormality is an elevated systolic pressure. The LVEDP may be elevated, but the LVEDV is not increased[81] (see Fig 7–5). Systolic work, expressed graphically as the area within the loop (Fig 7–17), is substantially increased, indicating that maintenance of normal cardiac performance is achieved only at a greater expenditure of energy. The ventricle has become inefficient. If stenosis worsens or contractile performance significantly decreases[61, 103] (decreased contractile state is a characteristic of hypertrophied heart muscle),[108] then the Starling mechanism is recruited and chamber dilatation occurs (Fig 7–18).

The disease now enters a decompensated phase, and heart failure eventually ensues. The LVEDV and LVEDP increase to maintain

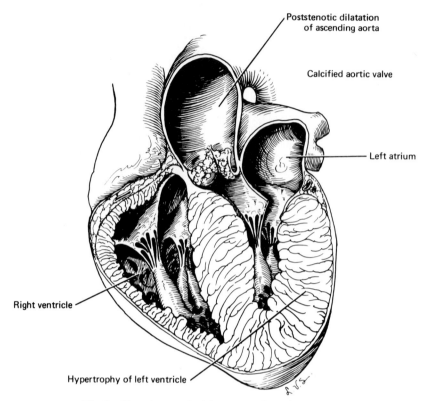

Fig 7–16.—Anatomical features of aortic stenosis. (From Sokolow and McIlroy.[105] Used by permission.)

stroke volume, but the ejection fraction decreases.[30, 81] Wall tension and stress increase with this increase in cavity volume, but further increases in wall thickness are ineffective in maintaining wall stress within normal limits. The pressure-volume loop has about the same area but is shifted to the right, indicating that the same stroke volume and work are now achieved at greater chamber volume. More energy and oxygen are required for a similar level of cardiac performance in this dilated state; that is, efficiency has further declined.

Aspects of Aortic Stenosis

LEFT ATRIAL FUNCTION.—During diastole, the ventricles normally receive about 20% of left ventricular stroke volume during atrial contraction; the remainder enters the ventricles in a passive fashion. Patients with aortic stenosis receive as much as 40% of the left ventricular stroke volume by the "booster-pump" mechanism of atrial contraction.[55, 114] The rate of left ventricular filling is more than doubled during atrial systole, although little increase in flow is seen in normal patients. Decreased left ventricular compliance as a result of hypertrophy explains the dependence on atrial contraction for the maintenance of adequate filling.[41] The contribution of coordinated atrial contraction to left ventricular filling becomes more important as left ventricular diastolic compliance decreases.[92] Ventricular hypertrophy lowers the rate of left ventricular filling by the passive reservoir and conduit functions of the left atrium, with flow from the atrium often having ceased before atrial systole begins. Atrial systole now continues the process of left ventricular filling, and because atrial contraction is brief, mean left atrial pressure is little increased. A high LVEDP can be generated without much increase in mean left atrial pressure, and in this way the pulmonary circulation is spared from congestion. The nondistensible ventricle needs a high LVEDP to maintain adequate LVEDV[61] and becomes critically dependent on atrial systole for mainte-

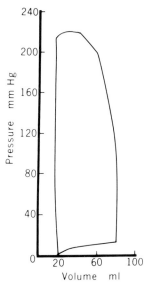

Fig 7–17.—Pressure-volume loop constructed for patient with compensated aortic stenosis. Work is increased because of high systolic pressure. Left ventricular end-diastolic volume at this stage of disease is normal. (From Brest A.N.: *Diagnostic Methods in Cardiology*. Philadelphia, F. A. Davis Co., 1975. Used by permission.)

nance of preload. Ventricular compliance is illustrated in Figure 7–5. Loss of sinus rhythm leads to a significant decrease in performance.[15]

Reduced distensibility limits the ability of the ventricle to compensate for reduced contractile performance by means of the Starling mechanism, but forceful atrial contraction somewhat overcomes this problem. Loss of sinus rhythm would necessitate high left atrial pressure, with associated pulmonary congestion, to maintain the same degree of preloading.

TACHYCARDIA.—When heart rate increases, cardiac output tends not to increase because stroke volume diminishes.[39] Tachycardia has a number of detrimental effects on the heart and its performance.[119] Systolic time is reduced, ejection time is shortened, and, in the absence of an increased pressure gradient to drive blood flow, the stroke volume (SV) decreases. This relationship can be appreciated from the following relationship:

$$SV \propto \text{aortic valve area} \times \text{duration of ejection} \times \sqrt{\text{pressure gradient}}$$

To maintain stroke volume, flow across the valve must increase, and this increase is achieved by an increase in the intraventricular pressure and gradient.

Increased pressure requires more oxygen but, at the same time, reduces coronary blood flow by compressing coronary vessels within the ventricular wall. Maximal left ventricular pressure seems to be between 250 and 300 mm Hg, higher pressures being prevented by the appearance of ischemia.[39]

Tachycardia reduces diastolic time per cycle, resulting in a decrease in the period available for ventricular filling by the passive function of the left atrium. Reduced diastolic time also less-

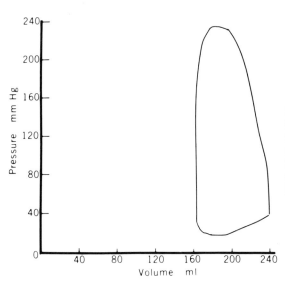

Fig 7–18.—Pressure-volume loop in patient with decompensated aortic stenosis has shifted to right, implying chamber dilatation. Both left ventricular end-diastolic volume and pressure are increased. Starling mechanism has been introduced to compensate for declining performance. (From Rackley and Hood.[81] Used by permission.)

ens the time available for blood flow in the coronary arteries. Thus, while oxygen demand is increased by more frequent contractions, oxygen delivery is reduced by diminished coronary blood flow.

Bradycardia has a pronounced deleterious effect, because aortic stenosis limits the extent to which stroke volume may be increased to compensate. Cardiac output and blood pressure may be very dependent on heart rate within a narrow range.

CONTRACTILITY.—Changes in contractile state with muscle hypertrophy have been discussed. Usually, contractile state is well maintained in the heart that has not dilated, and this preservation of contractile state is manifested by the often excellent cardiac performance observed after aortic valve replacement. Long-standing pressure overload eventually results in diminished contractile state[59, 61, 103] and, characteristically, dilatation as well as hypertrophy. Improved performance may not be so dramatic after valve replacement.

EXERCISE.—The LVEDP increases, and the change is more pronounced when the aortic stenosis is more severe. This increase in LVEDP during exercise signifies reduced myocardial compliance,[59] perhaps brought about by exercise-induced ischemia, and indicates depressed myocardial function. The ejection fraction decreases.

ANGINA.—Angina may be a symptom of aortic stenosis because the increased work necessitated by outflow obstruction is pressure work involving a high oxygen demand. Ventricular muscle mass increases, but the coronary arteriolar and capillary system may not have proliferated to the same extent as the muscle mass[97]; therefore, coronary vascular reserve may be diminished. As discussed, increased systolic pressure has a "throttling" effect on the intramyocardial vessels.[16] Oxygen supply may be further reduced by tachycardia and the accompanying shortened diastolic period.

A further contributor to ischemia is a low aortic diastolic pressure, reducing coronary perfusion pressure.

Thus, angina may occur even though the coronary system is free of atheromatous changes. A normal coronary system maximally dilated is still often unable to provide adequate perfusion.[17, 119] If coronary artery disease coexists with aortic stenosis, then angina occurs more readily.[17]

Aortic Regurgitation

Aortic regurgitation produces a volume overload on the left ventricle, but unlike the situation in mitral regurgitation, the extra volume must be moved against the high impedance of the arterial system. Aortic regurgitation is usually the result of rheumatic heart disease, but it also can be congenital in origin.[86] Other causes include hypertension, syphilitic aortitis, infective endocarditis, dissecting aortic aneurysm, and Marfan's syndrome. Regurgitation results from damage to the cusps or from dilatation of the aorta and the valve ring. Rheumatic endocarditis results in thickening and shortening of the cusps, and there may be some fusion of the commissures. Both stenosis and regurgitation may occur (Fig 7–19).

Symptoms

The initial symptom is usually dyspnea on exertion, but many years may elapse between acute rheumatic carditis and the emergence of symptoms. Angina may occur with severe aortic regurgitation.

Signs

The pulse pressure is wide, with a systolic pressure as high as 250 mm Hg and a diastolic pressure that may decrease to nearly zero. There is an early diastolic murmur, and it may be accompanied by a systolic flow murmur caused by the large total stroke volume. The Austin Flint murmur is a mid-diastolic murmur that probably results from the effect of the regurgitant flow on the aortic leaflet of the mitral valve that lies near the aortic valve orifice.

Investigations

Left ventricular hypertrophy is evident on the ECG, and the chest roentgenogram demonstrates left ventricular enlargement with dilatation of the ascending aorta.

Hemodynamics

This condition is one of volume overload of the left ventricle, with total cardiac output that

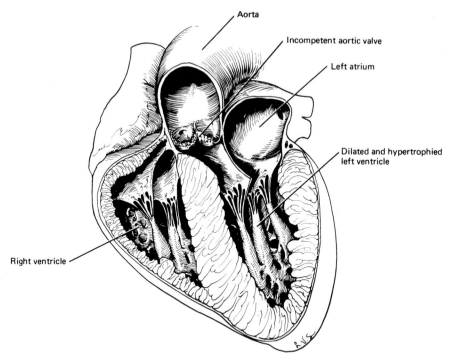

Fig 7–19.—Anatomical features of aortic incompetence. (From Sokolow and McIlroy.[105] Used by permission.)

may be as high as 30 L/minute.[30] The principal filling of the left ventricle occurs by regurgitation from the aorta. In pure aortic regurgitation, there is little or no pressure gradient across the valve. Aortic valve gradients do not develop, even though aortic flow is greatly increased. The LVEDV is increased and may be about 200 ml/sq m, although massively dilated ventricles may have a volume of 400 ml/sq m. This value is probably close to the largest possible left ventricular volume seen in man. Stroke volume increases in proportion to the degree of regurgitation. This stroke volume is divided into forward and regurgitant fractions. The total stroke volume may increase during aortic regurgitation to 110 ml/sq m and even higher volumes; for example, 200 ml/sq m may be seen.[30] Stroke volume decreases with the onset of failure.

The high total cardiac output is achieved by increased stroke volume, but the greater part of the total flow may regurgitate; for example, total output may be as high as 30 L/minute, but 24 L/minute regurgitates, leaving the remaining 6 L as forward cardiac output. Such enormous flows are achieved by substantial left ventricular dilatation and wall hypertrophy. As regurgitant stroke volume increases, so does LVEDV.

During diastole, even though the incompetent area of the valve may be small, the high pressure in the aorta and arterial system results in a large regurgitant volume rapidly filling the ventricle. Volume loading is also increased by the atrial contribution to ventricular end-diastolic volume. The total volume overload causes the ventricle to dilate. As regurgitation worsens, LVEDV tends to become elevated (Fig 7–20), but because wall compliance may be greater than normal, LVEDP does not increase proportionally (see Fig 7–5).

As was described, LVEDV and LVESV are much increased, but the ejection fraction remains normal. Although total stroke volume is increased, the effective stroke volume (that is, total LVESV minus regurgitant volume) remains normal. The condition at this stage is well compensated.[81]

As has been indicated previously, increase in cavity volume or cavity pressure results in an increase in wall stress, which is normalized by

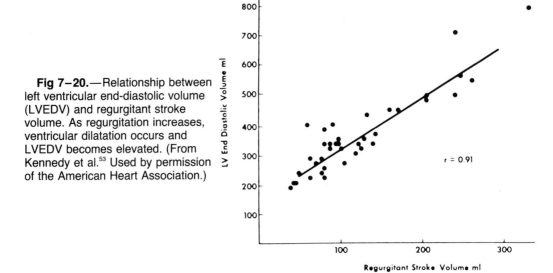

Fig 7-20.—Relationship between left ventricular end-diastolic volume (LVEDV) and regurgitant stroke volume. As regurgitation increases, ventricular dilatation occurs and LVEDV becomes elevated. (From Kennedy et al.[53] Used by permission of the American Heart Association.)

increased wall thickness. This principle applies, with resultant eccentric hypertrophy.

The pressure-volume loop for aortic regurgitation shows that LVEDP and left ventricular end-systolic pressure remain normal but the ventricle is dilated. Pressure-volume work is increased owing to the large stroke volume.

Cardiac output is maintained by the introduction of ventricular dilatation and hypertrophy, but these changes have a detrimental effect on the intrinsic contractile performance of the myocardium. Eventually, deterioration occurs and is manifested by an increase in LVEDV that is out of proportion to the increase in LVESV; that is, ejection fraction declines and eventually so does stroke volume.[30, 81] The hypertrophy mechanism fails, leading to increasing wall stress, loss of compliance, and an elevation of LVEDP. Elevated LVEDP results in dyspnea, and the patient is subjected to decreasing cardiac output and pulmonary congestion. Elevated LVEDP in association with aortic stenosis implies a reduced compliance in a stiff, concentrically hypertrophied ventricle rather than an onset of pulmonary congestion. The increase in LVEDP seen during deterioration of aortic regurgitation implies that the Starling mechanism is being actively used to support a poorly performing, enlarging but compliant ventricle. Mean left atrial pressure mirrors this increase in LVEDP.

Examination of a pressure-volume loop of the patient with deteriorating aortic regurgitation demonstrates some elevation of LVEDP but substantially increased LVEDV[81] (Fig 7–21). Stroke volume is maintained, but the ejection fraction has decreased significantly. Pressure-volume work is not much increased, but, at this degree of ventricular dilatation, it is performed very inefficiently, with high oxygen consumption.

Aspects of Aortic Regurgitation

REGURGITANT FLOW.—Regurgitant flow can be as high as 20 L/minute, resulting in a very high total ventricular output. Aortic regurgitation can be classified according to the degree of regurgitation: little, 0 to 1 L/minute; mild, 1 to 3 L/minute; moderate, 3 to 6 L/minute; and severe, greater than 6 L/minute.[30] A number of factors influence regurgitant flow: (1) aortic valve regurgitant area during diastole, (2) aortic-ventricular pressure gradient during diastole, and (3) duration of diastole. Aortic regurgitant flow is proportional to regurgitant valve area times diastolic period times heart rate times diastolic gradient.

HEART RATE.—It has been shown that, in patients with elevated LVEDP, when the heart rate is increased above the intrinsic rate by atrial pacing, then LVEDP, LVEDV, and total stroke volume are reduced[50] (Fig 7–22). Accom-

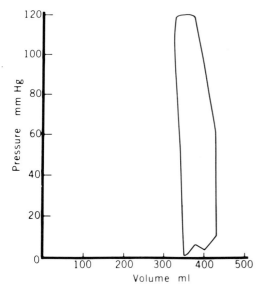

Fig 7–21.—Pressure-volume loop for patient with decompensated aortic regurgitation. Ventricular dilatation has resulted in shift of loop to right. Chamber is much enlarged, and left ventricular end-diastolic pressure is elevated. (From Rackley and Hood.[80] Used by permission.)

panying these decreases is a lowering in diastolic wall tension and stress.[50] (The decreased LVEDP insignificantly worsens the aortic gradient.) Tachycardia also reduces diastolic time, thus decreasing regurgitant flow. Although stroke volume and regurgitant flow per stroke are reduced, the total volume of regurgitation per minute is little altered. Forward cardiac output is usually increased with increase in rate. Bradycardia increases regurgitation because diastolic time is prolonged, resulting in an increase in LVEDV, LVEDP, and diastolic wall stress. These changes may induce pulmonary congestion and dramatically reduce forward cardiac output.

CONTRACTILITY.—The contractile state is often depressed, and if extensive myofibrillar slippage has occurred, this alteration in the inotropic state may not be reversed by valve replacement.[36, 65, 81]

AFTERLOAD.—Increased impedance to ejection worsens regurgitation.[9] Patients with pronounced regurgitation show a decline in stroke volume and an increase in LVEDP in response to afterload stress (for example, with angiotensin infusion) even though the ejection fraction may be normal at rest. Increased systemic vascular resistance becomes more detrimental to performance as heart function deteriorates (Fig 7–23).

Afterload reduction with vasodilators in severe aortic regurgitation improves cardiac performance,[7, 68] decreases LVEDV and LVEDP, and reduces regurgitant volume. Forward cardiac index is augmented and total stroke work index is diminished (Fig 7–24).

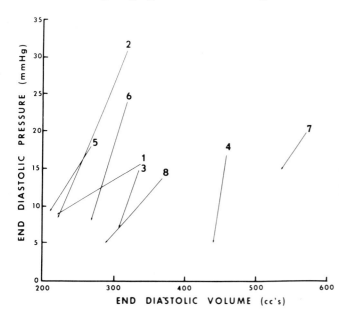

Fig 7–22.—Data on eight patients with aortic regurgitation undergoing atrial pacing at a more rapid rate show reduction in left ventricular end-diastolic pressure and volume. (From Judge et al.[50] Used by permission of the American Heart Association.)

Fig 7–23.—Ejection fraction in patients with compensated **(A)** and decompensated **(B)** aortic regurgitation when challenged by elevation of systemic vascular resistance with angiotensin. Group B patients demonstrate noticeable deterioration when impedance to ejection is elevated. (From Bolen et al.[9] Used by permission of the American Heart Association.)

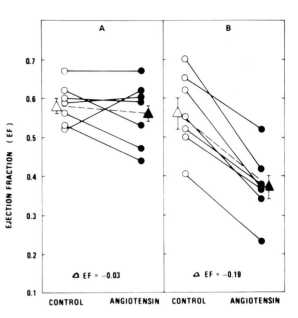

MYOCARDIAL OXYGEN BALANCE.—Aortic regurgitation is a condition of volume overload, and additional cardiac work is performed in moving increased volume.

Overall myocardial oxygen demand is increased because of greater muscle mass, but oxygen consumption and coronary blood flow per gram of myocardium are normal at rest. Chronic vasodilatation may be responsible for this normal coronary blood flow, but unlike that in the

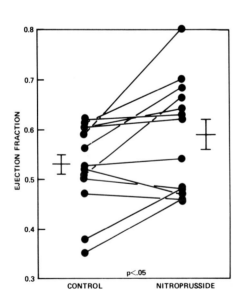

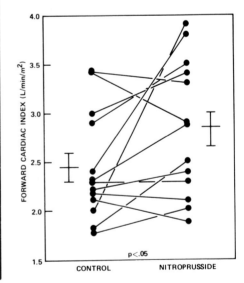

Fig 7–24.—**Left,** ejection fraction in control condition and during nitroprusside infusion in patients with aortic regurgitation. Patients showing most significant improvement had severe ejection fraction depression at rest. **Right,** forward cardiac index in control condition and during nitroprusside infusion, showing significant improvement in eight of 13 patients. (From Bolen and Alderman.[7] Used by permission of the American Heart Association.)

normal heart, further dilatation may not be possible during increased demand; that is, coronary blood flow reserve is diminished.[33]

ACUTE AORTIC REGURGITATION.—When aortic regurgitation develops gradually, the left ventricle dilates and becomes more distensible, with the result that the regurgitant volume is accepted with little increase in LVEDP. If aortic regurgitation develops abruptly, this adaptation is not possible. Acute aortic regurgitation or acute worsening of aortic regurgitation is associated with rapidly increasing LVEDP, rising diastolic pressure, pulmonary venous congestion, and sudden death.[73]

COMBINED AORTIC STENOSIS AND AORTIC REGURGITATION.—Rheumatic endocarditis involving the aortic valve frequently results in combined stenosis and regurgitation, and gradations between the two hemodynamic states occur. Stenosis usually predominates when aortic stenosis and aortic regurgitation are the result of congenital or atherosclerotic lesions. The overloads are both pressure and volume and lead to chamber dilatation and massive muscle hypertrophy. The pressure-volume loop demonstrates a much enlarged area, indicating that considerable work is involved in ejecting this increased total stroke volume against the severe resistance of the stenosed valve.[81]

TRICUSPID VALVE DISEASE

The tricuspid valve has three cusps but otherwise is structurally similar to the mitral valve. Isolated tricuspid valve disease is very unusual, occurring more frequently in association with mitral valve disease.[29, 120] Some tricuspid stenosis occurs in rheumatic mitral disease, although the tricuspid contribution to hemodynamic disturbance is rarely significant. The pathologic changes occurring in the tricuspid valve are similar to those involving the mitral valve.[6]

Tricuspid Stenosis

Tricuspid stenosis is nearly always rheumatic in origin.[19] Right ventricular filling is impaired by the stenotic obstruction to flow during diastole. There is volume underloading of the right ventricle. Right atrial pressure increases, and the right atrium dilates and hypertrophies.

A large venous "a" wave of atrial contraction is seen on catheterization of the right atrium, but this wave disappears with the onset of atrial fibrillation. There is a diastolic pressure gradient across the tricuspid valve. If the lesion is severe, cardiac output decreases and signs of "right-sided failure" develop (for example, ascites, hepatic enlargement, jaundice, and cachexia).[105]

Interestingly, a more frequent symptom is dyspnea, as a result of coexisting mitral valve disease. Tricuspid stenosis reduces right ventricular output. Thus, pulmonary congestion during coexisting mitral valve disease is less severe but occurs at the expense of systemic venous congestion and lowered cardiac output.

Tricuspid Insufficiency

Tricuspid insufficiency resembles mitral insufficiency in its etiology. Tricuspid insufficiency may have an organic cause, such as rheumatic heart disease, or may be functional, that is, as a result of right ventricular dilatation leading to distention of the valve ring and disturbance of the closing mechanism.[19, 29] Pulmonary hypertension may cause right ventricular hypertrophy and failure, and the accompanying right ventricular dilatation further reduces tricuspid valve competence.

The hemodynamic lesion is one of volume overload, with sequelae similar to those encountered in mitral regurgitation, that is, dilatation of the chamber with accompanying eccentric wall hypertrophy. Elevated blood flow occurs through the insufficient tricuspid valve during diastole and systole, and this flow is increased during spontaneous inspiration, when venous return to the heart is increased.

The right atrium and venae cavae are extremely compliant and therefore can accept the regurgitant volume without much increase in pressure, but large systolic waves from right ventricular contraction are transmitted to the peripheral venous system.

Tricuspid insufficiency is usually well tolerated, and complete removal of the tricuspid valve may have few adverse sequelae.[88] The disease may become significant if pulmonary hypertension coexists, because this condition imposes a pressure overload on a dilated ventricle that is principally accustomed to volume work. Forward stroke volume is reduced, while regurgitant fraction increases. Right ventricular dilatation may disturb left ventricular performance[52] because of the close anatomical relationship. Also, right ventricular hypertrophy may influence the left ventricle because some myocardial fibers are common to both ventricles.

ANESTHESIA

Anesthesia and surgery constitute, in biologic terms, a very unusual and artificial situation that in some aspects resembles strenuous exercise or the "fight or flight" response to environmental danger. Patients respond to surgical stimulation by activation of the sympathetic axis, with an immediate adrenergic nervous discharge, followed by numerous humoral changes. Release of endogenous catecholamines, renin-angiotensin, aldosterone, corticosteroids, prostaglandins, and vasopressin represents a response to stress.

The cardiovascular system is dramatically influenced by this altered autonomic and humoral background, manifest most obviously by an increase in heart rate, contractile state, and systemic vascular resistance. These changes may not be beneficial to the patient with valvular heart disease.

The anesthesiologist has a vantage point from which he can assess and influence circulatory performance. In simple terms, he has four roles[4]: (1) to maintain or to improve the preoperative cardiovascular performance, (2) to prevent the deleterious effects of the "stress" reaction to surgery, (3) to protect jeopardized organs, and (4) to provide sedation, analgesia, amnesia, or hypnosis.

The efficacy of interventions is directly related to the ability to gather accurate information on the state of the cardiovascular system. The four-lumen pulmonary artery balloon-tipped catheter, with an ability to measure cardiac output, provides an essential means of extending the assessment of circulatory function.[56,63] Now, not only can an estimate of left-sided filling pressure be obtained but rapid measurement of cardiac output also can be performed. Because central venous and arterial pressure are known, numerous derived values can be calculated. Systemic vascular resistance, pulmonary vascular resistance, stroke volume, and ventricular stroke work can be quickly obtained using a pocket calculator, and from the collected information, appropriate manipulations of the circulatory system may be introduced. These values are important within themselves, but trends evolving in response to therapy are further evidence of the efficacy of pharmacologic intervention.

Many patients, although suffering some limitation of function, remain in good health, and the use of a Swan-Ganz catheter is not essential. Monitoring of central venous pressure may be sufficient, and monitoring of pulmonary artery pressure may be unnecessary in patients with reasonable myocardial function. Insertion of a left atrial catheter by the surgeon before the termination of bypass provides a means of assessing left ventricular filling during the period after bypass. Cardiac output values may be obtained by the dye-dilution technique, but rapid sequential measurements are cumbersome. In summary, use of the Swan-Ganz catheter permits a more complete assessment of the state of the circulation and provides information that is useful even when few perioperative difficulties are encountered.

Principles of Manipulations During Anesthesia

The factors that govern cardiac performance are readily modified by techniques of anesthesia.

Preload

Preload should be manipulated to the optimal position on the ventricular function curve. It must be remembered that diastolic myocardial fiber length is better estimated by end-diastolic volume than by end-diastolic pressure (see Fig 7–5). The compliant ventricle shows large changes in volume during diastole but little change in LVEDP, whereas the stiff ventricle may undergo small changes in end-diastolic volume for a large change in end-diastolic pressure. During sinus rhythm, LVEDP is greater than left atrial pressure or pulmonary capillary wedge pressure, and this difference may be substantial when the ventricle is hypertrophied or noncompliant, as in aortic stenosis. The reverse is true of mitral stenosis, in which pulmonary capillary wedge pressure and left atrial pressure substantially exceed LVEDP. Also, the ventricular function curve becomes less linear or flattened at higher filling pressures, resulting in less increase in performance. The function curve of the hypertrophied or failing heart is less steep than that of the normal heart, and methods other than increase in preload may be necessary to achieve improvement in cardiac function. Acutely, there may be a descending limb to this curve, necessitating the exercise of caution when high filling pressures are reached.

Rapidly developing failure may elevate the filling pressure above threshold for the development of pulmonary edema, necessitating treatment—principally by venodilatation, inotropic augmentation, and reduction of afterload.

Preload can be increased by volume infusion. An adequate filling pressure should be achieved before inotropic agents are used. Augmented cardiac output from inotropic stimulation requires more oxygen than an equal increase from the preload mechanism. The Trendelenburg position provides a rapid means of increasing filling pressure. Likewise, the reverse Trendelenburg position will cause venous pooling and is useful prior to anesthesia in patients with mitral stenosis, if pulmonary edema is imminent. A more advantageous position for spontaneous respiration may be more responsible for improvement when the reverse Trendelenburg position is used. Mechanical ventilation also reduces venous return.[40]

Filling pressure can be reduced by a number of drugs. Nitroglycerin produces venodilatation and, to a lesser extent, so does nitroprusside, but both drugs also reduce arterial vascular resistance and blood pressure[13,69,70] (Fig 7–25). (Much of this decrease in preload may be achieved by enhanced ventricular emptying.) Morphine has venodilating properties[46] (probably due to histamine release) and has long been used in the therapy of acute pulmonary edema. Furosemide produces an early decrease in pulmonary artery pressure and pulmonary capillary wedge pressure before its diuretic action.[72]

Lastly, if the aortic or right atrial pump lines are in place when preload is inappropriately high, volume can be rapidly removed into the heart-lung machine.

Contractility

The hypertrophied, pressure- or volume-overloaded ventricle has a diminished contractile performance.[108] Decreased inotropic characteristics may be the final event that precipitates heart failure.

In clinical practice, most disease is recognized and surgical treatment is undertaken before the onset of frank heart failure, but reduced contractile performance may contribute significantly to the overall disturbance of circulatory function. Inotropic stimulation is indicated if conditions of preload (pulmonary capillary wedge pressure), afterload (represented in practice by systemic vascular resistance), and heart rate are optimal, yet the cardiac index remains at 1.8 L/minute/sq m or less. An alternative indication for inotropic support may be the inability to reduce elevated preload despite the use of vasodilators. In this situation, the use of an inotropic drug may be associated with diminution of preload, with a decrease in ventricular dilatation, and therefore with a reduction in diastolic wall stress, oxygen consumption, and pulmonary congestion. Available inotropic agents, while improving contractile performance, have various effects on preload, heart rate, afterload, and renal perfusion.

Dopamine has become a frequently used inotropic agent because it not only enhances the contractile state but, at low doses, also changes

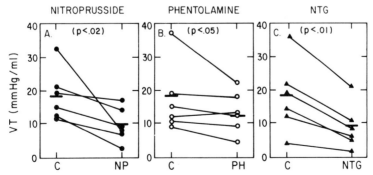

Fig 7–25.—Effects of nitroprusside *(NP)*, phentolamine *(PH)*, and nitroglycerine *(NTG)* on forearm venous tone *(VT)*. Control *(C)*. (From Miller et al.[70] Used by permission.)

heart rate or systemic vascular resistance very little while improving renal blood flow. Dobutamine,[98,117,118] a more recently introduced inotropic agent, has a number of attractive potential advantages. Contractile state is enhanced without much increase in heart rate, and both pulmonary and systemic vascular resistances are reduced. The importance of the pulmonary vasculature has frequently been ignored when an inotropic agent is selected, and yet the right ventricle may be failing at the same time as the left ventricle and may also benefit from afterload reduction. Furthermore, dobutamine tends to reduce an elevated filling pressure.

Unfortunately, the use of isoproterenol is strictly limited because of the accompanying tachycardia and a tendency to provoke ventricular ectopy. Epinephrine, although not as chronotropically active as isoproterenol, also may produce tachycardia and ventricular ectopy. Norepinephrine lacks these chronotropic disadvantages, and its property of elevating systemic vascular resistance may be antagonized by the simultaneous infusion of a vasodilator, for example, nitroprusside.

Many patients with valve disease remain free of serious hemodynamic disturbance, and their cardiac output is satisfactory at rest and during exercise. Surgical stimulation results in sympathetic discharge and an increased cardiac output. The heart performs more work than is required and does so at the expense of increased oxygen demand. Patients with aortic stenosis or those with coexistent coronary artery disease are at risk of developing acute myocardial ischemia under these conditions. Such inhalational anesthetic agents as halothane or enflurane may be advantageously introduced to depress the myocardium in a controlled fashion. Care must be exercised because these anesthetics depress the contractile state,[60,101,102,107] especially in the heart that has reduced inotropic reserve.

If an element of failure is induced, ventricular dilatation occurs, with increased wall tension and increased oxygen demand, thus defeating the rationale for the use of inhalational agents. Even so, patients with valvular heart disease can be anesthetized with such drugs, without detrimental cardiac depression.[26,112]

Impedance to Ejection

Impedance to ejection is clinically related to, and represented by, systemic vascular resistance. Five generalizations concerning systemic vascular resistance and performance can be made. The first is that elevated systemic vascular resistance increases regurgitant flow in mitral[11] and aortic[9] regurgitation and thus may detrimentally alter performance.[113] The second is that hypertrophied hearts frequently respond to afterload increase with a reduction in stroke volume and cardiac output.[20,23] The third is that, as valvular heart disease progresses to failure, elevated systemic vascular resistance is often observed and may be a late adaptive mechanism to maintain blood pressure, despite the unfavorable influence on cardiac output. This increase in systemic vascular resistance may be an inappropriate side effect of an otherwise beneficial increase in sympathetic activity.[20] The fourth is that laryngoscopy, endotracheal intubation, and surgical stimulation are stresses that increase the secretion of norepinephrine and other vasoactive substances, resulting in increased systemic vascular resistance. The fifth is that vasodilator drugs relax resistance vessels and thus reduce the impedance to ejection.

Vasodilators enable the ventricle to empty more completely. Thus, stroke volume is increased and wall tension is reduced so that, while cardiac output is augmented, there is a concomitant reduction in myocardial oxygen requirement.[20,42,67,70] This action is a physiologic bargain. Pressure work is converted to flow work and is accomplished more efficiently (see Fig 7–7). Using a vasodilator (for example, nitroprusside), the anesthesiologist may prevent an increase in systemic vascular resistance in a controlled way. These aspects can be outlined. First, anesthetic agents tend to have mild vasodilating properties, but their main usefulness is the prevention of an increase in systemic vascular resistance in response to surgical stimulation. Changes in systemic vascular resistance are mediated by the sympathetic nervous system and by various humoral factors. This activity may be suppressed by anesthetic agents. It has been suggested that 1.5 minimum alveolar concentration for halothane and enflurane or about 1.1 mg/kg morphine is needed to prevent an increase in release of norepinephrine in response to skin incision in ASA I or II adults.[89,90] Thus, a depth of anesthesia may be used that is sufficient to suppress adverse circulatory reflexes in response to surgical stimulation. Unfortunately, this dose of anesthetic may cause unacceptable hemodynamic side effects in patients whose circulations are impaired by valvular heart disease. However, in such patients, less anesthetic may be required to cause the same degree of reflex depression when compared with that in healthy patients. Anesthetic agents reduce arteriolar tone, predominantly by reduction in sympathetic outflow. Ketamine is an exception because systemic vascular resistance is increased, and nitrous oxide has a mixture of peripheral vascular actions, increased systemic vascular resistance being often reported in patients with heart disease.

Second, patients with mitral or aortic regurgitation respond favorably to a reduction in systemic vascular resistance.[7,21,43,68] The regurgitant fraction is reduced, and forward output is consistently improved by vasodilator therapy. Sodium nitroprusside infusion is an excellent means of reducing systemic vascular resistance in a controlled fashion.

Third, the hypertrophied or failing heart responds to increased impedance to ejection by a reduction in stroke volume. A parabolic relationship is believed to exist between stroke volume and outflow resistance[23] (see Fig 7-9), but recently the universality of this observation has been questioned.[96] Generally, patients with severe valvular disease have an inappropriately elevated systemic vascular resistance, which may be reduced by vasodilators. There is some inconsistency in the improvement of cardiac function with a reduction in systemic vascular resistance.[96] The efficacy of vasodilator therapy can be assessed by close observation of the accompanying changes in cardiac output. Vasodilators may be infused throughout the operative course to maintain the systemic vascular resistance within the most advantageous range.

Fourth, occasionally patients who need correction of valvular lesions have a pronounced depression in cardiac output that improves little with vasodilator therapy. An inotropic drug will improve performance but frequently does not lower the elevated filling pressures that accompany the low output state. Combined vasodilator-inotropic infusion may improve cardiac index more than either agent alone and also may reduce elevated filling pressure[71] (Fig 7-26).

Heart Rate

Heart rate is of crucial importance in the management of valvular heart disease, is readily altered by surgical stimulation, and may be adversely affected by inappropriate choice of anesthetic agents. Procedures performed in the operating room, such as insertion of a monitoring line, laryngoscopy, endotracheal intubation, bladder catheterization, and the surgical stimulation itself, increase adrenergic tone as well as the secretions of many vasoactive humoral factors. A result of such activity is tachycardia, although occasionally a sudden slowing of the heart rate may occur. Tachycardia shortens the

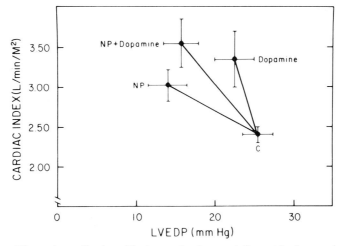

Fig 7-26.—Conditions in patients with low cardiac index and high filling pressure may be improved by vasodilators or inotropes. Usefulness of nitroprusside (NP) may be limited by decline in systemic pressure, while dopamine may fail to lower left-ventricular end-diastolic pressure (LVEDP). Combined vasodilator-inotrope therapy can overcome these problems, while further enhancing cardiac output. (From Miller et al.[71] Used by permission.)

diastolic period, reducing the time available during each cycle for coronary artery blood flow. A shorter diastolic period reduces left ventricular filling across the narrowed valve of mitral stenosis,[2,116] and a shorter systolic time increases the intraventricular pressure needed to generate flow through the narrowed valve in aortic stenosis.[119] Bradycardia permits greater backward flow in aortic regurgitation, thus lowering arterial diastolic pressure and reducing coronary artery perfusion pressure. This worsened regurgitation results in an increase in chamber volume, with an associated increase in wall tension and oxygen requirement. Slow heart rates are hazardous in aortic stenosis because stroke volume is limited, causing heart rate to gain greater importance in determining cardiac output. A sufficient depth of anesthesia will blunt the change in heart rate seen in response to surgical stimulation, but it would seem that only narcotics possess an intrinsic rate-reducing property. Reduction in heart rate during the administration of fentanyl has been described. Fentanyl probably causes such changes by a centrally mediated action.[35,58] Muscle relaxants also may alter heart rate. Pancuronium frequently causes tachycardia,[10] but despite this disadvantage, the drug remains in wide use because its lack of ganglion-blocking properties avoids the tendency to hypotension seen with curare.[47] Curare given in small, well-spaced increments permits muscle relaxation with little influence on the circulation. Metocurine may become accepted because it causes little chronotropic activity or autonomic ganglion blockade.[47,48,95,123]

Heart rate may be effectively slowed with small doses of propranolol, such increments rarely exerting a detrimental negative inotropic action. Edrophonium also can be used to reduce the rate. Currently, negative chronotropic substances that are free of side effects are not available. Prevention of tachycardia usually can be accomplished by adequate anesthetic depth. If tachycardia is anticipated, narcotics may be more useful than inhalational agents in achieving this goal. High-dose fentanyl may provide adequate blunting of the heart rate response to stressful stimulation yet alter contractility or peripheral vascular tone very little. The dose of morphine required to produce a similar degree of sensory blockade may be associated with adverse effects, such as histamine-mediated venodilatation and an unpredictable action on arterial tone. Tachycardia may be a compensatory response to a decline in cardiac performance. Treatment of heart failure may reduce the cardiac rate.

Increases in heart rate are frequently encountered during cardiac surgery, and much attention is directed to preventing or controlling this rate change, but bradycardia also may appear and may herald or cause significant impairment of circulatory function. To provide an adequate cardiac output, the diseased heart may require a rate within a narrow range, and decreases below this optimal rate can precipitate a decline in cardiac index and systemic blood pressure. Sinus bradycardia is the most commonly encountered slow rhythm, and the heart rate should be accelerated if blood pressure decreases adversely, output falls substantially, or ventricular ectopy appears.

Atropine usually corrects sinus bradycardia, but care should be exercised with dosage, as the response may be unpredictable. Junctional bradycardia may require a larger dose of atropine than does sinus bradycardia. Increments of ephedrine provide a short-duration increase in heart rate, but contractility and vascular tone also are altered. Careful infusion of isoproterenol may very occasionally be necessary if the bradycardia is unresponsive to atropine or ephedrine, but use of this potent β agonist must be approached with caution. Dopamine infusion may provide a more controlled and less startling increase in heart rate than does isoproterenol, but again contractility and peripheral vascular tone are simultaneously altered.

Swan-Ganz catheters with atrial and ventricular pacing capabilities are available and can be used to increase rate in a controlled way to the most optimal range. This catheter is especially useful for the patient with aortic stenosis, as a damaged bundle of His may become manifest during anesthesia and surgery and lead to a slow ventricular rhythm.

Rhythm

Dysrhythmias occur frequently during cardiac anesthesia and operation and may have adverse consequences when hemodynamic function is already jeopardized. For example, loss of sinus rhythm and atrial contraction greatly diminishes filling of the noncompliant ventricle. Factors that predispose to the development of dysrhythmias must be corrected (for example, acidosis or alkalosis, dysrhythmia-generating hypoxemia, ischemia, electrolyte imbalance, and digoxin toxicity).

Halothane and enflurane possess ventricular and supraventricular dysrhythmia-generating properties.[3, 25, 34, 84, 104, 121] In dogs, these agents alter atrial and atrioventricular nodal refractory periods and atrioventricular nodal conduction time.[3] Supraventricular dysrhythmias may result from the anesthetic effects on conduction and automaticity.[3] Ventricular dysrhythmias may occur more frequently with halothane than with enflurane.

A number of disturbances in cardiac rhythm may occur. Probably the most frequently encountered abnormality is sinus tachycardia. A search must be made for the cause, for example, hypovolemia, hypoxemia, hypercarbia, or heart failure. Sinus tachycardia usually responds to increased anesthetic depth. Small doses of propranolol are effective in slowing the rate, but the drug should be used cautiously if the contractile state is severely depressed. In this circumstance, tachycardia may be caused by heart failure, and inotropic support may increase stroke volume and cardiac output, with some abatement of the rapid rate.

Premature atrial contractions frequently do not require treatment but may lead to paroxysmal atrial tachycardia, atrial flutter, or atrial fibrillation. They may be evidence of underlying cardiac failure. Lidocaine has no effect on premature atrial contractions, but procainamide may be beneficial.

In paroxysmal supraventricular tachycardia, digitalis slows the ventricular response. Also, rapid atrial pacing may capture the atria and interrupt the tachycardia. Cardioversion will be necessary if the dysrhythmia brings about hemodynamic deterioration, induces myocardial ischemia, or is persistent.

In atrial fibrillation and flutter, the aim of treatment is to slow the ventricular rate, and this can be achieved by blocking the atrioventricular node with digoxin. Cardioversion also can be used.

Junctional rhythms are difficult to treat because several mechanisms may be involved in their production. If digitalis toxicity is not the cause, then digoxin may be given. Lidocaine may suppress automaticity of the junctional pacemaker. Direct-current conversion may be the only means of correcting this disturbance, although slow junctional rhythms often respond to a more rapid sinus rate induced by atropine, isoproterenol, or pacing.

Ventricular dysrhythmias are seen frequently, and most respond well to lidocaine. When the intrinsic heart rate is slow, ventricular ectopy may be abolished by atropine or by pacing at a faster rate. Lidocaine is an effective treatment for ventricular ectopic beats and ventricular tachycardia, but the latter may require immediate direct-current shock. Ventricular fibrillation requires direct-current shock as well as lidocaine treatment. Procainamide may suppress ventricular ectopy that is not abolished by lidocaine and can be used safely if given slowly, with constant hemodynamic observation. Bretylium tosylate is useful for the treatment of refractory or recurrent ventricular tachycardia or fibrillation.

Course of Anesthesia

Preoperative Assessment

Much information concerning anesthetic management can be obtained from a preoperative assessment of the patient and review of laboratory data.[115] Symptoms and signs of heart failure should be sought, because congestive heart failure indicates that the disease has progressed to a decompensated state and contributes to an increased operative risk. The cardiologist's opinion will be helpful in deciding if further medical therapy will improve the patient's preoperative condition.

Congestive failure may lead to disturbance of hepatic function, including vitamin K deficiency. Congestive changes in the liver may preclude the use of halothane and reduce the rate of metabolism of anesthetic drugs. Coexistent renal disease may be reason to discourage the use of enflurane,[66] and the excretion of anesthetic agents is also impaired.[109] Patients with cerebral manifestations of heart failure require little sedation and become unconscious readily with small doses of anesthetic drugs.

Of the laboratory investigations available, hematocrit and potassium levels are immediately important. Blood-free cardiopulmonary bypass pump prime should not be used if the patient is anemic. Potassium is the most important of the electrolytes because of its role in cardiac muscle excitability. A further consequence of potassium loss is metabolic alkalosis. Hypokalemia should be corrected before operation.

The findings on the ECG, chest roentgenogram, and echocardiogram and at cardiac catheterization should be reviewed. The cardiac catheterization report is probably the most useful preoperative investigation, and review of the cineangiography films with the radiologist and surgeon may be helpful in planning management. Swan-Ganz right heart catheterization performed by the anesthesia team in the operating area before the induction of anesthesia provides up-to-date information on cardiac performance, and these results may better reflect the state of the circulation at the time of surgery than does the laboratory catheterization report (see chap. 1).

Premedication

Anxiety, catecholamine secretion, tachycardia, hypertension, and increased oxygen demand are deleterious to the patient with valvular heart disease. Preoperative tranquility reduces these adverse effects and provides a more cooperative patient.

Management in the Operating Room

The anesthesiologist's goal is the maintenance or improvement of hemodynamic homeostasis and oxygen transport while providing organ protection. Abolition of consciousness is not always possible without infringement on these three goals, but sedation, amnesia, and analgesia can almost always be achieved without jeopardizing circulatory function.

Preinduction

The period before induction of anesthesia is hazardous because the patient may be suffering the detrimental effects of anxiety (for example, tachycardia and elevated systemic vascular resistance), but the hemodynamic consequences may go undetected until monitoring has been fully instituted. Before induction, the patient should breathe extra oxygen by face mask or nasal cannulas while peripheral intravenous infusions are begun, an arterial line is inserted, and access to the central venous system is established. The ECG must be monitored during this period. A pulmonary artery catheter can be introduced into the pulmonary circulation to permit baseline measurements of cardiac index, vascular resistance, and filling pressure. Once this information has been obtained, further thought can be given to manipulation of the circulation, for example, volume infusion in the presence of reduced preload or a vasodilator for the modification of systemic vascular resistance. A cardiac index less than 1.8 L/minute/sq m is a reliable indication for vasodilator or inotropic support before the induction of anesthesia because hypnosis or the rigors of laryngoscopy and intubation may further depress cardiac output.

Induction and Maintenance of Anesthesia

The conduct of the prebypass period is determined by the degree of hemodynamic disturbance; for example, severe mitral regurgitation with pulmonary edema may require inotropic support and a vasodilator, whereas the patient with aortic stenosis and good function will need controlled depression of the hypertrophied myocardium to prevent hypertension and increased myocardial oxygen demand. Anesthesia and operation impose a profound stress, resulting in a further disturbance in cardiac function and metabolism. The stress may be blunted by intervention at the target organ; for example, vasodilators may be used to directly reduce systemic vascular resistance by action on arterioles. Optionally, activity of the CNS may be dampened to depress the reflexes that bring about an adverse response to stress. A combination of target-organ control and manipulation of the CNS is the usual approach. Anesthetic agents may interrupt the stress response by activity within both the nervous and circulatory systems. Enflurane or halothane induces hypnosis, reduces sympathetic outflow, produces some decrease in systemic vascular resistance, and reduces contractile state, thus antagonizing the effects of surgical stimulation. Fentanyl, when administered in large doses, produces profound analgesia and hypnosis and blocks an increase in catecholamine release on surgical stimulation while exhibiting little intrinsic action on the contractile state.[110, 111]

In summary, some generalizations can help guide the conduct of anesthesia. Induction before intubation may be brought about by small repeated doses of thiopental or diazepam.[110, 111] Fentanyl in high doses produces hypnosis without cardiovascular instability and without the degree of venodilatation seen with morphine administration. The associated tendency toward decreased heart rate may be beneficial.

Succinylcholine as a bolus and by constant infusion offers excellent relaxation for intubation without cardiovascular alterations and, after intubation, may be followed by the use of a nondepolarizing relaxant. Anesthesia may be maintained with fentanyl, repeated small doses of diazepam, or enflurane or halothane if hemodynamics permit. Nitrous oxide, although a frequently used agent with little cardiovascular activity in healthy patients, may produce adverse effects in patients with valvular heart disease and when in combination with enflurane or narcotics. In this situation, systemic vascular resistance may be increased and cardiac output reduced.[57, 79, 122] Administration of nitrous oxide also necessitates that the FIO_2 be less than 1.0.

Mitral Stenosis

Preoperatively, adequate digitalization reduces ventricular rate during atrial fibrillation. The preoperative withdrawal of digitalis therapy, though helpful in eliminating digitalis-induced dysrhythmias during operation, may permit rapid ventricular responses to atrial fibrillation, necessitating small doses of edrophonium or propranolol to control the heart rate. Occasionally, cardioversion is necessary before bypass if rapid ventricular rates are accompanied by hemodynamic deterioration. Diuretics deplete total-body potassium, and this electrolyte should be replaced before operation, especially if serum levels are very low (3.0 mEq/L or less).

The supine position may increase the work of breathing or even precipitate orthopnea. The head of the bed, stretcher, and operating room table can be elevated to a comfortable position. Oxygen by mask may be necessary for patients with advanced pulmonary changes. Hypoxemia causes pulmonary vasoconstriction, further burdening the right ventricle. Care must be taken to avoid respiratory depression from premedication, but morphine produces some tranquility and venodilatation. Extra oxygen should be given after premedication.

The choice of anesthesia technique is determined principally by the extent of decline in cardiac function, pulmonary involvement, and presence of coexisting coronary artery disease.

It may be useful to place monitoring catheters and even induce anesthesia with the patient in the reverse Trendelenburg position if pulmonary congestion is causing respiratory distress.

Monitoring

The right ventricle may be more vulnerable to depressed function than the left, because pulmonary hypertension places a chronic pressure overload on the right side of the heart. Pulmonary artery catheterization permits the measurement of right ventricular preload and afterload, and a value for right ventricular end-diastolic pressure can be obtained during the introduction of the catheter. Pulmonary hypertension sometimes responds to vasodilator treatment, and changes in pulmonary vascular resistance may be followed with measurements obtained from the pulmonary artery catheter. When interpreting such data, one must remember that the particularly reactive pulmonary vasculature will cause varying gradients between the pulmonary artery diastolic and the pulmonary artery occluded pressures. Stenosis of the mitral valve causes the pulmonary artery occluded pressure to be a less reliable guide to left ventricular preload because pulmonary artery occluded pressure and left atrial pressure exceed LVEDP in a way that may be difficult to predict.

Rhythm and Rate

Atrial fibrillation is usually present in patients who undergo mitral valve replacement, but if sinus rhythm persists, care should be exercised in its preservation.

As has previously been emphasized, heart rate is of great importance, and every effort should be directed toward the prevention of tachycardia. Tachycardia frequently appears with the onset of surgical stimulation and may be ameliorated by depressing the nervous system with anesthesia (narcotics being particularly useful because of their tendency to reduce heart rate) or by intervention with direct-acting drugs. The ventricular rate may be reduced by the use of edrophonium, digoxin, or propranolol.

Preload

Left ventricular end-diastolic pressure is unlikely to be increased because mitral stenosis inhibits ventricular filling, but left atrial pressure and pulmonary artery occluded pressure may be elevated, as may right ventricular end-diastolic pressure and right atrial pressure. Mechanical ventilation, nitroglycerin, nitroprusside, or the reverse Trendelenburg position may help reduce these pressures.

Contractility

The left ventricle does not undergo hypertrophy or a depression of contractile state, but the "mitral complex" syndrome may reduce ventricular performance.[28,45] The right ventricle may be more vulnerable than the left ventricle to negative inotropic influences. If cardiac output is significantly reduced, the use of enflurane or halothane should be avoided and awareness and pain perception abolished by the use of narcotics or diazepam (or both). Inotropic support may be necessary before induction and throughout the procedure if cardiac index is low despite manipulation of preloading and afterloading conditions.

Systemic Vascular Resistance and Pulmonary Vascular Resistance

Because the left ventricle does not usually fail until the late stages of mitral stenosis, reduction of systemic vascular resistance may be of little value, but vasodilators may be beneficial in reducing pulmonary vascular resistance and unloading the right ventricle. Nitrous oxide may cause a further increase in pulmonary vascular resistance,[57] and avoidance of its use may be necessary.

Ventilation

An FIO_2 of 1.0 may be needed because oxygenation may be impaired and high oxygen concentrations may result in beneficial pulmonary vasodilatation, especially if a permanent change in the pulmonary vasculature has not occurred. Introduction of positive end-expiratory pressure also may be necessary if pulmonary congestion is severe.

Valve Replacement

Hemodynamic improvement occurs after mitral valve replacement, with an immediate decrease in elevated left atrial pressure, followed by a more gradual decline in pulmonary vascular resistance.[32] Replacement valves exhibit a diastolic pressure gradient that averages between 4 and 10 mm Hg, depending on the valve.

Mitral valve prostheses perform poorly when the diastolic flow period is reduced during tachycardia, the result being an increase in gradient and left atrial pressure.[74] Care must be taken to avoid tachycardia during the postbypass period as well.

Mitral Regurgitation

In recent years, reduction of impedance to ejection has become established therapy for mitral regurgitation.[21,43] Afterload reduction can be used during anesthesia, with considerable benefit.[114] Submitral valvular area and regurgitation are reduced by a decrease in LVEDV,[11] and this decrease may be achieved by enhanced ventricular emptying during the administration of inotropic drugs or vasodilators or a combination of both.

Monitoring

Pulmonary artery catheterization is valuable while vasodilators are being administered as the decrease in systemic vascular resistance is monitored. A large V wave of ventricular contraction is usually seen in the pulmonary artery occluded pressure tracing and frequently is reduced in magnitude or may disappear when regurgitation is lessened.[21]

Rhythm and Rate

Loss of atrial contraction is not particularly detrimental because regurgitant volume provides adequate left ventricular filling. Mild tachycardia is advantageous because LVEDV is decreased, and although overall regurgitation per minute may be only slightly improved, left ventricular wall tension is beneficially reduced.

Preload

Preload is elevated, and a decrease in LVEDV may reduce regurgitation. Nitroprusside and nitroglycerin offer a pharmacologic approach to this problem.

Contractility

Chronic volume overload results in dilatation and eccentric hypertrophy of the ventricular wall and is accompanied frequently by a decline in contractile state.[65, 80, 97, 108] An inotropic drug may be necessary before induction of anesthesia, and the resulting improved contractile performance may cause a more complete emptying of the left ventricle and reduction in LVEDV and the submitral valvular area, with a decrease in regurgitant fraction. Enflurane and halothane may precipitate an increase in chamber size and regurgitation, because of a depression of the contractile state.

Systemic Vascular Resistance and Pulmonary Vascular Resistance

Mitral regurgitation is particularly sensitive to changes in systemic vascular resistance and classically shows considerable improvement with vasodilator therapy[11, 21, 43, 113] (Fig 7–27). Reduced systemic vascular resistance brings about an increased forward cardiac output, decreased regurgitant volume, reduction in the height of the V wave seen on the pulmonary artery occluded pressure tracing, and even a decrease in intensity of the apical pansystolic murmur (Fig 7–28). The improved ventricular emptying reduces left ventricular chamber volume and enhances competence of the mitral valve, thus further reducing regurgitation. Particular care should be taken to ensure that the systemic vascular resistance does not become elevated. Anesthetic agents alone may be unable to maintain a reduced systemic vascular resistance or may

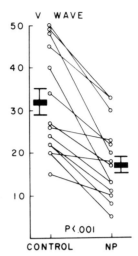

Fig 7–28.—Significant decrease in V wave is seen during nitroprusside *(NP)* infusion in patients with mitral regurgitation. (Heavy horizontal bars represent mean changes; lighter horizontal bars, SEM.) (From Goodman D.J., et al.: Effect of nitroprusside on left ventricular dynamics in mitral regurgitation. *Circulation* 50:1025, 1974. Used by permission of the American Heart Association.)

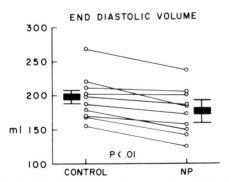

Fig 7–27.—Result of nitroprusside *(NP)* infusion on left ventricular end-diastolic volume in patients with mitral regurgitation. (Heavy horizontal bars indicate mean values; lighter horizontal bars, SEM.) (From Goodman D.J., et al.: Effect of nitroprusside on left ventricular dynamics in mitral regurgitation. *Circulation* 50:1025, 1974. Used by permission of the American Heart Association.)

do so only by depressing the contractile state. Constant infusion of nitroprusside, accompanied by small bolus doses in situations in which elevated systemic vascular resistance is anticipated, can achieve a constant, advantageously low impedance to ejection (Fig 7–29). A further benefit may be vasodilatation in the pulmonary circulation, as chronic mitral regurgitation may have resulted in pulmonary hypertension and right ventricular dysfunction. Thus, both ventricles are unloaded during nitroprusside infusion.

It may be desirable to omit nitrous oxide for five reasons: (1) FIO_2 of 1.0 is more likely to ensure adequate oxygenation if alveolar function is compromised by pulmonary congestion; (2) high oxygen concentration may reduce elevated pulmonary vascular resistance; (3) nitrous oxide tends to increase pulmonary vascular resistance[57]; (4) nitrous oxide may increase systemic vascular resistance in the presence of narcotics[122]; and (5) nitrous oxide has some negative inotropic properties.[79]

Valve Replacement

Mitral valve replacement poses a problem for the left ventricle, because the low-resistance ejection pathway into the left atrium is abolished by the new valve. The left ventricle, previously accustomed to a low afterload, is now confronted with only the higher-resistance aortic pathway, thus an increased afterload. The problem is magnified because chronic ventricular dilation frequently results in some disruption of the myofibrillar architecture and impaired contractile performance. Both an inotropic drug and a vasodilator may be needed to permit satisfactory performance after bypass. Again, the new valve exhibits a diastolic gradient of between 4 and 10 mm Hg,[74] and this difference between left atrial pressure and LVEDP must be considered when choosing the most appropriate filling pressure. Shortening of the diastolic flow period during tachycardia increases this gradient.

Aortic Stenosis

Patients with aortic stenosis tend to be seen for surgical correction of the valvular lesion at a time in the natural history of the disease when symptoms and signs of myocardial ischemia predominate over those of failure. The hypertrophied left ventricle is confronted with a substantial increase in pressure work; myocardial oxygen demand is elevated; and coronary perfusion may be unable to meet demands if the extra burdens imposed by anesthesia and operation are severe. Care must be taken to avoid unnecessary increases in myocardial oxygen demand, and planning should be directed toward the preservation of aerobic cardiac metabolism.

In this respect, enflurane and halothane offer a means of depressing contractile state and oxygen consumption in a controlled fashion. A potential disadvantage is a reported tendency for these agents to induce junctional tachydysrhythmias.[3] Of course, if aortic stenosis has resulted in significant depression of the contractile state,[108] high concentrations of these inhalational anesthetics should be avoided.

Rhythm

The thick-walled, hypertrophied, noncompliant ventricle is especially dependent on the booster-pump function of atrial contraction for the maintenance of preload. Without coordinated atrial systole, that is, sinus rhythm, preload decreases, even though a compensatory increase in left atrial pressure occurs. Maintenance of sinus rhythm is of great importance, and fac-

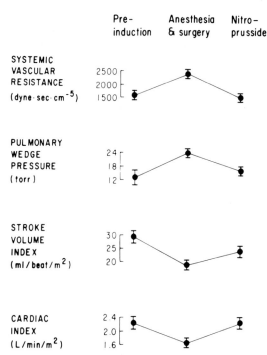

Fig 7–29.—Hemodynamic profile during pre-induction period, anesthesia, and surgery of patients with mitral regurgitation. Increases in systemic vascular resistance and pulmonary capillary wedge pressure with anesthesia and surgery are seen, with decrease in cardiac index. Nitroprusside, by reversing change in outflow impedance, improves ventricular performance. (From Stone et al.[113] Used by permission.)

tors that predispose to its disappearance must be avoided (for example, respiratory alkalosis, digitalis toxicity, and perhaps the anesthetic agents enflurane[3, 104] and halothane).

Rate

An adequate diastolic time is needed for filling the noncompliant left ventricle. Tachycardia reduces diastolic time per cycle, reducing time available for left atrial-to-left ventricular flow, bringing about a decrease in stroke volume.[39] Tachycardia has an undesirable effect on myocardial oxygen supply[17] because the time available for diastolic coronary artery flow is reduced. Tachycardia also decreases systolic time per cycle, necessitating a compensatory increase in pressure gradient to eject the stroke volume. Tachycardia has disadvantages for the hypertrophied ventricle, such as those noted with aortic stenosis. Tachycardia may bring about a change from myocardial lactate consumption to production, indicating ischemia-induced anaerobic metabolism.[119]

The anesthesiologist must protect the heart from the adverse effects of tachycardia. A sufficient depth of anesthesia before stimulation may prevent the development of an increased rate, and in this respect, the use of narcotic anesthesia is attractive because of a tendency toward drug-induced vagal stimulation, but such an advantage may be offset by the inability to depress contractility in a controlled fashion. A combination of narcotic and inhalational agent may be satisfactory. If tachycardia develops, cautious use of propranolol may reduce the rate, with an increase in stroke volume and little change in cardiac index. Bradycardia also poses a substantial threat to hemodynamic integrity. Because the stenosed valve limits the increase in stroke volume, a decrease in heart rate reduces cardiac output proportionately. This situation is especially hazardous, because an accompanying decrease in blood pressure reduces perfusion pressure in the coronary tree and may precipitate myocardial ischemia.

Preload

The characteristics of the left ventricular pressure volume are influenced by the decreased compliance that results from a thickened wall. A small-volume increment pushed into the left ventricle by atrial systole causes a substantial increase in pressure. This atrial contraction significantly elevates LVEDP and preload, with little effect on mean left atrial pressure. Preload must be maintained by adequate volume replacement, but the most effective way of ensuring adequate preload is the preservation of coordinated atrial contraction and sinus rhythm.

After bypass, the hypertrophied ventricle behaves as do all noncompliant ventricles. If pacing is required, atrial pacing is far more able to maintain or improve cardiac output than is ventricular pacing. If atrioventricular conduction is blocked, sequential atrioventricular pacing with an optimal P-R interval should be used rather than ventricular pacing.[44]

Contractility

A range of changes in the contractile state is seen, depending on the severity and duration of the aortic stenosis.[61] The pure pressure overload seen in aortic stenosis appears to have a less detrimental effect on ventricular performance than does the volume overload experienced during aortic regurgitation or even mitral regurgitation.[65] Ventricular function is well preserved, and occasionally the ejection fraction is greater than normal. Once the mechanical obstruction to ejection is replaced, the heart reverts to a normal performance.[99] It is often advantageous to depress the contractile state of the well-preserved, hypertrophied ventricle to reduce the oxygen demand, and in this situation halothane or enflurane is useful. Controlled depression of the contractile state, mild reduction in systemic vascular resistance, and blunted response to surgical stimulation can result in maintaining the circulatory system in a state in which demands and stresses are diminished. Enflurane or halothane can induce such conditions, but a potential disadvantage is an anesthetic agent-induced appearance of junctional rhythm at the expense of sinus rhythm.[3, 104]

If chronic or severe stenosis has resulted in failing compensation, then inhalational agents may exacerbate the failure. Narcotics would be preferable in such a situation.[62] Narcotic anesthesia is a well-established approach to aortic valve replacement,[62] but a disadvantage that must be recognized is an unpredictable decline in venous and arteriolar tone occasionally encountered with morphine. Hypotension is particularly dangerous for the patient with aortic stenosis, because coronary vasodilatation reserve may be exhausted and coronary perfusion becomes dependent on aortic diastolic pressure.

Systemic Vascular Resistance

Valvular stenosis is responsible for the major proportion of impedance to ejection. Vasodilatation may improve performance, if the diastolic pressure and coronary perfusion are not simultaneously reduced. An increase in aortic pressure must be avoided, because this change implies a detrimental increase in intraventricular pressure. Such increases in pressure can be prevented or controlled by anesthetic agents or vasodilators.

Aortic Valve Replacement

A gradient persists between the ventricle and the aorta after valve replacement, with the peak-to-peak systolic pressure gradient varying between 7 and 19 mm Hg, depending on the valve used in replacement.[74] Eventually, left ventricular pump function returns to normal after valve replacement, if the disease has not resulted in substantial dilatation of the ventricular chambers.

Aortic Regurgitation

When planning the anesthetic management of the patient with aortic regurgitation, one must consider the factors that improve and those that worsen regurgitation. Especially important is the influence of systemic vascular resistance on forward stroke volume, regurgitant fraction, and left ventricular chamber size.[7, 9, 68] Manipulation of the systemic vascular resistance offers a means of improving cardiac performance. The anesthesiologist is confronted by a number of abnormalities of function. Aortic regurgitation results in greater depression of contractile state than aortic stenosis, probably because eccentric hypertrophy causes slippage of myofibrils.[80] Left ventricular performance is maintained by use of the preload mechanism, but a hazardous consequence is pulmonary congestion.

Problems of imbalance in the myocardial oxygen supply and demand arise, because demand increases with progression of hypertrophy but supply may not meet demand, particularly since a low aortic diastolic pressure is a characteristic of the disease.

Rate

Mild tachycardia results in some decrease in diastolic chamber volume and wall tension, although minute regurgitant volume may be little changed[50] (see Fig 7–22). Mild tachycardia maintains diastolic arterial pressure and coronary perfusion pressure. Unlike that in aortic stenosis, tachycardia is not associated with myocardial lactate production.[119]

Slow heart rates are hazardous because diastolic left ventricular volume and pressure tend to increase, and forward cardiac output may be dangerously reduced. Also, bradycardia causes a further decrease in the already lowered aortic diastolic pressure. From these points, it can be seen that mild tachycardia is advantageous.

Rhythm

Left ventricular filling is not crucially dependent on atrial contraction and sinus rhythm because left ventricular compliance is not significantly decreased.

Systemic Vascular Resistance

Anesthetic management must include careful control of the systemic vascular resistance. Volatile drugs such as halothane and enflurane or narcotics may not prevent an increase in systemic vascular resistance, but nitroprusside infusion will effectively control such an increase. The efficacy of vasodilators has been well demonstrated[7, 68] (see Fig 7–24). Great care must be exercised in reducing the afterload because an already low diastolic aortic pressure may be further reduced.

Contractility

The myocardium may have undergone a significant decrease in contractile state, as has been described. If inhalational agents are used, further decrease in contractile performance may not be compensated for by an anesthetic-induced decrease in systemic vascular resistance. Narcotics have little measurable effect on myocardial performance.[62] Emphasis must be placed on the importance of supporting the performance of an impaired left ventricle. Early introduction of a vasodilator or inotrope or a combination of both may provide greater circulatory stability during the prebypass period. It is frequently necessary to continue this vasodilator-inotrope combination on emergence from bypass. Rational application of this therapy can be achieved only with hemodynamic monitoring by a Swan-Ganz catheter and sequential cardiac output determinations.

Aortic Valve Replacement

Unfortunately, chronic volume overload may result in permanent alteration in ventricular muscle structure, and valve replacement may not produce the dramatic improvement often seen in aortic valve replacement for aortic stenosis. Left ventricular mass and LVEDV decrease but do so less consistently than in patients with aortic stenosis. Ejection fraction and velocity of fiber shortening may improve, but probably not to the same extent as in aortic stenosis. For these reasons, inotropic support may be necessary after valve replacement.

REFERENCES

1. Ahmed S.S., et al.: The state of the left ventricular myocardium in mitral stenosis. *Am. Heart J.* 94:28, 1977.
2. Arani D.T., Carleton R.A.: The deleterious role of tachycardia in mitral stenosis. *Circulation* 36:511, 1967.
3. Atlee J.L., et al.: Supraventricular excitability in dogs during anesthesia and halothane and enflurane. *Anesthesiology* 49:407, 1978.
4. Balakrishnan R., et al.: *Cardiac Anesthesia Workshop*. Baltimore, Johns Hopkins Hospital, 1979.
5. Baxley W.A., et al.: Hemodynamics in ruptured chordae tendineae and chronic rheumatic mitral regurgitation. *Circulation* 48:1288, 1973.
6. Baxter R.H., et al.: Tricuspid valve replacement: A five-year appraisal. *Thorax* 30:158, 1975.
7. Bolen J.L., Alderman E.L.: Hemodynamic consequences of afterload reduction in patients with chronic aortic regurgitation. *Circulation* 53:879, 1976.
8. Bolen J.L., et al.: Analysis of left ventricular function in response to afterload changes in patients with mitral stenosis. *Circulation* 52:894, 1975.
9. Bolen J.L., et al.: Evaluation of left ventricular function in patients with aortic regurgitation using afterload stress. *Circulation* 53:132, 1976.
10. Bonta I.L., et al.: Pharmacological interaction between pancuronium bromide and anaesthetics. *Eur. J. Pharmacol.* 4:83, 1968.
11. Borgenhagen D.M., et al.: The effects of left ventricular load and contractility on mitral regurgitant orifice size and flow in the dog. *Circulation* 56:106, 1977.
12. Braunwald E.: Mitral regurgitation: Physiologic, clinical and surgical considerations. *N. Engl. J. Med.* 281:425, 1969.
13. Braunwald E.: Vasodilator therapy: A physiologic approach to the treatment of heart failure, editorial. *N. Engl. J. Med.* 297:331, 1977.
14. Braunwald E.: Heart failure: An overview, in Fishman A.P. (ed.): *Heart Failure*. Washington, D.C., Hemisphere Publishing Corporation, 1978, p. 55.
15. Braunwald E., Frahm C.J.: Studies on Starling's law of the heart: IV. Observations on the hemodynamic functions of the left atrium in man. *Circulation* 24:633, 1961.
16. Braunwald E., Ross J. Jr., Sonnenblick E.H.: *Mechanisms of Contraction of the Normal and Failing Heart*, ed. 2. Boston, Little, Brown & Co., 1976.
17. Buckberg G., et al.: Ischemia in aortic stenosis: Hemodynamic prediction. *Am. J. Cardiol.* 35:778, 1975.
18. Byrne J.P., et al.: Replacement of heart valves by prosthetic devices. *Pathobiol Ann.* 7:83, 1977.
19. Carpentier A., et al.: Surgical management of acquired tricuspid valve disease. *J. Thorac. Cardiovasc. Surg.* 67:53, 1974.
20. Chatterjee K., Parmley W.W.: The role of vasodilator therapy in heart failure. *Prog. Cardiovasc. Dis.* 19:301, 1977.
21. Chatterjee K., et al.: Beneficial effects of vasodilator agents in severe mitral regurgitation due to dysfunction of subvalvar apparatus. *Circulation* 48:684, 1973.
22. Cohn J.N.: Blood pressure and cardiac performance. *Am. J. Med.* 55:351, 1973.
23. Cohn J.N., Franciosa J.A.: Vasodilator therapy of a cardiac failure. *N. Engl. J. Med.* 297:27, 1977.
24. Cohn P.F., Gorlin R.: Abnormalities of left ventricular function associated with the anginal state. *Circulation* 46:1065, 1972.
25. Collins V.J.: *Principles of Anesthesiology*, ed. 2. Philadelphia, Lea & Febiger, 1976, p. 1471.
26. Conahan T.J. III, et al.: A prospective random comparison of halothane and morphine for open-heart anesthesia: One year's experience. *Anesthesiology* 38:528, 1973.
27. Cortese D.A.: Pulmonary function in mitral stenosis. *Mayo Clin. Proc.* 53:321, 1978.
28. Currey G.C., Elliott L.P., Ramsey H.W.: Quantitative left ventricular angiocardiographic findings in mitral stenosis: Detailed analysis of the anterolateral wall of the left ventricle. *Am. J. Cardiol.* 29:621, 1972.
29. Danielson G.K.: Tricuspid insufficiency, in Hardy J.D. (ed.): *Rhoads Textbook of Surgery: Principles and Practice*, ed. 5. Philadelphia, J.B. Lippincott Co., 1977, p. 1648.
30. Dodge H.T., Kennedy J.W., Peterson J.L.: Quantitative angiocardiographic methods in the evaluation of valvular heart disease. *Prog. Cardiovasc. Dis.* 16:1, 1973.
31. Eckberg D.L., et al.: Mechanics of left ventricular contraction in chronic severe mitral regurgitation. *Circulation* 47:1252, 1973.

32. Ellis F.H. Jr.: Mitral valve prostheses: Hemodynamics, in Davila J.C. (ed.): *Second Henry Ford Hospital Symposium on Cardiac Surgery,* New York, Appleton-Century-Crofts, 1975, section X, p. 432.
33. Feldman R.L., et al.: Influence of aortic insufficiency on the hemodynamic significance of a coronary artery narrowing. *Circulation* 60:259, 1979.
34. Foëx P., Prys-Roberts C.: Anaesthesia and the hypertensive patient. *Br. J. Anaesth.* 46:575, 1974.
35. Gardocki J.F., Yelnosky J.: A study of some of the pharmacologic actions of fentanyl citrate. *Toxicol. Appl. Pharmacol.* 6:48, 1964.
36. Gault J.H., et al.: Left ventricular performance following correction of free aortic regurgitation. *Circulation* 42:773, 1970.
37. Goodwin J.F.: The indications for surgery in acquired heart disease. *Proc. R. Soc. Med.* 60:1009, 1967.
38. Gorlin R., Gorlin S.G.: Hydraulic formula for calculation of the area of the stenotic mitral valve, other cardiac valves, and central circulatory shunts: I. *Am. Heart J.* 41:1, 1951.
39. Gorlin R., et al.: Dynamics of the circulation in aortic valvular disease. *Am. J. Med.* 18:855, 1955.
40. Gracey D.: Personal communication.
41. Grossman W., McLaurin L.P.: Diastolic properties of the left ventricle. *Ann. Intern. Med.* 84:316, 1976.
42. Guiha N.H., et al.: Treatment of refractory heart failure with infusion of nitroprusside. *N. Engl. J. Med.* 291:587, 1974.
43. Harshaw C.W., et al.: Reduced systemic vascular resistance as therapy for severe mitral regurgitation of valvular origin. *Ann. Intern. Med.* 83:312, 1975.
44. Hartzler G.O., et al.: Hemodynamic benefits of atrioventricular sequential pacing after cardiac surgery. *Am. J. Cardiol.* 40:232, 1977.
45. Heller S.J., Carleton R.A.: Abnormal left ventricular contraction in patients with mitral stenosis. *Circulation* 42:1099, 1970.
46. Hsu H.O., Hickey R.F., Forbes A.R.: Morphine decreases peripheral vascular resistance and increases capacitance in man. *Anesthesiology* 50:98, 1979.
47. Hughes R., Chapple D.J.: Effects of non-depolarizing neuromuscular blocking agents on peripheral autonomic mechanisms in cats. *Br. J. Anaesth.* 48:59, 1976.
48. Hughes R., Ingram G.S., Payne J.P.: Studies on dimethyl tubocurarine in anaesthetized man. *Br. J. Anaesth.* 48:969, 1976.
49. Hurst J.W.: *The Heart, Arteries and Veins,* ed. 4. New York, McGraw-Hill Book Co., 1978.
50. Judge T.P., et al.: Quantitative hemodynamic effects of heart rate in aortic regurgitation. *Circulation* 44:355, 1971.
51. Kalmanson D.: *The Mitral Valve: A Pluridisciplinary Approach.* Acton, Mass., Publishing Sciences Group, 1976.
52. Kelly D.T., et al.: Effects of chronic right ventricular volume and pressure loading on left ventricular performance. *Circulation* 44:403, 1971.
53. Kennedy J.W., et al.: Quantitative angiocardiography: IV. Relationships of left atrial and ventricular pressure and volume in mitral valve disease. *Circulation* 41:817, 1970.
54. Kramer R.S., Mason D.T., Braunwald E.: Augmented sympathetic neurotransmitter activity in the peripheral vascular bed of patients with congestive heart failure and cardiac norepinephrine depletion. *Circulation* 38:629, 1968.
55. Kroetz F.W., et al.: The effect of atrial contraction on left ventricular performance in valvular aortic stenosis. *Circulation* 35:852, 1967.
56. Lappas D., et al.: Indirect measurement of left-atrial pressure in surgical patients: Pulmonary-capillary wedge and pulmonary-artery diastolic pressures compared with left-atrial pressure. *Anesthesiology* 38:394, 1973.
57. Lappas D.G., et al.: Left ventricular performance and pulmonary circulation following addition of nitrous oxide to morphine during coronary-artery surgery. *Anesthesiology* 43:61, 1975.
58. Laubie M., et al.: Centrally mediated bradycardia and hypotension induced by narcotic analgesics: Dextromoramide and fentanyl. *Eur. J. Pharmacol.* 28:66, 1974.
59. Lee S.J.K., et al.: Hemodynamic changes at rest and during exercise in patients with aortic stenosis of varying severity. *Am. Heart J.* 79:318, 1970.
60. Levesque P.R., et al.: Circulatory effects of enflurane in normocarbic human volunteers. *Can. Anaesth. Soc. J.* 21:580, 1974.
61. Liedtke A.J., et al.: Determinants of cardiac performance in severe aortic stenosis. *Chest* 69:192, 1976.
62. Lowenstein E., et al.: Cardiovascular response to large doses of intravenous morphine in man. *N. Engl. J. Med.* 281:1389, 1969.
63. Mangano D.T.: Personal communication.
64. Mangano D.T., van Dyke D.C., Ellis R.J.: Optimal filling pressures following cardiopul-

monary bypass, abstracted. *Anesthesiology* 51(suppl.):S165, 1979.
65. Mason D.T.: *Congestive Heart Failure: Mechanisms, Evaluation and Treatment.* New York, Yorke Medical Books, 1976, p. 111.
66. Mazze R.I., Calverley R.K., Smith N.T.: Inorganic fluoride nephrotoxicity: Prolonged enflurane and halothane anesthesia in volunteers. *Anesthesiology* 46:265, 1977.
67. Miller R.R., Mason D.T.: Ventricular afterload reducing agents in congestive heart failure therapy, in Mason D.T. (ed.): *Congestive Heart Failure: Mechanisms, Evaluation and Treatment.* New York, Yorke Medical Books, 1976, p. 343.
68. Miller R.R., et al.: Afterload reduction therapy with nitroprusside in severe aortic regurgitation: Improved cardiac performance and reduced regurgitant volume. *Am. J. Cardiol.* 38:564, 1976.
69. Miller R.R., et al.: Pharmacological mechanisms for left ventricular unloading in clinical congestive heart failure: differential effects of nitroprusside, phentolamine, and nitroglycerin on cardiac function and peripheral circulation. *Circ. Res.* 39:127, 1976.
70. Miller R.R., et al.: The concept of afterload reduction therapy in congestive heart failure: Clinical application and spectrum of peripheral vasodilator drugs. *Adv. Heart Dis.* 1:25, 1977.
71. Miller R.R., et al.: In-hospital and outpatient use of systemic vasodilator therapy in congestive heart failure. *Adv. Heart Dis.* 2:419, 1978.
72. Mond H., Hunt D., Sloman G.: Haemodynamic effects of frusemide in patients suspected of having acute myocardial infarction. *Br. Heart J.* 36:44, 1974.
73. Morganroth J., et al.: Acute severe aortic regurgitation: pathophysiology, clinical recognition, and management. *Ann. Intern. Med.* 87:223, 1977.
74. Murphy E.S., Kloster F.E.: Late results of valve replacement surgery: I. Clinical and hemodynamic results. *Mod. Concepts Cardiovasc. Dis.* 48:53, 1979.
75. Noble M.I.M., Pollack G.H.: Molecular mechanisms of contraction. *Circ. Res.* 40:333, 1977.
76. Paquay P.A., et al.: Chest pain as a predictor of coronary artery disease in patients with obstructive aortic valve disease. *Am. J. Cardiol.* 38:863, 1976.
77. Patterson S.W., Starling E.H.: On the mechanical factors which determine the output of the ventricles. *J. Physiol.* 48:357, 1914.
78. Perloff J.K., Roberts W.C.: The mitral apparatus: Functional anatomy of mitral regurgitation. *Circulation* 46:227, 1972.
79. Price H.L.: Myocardial depression by nitrous oxide and its reversal by Ca^{++}. *Anesthesiology* 44:211, 1976.
80. Rackley C.E., Hood W.P. Jr.: Quantitative angiographic evaluation and pathophysiologic mechanisms in valvular heart disease. *Prog. Cardiovasc. Dis.* 15:427, 1973.
81. Rackley C.E., Hood W.P. Jr.: Aortic valve disease, in Levine H.J. (ed.): *Clinical Cardiovascular Physiology.* New York, Grune & Stratton, 1976, p. 493.
82. Rackley C.E., et al.: Management of acute myocardial infarction, in Rackley C.E., Russell R.O. Jr. (eds.): *Coronary Artery Disease: Recognition and Management.* Mount Kisco, N.Y., Futura Publishing Co., 1979, p. 371.
83. Rapaport E.: Natural history of aortic and mitral valve disease. *Am. J. Cardiol.* 35:221, 1975.
84. Raventós J.: The action of fluothane—A new volatile anaesthetic. *Br. J. Pharmacol.* 11:394, 1956.
85. Reichek N., Shelburne J.C., Perloff J.K.: Clinical aspects of rheumatic valvular disease. *Prog. Cardiovasc. Dis.* 15:491, 1973.
86. Roberts W.C.: The structural basis of abnormal cardiac function: A look at coronary, hypertensive, valvular, idiopathic myocardial, and pericardial heart disease, in Levine H.J. (ed.): *Clinical Cardiovascular Physiology.* New York, Grune & Stratton, 1976, p. 1.
87. Roberts W.C., Perloff J.K.: Mitral valvular disease: A clinicopathologic survey of the conditions causing the mitral valve to function abnormally. *Ann. Intern. Med.* 77:939, 1972.
88. Robin E., et al.: Hemodynamic consequences of total removal of the tricuspid valve without prosthetic replacement. *Am. J. Cardiol.* 35:481, 1975.
89. Roizen M.F., Horrigan R.W.: Anesthetic dose that blocks adrenergic response to incision, abstracted. *Anesthesiology* 51(suppl.):S141, 1979.
90. Roizen M.F., et al.: Effects of general anesthetics on handling- and decapitation-induced increases in sympathoadrenal discharge. *J. Pharmacol. Exp. Ther.* 204:11, 1978.
91. Ross J. Jr., et al.: Diastolic geometry and sarcomere lengths in the chronically dilated canine left ventricle. *Circ. Res.* 28:49, 1971.
92. Ruskin J., et al.: Contribution of atrial systole to ventricular stroke volume in man, abstracted. *Circulation* 38(suppl. 6):168, 1968.
93. Ryan T.J.: Mitral valve disease, in Levine H.J. (ed.): *Clinical Cardiovascular Physiol-*

ogy. New York, Grune & Stratton, 1976, p. 523.
94. Sandler H., Dodge H.T.: Left ventricular tension and stress in man. *Circ. Res.* 13:91, 1963.
95. Savarese J.J., Ali H.H., Antonio R.P.: The clinical pharmacology of metocurine: Dimethyltubocurarine revisited. *Anesthesiology* 47:277, 1977.
96. Schauble J.F., et al.: Sensitivity of the left ventricle to outflow resistance, abstracted. *Anesthesiology* 51(suppl.):S107, 1979.
97. Schlant R.C., Nutter D.O.: Heart failure in valvular heart disease. *Medicine* 50:421, 1971.
98. Schneider R.C., et al.: Hemodynamic effects of dobutamine in cardiac surgical patients, abstracted. *Anesthesiology* 51(suppl.):S110, 1979.
99. Schwarz F., et al.: Correlation between myocardial structure and diastolic properties of the heart in chronic aortic valve disease: Effects of corrective surgery. *Am. J. Cardiol.* 42:895, 1978.
100. Selzer A., Cohn K.E.: Natural history of mitral stenosis: A review. *Circulation* 45:878, 1972.
101. Shimosato S., Etsten B.E.: Effect of anesthetic drugs on the heart: A critical review of myocardial contractility and its relationship to hemodynamics. *Clin. Anesth.* 3:17, 1969.
102. Shimosato S., et al.: The effect of Ethrane on cardiac muscle mechanics. *Anesthesiology* 30:513, 1969.
103. Simon H., et al.: The contractile state of the hypertrophied left ventricular myocardium in aortic stenosis. *Am. Heart J.* 79:587, 1970.
104. Smith N.T., et al.: The hemodynamic impact of atrial arrhythmias during enflurane anesthesia in man. Abstracted, Scientific Papers, American Society of Anesthesiologists Annual Meeting, 1977, p. 99.
105. Sokolow M., McIlroy M.B.: *Clinical Cardiology.* Los Altos, Calif., Lange Medical Publications, 1977.
106. Sonnenblick E.H., et al.: The ultrastructure of the heart in systole and diastole: Changes in sarcomere length. *Circ. Res.* 21:423, 1967.
107. Sonntag H., et al.: Left ventricular function in conscious man and during halothane anesthesia. *Anesthesiology* 48:320, 1978.
108. Spann J.F. Jr., et al.: Contractile state of cardiac muscle obtained from cats with experimentally produced ventricular hypertrophy and heart failure. *Circ. Res.* 21:341, 1967.
109. Stanley T.H., Lathrop G.D.: Urinary excretion of morphine during and after valvular and coronary-artery surgery. *Anesthesiology* 46:166, 1977.
110. Stanley T.H., Webster L.R.: Fentanyl-oxygen anesthesia for patients with mitral valve disease, stress free anesthesia, in Wood C. (ed.): *The Royal Society of Medicine, International Congress and Symposium Series No. 3.* New York, Academic Press, 1978.
111. Stanley T.H., et al.: Fentanyl-oxygen anesthesia for coronary artery surgery: Plasma catecholamine and cortisol responses, abstracted. *Anesthesiology* 51(suppl.):S139, 1979.
112. Stoelting R.K., Reis R.R., Longnecker D.E.: Hemodynamic responses to nitrous oxide-halothane and halothane in patients with valvular heart disease. *Anesthesiology* 37:430, 1972.
113. Stone J.G., Faltas A.N., Hoar P.F.: Sodium nitroprusside therapy for cardiac failure in anesthetized patients with valvular insufficiency. *Anesthesiology* 49:414, 1978.
114. Stott D.K., et al.: The role of left atrial transport in aortic and mitral stenosis. *Circulation* 41:1031, 1970.
115. Tarhan S., White R.D., Moffitt E.A.: Anesthesia and postoperative care for cardiac operations. *Ann. Thorac. Surg.* 23:173, 1977.
116. Thompson M.E., Shaver J.A., Leon D.F.: Effects of tachycardia on atrial transport in mitral stenosis. *Am. Heart J.* 94:297, 1977.
117. Tinker J.H., et al.: Dobutamine for inotropic support during emergence from cardiopulmonary bypass. *Anesthesiology* 44:281, 1976.
118. Tinker J.H., et al.: Efficacy of dopamine, dobutamine and epinephrine during emergence from cardiopulmonary bypass in man, objective monitoring. Abstracted, Scientific Papers, American Society of Anesthesiologists Annual Meeting, 1977, p. 515.
119. Trenouth R.S., Phelps N.C., Neill W.A.: Determinants of left ventricular hypertrophy and oxygen supply in chronic aortic valve disease. *Circulation* 53:644, 1976.
120. Willerson J.T., Sanders C.A.: *Clinical Cardiology.* New York, Grune & Stratton, 1977.
121. Williams H.D., Sone L. Jr.: Cardiac arrhythmias during coronary-artery operations with halothane and enflurane anesthesia. *Anesthesiology* 50:551, 1979.
122. Wong K.C., et al.: The cardiovascular effects of morphine sulfate with oxygen and with nitrous oxide in man. *Anesthesiology* 38:542, 1973.
123. Zaidan J.R., Kaplan J.A., Sumpter R.M.: Cardiovascular effects of dimethyl tubocurarine in patients with aortic valvular disease during morphine-diazepam-oxygen anesthesia, abstracted. *Anesthesiology* 51(suppl.): S137, 1979.

8 / Coronary Circulation and Anesthesia for Coronary Artery Bypass Graft Surgery

SAIT TARHAN
HUGO S. RAIMUNDO

CORONARY CIRCULATION

Coronary blood flow is related directly to the perfusion pressure gradient, which is the difference between the pressure in the proximal segments of the large coronary arteries and that in the right atrium. Resistance in the coronary artery system, which is influenced by several factors,[31] also decreases coronary blood flow. With the onset of isovolemic contraction, the coronary arteries that supply the left ventricle are compressed by the actively contracting myocardium, and, because of this, blood flow going through the left coronary artery decreases suddenly.[16] The perfusion pressure in the coronary arteries then increases quickly, and coronary blood flow is slightly higher in late systole than during isovolemic contraction.

During isovolemic relaxation, coronary blood flow increases greatly; throughout the remainder of diastole, coronary blood flow declines gradually as coronary artery perfusion pressure slowly falls. Yet these differences are not as prominent in the right coronary artery as they are in the left coronary artery, because right ventricular myocardium exerts little extravascular compression. Quantitatively, blood flow in the coronary arteries to the left ventricular myocardium during systole ranges from 7% to 45% of coronary flow during diastole.[24]

During rest, almost 25% of the total resistance to coronary blood flow is caused by extravascular compression.[70] But during tachycardia, this resistance increases to about 55%, because, at faster heart rates, the fraction of the cardiac cycle taken up by systole is also increased.[49] Resistance to the coronary blood flow caused by systolic contraction is highest in the endocardium and lowest in the epicardium.[31] Because of this difference, endocardium is more likely than epicardium to be damaged by ischemia.[31]

Factors Limiting Coronary Artery Blood Flow

Latham[46] and Osler[64] and others suggested that coronary vasospasm might be a cause of typical angina pectoris, but this functional hypothesis fell into disrepute when it was shown that almost all patients with angina had severe organic coronary artery atherosclerotic obstructions.[4] A new concept then arose that stenosis of the coronary artery sets a fixed limit to the possible increase of coronary blood flow, and angina ensues whenever the oxygen supply is short of myocardial metabolic demand. This concept set the guidelines for medical and surgical therapy of angina for several years. Also, experimental studies, most often performed on anesthetized, open-chest animals, showed that the metabolic requirements of the myocardium, and not neural mechanisms of coronary vascular control, were the principal determinants of coronary blood flow.[31] Some studies suggested that a product of myocardial metabolism may affect the local control of coronary vascular tone. Therefore, whenever the coronary blood flow is reduced or myocardial metabolism is increased, local concentrations of metabolites also increase, which in turn relaxes the smooth muscles of the precapillary arterioles (resistance vessels), reduces coronary vascular resistance, and increases coronary blood flow. Several substances and combinations have been mentioned as affecting the myocardial metabolic activity, such as reduced oxygen and increased partial pressures of carbon dioxide in blood and increased levels of hydrogen and potassium ions, adenine nucleotides, adenosine, and lactic acid, as well as prostaglandin-increased osmolarity.[31]

However, different segments of the coronary arterial bed give different responses to various metabolic stimuli and pharmacologic agents.[8]

Extramural-Intramural Coronary Arteries

Larger coronary arteries (extramural or conductance vessels) are found on the epicardial surface, yet smaller precapillary vessels (intramuscular resistance vessels) are located within the myocardium. Under normal conditions, large vessels contribute little to coronary vascular resistance. However, resistance primarily reflects changes in the caliber of the intramural vessels.[6] Therefore, the reduction of coronary vascular resistance caused by an accumulation of myocardial metabolites results from dilatation of the small precapillary intramural (resistance) vessels. The extramural coronary stem arteries are shielded from heart muscle by the surrounding fat and connective tissue, so that, particularly in their proximal part where, in man, the arteriosclerotic process can develop, blood flow cannot be improved locally by the presence of myocardial metabolites.[63]

Prinzmetal's Angina

Classic angina, as described by Heberden, is a distinct syndrome with two major characteristics.[65] First, pain can be provoked with the increase of the work of the heart and is relieved by rest or the administration of nitroglycerin (or both), and second, an ECG taken during pain generally shows depression of the ST segment in standard test leads I, II, III, and V_4, without a reciprocal elevation (Fig 8–1,A). However, there is another type of angina pectoris that appears to be a separate entity. This type does not show the two major characteristics of the classic form. In this variant type, pain begins with the subject at rest or at ordinary activity during the day or night—it is not brought on by effort.[65] During an attack, the ST segments are transiently and often significantly elevated, and there are reciprocal ST depressions in the standard leads[65] (Fig 8–1,B). The anginal attack usually terminates spontaneously but may lead to myocardial infarction if it continues long. Coro-

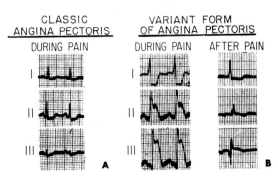

Fig 8–1.—Comparison of ECG differences between classic angina pectoris and Prinzmetal's variant angina. **A,** classic angina pectoris. After exercise, ECG shows ST-segment depression without reciprocal ST-segment elevation. **B,** Prinzmetal's angina, spontaneous pain. Elevation of ST segment in leads II and III with reciprocal ST depression in lead I. Immediately after pain, ECG returns to normal or to pattern before pain. (From Prinzmetal et al.[65] Used by permission.)

nary arteriosclerosis is also common to both forms of angina pectoris.[65]

Prinzmetal and his co-workers[65] postulated that coronary artery spasm was associated with this syndrome, and more recent studies have confirmed this.[82] The wide application of coronary arteriography has provided important evidence of the existence of coronary artery spasm in man.

Prinzmetal's variant angina can be provoked either spontaneously or pharmacologically.[29] It can occur among patients with no abnormalities on coronary angiograms and can produce myocardial ischemia sufficient to cause angina or myocardial infarction or both.[29] Total or near-total occlusion of major coronary arteries at sites far removed from a catheter's tip can occur spontaneously.[29] Spasm can be localized to a single coronary artery,[29] yet different branches of the coronary artery system can show the same phenomenon.

Provocation of coronary artery spasm is a relatively new angiographic technique and apparently is dependent on the hypersensitivity of localized arterial segments to the direct vascular constricting actions of ergonovine maleate.[29] The drug has two known actions on blood vessels: a direct action on vascular smooth muscle, causing vasoconstriction, and an effect on the cardiovascular center of the medulla, increasing the parasympathetic tone.[23] Ergonovine can provoke spasm at the site of low-grade stenosis (>30% reduction in cross-sectional diameter) of the right coronary artery (Fig 8–2). Alterations can be rapidly abolished after the sublingual administration of nitroglycerin.

Effects of Parasympathomimetic Agents on Coronary Arteries

Another pharmacologic agent capable of reproducing coronary artery spasm in patients with Prinzmetal's angina is the parasympathomimetic agent methacholine.[81] In contrast, the parasympatholytic drug atropine induces vasodilatation.[81] Methacholine can be administered either intramuscularly or subcutaneously. Coronary artery spasm caused by methacholine is promptly relieved by nitroglycerin.

Effects of Hyperventilation on Coronary Arteries

Coronary blood flow decreases with hyperventilation in man.[69] More recently, in another study,[82] vigorous hyperventilation was induced for five minutes immediately after a five-minute infusion of 100 ml of tris buffer (pH 10) in nine patients with Prinzmetal's variant angina. In

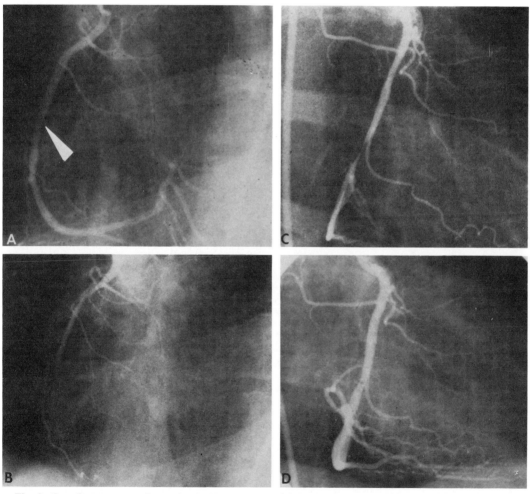

Fig 8–2.—Coronary angiography in Prinzmetal's angina showing production of coronary vasospasm with ergonovine. **A**, note stenosis of 20% *(arrowhead)* in right coronary artery (left anterior oblique view). **B**, after intravenous injection of 0.1 mg of ergonovine, there is complete occlusion. **C**, right anterior oblique view 2 minutes later shows partial resolution of spasm. **D**, after oral nitroglycerin, there is complete abolishment of vasospasm. (Courtesy of Dr. R. E. Vlietstra.)

eight patients, chest pain and ischemic changes seen on the ECG occurred during this procedure or within five minutes after it was terminated. Coronary vasospasm was documented with coronary cinearteriography after the procedure within five minutes after hyperventilation. The spasm was relieved by the administration of nitroglycerin in these patients. The oral administration of 90 mg of diltiazem, a calcium antagonistic drug, two hours before hyperventilation and infusion of tris buffer, suppressed the attack.[82]

Effects of Calcium and Hydrogen Ions on Coronary Arteries

The contraction of vascular smooth muscle depends quantitatively on calcium ions, whose presence is required for activation of myofibrillar adenosine triphosphatase. A highly potent calcium antagonistic action is exerted by hydrogen ions, which seem to compete with calcium ions for the same sites, both in the transmembrane calcium transport system and at the myofibrillar adenosine triphosphatase.[63] This effect causes vasoconstriction if calcium ion concentration increases or hydrogen ion concentration decreases. However, vasodilatation is produced by either calcium deficiency or increased hydrogen ion concentration.[63] Therefore, if hydrogen ion is decreased by hyperventilation and by tris buffer infusion, ischemic changes in the ECG can be induced among patients with known Prinzmetal's angina, and vasoconstriction also can occur both in normal subjects and in patients with stable exertional angina pectoris.[82]

Myocardial Infarction With Normal Coronary Arteries

Myocardial infarctions with normal and near-normal coronary arteries on cineangiography and without any other type of heart disease also have been reported.[41] Prolonged localized coronary artery spasm or platelet thrombi that subsequently resolved were considered part of the pathogenic mechanism. Later, those assumptions were confirmed, and, in one study, the sequence of events suggested that vasospasm initiated the infarction and the platelet aggregation or the coronary thrombosis.[56] Thromboxane A_2 released from platelet aggregation may further potentiate coronary vasospasm.[18] Atherosclerotic lesions are not essential for the development of coronary vasospasm and myocardial infarctions.[56]

Drug Therapy and Its Effect on Anesthetic Management

The implications of recent reports are important in the management and anesthetic care of the patient undergoing surgery. When thrombosis is the principal cause of infarction, anticoagulants are the logical choice for prophylaxis and treatment. Yet, these have not been uniformly successful. Coronary artery spasm superimposed on an atherosclerotic plaque opens up a wide range of therapeutic possibilities. Coronary vasodilators such as nitroglycerin may be helpful in acute myocardial infarction. Nifedipine is another drug that produces pronounced coronary artery dilatation with blocking of the slow calcium currents that are responsible for the action potential and for contraction of smooth muscle cell.[5] Also, α-adrenergic receptor blocking agents can prevent coronary spasm. Studies have shown that phenoxybenzamine can block the reflex coronary vasoconstriction.[5] Finally, vasodilator factors acting on the coronary vascular bed should not be blocked. $β_2$-Adrenergic receptors, if stimulated, induce vasodilatation in coronary vessels. Their blocking by propranolol may lead to an unopposed influence of coronary vasoconstrictor impulses, causing coronary spasm and ischemia.[5] Therefore, a cardioselective β-adrenergic blocking agent that does not block the $β_2$-adrenergic receptors might be beneficial in patients with acute myocardial ischemia.

The occurrence of Prinzmetal's variant angina during the immediate postanesthetic state has been reported.[1] Unquestionably, coronary artery spasms occur much more frequently than is presently appreciated. Some of the conditions that commonly occur during anesthesia and should be considered as possibly capable of producing coronary artery spasm, and even myocardial infarction, are the intravenous injection of calcium salts, the high incidence of vasovagal reflexes during abdominal and thoracic surgery, and hypothermia created intentionally (hypothermia during bypass) or unintentionally (body heat loss during anesthesia and surgery). Also ST-segment elevations observed during anesthesia and surgery are no rarity. Awareness of this entity (coronary vasospasm) is a must and may decrease the mortality and morbidity of the patients undergoing anesthesia and surgery.

ANESTHESIA FOR CORONARY ARTERY BYPASS GRAFT SURGERY

The first aorta-coronary artery bypass graft surgery was performed in 1964 and was considered a breakthrough in therapy for coronary artery disease. By 1974 more than 100,000 patients had undergone this operation, and by the summer of 1977, the number was between 280,000 and 300,000.[58] Since ischemic heart disease is the most frequent cause of death in the United States, and approximately 1.3 million patients sustain myocardial infarctions each year,[30] the number of operations performed on patients to correct their ischemic heart disease will increase. Yet after extensive experience spanning more than a decade, the procedure is still surrounded by controversy. The procedure itself can result in perioperative myocardial infarction. The incidence of such infarcts has been reported as ranging from 4%[20] to 46%,[58] as evidenced by ECG changes, vectorcardiogram, serum enzyme levels, and radioisotope myocardial imaging. Because radioisotope scintigraphy probably is more precise in determining myocardial damage, the percentage of myocardial infarctions could be higher than previously reported.[20] Aorta-coronary artery bypass graft surgery itself is now associated with a low operative mortality. Most cardiovascular centers report a mortality of 2% or less for revascularization alone.[20] However, several different factors may increase the risk.

Extensive efforts to protect the myocardium during and after surgery undoubtedly reduce the incidence of perioperative myocardial infarction and mortality. Greater understanding of the pathophysiology of ischemic events and constant attention to the balance between myocardial oxygen supply and demand are crucial in this setting. Myocardial oxygen demand increases with the cardiac work occasioned by increases of arterial blood pressure (afterload) and by increases of left ventricular filling pressure (preload).

One of the most important determinants of oxygen demand of the myocardium is the heart rate.[9] In one study, myocardial oxygen consumption was increased similarly with atrial pacing (increase of heart rate) and infusion of methoxamine (increased blood pressure), and increased heart rate produced more myocardial ischemia than did the stress of increased afterload, which was documented by chest pain and ischemic ST-segment changes.[50]

Myocardial oxygen supply depends on coronary blood flow, which in turn is affected by the diastolic arterial blood pressure or by the patency of the coronary arteries. Obviously, the oxygen supply to the myocardium would be decreased with hypoxemia or with a decreased oxygen-carrying capacity of blood due to any cause (Fig 8-3).

Some of these factors can be controlled pharmacologically. Medical management of ischemic heart disease generally can be achieved by reducing the myocardial oxygen demand rather than by increasing the coronary blood flow. However, recent studies have shown that coronary artery spasm also can cause myocardial ischemia, which can be relieved by nitroglycerin or other coronary vasodilating agents, such as nifedipine or verapamil, therefore increasing coronary blood flow. A different group of drugs, that is, vasodilator drugs such as nitroglycerin, mainly reduce the preload. Phentolamine (which reduces afterload) and nitroprusside (which reduces both afterload and preload[9]) lessen cardiac work and decrease myocardial oxygen consumption. However, drugs such as propranolol decrease the heart rate and reduce myocardial contractility and thus indirectly reduce myocardial oxygen consumption.[37]

Few data are available on the relationship between myocardial oxygen demand and supply as influenced by anesthetic drugs, especially in patients with myocardial ischemia. Enthusiasm for revascularization surgery has given enormous impetus to laboratory and clinical studies of this subject. In the normal dog heart, anesthetics such as halothane reduce myocardial oxygen consumption by decreasing preload, afterload, and the inotropic state.[77] Also, in the absence of ventricular failure, halothane favorably influences the relationship between myocardial oxygen supply and demand when coronary artery blood flow is limited. However, its effect on the failing heart is not known. Halothane anesthesia may have adverse effects and cause further elevation of left ventricular end-diastolic pressure with increased wall tension and myocardial oxygen consumption, which in turn may lead to impaired subendocardial blood flow.[3]

Anesthetic agents such as ketamine have been

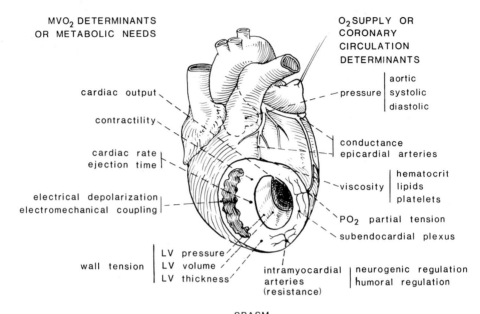

Fig 8–3.—Factors determining myocardial perfusion and myocardial oxygen consumption *(MVO₂)*. Spasm and collateral circulation have important role. (Modified from Favaloro.[20])

recommended as suitable during cardiovascular surgery because they permit cardiovascular stability while maintaining anesthesia; however, recent studies have shown that ketamine doubles or triples coronary blood flow and myocardial oxygen consumption, probably by increasing the arterial blood pressure and heart rate. Because of the effect on myocardial oxygen consumption, the drug has been considered to be contraindicated in patients with fixed hypertension, ischemic heart disease, or mitral valve disease.[73] Ketamine also is a potent pulmonary vasoconstrictor, even in relatively low dosage.[13]

In the past, nitrous oxide has been used as an analgesic agent for pain of myocardial ischemia and infarction; recent studies have shown that nitrous oxide also favorably influences oxygen demand without inducing left ventricular dysfunction.[80] This effect may be a particular advantage in the anesthetic management of patients with ischemic heart disease.

Neuroleptanalgesia, achieved by a combination of droperidol and fentanyl, has been used extensively for cardiac surgery. In one study, droperidol alone (0.33 mg/kg) increased the heart rate significantly, with a slight decrease in arterial blood pressure, owing to reduction in peripheral resistance. Because of the increase of heart rate, myocardial oxygen consumption also increased by 38%. Subsequent injection of fentanyl (0.0067 mg/kg) antagonized all the hemodynamic changes induced by droperidol, and coronary blood flow and myocardial oxygen consumption returned to control levels.[73]

Similar studies with other anesthetic agents and drugs administered during surgery (such as muscle relaxants and adrenergic agonists and antagonists) and on their effects on myocardial oxygen supply and demand are still scarce. Anesthetics and drugs presently available can be used in combination to protect the myocardium during and after surgery, especially in ischemic heart disease. Therefore, the proper choice of anesthetics may be of crucial importance for preventing perioperative myocardial infarction and death.

Preoperative Evaluation

The preoperative evaluation of the patient and his cardiopulmonary status may determine the management. Data from pulmonary function tests and arterial blood gas determinations are useful in the selection of ventilatory patterns to be used during and after surgery. Symptoms of cardiac failure can be a warning signal for the need of special supportive measures after surgery, such as endotracheal intubation, prolonged mechanical ventilation, and vasodilator or inotropic therapy.

Cigarette Smoking

Cigarette smoking produces chronic bronchitis and emphysema,[36] and the anesthetic implications of these conditions are commonly known. Cigarette smoking also contributes to death from myocardial infarction and coronary heart disease, especially sudden death[35] (see chap. 1). Therefore, cigarette smoking should be stopped long before surgery is undertaken.

Preoperative Drug Intake

Drugs that patients take before surgery also may influence the management during and after the procedure. Digitalis, diuretics, corticosteroids, β-adrenergic blocking agents, and monoamine oxidase inhibitors are especially important to consider.

CARDIAC GLYCOSIDES AND DIURETICS.—Prolonged therapy with cardiac glycosides and diuretics may diminish the total amount of body potassium, with or without lowering the serum concentration of potassium.[53]

Potassium is the electrolyte that most likely influences the electrophysiologic properties of the heart.[21] In a clinical setting, altered concentrations of potassium are the cause of the vast majority of arrhythmias.[21] Clinical evidence of hypokalemia usually does not appear until potassium concentrations are less than 2.5 mEq/L. Prolongation of the S-T interval and sagging of the ST segment are typical. Occasionally, a low-amplitude T wave can be seen. Hypokalemia also aggravates digitalis-induced arrhythmia, even with therapeutic serum concentrations of digitalis during and after operation.[21] Hypokalemia should be corrected before surgery begins. The oral administration of potassium is preferable. If potassium is administered rapidly or in large doses intravenously, the rate of increase in plasma potassium may induce a second- or third-degree block. Effects on a potassium-depleted animal or human being are even more serious and include bradycardia, cardiac arrest, and depression of conduction.[21] Therefore, caution is important with the intravenous administration of potassium. In an adult, a maximal replacement rate of 20 mEq of potassium chloride per hour is preferable.

Myocardial sensitivity to digitalis may be increased during the first 24 hours after cardiopulmonary bypass, even if the serum potassium level is normal.[61, 67] The use of digoxin should be stopped 36 to 48 hours before operation and that of digitoxin should be stopped 72 hours before operation. Being usually confined to bed before surgery, patients seem to tolerate well the temporary withdrawal of digitalis.

β-ADRENERGIC BLOCKERS.—β-Adrenergic blockade is an important therapeutic modality in the management of angina pectoris, and propranolol hydrochloride is the agent most frequently used. Propranolol decreases the frequency of anginal episodes because it decreases myocardial oxygen consumption. Theoretically, if administration is continued to the time of operation, propranolol may depress the myocardium during the surgical and postperfusion periods, causing left ventricular failure. Therefore, its discontinuation up to two weeks before surgery has been recommended.[38] Yet several reports have indicated the occurrence of acute myocardial infarction, severe angina, and ventricular arrhythmias shortly after the abrupt withdrawal of propranolol or other β-adrenergic blocking drugs in patients with coronary artery disease.[26] The onset of rebound angina correlates well with physiologic data on the disappearance of propranolol from myocardial tissue. Measurements of both myocardial propranolol and residual radioactivity from ^{14}C-labeled propranolol have shown that neither residual propranolol nor its metabolites persist more than 24 hours after withdrawal of the drug.[26]

Usually, propranolol therapy can be continued until the day before cardiac surgery. For patients whose ischemic symptoms are severe before therapy, the use of propranolol should be continued until the day of surgery. In some patients whose propranolol dosage was halved, anginal symptoms were increased and the hazards of withdrawal from propranolol were not completely eliminated.[72] In the same study, the hypotension and bradycardia anticipated from the interaction of propranolol with general anesthesia were not apparent among the patients who had taken propranolol up until the day of surgery. Also, hypertension and tachycardia leading to ventricular arrhythmias and ST-segment depression were considerably less frequent in those patients.[72] Rate-pressure product (an index of myocardial oxygen demand) before intubation and its significantly smaller increase after intubation also were considered to be due to propranolol's protecting the patient with ischemic heart disease who received narcotic general anesthesia. One of the major hazards during this operation was excessive sympathetic stimulation from intubation, especially during light anesthesia. Therefore, it was concluded that persisting β-adrenergic blockade may provide a protective effect against excessive responses.[72]

For patients with unstable angina, continuation of the therapy until the time of surgery is especially important.

Cardiac Catheterization and Coronary Angiographic Data

The preoperative evaluation of the patient also includes consideration of data obtained from cardiac catheterization and coronary angiography. This information may be predictive of the outcome of surgery. Patients undergoing coronary artery bypass graft surgery who have severe depression of left ventricular performance (manifested by an ejection fraction ≤33%, an end-diastolic volume ≥103 ml/sq m, or left ventricular end-diastolic pressure ≥18 mm Hg) have a significantly higher risk of postoperative death.[25]

A patient who has a normal left ventricle with evidence of good distal runoff on coronary angiography is an ideal candidate for surgery. Such patients have a mortality of 2% or less. If patients have a normal left ventricle and the damage is moderate, surgery can be accomplished with a mortality of about 5%. However, patients with severely deteriorated left ventricular function and angina pectoris have a mortality of 12%.[20]

In addition to these considerations, the following factors also increase the risk: operation in patients with left main coronary artery obstruction; the number of grafts inserted; combined procedures, such as left ventricular reconstruction or valve replacement in addition to coronary artery bypass graft; surgery performed on elderly patients (if they have a good left ventricular function, chances slightly improved); and ventricle deteriorated from previous myocardial infarction. Severe hypertension is the most important risk factor. Patients with long-standing severe hypertension should be operated on only if they are totally disabled.[20] The presence of diabetes alone does not increase mortality.[20]

A syndrome of sudden death in patients awaiting coronary artery surgery has been described.[48] Patients who had recent onset of severe angina pectoris caused by critical narrowing of 90% or more of a major coronary artery supplying a large portion of the left ventricular myocardium are liable to sudden death and require urgent myocardial revascularization.

Acute myocardial infarction has been considered an absolute contraindication to myocardial revascularization. However, recent clinical reports indicate that acute revascularization of an evolving myocardial infarction seems to be beneficial in terms of preserving viable myocardium and reducing mortality and morbidity.[62] The clinical use of effective mechanical circulatory-assistance devices has greatly increased the rate of survival of these patients.

Subendocardial infarction is usually considered to be a benign entity; yet one study revealed that subendocardial infarction was followed by an incidence of unstable angina of 46%, and ultimately 21% of patients suffered transmural infarctions after a follow-up period of 10.6 months.[54] Late follow-up has shown that the incidence of sudden death, angina, and recurrent infarction is higher in these patients than in patients with transmural infarctions.[47] A large percentage of patients who are medically treated for their subendocardial infarction develop transmural infarctions.[25] To prevent this, such patients can undergo coronary artery bypass graft surgery early after their subendocardial infarction, especially those with unstable angina. These patients can undergo saphenous vein bypass graft surgery, with an incidence of perioperative infarction and a death rate comparable to that experienced by patients undergoing surgery for unstable angina alone.[55] In one study from the Mayo Clinic, the incidence of perioperative myocardial infarction, defined as the appearance of new Q waves on the ECG, was 10.7% among patients with subendocardial infarction. In the same study, the mortality for these patients undergoing coronary artery bypass graft surgery was 3.6%,[55] therefore making the surgery a worthwhile risk.

Routines Closely Related to Operation

Premedication

Previously, in premedication for any kind of surgery, profound sedation and respiratory and circulatory depression were to be avoided. This concept, however, cannot be applied to coronary artery bypass graft surgery, especially when ventricular function is not impaired. Increased amounts of premedication are justified because patients have severe apprehension before coronary artery bypass graft surgery, usually leading to tachycardia and hypertension, which in turn increase the myocardial oxygen demand.

Although different combinations of sedatives, tranquilizers, and opiates can be used successfully, pentobarbital and morphine are the most frequently used agents for premedication in our institution. Pentobarbital is given orally in doses of 2 mg/kg (to a maximum of 100 mg) two hours before surgery, and morphine in doses of 1 mg/5 kg (to a maximum of 10 mg) is administered intramuscularly one hour before surgery.

Belladonna derivatives and related drugs are not used as part of premedication because they may increase the heart rate and the incidence of arrhythmias.[17] If a vagolytic drug is needed during anesthesia, atropine can be given intravenously in small controlled increments until the desired effect is achieved.

Nitroglycerin

One of the recent useful additions to premedication for patients undergoing coronary artery bypass graft surgery is the application of 2% nitroglycerin ointment to the chest before the patient is brought to the operating room.[60] However, it has recently been reported that sublingual nitroglycerin adversely affects the Pao_2 levels in patients with coronary artery disease breathing room air.[44] Nitroglycerin ointment probably has the same effect. The drug does not change the $Paco_2$ levels. Therefore, it does not affect the alveolar ventilation. The reduction of Pao_2 after application of nitroglycerin seems to be related to hemodynamic changes, such as vasodilatation in poorly ventilated or nonventilated areas, opening of arteriovenous anastomoses, and decreases in pulmonary artery pressure, favoring the perfusion of less dependent ventilated lung areas. A clinical implication of these is myocardial hypoxia, which may still result from a decrease in available oxygen. Therefore, when nitroglycerin and narcotics are used in combination for the treatment of anginal pain before surgery, a high inspired oxygen concentration should be initiated.[44]

Induction

In patients with coronary artery disease, induction is increasingly recognized as a critical phase of anesthetic management. As soon as the patient is placed on the operating table, the ECG electrodes, including a V_5 lead, are attached. After the leads are placed, a plastic needle is inserted into a vein of each arm (usually 14- or 16-gauge Teflon). Each needle is attached to an intravenous infusion set containing 250 ml of 5% glucose in water. The patient then breathes 100% oxygen by face mask. Induction is started with 5 to 10 mg of diazepam, followed by the use of small increments of thiopental (50 to 75 mg), as tolerated and as needed. Pancuronium in doses of 0.1 to 0.12 mg/kg is added intravenously, and this treatment is followed quickly with thiopental; thus, three to four minutes can elapse to allow adequate time for relaxation before intubation. Circulatory stability and longer duration of action make pancuronium reasonably suitable for coronary artery bypass graft surgery, although tachyarrhythmias occasionally occur.

If induction is started with diazepam, the drug, in addition to its central sedative effects, has a nitroglycerin-like action on the coronary and systemic circulations. It decreases the left ventricular end-diastolic pressure, probably by reducing the afterload or venous return (preload) or both. The combination of these effects reduces intracavitary volume, myocardial wall tension, and left ventricular myocardial oxygen consumption.[10]

Before intubation, the trachea is sprayed with 4% topical lidocaine in an effort to prevent arrhythmias, as well as to provide anesthetic tracheal block. This prevention of arrhythmias (if achieved) is likely a result of the rapid absorption of lidocaine across the tracheal mucosa. It may also be due to obtundation of tracheal reflexes, especially when a suitable time elapses before the insertion of the endotracheal tube (about 30 seconds to one minute).

Maintenance

Maintenance is achieved with nitrous oxide (50% to 60%) and oxygen supplemented with other drugs, such as narcotic analgesics (meperidine, fentanyl, or morphine) or a volatile agent (either halothane or enflurane). If meperidine is chosen, 20-mg increments are given intravenously up to a total dose of 200 to 300 mg.

Morphine anesthesia has been widely accepted for cardiac surgery because of its relatively benign effects on the cardiovascular system. However, morphine can cause release of endogenous norepinephrine or epinephrine in man, resulting in an increase of blood pressure. It can produce profound analgesia without consistently providing loss of consciousness.[51] Therefore, morphine often needs to be supplemented with nitrous oxide to achieve amnesia; yet such a combination reduces cardiac output significantly during morphine anesthesia.[75] Recent studies[43] comparing morphine–nitrous oxide–oxygen with halothane–nitrous oxide–oxygen indicated that myocardial oxygen demand was greater in patients who received morphine than in those who received halothane. Myocardial depression with halothane was not detrimental, and the myocardial oxygen supply-to-demand ratio may have been preserved better during the crucial precardiopulmonary bypass period with halothane.

Halothane is of value in patients who do not have severely compromised left ventricular function and do not have hepatic disease. Preferably, halothane should not be used in patients who have received it during the previous six months. The inspired concentration of halothane is seldom higher than 1.0% with 50% nitrous oxide. If the systolic pressure becomes less than 90 mm Hg in a previously normotensive patient, the halothane concentration is decreased or its use is discontinued, and the anesthetic is supplemented with a narcotic such as meperidine (in increments of 10 to 20 mg).

Halothane sensitizes the heart to both exogenous and endogenous catecholamines, and halothane-induced conduction defects have been assumed to result in arrhythmias. However, according to recent studies,[42] halothane sensitizes muscle cells directly to epinephrine.

Enflurane is a recent addition to anesthetic practice. A dose of 0.5% to 2.0% is used with a 50% nitrous oxide–oxygen mixture. No available evidence indicates that enflurane has a hepatotoxic effect, and clinical impression suggests that it produces less myocardial sensitization to catecholamines, thus perhaps resulting in fewer arrhythmias.

In recent years, emphasis has been placed on hypertension and its effects on the oxygen supply and demand of the myocardium during and after coronary artery bypass graft surgery. Perhaps the importance of hypotension has not been appreciated, but serious consequences of hypotension cannot be ignored. Diminished arterial pressure may have a part in the vicious cycle of decreasing coronary perfusion pressure, greater ischemic injury, and more severe hypotension. In addition, a baroreceptor-mediated increase in heart rate would tend to increase myocardial oxygen demand[19] and cause further ischemic injury. The precise level of decreased arterial blood pressure or coronary perfusion pressure that may jeopardize the myocardium cannot be established in the operating room because it varies from patient to patient. However, a decrease in systolic blood pressure of 10% to 20% is considered acceptable by most anesthesiologists.[52]

Monitoring

Arterial and external jugular or right atrial pressures (in some patients, left atrial pressure) are monitored routinely. The ECG, heart sounds, and temperature are also monitored. Indirect monitoring of arterial pressure is unreliable, especially if there is hypotension; therefore, direct measurement of arterial pressure is essential in cardiac operations. Percutaneous insertion of an 18- or a 20-gauge Teflon catheter into the radial artery is relatively simple. If ulnar arterial pulses cannot be palpated and adequate collateral circulation cannot be demonstrated (Allen's test), the femoral or the dorsalis pedis artery can be used.

The venous pressure is measured through a large-bore plastic needle placed in the right internal or external jugular vein. The external jugular vein may accurately reflect right atrial pressure during anesthesia with controlled or spontaneous respiration, and it has the advantages of simplicity and safety; however, its function can be nullified by certain positions of the patient. The internal jugular vein catheter can function in all positions, and it provides direct access to right atrial blood for gas analysis.[74]

Because the determinants of myocardial oxygen supply and demand are of the utmost importance during and after coronary artery bypass graft surgery, these factors should be considered during monitoring. A continuous display of arterial pressure and heart rate is essential.

RATE-PRESSURE PRODUCT.—In the dog, heart rate, ejection time, and arterial pressure are major determinants of myocardial oxygen consumption. Demand for oxygen has been successfully correlated with the product of heart rate and systolic arterial pressure[22] (this product is referred to as rate-pressure product) and is calculated by multiplying the heart rate by the systolic blood pressure and dividing the product by 100 to reduce the value to convenient units.[66] When heart rate and peak systolic pressure are held constant, myocardial oxygen consumption varies with alterations in the ejection time.[71] This relationship suggests that, in addition to heart rate and systolic pressure, ejection time determines the myocardial oxygen consumption. However, peak systolic pressure itself correlates well with left ventricular oxygen consumption and is the basis of many of the double product values (systolic pressure times heart rate) used in human studies.[32] This product is easy to calculate in the operating room and can be a valuable addition to the monitoring of myocardial oxygen consumption in patients undergoing coronary artery surgery. The product of rate and pressure also is more nearly constant at the onset of each attack of anginal pain in awake patients, indicating a consistent relationship between the level of cardiac work and the onset of pain.[66]

ECG.—The ECG should be used to identify myocardial ischemia and arrhythmias that may occur during the induction of anesthesia and throughout the surgery. It has been shown that 89% of the changes in the ST segment can be documented with lead V_5[2] (Fig 8–4). Therefore, this lead is also monitored in addition to the standard limb leads and leads aV_R, aV_L, and aV_F. The ECG should be recorded before the induc-

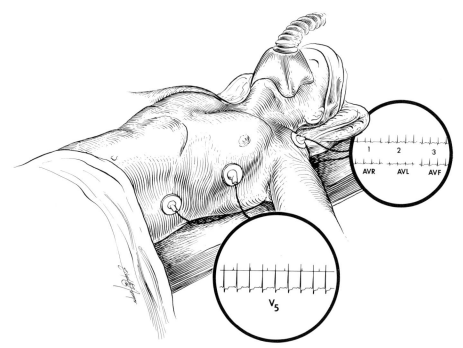

Fig 8–4.—Monitoring of ECG with lead V_5. (From Tarhan S., White R.D., Raimundo H.S.: Anesthetic considerations for aortocoronary bypass graft surgery. *Ann. Thorac. Surg.* 27:376, 1979. Used by permission.)

tion of anesthesia to provide a good baseline for changes taking place during and after surgery and to make comparisons easy. The ECG is standardized with 1 mV (10 mm). It has been suggested that 1 mm horizontally or a downsloping depression of the ST segment from baseline is a significant indicator of myocardial ischemia,[39] and such ischemic changes could go undiagnosed if the V_5 lead was not used.

LEFT VENTRICULAR END-DIASTOLIC PRESSURE.—Left ventricular end-diastolic pressure is the result of left ventricular content and associated wall stress. Left atrial pressure closely approximates left ventricular end-diastolic pressure, and left atrial pressure can be estimated accurately from pulmonary capillary wedge pressure,[19] which in turn can be measured with relative ease by means of a balloon-tipped, flow-directed catheter.[76] However, there is still a preference for the direct measurement of left atrial pressures with a catheter left in place after bypass. This catheter can be removed without difficulty on the third or fourth postoperative day, and bleeding after removal has not been a problem.

BODY TEMPERATURE.—The monitoring of temperature also is essential. A probe thermistor placed in the nasopharynx or oropharynx provides a more reliable guide to the temperature of the brain than do rectal and esophageal thermometers. Aortic blood temperature is usually measured if the temperature probe is placed in the esophagus. Since the recent advent of hypothermic cardioplegic solutions, needle thermistor probes have been used to monitor myocardial temperature.

Special Problems and Techniques

Protection of Myocardium During Ischemic Cardiac Arrest

During open-heart surgery with cardiopulmonary bypass, ischemic arrest is often used as a convenient way to provide the surgeon with a nonbleeding, bloodless, relaxed heart. Nevertheless, ischemic cardiac arrest may initiate deleterious cellular changes that may lead to irreversible cell damage. The suggestion that this damage might be reduced by specially formulated solutions has attracted considerable attention.

Composition of these solutions may vary widely, but the basic ingredients are similar. They include agents that can cause rapid diastolic arrest (cardioplegia), and they may contain some protective agents to combat one or more harmful effects of ischemia.[34] For example, hyperosmolar agents have been used to counteract cell swelling, β-adrenergic blocking drugs have been used to reduce cellular energy demands, glucose has been used to enhance cellular energy production, and steroids have been used to stabilize the cell membrane.[28] The length of the interval from the beginning of ischemia to the occurrence of irreversible damage is determined by energy-rich phosphates. Apparently, coronary perfusion with hypothermic solutions or solutions containing high concentrations of potassium chloride, which induce arrest without excessively depleting myocardial adenosine triphosphate, protects the heart during such periods and enables the myocardium to respond better at the end of ischemic cardiac arrest.[27] However, little is presently understood about the mechanisms involved in both protection and damage.

Circulatory Care

Proper intraoperative anesthetic management of a patient with ischemic heart disease dictates careful regulation of hemodynamics. Patients may have a certain degree of heart failure related to coronary artery disease, and the heart may have been performing on a depressed Frank-Starling curve (Fig 8–5). In the clinical setting, cardiac failure traditionally is treated by the administration of inotropic drugs to increase the contractile force and by diuretics to increase the excretion of salt and water. Mild congestive heart failure responds satisfactorily to this therapy, but the conventional measures may be inadequate if the failure is more severe. In recent years, it has been recognized that pharmacologically induced peripheral vasodilatation can shift the function curve upward and to the left (see Fig 8–5), relieving the signs of both circulatory congestion and low cardiac output. Improvement of pump performance produced by vasodilator drugs is often accompanied by reduction of myocardial oxygen consumption.[9] (Arterial vasodilatation reduces afterload and decreases the tension generated in the left ventricle. Venous vasodilatation causes pooling of blood, which de-

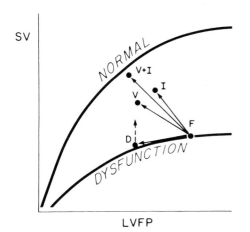

Fig 8–5.—Frank-Starling left ventricular function curve; left ventricular filling pressure *(LVFP)* and stroke volume *(SV)*. Depressed curve can be shifted to left by inotropic drugs *(I)* or by vasodilator drugs *(V)*. Effects would be complementary if drugs were infused together *(V + I)*. Diuretics *(D)* reduce filling pressure *(F)* without increasing output. Stroke volume may later increase *(broken line)*, probably because of gradual improvement of ventricular function. (From Cohn and Franciosa.[9] Used by permission.)

creases venous return or preload and left ventricular end-diastolic pressure, thus reducing myocardial oxygen consumption.) Conversely, an inotropic drug would increase arterial pressure and the velocity of fiber shortening and increase myocardial oxygen consumption. The metabolic consequences of these two forms of therapy are of great importance to patients with ischemic heart disease.

A lightly anesthetized patient, especially a patient receiving morphine as an anesthetic, may sustain increased blood pressure or heart rate and an increase in myocardial oxygen consumption. Also, hypertension occasionally develops after coronary artery bypass graft surgery, possibly because of reflexes originating from the heart or great vessels or both.[21] In these circumstances, pharmacologic vasodilatation may be needed.

SODIUM NITROPRUSSIDE AND NITROGLYCERIN.—The drugs most commonly used for the treatment of hypertension are sodium nitroprusside and nitroglycerin. Nitroprusside is administered intravenously in a concentration of 50 mg/250 ml of 5% dextrose in water. The agent is extremely potent, and its action is rapid but brief. One drawback is its potential for cyanide toxicity with overdosage. Nitroprusside reduces arterial impedance and causes some venous pooling.[9] When left ventricular function is severely impaired, the response to the drug may include an increase in cardiac output. In normal persons, lowering the blood pressure with sodium nitroprusside increases the heart rate, yet in heart failure, it usually does not alter the rate significantly—indeed, the rate may actually decrease. Pulmonary vascular resistance also decreases with the infusion of nitroprusside.

Nitroglycerin is remarkably effective for angina pectoris. It primarily reduces myocardial oxygen consumption by dilating the venous capacitance vessels, thereby reducing venous return and producing a sharp decrease in cardiac filling pressure (preload) and pulmonary arterial pressure.[9] It has long been used as a sublingual medication, but its intravenous form is relatively new and is not commercially available. The intravenous route has advantages, such as easy reversal and control of the dose. Nitroglycerin has no cyanide toxicity. The solution must be prepared under sterile conditions: 8 mg of nitroglycerin are dissolved in 250 ml of dextrose in water, resulting in a concentration of 32 µg/ml. A reasonable standard dosage is 1.0 µg/kg per minute. Although nitroglycerin and nitroprusside produce basically similar hemodynamic effects, nitroglycerin may reduce ischemic injury, partly by increasing perfusion of ischemic areas. However, nitroprusside may worsen ischemic injury, in part by reducing regional perfusion. Therefore, nitroglycerin seems preferable to nitroprusside for reducing preload and afterload in patients during the early phase of acute myocardial infarction.[7] This experimental evidence seems to be immediately applicable in the operating room.

PHENTOLAMINE.—The other drug used for vasodilator therapy is phentolamine. This agent blocks α-adrenergic receptors and has an effect predominantly on the arterial vascular bed, yet it produces more prominent tachycardia than does nitroprusside. Because of this effect and the cost of continuous infusion of this drug, it has not achieved wide use in the treatment of severe heart failure.[9]

INOTROPES.—The heart with impaired function (pump failure) may require pharmacologic inotropic support. All known positive inotropic substances increase myocardial oxygen consumption by increasing preload and afterload (or both), as well as by increasing contractility and heart rate. Epinephrine (0.02 to 0.04 µg/kg/minute) is often helpful. Dopamine, a norepinephrine precursor, increases cardiac output by augmenting stroke volume, with a somewhat lesser effect on heart rate than epinephrine. This agent also decreases renal vascular resistance and increases renal blood flow and sodium excretion.[68] Dopamine in an amount of 200 to 400 mg in 250 ml of 5% glucose in water is prepared and is infused intravenously in doses of 5 to 20 µg/kg/minute.

A relatively new inotropic agent is dobutamine, a derivative of dopamine. It has been reported to have less arrhythmogenicity and less chronotropic effect than isoproterenol, yet it has a potent inotropic effect. In a clinical study, a dose of 10 µg/kg/minute increased cardiac output by 27%, with little increase in heart rate during emergence from bypass, and few arrhythmias were noted.[78]

Because potent inotropic agents may increase cardiac output (often at the expense of increased myocardial oxygen consumption) and because vasodilator therapy reduces elevated left ventricular filling pressure and myocardial oxygen consumption and augments cardiac output,[9] the combination of dobutamine or dopamine with a vasodilator in refractory congestive heart failure may produce better ventricular performance than is obtained with either vasodilators or inotropic agents alone. The vasodilators can be titrated to produce maximal tolerated reduction of impedance, while inotropic drugs are titrated to effect optimal cardiac stimulation. In contrast to isoproterenol, an inotropic-vasodilator drug combination usually does not increase heart rate.[9] Combined dopamine and nitroprusside treatment increases the cardiac index considerably while reducing elevated left ventricular end-diastolic pressure, and it provides a useful pharmacologic modality for the treatment of severe congestive heart failure.[59]

In the absence of specific contraindications, cardiac glycosides also can be given to patients with postoperative low cardiac output. Digoxin is our choice because of its rapid effect and relatively short biologic half-life. The digitalizing dose is estimated to be 0.9 mg/sq m of body surface area. Initially, one half of the estimated total dose is administered intravenously, and then one fourth or one eighth is added intravenously every one to two hours during continuous ECG monitoring, until the desired effect is obtained or adverse effects appear. A maintenance dose of approximately one eighth of the digitalizing dose is given daily, beginning on the day after digitalization has been achieved.

Usually, however, patients have been given digitalis previously, and, in this situation, redigitalization must be monitored with determinations of the blood level of digitalis.

Calcium chloride is commonly administered intravenously as an inotropic agent to critically ill patients, yet reports on its effectiveness have been controversial.[14] Clinically, an increase of blood pressure is often seen after intravenous administration. In a comparative study of three calcium salts, plasma ionic calcium levels were higher after the administration of calcium chloride than after the administration of either gluconate or gluceptate salts.[79]

INTRA-AORTIC BALLOON ASSIST.—The duration of cardiopulmonary bypass and induced myocardial ischemia is related to the possibility of maintaining cardiac output after operation. Studies have shown that cardiopulmonary bypass longer than one hour increases the incidence of perioperative infarcts significantly.[45] In some patients, extracorporeal circulation cannot be terminated because of inadequate myocardial performance and impaired coronary blood flow. If other methods to support hemodynamics fail, an intra-aortic balloon assist can be used for circulatory support. During the preoperative and immediate postoperative period, this technique to support the failing circulation is sometimes lifesaving. The usual pharmacologic agents in the treatment of patients with intraoperative and postoperative cardiogenic shock are vasopressors and inotropic drugs; however, these drugs increase myocardial oxygen requirements during a time when total oxygen availability and delivery may be decreased. Intra-aortic balloon assist lowers myocardial oxygen requirements[33] by reducing systolic blood pressure and thus reducing left ventricular work. At the same time, it increases the diastolic pressure, thus increasing coronary blood flow and achieving greater oxygen availability[33] (see chap. 19).

FEMORAL ARTERY TO FEMORAL VEIN BYPASS.—An alternative method for the anesthetic management of a patient with unstable hemodynamics is to establish extracorporeal circulation before the induction of anesthesia. The femoral artery and veins can be cannulated under local anesthesia and connected to the oxygenator (Fig 8–6); bypass then can be started if the circulation fails.[12]

Arrhythmias

Arrhythmias occur in many patients, even with good management (see chap. 17). In general, slow supraventricular rhythms, such as atrial rhythm, atrioventricular junctional rhythm, and wandering pacemaker, are benign and do not require treatment.[40] However, some may be deleterious to myocardial performance,

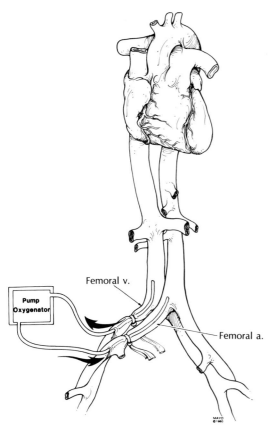

Fig 8–6.—Cannulation of femoral vein and artery (established under local anesthesia). Note position of cannula in femoral vein. In some patients, cannulation of one femoral vein may provide sufficient venous return to oxygenator to keep flow at 2 L/minute/sq m.

and they may be warning signals of the development of more serious problems. For example, an episode of ventricular extrasystoles or bigeminy may presage ventricular tachycardia and fibrillation. Therefore, ventricular arrhythmia should be considered a sign of serious derangement until proved otherwise.

The mechanism of myocardial excitation is complex, but factors that cause ectopic activity during and after operation are fairly well understood. These entities include myocardial ischemia, hypoxemia, alterations in serum potassium concentration, and high blood concentration of certain drugs, such as digitalis. Therefore, before antiarrhythmic therapy is undertaken, the type of arrhythmia should be identified. Its cause should be investigated and then therapy should be started. Treatment may consist in the intravenous administration of lidocaine for frequent and multiform premature ventricular beats or ventricular tachycardia or the use of β-adrenergic blocking agents, such as propranolol, to terminate the tachyarrhythmias caused by an excess of catecholamines or increased sympathetic tone. The drug slows the ventricular rate in patients with atrial fibrillation or flutter when it cannot be controlled by digitalis. It is also effective in treating digitalis-induced tachyarrhythmias of supraventricular or ventricular origin.[15] If arrhythmias are caused by low total-body potassium concentration, the intravenous infusion of potassium chloride is warranted. Digitalis overdosage can produce any type of cardiac arrthythmias.[40] Therefore, when arrhythmias occur in patients receiving digitalis, toxicosis should be suspected and can be treated by withholding the digitalis, administering potassium salts, or, in some patients, using antiarrhythmic drugs, especially phenytoin. If there is a doubt about the digitalis toxicity, serum levels should be determined. Levels above 2.0 ng/ml indicate a need for caution.

Another specific method of treating arrhythmias is cardiac pacing,[11] with temporary epicardial electrodes placed during the operation. The heart should be paced at a rate sufficient to suppress ectopic beats and to correct bradycardia. The pacing wires are carried externally anterior to the sternum[57] and are attached to an external temporary pacemaker. Care must be taken with electrocautery, because current that may be induced in the wires may cause ventricular fibrillation (see chap. 21).

REFERENCES

1. Balagot R.C., et al.: Prinzmetal's variant angina in the immediate postanesthetic state. *Anesthesiology* 46:355, 1977.
2. Blackburn H., Taylor H.L., Okamoto N., et al.: Standardization of the exercise electrocardiogram: A systematic comparison of chest lead configurations employed for monitoring during exercise, in Karvonen M., Barry A.J. (eds.): *Physical Activity and the Heart*. Springfield, Ill., Charles C Thomas, Publisher, 1966.
3. Bland J.H.L., Lowenstein E.: Halothane-induced decrease in experimental myocardial ischemia in the nonfailing canine heart. *Anesthesiology* 45:287, 1976.
4. Blumgart H.L., Schlesinger M.J., Davis D.: Studies on the relation of the clinical manifestations of angina pectoris, coronary thrombosis, and myocardial infarction to the pathologic findings: With particular reference to the significance of the collateral circulation. *Am. Heart J.* 19:1, 1940.
5. Braunwald E.: Coronary spasm and acute myocardial infarction—new possibility for treatment and prevention, editorial. *N. Engl. J. Med.* 299:1301, 1978.
6. Braunwald E., Ross J. Jr., Sonnenblick E.H.: *Mechanisms of Contraction of the Normal and Failing Heart*, ed. 2. Boston, Little, Brown & Co., 1976, p. 200.
7. Chiariello M., et al.: Comparison between the effects of nitroprusside and nitroglycerin on ischemic injury during acute myocardial infarction. *Circulation* 54:766, 1976.
8. Cohen M.V., Kirk E.S.: Differential response of large and small coronary arteries to nitroglycerin and angiotensin: Autoregulation and tachyphylaxis. *Circ. Res.* 33:445, 1973.
9. Cohn J.N., Franciosa J.A.: Vasodilator therapy of cardiac failure: I, II. *N. Engl. J. Med.* 297:27 and 254, 1977.
10. Côté P., Guéret P., Bourassa M.G.: Systemic and coronary hemodynamic effects of diazepam in patients with normal and diseased coronary arteries. *Circulation* 50:1210, 1974.
11. Danielson G.K., Ellis F.H. Jr.: Low cardiac output and cardiac arrhythmias after open-heart surgery, in Hardy J.D. (ed.): *Critical Surgical Illness*. Philadelphia, W.B. Saunders Co., 1971, p. 587.
12. Danielson G.K., Hasbrouck J.D., Bryant L.R.: Cannulation under local or regional anesthesia for the 'salvage' cardiac patient. *J. Thorac. Cardiovasc. Surg.* 55:864, 1968.
13. De Master R.J., Fogdall R.P.: The effects of ketamine on the pulmonary and systemic circulations in patients with coronary artery disease. Abstracted in the Scientific Papers of the American Society of Anesthesiologists Annual Meeting, 1977, p. 721.
14. Denlinger J.K., et al.: Cardiovascular responses to calcium administered intravenously to man during halothane anesthesia. *Anesthesiology* 42:390, 1975.
15. Department of Drugs: Current status of propranolol hydrochloride (Inderal). *J.A.M.A.* 225:1380, 1973.
16. Downey J.M., Kirk E.S.: Inhibition of coronary blood flow by a vascular waterfall mechanism. *Circ. Res.* 36:753, 1975.
17. Eger E.I. II: Atropine, scopolamine, and related compounds. *Anesthesiology* 23:365, 1962.
18. Ellis E.F., et al.: Coronary arterial smooth muscle contraction by a substance released from platelets: Evidence that it is thromboxane A_2. *Science* 193:1135, 1976.
19. Epstein S.E.: Hypotension, nitroglycerin, and acute myocardial infarction, editorial. *Circulation* 47:217, 1973.
20. Favaloro R.G.: Direct myocardial revascularization: A ten-year journey; myths and realities. *Am. J. Cardiol.* 43:109, 1979.
21. Fisch C.: Relation of electrolyte disturbances to cardiac arrhythmias. *Circulation* 47:408, 1973.
22. Gerola A., Feinberg H., Katz L.N.: Oxygen cost of cardiac hemodynamic activity, abstracted. *Physiologist* 1:31, 1957.
23. Goodman L.S., Gilman A.Z.: *The Pharmacological Basis of Therapeutics: A Textbook of Pharmacology, Toxicology, and Therapeutics for Physicians and Medical Students*, ed. 3. New York, Macmillan Publishing Co., 1965, p. 554.
24. Gregg D.E., Khouri E.M., Rayford C.R.: Systemic and coronary energetics in the resting unanesthetized dog. *Circ. Res.* 16:102, 1965.
25. Hammermeister K.E., Kennedy J.W.: Predictors of surgical mortality in patients undergoing direct myocardial revascularization. *Circulation* 50 (suppl. 2):112, 1974.
26. Harrison D.C., Alderman E.L.: Discontinuation of propranolol therapy: Cause of rebound angina pectoris and acute coronary events, editorial. *Chest* 69:1, 1976.
27. Hearse D.J., Stewart D.A., Braimbridge M.V.: Hypothermic arrest and potassium arrest: Metabolic and myocardial protection during elective cardiac arrest. *Circ. Res.* 36:481, 1975.
28. Hearse D.J., Stewart D.A., Braimbridge M.V.: Myocardial protection during bypass

and arrest: A possible hazard with lactate-containing infusates. *J. Thorac. Cardiovasc. Surg.* 72:880, 1976.
29. Higgins C.B., et al.: Spontaneously and pharmacologically provoked coronary arterial spasm in Prinzmetal variant angina. *Radiology* 119:521, 1976.
30. Hillis L.D., Braunwald E.: Myocardial ischemia. *N. Engl. J. Med.* 296:971, 1977.
31. Hillis L.D., Braunwald E.: Coronary-artery spasm. *N. Engl. J. Med.* 299:695, 1978.
32. Hoffman J.I.E., Buckberg G.D.: The myocardial supply: Demand ratio—a critical review. *Am. J. Cardiol.* 41:327, 1978.
33. Housman L.B., et al.: Counterpulsation for intraoperative cardiogenic shock: Successful use of intra-aortic balloon. *J.A.M.A.* 224:1131, 1973.
34. Jynge P., Hearse D.J., Braimbridge M.V.: Myocardial protection during ischemic cardiac arrest: A possible hazard with calcium-free cardioplegic infusates. *J. Thorac. Cardiovasc. Surg.* 73:848, 1977.
35. Kannel W.B., et al.: Report of the Ad Hoc Committee on Cigarette Smoking and Cardiovascular Diseases for health professionals. *Circulation* 57:404A, 1978.
36. Kannel W.B., et al.: American Heart Association report of Ad Hoc Committee on Cigarette Smoking and Cardiovascular Diseases. *Circulation* 57:406A, 1978.
37. Kaplan J.A.: The pharmacological treatment of the cardiovascular system, in *28th Annual Refresher Course Lectures*, American Society of Anesthesiologists, 1977, Lecture 212, p. 1.
38. Kaplan J.A., et al.: Propranolol and cardiac surgery: A problem for the anesthesiologist? *Anesth. Analg.* 54:571, 1975.
39. Kaplan J.A., King S.B. III: The precordial electrocardiographic lead (V_5) in patients who have coronary-artery disease. *Anesthesiology* 45:570, 1976.
40. Katz R.L., Bigger J.T. Jr.: Cardiac arrhythmias during anesthesia and operation. *Anesthesiology* 33:193, 1970.
41. Khan A.H., Haywood L.J.: Myocardial infarction in nine patients with radiologically patent coronary arteries. *N. Engl. J. Med.* 291:427, 1974.
42. Khan A.A., Miletich D.J., Albrecht R.F.: Direct "sensitization" of myocardial muscle cells to epinephrine by halothane. Abstracted in the Scientific Papers of the American Society of Anesthesiologists Annual Meeting, 1977, p. 93.
43. Kistner J.R., et al.: Indices of myocardial oxygenation during coronary revascularization with morphine versus halothane anesthesia in man. Abstracted in the Scientific Papers of the American Society of Anesthesiologists Annual Meeting, 1977, p. 509.
44. Kopman E.A., et al.: Arterial hypoxemia following the administration of sublingual nitroglycerin. *Am. Heart J.* 96:444, 1978.
45. Langou R.A., et al.: Incidence and mortality of perioperative myocardial infarction in patients undergoing coronary artery bypass grafting. *Circulation* 56 (suppl. 2):54, 1977.
46. Latham P.: Cited by Hillis, Braunwald.[31]
47. Levy W.K., Cannom D.S., Cohen L.S.: Prognosis of subendocardial myocardial infarction, abstracted. *Circulation* 52 (suppl. 2):107, 1975.
48. Lewis B.S., Gotsman M.S.: Sudden death in patients awaiting coronary artery surgery. *Thorax* 29:209, 1974.
49. Lewis F.B., Coffman J.D., Gregg D.E.: Effect of heart rate and intracoronary isoproterenol, levarterenol, and epinephrine on coronary flow and resistance. *Circ. Res.* 9:89, 1961.
50. Loeb H.S., et al.: Effects of pharmacologically-induced hypertension on myocardial ischemia and coronary hemodynamics in patients with fixed coronary obstruction. *Circulation* 57:41, 1978.
51. Lowenstein E.: Morphine "anesthesia"—a perspective, editorial. *Anesthesiology* 35:563, 1971.
52. Lowenstein E.: Anesthetic considerations in coronary artery disease, in Hershey S.G. (ed.): *Refresher Courses in Anesthesiology*. Philadelphia, American Society of Anesthesiologists, 1976, vol. 4, p. 51.
53. Lown B., Black H., Moore F.D.: Digitalis, electrolytes and the surgical patient. *Am. J. Cardiol.* 6:309, 1960.
54. Madigan N.P., Rutherford B.D., Frye R.L.: The clinical course, early prognosis and coronary anatomy of subendocardial infarction. *Am. J. Med.* 60:634, 1976.
55. Madigan N.P., et al.: Early saphenous vein grafting after subendocardial infarction: Immediate surgical results and late prognosis. *Circulation* 56 (suppl. 2):1, 1977.
56. Maseri A., et al.: Coronary vasospasm as a possible cause of myocardial infarction: A conclusion derived from the study of "preinfarction" angina. *N. Engl. J. Med.* 299:1271, 1978.
57. McGoon D.C., Pluth J.R.: Postoperative care of the open-heart patient: General considerations, in Burford T.H., Ferguson T.B. (eds.): *Cardiovascular Surgery: Current Practice*. St. Louis, C.V. Mosby Co., 1969, vol. 1, p. 33.

58. McIntosh H.D.: Benefits from aortocoronary bypass graft. *J.A.M.A.* 239:1197, 1978.
59. Miller R.R., et al.: Combined dopamine and nitroprusside therapy in congestive heart failure: Greater augmentation of cardiac performance by addition of inotropic stimulation to afterload reduction. *Circulation* 55:881, 1977.
60. Miner J.A., Conti C.R.: Topical nitroglycerin for ischemic heart disease. *J.A.M.A.* 239:2166, 1978.
61. Morrison J., Killip T.: Serum digitalis and arrhythmia in patients undergoing cardiopulmonary bypass. *Circulation* 47:341, 1973.
62. Mundth E.D., Austen W.G.: Surgical measures for coronary heart disease. *N. Engl. J. Med.* 293:124, 1975.
63. Nakayama K., et al.: Fundamental physiology of coronary smooth musculature from extramural stem arteries of pigs and rabbits. *Eur. J. Cardiol.* 8:319, 1978.
64. Osler W.: Cited by Hillis, Braunwald.[31]
65. Prinzmetal M., et al.: Angina pectoris: I. A variant form of angina pectoris: Preliminary report. *Am. J. Med.* 27:375, 1959.
66. Robinson B.F.: Relation of heart rate and systolic blood pressure to the onset of pain in angina pectoris. *Circulation* 35:1073, 1967.
67. Rose M.R., Glassman E., Spencer F.C.: Arrhythmias following cardiac surgery: Relation to serum digoxin levels. *Am. Heart J.* 89:288, 1975.
68. Rosenblum R., Frieden J.: Intravenous dopamine in the treatment of myocardial dysfunction after open-heart surgery. *Am. Heart J.* 83:743, 1972.
69. Rowe G.G., Castillo C.A., Crumpton C.W.: Effects of hyperventilation on systemic and coronary hemodynamics. *Am. Heart J.* 63:67, 1962.
70. Sabiston D.C. Jr., Gregg D.E.: Effect of cardiac contraction on coronary blood flow. *Circulation* 15:14, 1957.
71. Sarnoff S.J., et al.: Determinants of oxygen consumption of the heart with special reference to the tension-time index. *Am. J. Physiol.* 192:148, 1958.
72. Slogoff S., Keats A.S., Ott E.: Preoperative propranolol therapy and aortocoronary bypass operation. *J.A.M.A.* 240:1487, 1978.
73. Sonntag H., et al.: Über die Myokarddurchblutung und den myokardialen Sauerstoffverbrauch bei Patienten während Narkoseeinleitung mit Dehydrobenzperidol/Fentanyl oder Ketamine. *Z. Kreislaufforsch.* 61:1092, 1972.
74. Stoelting R.K.: Evaluation of external jugular venous pressure as a reflection of right atrial pressure. *Anesthesiology* 38:291, 1973.
75. Stoelting R.K., Gibbs P.S.: Hemodynamic effects of morphine and morphine–nitrous oxide in valvular heart disease and coronary-artery disease. *Anesthesiology* 38:45, 1973.
76. Swan H.J.C., et al.: Catheterization of the heart in man with use of a flow-directed balloon-tipped catheter. *N. Engl. J. Med.* 283:447, 1970.
77. Theye R.A.: Myocardial and total oxygen consumption with halothane. *Anesthesiology* 28:1042, 1967.
78. Tinker J.H., et al.: Dobutamine for inotropic support during emergence from cardiopulmonary bypass. *Anesthesiology* 44:281, 1976.
79. White R.D., et al.: Plasma ionic calcium levels following injection of chloride, gluconate, and glucepate salts of calcium. *J. Thorac. Cardiovasc. Surg.* 71:609, 1976.
80. Wynne J., et al.: Beneficial effects of nitrous oxide in patients with ischemic heart disease, abstracted. *Circulation* 56 (suppl. 3):8, 1977.
81. Yasue H., et al.: Role of autonomic nervous system in the pathogenesis of Prinzmetal's variant form of angina. *Circulation* 50:534, 1974.
82. Yasue H., et al.: Coronary arterial spasm and Prinzmetal's variant form of angina induced by hyperventilation and tris-buffer infusion. *Circulation* 58:56, 1978.

ง # 9 / Oxygenators and Hemodilution in Cardiopulmonary Bypass

ANDREW J. KULESZA
ROGER D. WHITE

OXYGENATORS

There are basically four types of oxygenators used for cardiopulmonary bypass: vertical screen, disk, bubble, and membrane.[16] Gas comes into direct contact with the perfusate in the screen, disk, and bubble types, whereas in the membrane type, blood and gas are separated by a membrane interface.

Types of Oxygenators

Vertical Screen

The stationary vertical screen oxygenator[13] was developed by Gibbon and modified by the Mayo Clinic Section of Engineering in the early 1950s (Fig 9–1). Although the instrument is no longer in use, it is of considerable historical interest. This type was used extensively in earlier years, and much of what is known about extracorporeal perfusion evolved from many clinical studies in which it was used. The oxygenating chamber consisted of a series of 3 to 14 Mylar-coated, vertically oriented screens. The perfusate flowed in a thin film down the screens and was exposed to oxygen during its passage over the screens. The perfusate entered the oxygenating chamber from an upper reservoir through a slit along the upper edge of each screen. It then passed from the bottom of the screens into a lower reservoir. Two pumps were necessary: one to move blood to the upper reservoir and the other, an arterial pump, to perfuse the patient from the lower reservoir. Flow rates of 500 to 3,500 ml/minute were possible, with an oxygen saturation of 95% to 100%. Such a range of flow rates permitted its use in the perfusion of small infants and children as well as adults. This type of oxygenator required disassembly and cleaning of the screens and resterilization after each use. Blood required was 215 ml for the upper reservoir, 300 to 500 ml for the lower reservoir, and 70 ml for each screen.[16]

Disk

The disk oxygenator was originally designed by Björk[2] in 1948, and there have been several modifications of his design, including those by Melrose[22] in 1953 and Cross and Kay[5] in 1957. The Kay-Cross oxygenator is composed of a series of 60 to 120 stainless steel disks coated with fiber and siliconized. These disks rotate at a rate of 120 revolutions per minute inside a horizontal cylinder that is 33 to 64 cm long. Venous blood comes into contact with the upper two thirds of the disks, where the exchange of oxygen and carbon dioxide occurs. The exchange of gases depends on the following factors: the flow rate of perfusate and gases, the rotational speed of the disks, the blood level, and the temperature of the system. At an oxygen flow rate of 5 L/minute, the P_{CO_2} of the perfusate will be too low, and it is therefore necessary to add 1% to 3% carbon dioxide.

The disk-type oxygenator is relatively atraumatic to blood constituents and has a good oxygenating capacity, but it requires a relatively large priming volume. In 1963, a presterilized disposable model, constructed of polycarbonate and requiring a lower priming volume, was made available.

Bubble

The bubble-type oxygenator was originally designed by DeWall et al.[7] in 1956 and, with

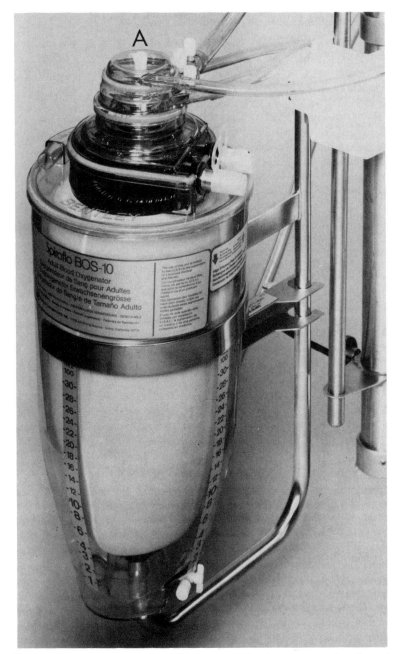

Fig 9–3.—A, exterior view of BOS-10 adult blood oxygenator (continued).

the Lande-Edwards membrane oxygenator. They noted that damage to erythrocytes and platelets was less with the membrane type and that postoperative bleeding decreased (this also was one of the findings of Liddicoat et al.[17]). Platelet counts were similar with both oxygenators, but platelet adhesiveness, as measured by the Salzman technique, was not as depressed with the membrane oxygenator. Plasma hemoglobin level was also lower with the membrane oxygenator.

Siderys et al.[27] noted similar results, that is,

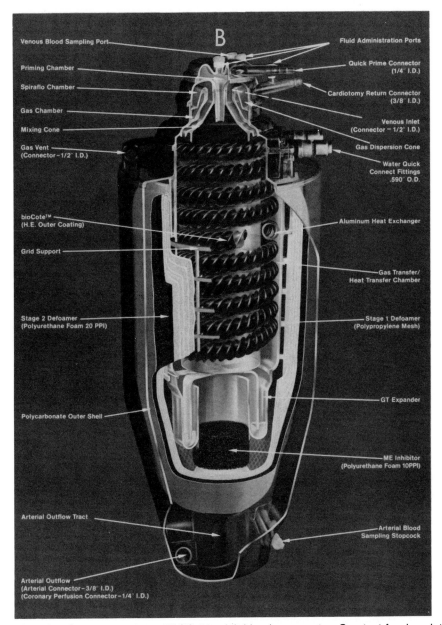

Fig 9–3 (Cont.).—**B,** cutaway view of BOS-10 adult blood oxygenator. See text for description of pathway followed by perfusate within oxygenator. (Photographs courtesy of Bentley Laboratories.)

more hemolysis with the bubble oxygenator. In addition, they observed a greater decrease in platelet count with the bubble oxygenator. They also noted that blood touching the pericardium undergoes more hemolysis than blood not in contact with the pericardial surface; therefore, they did not return blood to the pump from the pericardial cavity. Hemolysis was also related to the degree of pump head occlusion, the degree of intracardiac suctioning, and the size of the cannulas.

Subramanian and Berger[31] similarly observed a greater decrease in the number of platelets and a higher level of plasma hemoglobin in dogs with the bubble oxygenator. They noted an increase in fibrinolytic activity with the bubble oxygenator but not with the membrane oxygenator. Thus, for prolonged bypass durations, the bubble-type oxygenator may be more traumatic to blood constituents, although it is suitable for the management of intraoperative cardiopulmonary bypass. When a bypass of prolonged duration is anticipated, such as in the management of severe respiratory failure, the membrane oxygenator has some definite advantages.

COMPLICATIONS

A number of complications occur with the use of oxygenators: destruction of erythrocytes, with resulting increased plasma hemoglobin level; microemboli; protein denaturation; destruction of platelets and inhibition of their function; coagulation abnormalities; hyperoxygenation; and hypocapnia. A number of studies have been performed with various oxygenators to assess these adverse effects.[1, 6, 10, 23, 24, 26]

Microemboli

The production of microemboli has been investigated by several groups. Solis et al.[30] analyzed particle size of microemboli in both membrane and bubble oxygenators and observed that the amount of microemboli in the cardiotomy reservoir increased with both types, compared with that in arterial blood. With the bubble oxygenator, they also noted a small increase in number of microemboli in arterial blood compared with the number in venous blood, but this change was not noted with the membrane oxygenator. Platelet adhesiveness was also decreased with the bubble oxygenator.

Blood Filter

The effectiveness of a blood filter in the arterial line has been questioned. Heimbecker et al.[11] obtained scanning electron micrographs of the mesh removed from blood filters and found deposition of platelets and fibrin. They suggested that excessive turbulence and high-frequency vibrations of the filter mesh were possible causes. When the filter was placed in the cardiotomy reservoir system, the deposition of fibrin and platelets was not observed, possibly because of the lower flow rate as compared with the flow rate in the arterial line. They also noted that platelet counts measured after operation were improved by 260% and that the amount of chest-tube drainage was reduced significantly when the arterial line filter was not used. They postulated that perhaps a consumptive coagulopathy may result from blood flow through an arterial line filter.

Dutton et al.[8] studied the effects of a filter with a pore size of 27 μm and observed that it removed particles greater than 50 μm but not those less than 50 μm, thus suggesting that the filter may actually produce small microemboli. They noted no difference in platelet concentrations, fibrinogen levels, fibrin split products, and plasma hemoglobin levels between the membrane and bubble oxygenator—a finding different from that of other similar studies.

Simmons et al.[29] noted an increase in the number of microparticles as oxygen and perfusate flow rates increased. None of the three types of oxygenators has been proved to be harmless to blood constituents, and the differences noted among them have not always been consistent.[29] Kessler and Patterson[15] observed that fewer microemboli were generated by the disk oxygenator than by the bubble and membrane types. Tamari et al.[32] studied changes in platelets and found that with the membrane oxygenator not only did the number of platelets decrease but their function also decreased.

Air Bubbles

Air bubbles may form if the Po_2 of the perfusate increases to a high level. This problem may also occur in the Bentley Temptrol Q-130 infant oxygenator when a high ratio of gas flow to blood flow is present. In a study in dogs, Fisk et al.[9] noted that air bubbles were present when the level of blood in the reservoir was below the maximal level and when the temperature of the heat exchanger reservoir was higher than venous blood temperatures by 5 C. These findings did not occur with the Q-110 pediatric model. They recommended that, with the Q-130 model, if low perfusate flows are used, the reservoir level should be kept high and the flow of gas should be as low as possible.

HEMODILUTION

Historical Development

In the early days of cardiopulmonary bypass, the oxygenators were primed with fresh heparinized blood, which led to a large demand on blood banks that served to limit procedures on patients with rare blood types. Serum hepatitis was also a problem at that time. Another difficulty was the development of the "homologous blood syndrome," which comprises the following manifestations: hepatic congestion, portal hypertension, coagulation defects, pulmonary congestion, renal failure, and cerebral insufficiency. The hepatic changes were believed to be secondary to the pooling of blood in the splanchnic circulation. This syndrome was not observed when other types of primes were used.

In 1959, Panico and Neptune[25] reported the use of a normal saline prime. This report was followed by that of Cooley et al.[4] in 1961 of the successful use of 5% dextrose in water as the prime in 100 patients at normothermia. One of the difficulties with the use of "clear primes" was the large volume required by the oxygenators being used at that time, which resulted in much hemodilution and low hematocrit values.

There was further investigation into the use of blood-electrolyte mixtures employing acid-citrate-dextrose blood, 5% dextrose with lactated Ringer's solution, and albumin. Fewer pulmonary and coagulation dysfunctions were observed with the hemodiluted primes.

The use of low-molecular-weight dextran was also investigated in combination with electrolyte solutions. Urine output was maintained, and there was less hemolysis. Coagulation abnormalities were not detectable if the quantity of dextran solution was less than 20 ml/kg.[21] The acid-base balance and electrolytes were not significantly disturbed. There were some reports[12] of increased bleeding, even with normal coagulation studies.

As previously mentioned, the use by Cooley et al.[4] of 5% dextrose as a prime with a bubble oxygenator was another choice. They noted good urinary outputs and satisfactory tissue perfusion, with recovery of normal cerebral, renal, and pulmonary functions. The reported disadvantages included dilutional hyponatremia (up to ten days after operation), hemolysis, and increased levels of plasma hemoglobin.

In addition to these studies, investigations were done on the effects of adding mannitol, albumin, and fresh-frozen plasma to the prime. Mannitol was used if hemolysis occurred or if renal dysfunction was suspected. The use of albumin and fresh-frozen plasma increased the risk of hepatitis.

Alterations were observed in renal function, acid-base status, and fluid balance with the use of hemodilution. Renal tubular cell damage occurred in dogs on bypass if they had low urinary outputs. The pathologic changes were prevented when higher urinary outputs were achieved by the use of osmotic diuretics. The use of hemodilution primes also served to maintain urinary output and helped to alleviate subsequent problems with hematuria, oliguria, and anuria. (Renal considerations of cardiopulmonary bypass are discussed in chap. 16.)

The alterations in acid-base status depended on the volume of priming solutions used. If more than 100 ml/kg was used, severe metabolic acidosis resulted. With 70 to 100 ml/kg, acidosis occurred that could be partially corrected by the administration of bicarbonate, and if 50 to 70 ml/kg was used, the acidosis was completely correctable with bicarbonate. There seemed to be less acidosis associated with lactated Ringer's solution.

As a result of the use of clear primes, patients required additional fluids during the bypass period and thus increased their extracellular fluid volume and subsequently gained weight. This situation was corrected by fluid restriction or the use of diuretic agents (or both).

A number of studies followed that compared the effects of blood, blood crystalloid, and crystalloid priming solutions. Moffitt et al.[23] compared the results of blood with blood (60%) and crystalloid primes and found that there were the expected changes from dilution in sodium, chloride, potassium, and blood urea nitrogen during bypass and after the operation. Blood glucose levels increased because of the glucose in the priming solutions. They also noted a trend toward hypokalemia after bypass.

Lilleaasen and Stokke[19, 20] have reported the effects of moderate (hematocrit, 27%) to extreme (hematocrit, 18%) hemodilution on postoperative bleeding, diuresis, and pulmonary function. They observed a decrease of 71% in the requirement for donor blood and a decrease of 47% in the amount of chest-tube drainage in the group with extreme hemodilution. The group with moderate hemodilution had a greater decrease in platelet counts. These authors were able to maintain adequate arterial and venous oxygen tensions in the group with extreme hemodilution, and this group also reported higher postoperative PaO_2, thus suggesting better overall pulmonary function. As would be expected, the patients with extreme hemodilution had a greater degree of diuresis.

In addition to Cooley's group, in 1965 Silvay et al.[28] reported successful results with a prime of 5% dextrose in water. In 1975 Lee et al.[18] compared three types of clear primes, including 5% dextrose, lactated Ringer's solution with dextran 40, and lactated Ringer's solution with hydroxyethyl starch, and they found no significant differences in flow rates, pressures, urinary volume, hematocrit, blood urea nitrogen, blood loss, coagulation function, and pulmonary and neurologic complications.

In his discussion of hemodilution, Keats[14] pointed out some other considerations such as viscosity changes, oxygenation, and tolerance to stress. If the temperature decreases by 10 C, viscosity increases 20% to 25%. To maintain viscosity constant during hypothermia to 20 C, the hematocrit value must decrease from 45% to 25%. If the hematocrit is lowered to between 10% and 15%, subendocardial and renal cortical ischemia may occur in the intact organism. In the absence of stress, a hematocrit near 20% can provide an adequate myocardial oxygen supply, but if hemorrhage, fever, hypotension, or acute myocardial infarction occurs, this level would be potentially harmful. This situation is obviously of concern during the postoperative period and after hemodilution; the hematocrit value should be returned toward normal as soon as possible.[14]

TABLE 9–1.—PRIMES USED FOR BENTLEY BOS-10 OXYGENATOR

TOTAL FLOW 3.0 TO 4.8 L/MIN	
At 2.0 L/min/sq m for patients between 1.50 and 2.4 sq m (≈50.0 to 106.0 kg)	
At 2.4 L/min/sq m for patients between 1.25 and 2.0 sq m (≈37.5 to 81.0 kg)	
Packed RBCs (2 units)	600.0 ml
Plasmalyte-148 (pH 7.4)	1,400.0 ml
Heparin sodium (1,000 USP units/ml)	9.0 ml
Sodium bicarbonate (8.4%)	20.0 ml
Mannitol (15%)	100.0 ml
Calcium chloride (10%)	10.0 ml
Priming volume	2,139.0 ml
ADDITION	
No. 1	
Citrate-phosphate-dextrose blood (1 unit)	500.0 ml
Heparin sodium (1,000 USP units/ml)	3.0 ml
Sodium bicarbonate (8.4%)	10.0 ml
Calcium chloride (10%)	5.0 ml
	518.0 ml
No. 2	
Plasmalyte-148 (pH 7.4)	500.0 ml
Heparin sodium (1,000 USP units/ml)	1.5 ml
	501.5 ml
Sequence of addition: For patients between 1.25 and 1.50 sq m, use addition 1 first, then addition 2. For patients larger than 1.50 sq m, use addition 2 first, then addition 1. Repeat in sequence as needed	

TABLE 9–2.—PRIMES USED FOR BENTLEY BOS-10 OXYGENATOR (SHORT PERFUSIONS)*

TOTAL FLOW >3.0 L/MIN	
At 2.0 to 2.4 L/min/sq m for patients >1.25 sq m (≈37.5 kg)	
Plasmalyte-148 (pH 7.4)	1,500.0 ml
Heparin sodium (1,000 USP units/ml)	4.5 ml
Priming volume	1,504.5 ml
Add to this initial priming volume 30 ml of Plasmalyte per kilogram body weight for each kilogram above 37.5 kg	
ADDITION	
No. 1	
Plasmalyte-148 (pH 7.4)	500.0 ml
Heparin sodium (1,000 USP units/ml)	1.5 ml
	501.5 ml
No. 2	
Packed RBCs (1 unit)	300.0 ml
Plasmalyte-148 (pH 7.4)	200.0 ml
Heparin sodium (1,000 USP units/ml)	3.0 ml
Sodium bicarbonate (8.4%)	10.0 ml
Calcium chloride (10%)	5.0 ml
	518.0 ml
No. 3	
Citrate-phosphate-dextrose blood (1 unit)	500.0 ml
Heparin sodium (1,000 USP units/ml)	3.0 ml
Sodium bicarbonate (8.4%)	10.0 ml
Calcium chloride (10%)	5.0 ml
	518.0 ml
If patient is less than 1.70 sq m, use addition 1 first, then addition 2 or 3, depending on the availability of packed RBCs. Repeat in sequence additions 1 and 2 or additions 1 and 3	
If patient is larger than 1.70 sq m, use addition 1 first and repeat if necessary; if a third addition is required, add addition 2 if packed RBCs are available or addition 3 if such cells are not available. Check hematocrit value of perfusate before any other additions	

*For patients with atrial septal defect, pulmonary valve stenosis, open mitral commissurotomy, single aortocoronary artery vein bypass graft, or other indications for clear prime.

Techniques of Cardiopulmonary Bypass

Primes

The presently used hemodilution techniques at the Mayo Clinic involve the Bentley Spiraflo oxygenators and various primes (Tables 9–1 through 9–4). For perfusion of infants with total flows less than 1.25 L/minute, the Shiley S-70 oxygenator is used (Table 9–5). This oxygenator appears to provide ideal oxygenation of blood at these low blood flow rates. For children less than 2 years of age, citrate-phosphate-dextrose blood less than 48 hours old is used. For adults, 1 or 2 units may be added to the priming mixture, and 200 to 250 ml of diluent are added for each unit of packed cells. After the addition of

TABLE 9-3.—PRIMES USED FOR BENTLEY BOS-5 OXYGENATOR*

TOTAL FLOW 1.25 TO 2.4 L/MIN	
At 2.0 L/min/sq m for patients between 0.52 and 1.20 sq m (≈12.0 kg to 36.5 kg)	
At 2.4 L/min/sq m for patients between 0.52 and 1.00 sq m (≈12.0 kg to 27.5 kg)	
Citrate-phosphate-dextrose blood (2 units)	1,000.0 ml
Plasmalyte-148 (pH 7.4)	250.0 ml
Heparin sodium (1,000 USP units/ml)	7.0 ml
Sodium bicarbonate (8.4%)	10.0 ml
Mannitol (15%)	25.0 ml
Calcium chloride (10%)	10.0 ml
Priming volume†	1,302.0 ml
ADDITION	
No. 1	
Citrate-phosphate-dextrose blood (1 unit)	500.0 ml
Heparin sodium (1,000 USP units/ml)	3.0 ml
Sodium bicarbonate (8.4%)	5.0 ml
Calcium chloride (10%)	5.0 ml
	513.0 ml
No. 2	
Plasmalyte-148 (pH 7.4)	500.0 ml
Heparin sodium (1,000 USP units/ml)	1.5 ml
	501.5 ml

*Prime with citrate-phosphate-dextrose blood less than 4 days old.
†For patient with cyanotic congenital heart disease and hemoglobin concentration higher than 15.0 gm/dl, add to priming volume 50 ml of Plasmalyte-148 (pH 7.4), for each 1 gm of hemoglobin above 15 gm. Choice of addition should be determined by hematocrit of perfusate.

TABLE 9-5.—PRIMES USED FOR SHILEY S-70 OXYGENATOR IN INFANTS*

TOTAL FLOW <1.25 L/MIN	
At 2.4 L/min/sq m for patients <0.52 sq m (<12.0 kg)	
Fresh citrate-phosphate-dextrose blood (1½ unit)	750.0 ml
Heparin sodium (1,000 USP units/ml)	4.5 ml
Sodium bicarbonate (8.4%)	7.5 ml
Mannitol (15%)	10.0 ml
Calcium chloride (10%)	7.5 ml
Priming volume	779.5 ml
To this priming volume, add Plasmalyte-148 (pH 7.4), in amounts as follows: (1) 15 ml/kg body weight for infants weighing less than 8.0 kg and 20 ml/kg body weight for infants weighing more than 8.0 kg; (2) 50 ml for each 1 gm of hemoglobin above 15 gm/100 ml of blood in cyanotic patients	
ADDITION	
No. 1	
Fresh citrate-phosphate-dextrose blood	100.0 ml
Heparin sodium (1,000 USP units/ml)	0.6 ml
Sodium bicarbonate (8.4%)	1.0 ml
Calcium chloride (10%)	1.0 ml
	102.6 ml
No. 2	
Plasmalyte-148 (pH 7.4)	100.0 ml
Check hematocrit value of perfusate during perfusion to determine whether to use when necessary an addition of blood or diluent	

*Prime with fresh citrated blood. Use citrate-phosphate-dextrose blood less than 48 hours old.

citrate-phosphate-dextrose blood, heparin is added (3,000 units per unit of packed cells or whole blood), followed by the addition of calcium chloride (500 mg/unit of blood); this is done to restore ionized calcium levels toward normal. The desired hematocrit value of the perfusate is between 25% and 30%. Sodium bi-

TABLE 9-4.—PRIMES USED FOR BENTLEY BOS-5 OXYGENATOR (SHORT PERFUSIONS)*

TOTAL FLOW 1.5 TO 3.0 L/MIN	
At 2.0 L/min/sq m for patients between 0.78 and 1.50 sq m (≈20.0 kg to 50.0 kg)	
At 2.4 L/min/sq m for patients between 0.78 and 1.25 sq m (≈20.0 kg to 37.5 kg)	
Plasmalyte-148 (pH 7.4)	1,500.0 ml
Heparin sodium (1,000 USP units/ml)	4.5 ml
Priming volume	1,504.5 ml
ADDITION	
No. 1	
Plasmalyte-148 (pH 7.4)	250.0 ml
No. 2	
Citrate-phosphate-dextrose blood (½ unit)†	250.0 ml
Heparin sodium (1,000 USP units/ml)	1.5 ml
Sodium bicarbonate (8.4%)	2.5 ml
Calcium chloride (10%)	2.5 ml
	256.5 ml

*For patients with atrial septal defect, pulmonary valve stenosis.
†Use citrate-phosphate-dextrose blood less than 4 days old.

carbonate is also added: 5 mEq/unit for blood less than 4 days old and 10 mEq/unit for blood more than 4 days old. The balanced electrolyte solutions used are either Normosol-R or Plasmalyte.

Equipment

The pump oxygenator assembly presently in use is composed of a Bentley Spiraflo oxygenator and a Sarns pump console (Fig 9-4). The built-in heat exchanger in the Bentley Spiraflo oxygenator has been found to be efficient in terms of the rapidity with which both cooling and rewarming can be effected, even in large patients. A Sarns bubble trap is placed on the arterial line just proximal to the arterial return to the patient. An arterial blood filter is occasionally used.

During bypass the inflow gas (composed of 98% oxygen and 2% carbon dioxide) is delivered at a rate of 1 to 2 L/L of blood per minute. Perfusate oxygen tension is continuously monitored during bypass on the arterial side.

The Bentley Q-220F disposable cardiotomy reservoir with filter is composed of a rigid polycarbonate outer shell (Fig 9-5). Its negative surface charge repels the hemoglobin molecule and decreases the degree of hemolysis that would otherwise occur. It has a polypropylene mesh

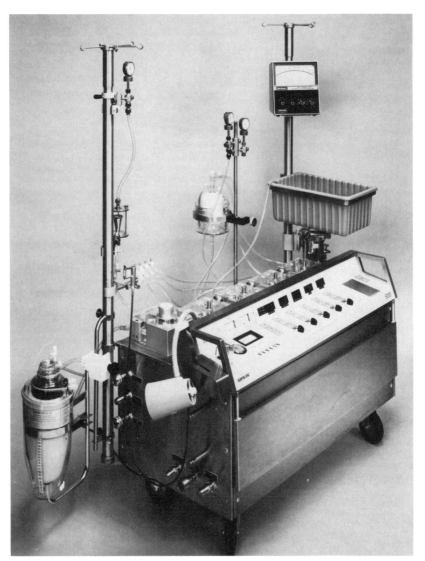

Fig 9-4.—Sarns pump assembly with Bentley Spiraflo BOS-10 oxygenator. Note ice bucket for cardioplegic solution bottle (above anesthetic vaporizor) and in-line Po_2 monitor mounted near top of pole on right.

that is coated with silicone antifoam, which is capable of defoaming and filtering blood at a rate of 3 L/minute.

Cannulation

Arterial cannulation is established either through the right or left femoral artery or the ascending aorta. A right-angle metal cannula is used for aortic cannulation, and a Bardic cannula is used for cannulation of the femoral artery; a pressure gradient of slightly less than 100 mm Hg across the cannula is considered acceptable, and this gradient determines the size of the cannula.

Heparinization and Neutralization

Before cannulation, systemic heparinization is accomplished by injecting heparin into the right atrium or a central venous cannula. Heparin is administered in a dose of 9,000 units/sq m, and

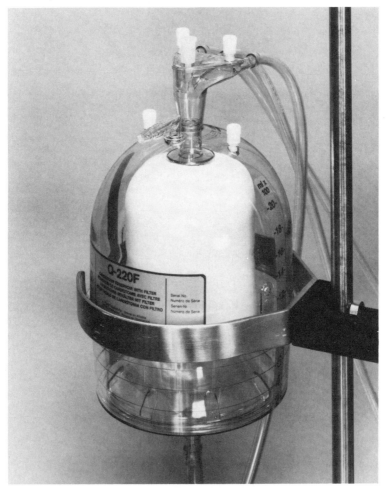

Fig 9–5.—Exterior view of disposable Bentley Q-22OF cardiotomy reservoir with filter.

for patients with less than 1 sq m of body surface area, 300 units/kg are used. One half the initial dose is repeated one hour after administration of the initial dose, and one fourth the initial dose is used at two hours. Another method for determining heparin requirements that is being used more frequently is the measurement of the activated clotting time using the Hemochron instrument. Heparin is neutralized at the end of bypass by the use of protamine sulfate. The dose of protamine is based on the principle that 1.3 mg of protamine will neutralize 1 mg of heparin. The total amount of heparin given intravenously and into the oxygenator can be converted to milligrams, and this value is then multiplied by 1.3 to determine the number of milligrams of protamine needed to neutralize all of the administered heparin. Additional doses of protamine may be needed, empirically in increments of 10 to 50 mg or as determined by the measurement of the activated clotting time (technique is discussed in chap. 20).

ACKNOWLEDGMENT

We wish to thank Burton Elfrink for his assistance in the preparation of the material in this chapter.

REFERENCES

1. Ashmore P.G., Svitek V., Ambrose P.: The incidence and effects of particulate aggregation and microembolism in pump-oxygenator systems. *J. Thorac. Cardiovasc. Surg.* 55:691, 1968.

2. Björk V.O.: An artificial heart or cardiopulmonary machine: Performance in animals. *Lancet* 2:491, 1948.
3. Clowes G.H.A. Jr., Neville W.E.: The membrane oxygenator, in Allen J.G. (ed.): *Extracorporeal Circulation*. Springfield, Ill., Charles C Thomas, Publisher, 1958, p. 81.
4. Cooley D.A., Beall A.C. Jr., Alexander J.K.: Acute massive pulmonary embolism: Successful surgical treatment using temporary cardiopulmonary bypass. *J.A.M.A.* 177:283, 1961.
5. Cross F.S., Kay E.B.: Direct vision repair of intracardiac defects utilizing a rotating disc reservoir-oxygenator. *Surg. Gynecol. Obstet.* 104:711, 1957.
6. Derman U.M., Rand P.W., Barker N.: Fibrinolysis after cardiopulmonary bypass and its relationship to fibrinogen. *J. Thorac. Cardiovasc. Surg.* 51:223, 1966.
7. DeWall R.A., et al.: Total body perfusion for open cardiotomy utilizing the bubble oxygenator: Physiologic responses in man. *J. Thorac. Surg.* 32:591, 1956.
8. Dutton R.C., et al.: Platelet aggregate emboli produced in patients during cardiopulmonary bypass with membrane and bubble oxygenators and blood filters. *J. Thorac. Cardiovasc. Surg.* 67:258, 1974.
9. Fisk G.C., et al.: Bubbles in an infant oxygenator at very low flow rates. *J. Thorac. Cardiovasc. Surg.* 64:98, 1972.
10. Hammond G.L., Bowley W.W.: Bubble mechanics and oxygen transfer. *J. Thorac. Cardiovasc. Surg.* 71:422, 1976.
11. Heimbecker R., Robert A., McKenzie F.N.: The extracorporeal pump filter—saint or sinner? *Ann. Thorac. Surg.* 21:55, 1976.
12. Hepps S.A., et al.: Amelioration of the pulmonary post-perfusion syndrome with hemodilution and low molecular weight dextran. *Surgery* 54:32, 1963.
13. Ionescu M.I., Wooler G.H.: *Current Techniques in Extracorporeal Circulation*. London, Butterworth & Co., 1976.
14. Keats A.S.: Hemodynamic consequences of hemodilution. *Cleve. Clin. Q.* 45:39, 1978.
15. Kessler J., Patterson R.H. Jr.: The production of microemboli by various blood oxygenators. *Ann. Thorac. Surg.* 9:221, 1970.
16. Kirklin J.W., Theye R.A., Patrick R.T.: The stationary vertical screen oxygenator, in Allen J.G. (ed.): *Extracorporeal Circulation*. Springfield, Ill., Charles C Thomas, Publisher, 1958, p. 57.
17. Liddicoat J.E., et al.: Membrane vs. bubble oxygenator: Clinical comparison. *Ann. Surg.* 181:747, 1975.
18. Lee W.H. Jr., Rubin J.W., Huggins M.P.: Clinical evaluation of priming solutions for pump oxygenator perfusion. *Ann. Thorac. Surg.* 19:529, 1975.
19. Lilleaasen P.: Moderate and extreme haemodilution in open-heart surgery: Blood requirements, bleeding and platelet counts. *Scand. J. Thorac. Cardiovasc. Surg.* 11:97, 1977.
20. Lilleaasen P., Stokke O.: Moderate and extreme hemodilution in open-heart surgery: Fluid balance and acid-base studies. *Ann. Thorac. Surg.* 25:127, 1978.
21. Long D.M. Jr., et al.: Clinical use of dextran-40 in extracorporeal circulation: A summary of 5 years' experience. *Transfusion* 6:401, 1966.
22. Melrose D.G.: A mechanical heart-lung for use in man. *Br. Med. J.* 2:57, 1953.
23. Moffitt E.A., Maher F.T., Kirklin J.W.: Effect of cardiopulmonary bypass and haemodilution on some constituents of blood. *Can. Anaesth. Soc. J.* 12:458, 1965.
24. O'Neill J.A. Jr., Collins H.A.: The effect of various blood additives on hemolysis during extracorporeal circulation. *Ann. Thorac. Surg.* 1:769, 1965.
25. Panico F.G., Neptune W.B.: A mechanism to eliminate the donor blood prime from the pump-oxygenator. *Surg. Forum* 10:605, 1959.
26. Reed C.C., et al.: Particulate matter in bubble oxygenators. *J. Thorac. Cardiovasc. Surg.* 68:971, 1974.
27. Siderys H., et al.: A comparison of membrane and bubble oxygenation as used in cardiopulmonary bypass in patients: The importance of pericardial blood as a source of hemolysis. *J. Thorac. Cardiovasc. Surg.* 69:708, 1975.
28. Silvay J., et al.: Clinical use of hemodilution in extracorporeal circulation. *J. Cardiovasc. Surg.* 6:447, 1965.
29. Simmons E., et al.: A comparison of the microparticles produced when two disposable-bag oxygenators and a disc oxygenator are used for cardiopulmonary bypass. *J. Thorac. Cardiovasc. Surg.* 63:613, 1972.
30. Solis R.T., et al.: Cardiopulmonary bypass: Microembolization and platelet aggregation. *Circulation* 52:103, 1975.
31. Subramanian V.A., Berger R.L.: Comparative evaluation of a new disposable rotating membrane oxygenator with bubble oxygenator. *Ann. Thorac. Surg.* 21:48, 1976.
32. Tamari Y., et al.: Functional changes in platelets during extracorporeal circulation. *Ann. Thorac. Surg.* 19:639, 1975.
33. Wright J.S., et al.: Some advantages of the membrane oxygenator for open-heart surgery. *J. Thorac. Cardiovasc. Surg.* 69:884, 1975.

10 / Anesthesia for Closed Cardiac Operations in Adults

HUGO S. RAIMUNDO
SAIT TARHAN

CLOSED MITRAL COMMISSUROTOMY

General Information

In most patients with mitral stenosis, symptoms develop during the fourth and fifth decades, yet symptoms remain unchanged for variable periods of time before worsening.[13] The most common cause of mitral valve disease appears to be typical rheumatic mitral valvulitis. The process causes thickening of the valves, fusion of commissures, chordal shortening and fusion, and valve calcification.[14] Structural architecture and pliability of the cusps of the stenosed mitral valve, the condition of the subvalvular area, and the degree of the associated incompetence are the major factors that influence the surgical decision regarding commissurotomy or valve replacement. Before surgery, these factors are evaluated by physical examination. Cardiac catheterization in patients with mitral stenosis always shows an elevated left atrial pressure, and, in turn, pulmonary capillary wedge pressure also will be increased. However, left ventricular end-diastolic pressure will be normal. In addition to having elevated left atrial pressure, patients with mitral stenosis will have pulmonary hypertension ranging up to systemic levels—the hypertension being directly related to the severity and duration of the stenosis. There also is a pressure gradient across the mitral valve during diastole.

In addition to cardiac laboratory data, radiologic techniques also are helpful in determining the amount of calcification on the valve, which is assessed with conventional fluoroscopy, whereas evaluation of the mobility of the cusps requires selective angiocardiography.[9] Ultrasound also has been used to evaluate these parameters. Being harmless and noninvasive, ultrasound has become an attractive tool for this purpose. Recently, echocardiographic evaluation of mitral valve calcification and mobility has become valuable in planning the surgical approach in patients with pure or predominant mitral stenosis.[9]

Many factors affect the mobility of the stenosed mitral valve. Reduced mobility may be due to the fusion of commissures, fibrous and calcific thickening of the cusps, fusion and shortening of the subvalvular apparatus, or some combination of these.[15]

Mitral valvotomy continues to be the operation of choice for pure or predominant mitral stenosis. In spite of progressive reduction in the operative mortality for valve replacement and continued improvement in prosthetic design, valve replacement may not be the primary surgical procedure for most patients with uncomplicated mitral stenosis.[15] Operative risk of valve replacement probably is similar to that of valvotomy (operative mortality, 2%).[14] However, prosthetic valves add the risk of late complications, such as thromboembolic phenomena, periannular leaks, ball variance, and hemolysis.[9]

Valvotomy can be done by two techniques: open and closed. The open technique has its advantages, such as careful dissection of the commissures and splitting of papillary muscles, ensuring an adequate opening of the valve, and complete control of the patient's hemodynamics with cardiopulmonary bypass; yet a closed valvotomy does not have the well-known drawbacks of cardiopulmonary bypass techniques. Therefore, it is still the preferred method by some.[8]

However, closed mitral commissurotomy is

most likely to restore the patient to an asymptomatic state without the need for cardiac medication and anticoagulation. Restenosis may occur, yet patients may have 10 years or more of being free of symptoms.[14]

Anesthetic Management

Induction for mitral commissurotomy is no different from induction for open commissurotomy or mitral valve replacement. As soon as the patient is placed on the operating table, ECG electrodes are attached and a plastic catheter, usually a 14-gauge Teflon, is inserted into a vein of each arm and is attached to an intravenous infusion set containing 250 ml of 5% glucose in water. Induction then is achieved by using small increments of thiopental (50 to 75 mg), as tolerated and needed. Intubation is facilitated either with pancuronium (0.1 mg/kg) or with succinylcholine (100 mg) intravenously. As soon as induction is completed, direct arterial pressure monitoring is started. Maintenance can be accomplished with any anesthetic agent, such as enflurane, halothane, or a narcotic agent, as long as the anesthesiologist is familiar with the hemodynamic effects of the particular agent.

The operation is performed with the patient supine but with the left side elevated 30 degrees. A left thoracotomy, generally near the fifth interspace, gives access to the heart. A heavy silk, felt-backed mattress suture is placed at the apex of the left ventricle and is held by a Rummel clamp. A sizable incision is then made in the left atrial appendage while the lungs are hyperinflated, and 100 to 200 ml of blood is allowed to escape from the heart. Any nonadherent thrombus in the appendage should be removed from the atrium by this maneuver. The appendage is then clamped, and a second Prolene pursestring suture is inserted around the neck of the appendage, and control is achieved with a Rummel tourniquet.[14] The index finger of the surgeon is then inserted into the atrium. The valve is palpated. If digital pressure does not release the fused commissures, then an incision is made at the apex of the left ventricle (through the mattress suture at the apex), and the hole is dilated to the size of the Tubbs dilator, which is then inserted through the hole and

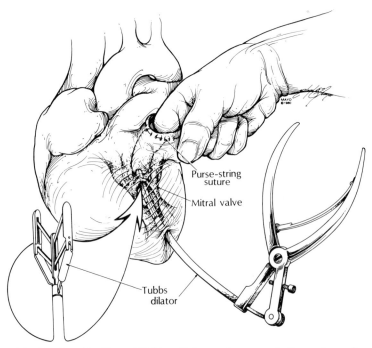

Fig 10–1.—Position of Tubbs dilator and surgeon's finger through appendage of left atrium. (Redrawn from Tyers et al.[14] Used by permission.)

passed retrograde through the mitral valve. The dilator is positioned with the index finger in the atrium at the level of the valve and is opened up, dilating and tearing the fused commissures of the leaflets (Fig 10–1).

A patient with mitral stenosis usually has a low cardiac output that is easily depressed further during intracardiac manipulation of the heart. Injection of an inotropic agent such as ephedrine (25 mg intravenously) before manipulation may prevent a large decrease in blood pressure. Because bradycardia is also common during this phase of the operation, vagal blocking with atropine may prevent the slowing of the heart rate. If cardiac arrest occurs before the commissurotomy is completed, resuscitation should be attempted after rapid dilation of the valve, because the stenosed valve will not allow an increase in cardiac output and will make resuscitation difficult. Another serious complication of closed commissurotomy is embolization, either from a clot or from calcium deposits, which is difficult to prevent.

If a thrombus is felt within the left atrium or if the valve is torn or commissurotomy is inadequate, the patient can be placed on cardiopulmonary bypass, and open commissurotomy, annuloplasty, or valve replacement can be performed. The inadvertent creation of significant mitral regurgitation may significantly affect the cardiac output and blood pressure. If this condition occurs, the surgeon can try to reduce the insufficiency by placing a finger on the mitral valve during systole through the left atrial appendage while the rest of the team prepares for emergency extracorporeal circulation. Cardiopulmonary bypass can be accomplished using a chest incision across the sternum. After heparin is administered intravenously, a large, single cannula is inserted into the right atrium through the atrial appendage, and the aorta is cannulated for the return of the blood from the pump.[14] The operation can then proceed with cardiopulmonary bypass.

After mitral valvotomy, a favorable change in pulmonary vascular resistance and a reduction of central blood volume may require many months (approximately six months). However, there may be an immediate decrease in right heart energy output per milliliter of pulmonary blood flow after mitral commissurotomy because of the relief of the mitral obstruction.[16]

PERICARDITIS

General Information

The causes of pericarditis are numerous, yet the reactions of the pericardium to these causes are similar. These reactions are acute inflammation, pericardial effusion with or without cardiac tamponade, and fibrosis with or without cardiac constriction. Recurrent acute pericarditis is seldom severe enough to justify surgery.[17] However, if the patients have incapacitating pain, surgery may be indicated. In these patients, removal of as much pericardium as is possible may give better relief than a limited resection. Pericarditis with effusion also can be treated in the same manner. Many patients with pericarditis and chronic effusion would eventually have constrictive pericarditis. Therefore, early operation and extensive resection of the pericardium would be safer for these patients.[17]

Constrictive pericarditis requires considerable expertise during anesthesia and the postoperative period. These patients are likely to have hemodynamic problems because of restriction of diastolic relaxation of the ventricles by the constricting pericardium. Venous pressure, as judged by the distention of the neck veins, is elevated in all patients (average, 25 cm H_2O). Most patients have a palpable liver and pleural effusion. Also, these patients may have a paradoxical pulse, that is, an inspiratory decline of greater than 10 mm Hg in systolic blood pressure during normal breathing.[17]

Cardiac catheterization reveals an elevated right atrial pressure equal to that in the vena cava.[17] The pulse contour taken from the right ventricle may give a "square-root sign" because of the early diastolic dip in pressure, followed by a rapid increase (with a plateau effect) to a high end-diastolic pressure. Pulmonary artery wedge pressure is usually elevated, and cardiac output is low in most patients.[17]

Anesthetic Management

The induction, monitoring, and maintenance in patients with pericarditis are similar to those in patients with other types of cardiac surgery. Direct arterial and venous pressure monitoring are helpful in detecting the hemodynamic changes during and after operation. Because

TABLE 10–1.—CAUSES OF HOSPITAL DEATHS IN 145 CASES (137 PATIENTS) OF CHRONIC CONSTRICTIVE PERICARDITIS*

| | PERICARDITIS | |
CAUSE	NONCALCIFIC	CALCIFIC
Congestive cardiac failure	3	5
Hemorrhage	1	2
Pulmonary embolus	2	1
Bronchopneumonia	1	1
Cardiac dysrhythmia	1	1
Generalized tuberculosis	1	0
Total	9	10

*From Wychulis et al.[17] Used by permission.

cardiac filling and stroke volume are severely limited in constrictive pericarditis,[4] manipulation of the heart or the anesthetic may depress the myocardium during operation and may cause severe hypotension. Widespread resection of the constricting pericardium, including the epicardium, is essential in these patients. Rarely the constriction may involve mainly the left ventricle and produce symptoms of pulmonary edema. Usually the ventricles are equally involved, and the elevation of ventricular end-diastolic pressure is approximately equal and, therefore, so are the right and left atrial pressures.[17] After extensive removal of the constricting pericardium and decortication, dilatation of the ventricles may result, thus leading to myocardial failure (Table 10–1) and low cardiac output, which can cause death. These patients also may bleed profusely from raw surfaces of decorticated areas and require a massive blood transfusion, which presents a serious situation.

ADULT COARCTATION

General Information

Coarctation of the aorta occurs in approximately 0.01% of the population.[10] It has resulted in significant hypertension and represents a distinct potential threat to health. Surgical correction of the coarctation on an elective basis should be undertaken. At our institution, surgery is usually accomplished through a left posterolateral thoracotomy approach in the bed of the nonresected fifth rib.[7]

Most coarctations of the aorta are diagnosed incidentally, such as at physical examination. Symptoms of hypertension or endocarditis may be the first signs to be detected. An angiocardiogram may reveal the site and degree of the coarctation and may further aid in the assessment of the collateral circulation. These patients might be receiving antihypertensive therapy, including β-adrenergic receptor blocking agents,[3] which can be continued up to the day of operation. In patients with severe hypertension who have not been receiving β-adrenergic blocking agents, severe hypertensive responses to the intubation are seen frequently.[11] Also, premedication given to those patients should provide good sedation.

Anesthetic Management

Venous cannulation is achieved (two 14-gauge intravenous lines and a jugular line, the first line inserted before induction). Induction starts with thiopental, in increments of 25 to 50 mg, as frequently as needed. Our group uses pancuronium, 0.1 mg/kg, for intubation. After induction and intubation, the right radial artery is cannulated with a No. 18 or No. 20 Teflon catheter for direct arterial monitoring. Circulation to the left arm may be occluded during aortic cross-clamping. Therefore, any arterial cannulation on the left radial artery would be useless during cross-clamping of the aorta.

Monitoring of arterial pressure below the coarctation during cross-clamping of the aorta has been recommended.[3] Direct measurement of aortic pressure can be done after thoracotomy, with an 18-gauge needle placed into the distal aortic segment and connected to the strain gauge. This line is required only during aortic cross-clamping and can be removed after the correction of the coarctation.

Maintenance of anesthesia usually is continued with halothane or enflurane. Halothane has an advantage over other anesthetic agents. After cross-clamping of the aorta, arterial pressure above the clamp may show a large increase and may cause dysrhythmias, left heart failure, or cerebrovascular accidents. With halothane[3] and intermittent positive-pressure ventilation, the blood pressure can be kept at acceptable levels. However, if the patient has well-formed collateral circulation, cross-clamping may not produce excessively high blood pressure.

The other method of reducing high blood pressure is the use of sodium nitroprusside by intravenous drip. This therapy is effective when the blood pressure cannot be reduced with halothane. Although a reasonable level of hypotension is an aid in surgery, control of the arterial pressure distal to the clamp must never be lost. Perfusion of the spinal cord below the coarctation is dependent on the blood flow developed in the collateral circulation by the branches of the subclavian arteries.[2] A mean blood pressure of 50 mm Hg in the distal segment is regarded as the critical pressure. Below that level, perfusion becomes inadequate and circulatory support of the distal segment may be necessary.[6] In such a situation, the use of a heparin-bonded cannula as a temporary bypass shunt from the ascending to the descending aorta is simpler and adequate. Without such precautions, postoperative neurologic sequelae occur (0.5%).[1]

Resection of the coarctated segment and end-to-end anastomosis are the usual forms of surgery. However, some patients may need grafts if segment resection is wider.

Postoperative Phase

Patients should be placed in intensive care units for observation and monitoring of arterial and central venous pressures. Reduction of a patient's arterial pressure to nearly normal levels can be anticipated during the several days or first few weeks after operation.[7] Immediately after the correction of the coarctation, the arterial pressure usually decreases to normal levels, yet 20% to 60% of the patients may have increased blood pressure within 24 hours. The level would gradually increase to preoperative levels or higher.[12] This increase of blood pressure in patients with coarctation is probably due to overactivity of the sympathetic nervous system, as evidenced by increasing secretion of catecholamines, especially norepinephrine, within 12 hours of surgery.[3] This sevenfold increase or more in the plasma levels of norepinephrine is interpreted as being due to sympathetic nervous activity, possibly related to baroreceptor mechanisms. These receptors are assumed to be situated near the aortic constriction and are adapted to hypertension before surgery. However, they react to lowered pressure in the proximal aortic segment after surgery. This theory is supported by the finding of concentrations of plasma norepinephrine 12 hours after resection, which correlates positively with the preoperative peak pressure gradient across the coarctation (Fig 10–2). The high blood pressure occurring immediately after surgery should be controlled. Use of a short-acting α-adrenergic blocking drug, such as intravenously administered phentolamine, for control of arterial pressure and a cardioselective β-adrenergic blocking agent or a drip of sodium nitroprusside should be sufficient to control the increase of blood pressure after operation.

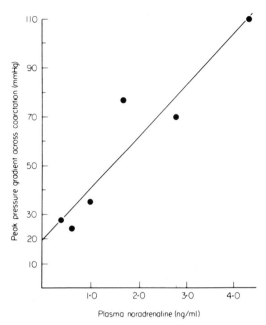

Fig 10–2.—Peak pressure gradient across coarctation and its relation to 12-hour postcorrection plasma concentrations of norepinephrine ($r = .94$, $P < .01$). (From Fisher and Benedict.[3] Used by permission.)

REOPERATION IN THE EARLY POSTOPERATIVE PERIOD ("REOPENING")

General Information

The most common cause of reoperation during the early postoperative period ("reopening") is persistent hemorrhage. Most patients have an intact clotting mechanism before operation, and it is impossible to predict who will bleed excessively after extracorporeal circulation.

In one study from our institution,[5] the average total bleeding of 656 patients was 513 ml/sq m per 24 hours, and the losses ranged from 72

TABLE 10-2.—CUMULATIVE BLEEDING AND TYPE
OF OPEN-HEART OPERATION*

TYPE OF OPERATION	NO. OF PATIENTS	BLEEDING (ML/SQ M) DURING FIRST 24 HR			
		MEAN	SD	RANGE	MEDIAN
Repair of tetralogy of Fallot	55	900	830	178–4,144	598
Miscellaneous (congenital diseases)	99	587	492	112–3,368	443
Multiple valve replacement	64	565	332	189–1,741	461
Aortic valve replacement	180	508	417	117–3,097	363
Miscellaneous (acquired diseases)	32	482	362	126–2,127†	377
Mitral valve replacement	104	449	363	98–2,275	347
Closure of ventricular septal defect	68	396	240	130–1,220	330
Closure of atrial septal defect	54	323	231	72–1,663	270
Total	656	513	686	72–4,144	374

*From Gomes and McGoon.[5] Used by permission.
†One patient lost more than 9,000 ml/sq m/24 hr and has been omitted from analysis.

to 4,144 ml. Averages ranged from 323 ml in the group that had repair of atrial septal defect to 900 ml in the group that underwent correction of tetralogy of Fallot (Table 10–2). The amount of bleeding was greatest during the first two postoperative hours and seemed to be related to the bypass time. The mean amount of bleeding was 450 ml/sq m per 24 hours for patients with one hour of bypass or less, 510 ml for patients with bypass times between one and two hours, and 585 ml for patients with more than two hours of bypass.[5] Excessive bleeding in itself is a serious postoperative complication and should be treated promptly to avoid additional complications, such as arrhythmias, low cardiac output, cardiac failure, and death.

At reoperation, the bleeding may be related to the surgery, although the exact cause may be difficult to determine (Table 10–3).

TABLE 10-3.—SOURCES OF
BLEEDING AT REOPERATION AFTER
OPEN-HEART SURGERY*

SOURCE OF BLEEDING	NO. OF PATIENTS†
Aortotomy	8
Pericardial fat	2
Branch of right coronary artery	2
Atriotomy	2
Sternum	2
No specific point of bleeding	5

*From Gomes and McGoon.[5] Used by permission.
†A total of 656 patients had operation; 21 (3%) of them had reoperation.

Anesthetic Management

During the early postoperative period, the anesthetic management is greatly facilitated if the patient is still intubated. In these patients, progressive analgesia-amnesia and muscle relaxation are used as needed, after all infusion lines are confirmed to be adequate and the usual monitoring has been established.

If the patient is not intubated, anesthesia should not be induced until the patient is fully draped and the surgeon is ready to make the skin incision. Most patients have significantly compromised ventricular function (usually due to existing cardiac tamponade, which would be relieved immediately after opening the chest and pericardium, leading to increase of systemic blood pressure), and high doses of almost any anesthetic agent should be avoided at this stage. Usually, our group preoxygenates and induces anesthesia with small increments of thiopental (25 to 50 mg) and diazepam (2.5 to 5 mg) given very slowly until the lid reflex is abolished. A large dose of succinylcholine is given intravenously to facilitate tracheal intubation and to prevent the patient from straining during and after intubation and thus avoiding even further impairment of the venous return to the heart. For maintenance of anesthesia, our group usually uses nitrous oxide with 50% oxygen and supplements this mixture with a narcotic analgesic, such as meperidine, fentanyl, or morphine, in small doses, and with muscle relaxants as needed.

Occasionally, the bleeding source may not be

accessible surgically without significantly compromising the hemodynamics. If this is the situation, the patient should be fully heparinized and should go on cardiopulmonary bypass.

REFERENCES

1. Brewer L.A. III, et al.: Spinal cord complications following surgery for coarctation of the aorta: A study of 66 cases. *J. Thorac. Cardiovasc. Surg.* 64:368, 1972.
2. Edwards J.E., et al.: The collateral circulation in coarctation of the aorta. *Proc. Staff Meet. Mayo Clin.* 23:333, 1948.
3. Fisher A., Benedict C.R.: Adult coarctation of the aorta: Anaesthesia and postoperative management. *Anaesthesia* 32:533, 1977.
4. Gilston A.: Anaesthesia for cardiac surgery. *Br. J. Anaesth.* 43:217, 1971.
5. Gomes M.M.R., McGoon D.C.: Bleeding patterns after open-heart surgery. *J. Thorac. Cardiovasc. Surg.* 60:87, 1970.
6. Hughes R.K., Reemtsma K.: Correction of coarctation of the aorta: Manometric determination of safety during test occlusion. *J. Thorac. Cardiovasc. Surg.* 62:31, 1971.
7. McGoon D.C.: Comments. *Chest* 63:87, 1973.
8. Mullin E.M. Jr., et al.: Current results of operation for mitral stenosis: Clinical and hemodynamic assessments in 124 consecutive patients treated by closed commissurotomy, open commissurotomy, or valve replacement. *Circulation* 46:298, 1972.
9. Nanda N.C., et al.: Mitral commissurotomy versus replacement: Preoperative evaluation by echocardiography. *Circulation* 51:263, 1975.
10. Perlman L.: Coarctation of the aorta: Clinical and roentgenologic analysis of thirteen cases. *Am. Heart J.* 28:24, 1944.
11. Prys-Roberts C., et al.: Studies of anaesthesia in relation to hypertension: V. Adrenergic beta-receptor blockade. *Br. J. Anaesth.* 45:671, 1973.
12. Sealy W.C., et al.: Paradoxical hypertension following resection of coarctation of aorta. *Surgery* 42:135, 1957.
13. Selzer A., Cohn K.E.: Natural history of mitral stenosis: A review. *Circulation* 45:878, 1972.
14. Tyers G.F.O., et al.: Present status of cardiac valve replacement. *Curr. Probl. Surg.* 14:44, Oct. 1977.
15. Wharton C.F.P., Bescos L.L.: Mitral valve movement: A study using an ultrasound technique. *Br. Heart J.* 32:344, 1970.
16. Wilcox B.R., et al.: Effect of mitral commissurotomy on right-heart work. *Circulation* 50 (suppl. 2):193, 1974.
17. Wychulis A.R., Connolly D.C., McGoon D.C.: Surgical treatment of pericarditis. *J. Thorac. Cardiovasc. Surg.* 62:608, 1971.

11 / Anesthesia for Abdominal Aortic Aneurysm

SAIT TARHAN
HUGO S. RAIMUNDO

THE FIRST RESECTION of an abdominal aortic aneurysm with a homograft replacement was performed almost 30 years ago.[10] Since then, the operation has become a standard surgical procedure. When the surgical treatment was new, the operation approximately doubled the life expectancy.[28]

Rupture of the aneurysm is the principal cause of death in patients treated medically. The disease is primarily seen among older people. According to Bergan and Yao,[4] 10 to 40 per 1,000 of the population more than the age of 50 years have abdominal aortic aneurysm.

A decision should be made for the surgical management of abdominal aortic aneurysm, with consideration given to the medical status of the patient. In patients who are more than 70 years of age, the decision of whether to operate often involves many factors, including age, size of the aneurysm, and associated medical conditions.[22]

Patient age in itself is not a contraindication. In very old patients, age is relatively more important because multiple chronic degenerative diseases significantly reduce the homeostatic reserve of the body. The size of the aneurysm has some importance. Patients with an aneurysm 6 cm or less in diameter have survived one year from the time of diagnosis, and 47.8% of them have lived for five years.[27] However, of patients with aneurysms bigger than 6 cm, only 50% survived for one year, only 6% were still alive after five years, and 43% of the larger aneurysms ruptured.[27]

Associated medical conditions have an important influence on the surgical decisions as the age of the patient increases. Contraindications to surgery may include recent acute myocardial infarction, intractable congestive heart failure, chronic heart disease, and advanced cancer. Therefore, incidental diseases as a cause of mortality must be considered. Diseases associated with abdominal aortic aneurysm vary[23] (Table 11–1).

Mortality in elective resections of aneurysms has decreased to between 3% and 7% in some centers.[30] However, the mortality for patients with ruptured aneurysms remains at approximately 50%,[16,25] and 28% of the 50% are patients who had undergone aneurysmectomy.[23] The reasons for the reduced mortality for patients who have elective surgery are careful preoperative preparation with correction or stabilization of associated disorders, improved anesthetic techniques, and careful monitoring of fluids and acid-base balance, as well as of central venous pressure, arterial pressure, and cardiac function. However, with patients who have ruptured abdominal aneurysm, there is no time for preoperative preparation. The patient is rushed from the emergency room to the operating room, where he undergoes surgery immediately. This type of patient will be considered separately in this chapter.

PREOPERATIVE ASSESSMENT

The mortality for patients undergoing aortic aneurysm surgery has decreased because surgery is done earlier in the course of the disease, when the aneurysms are smaller and less often symptomatic. Pulmonary disease is frequent among these patients (see Table 11–1). Such problems should be closely checked, and respiratory function tests should be done when necessary. The patient also should receive intensive preoperative physical and drug therapy.

TABLE 11–1.—ASSOCIATED DISEASES IN PATIENTS WITH ABDOMINAL AORTIC ANEURYSM*

ASSOCIATED DISEASE	% OF PATIENTS†
Coronary artery disease	65
Previous myocardial infarction	50‡
Angina	25‡
Hypertension	37
Peripheral vascular disease	33
Pulmonary disease	27
Renal or genitourinary disease	22
Cerebrovascular insufficiency	13
Gastrointestinal or liver disease	13
Diabetes	7
Other	8

*From Scobie et al.[23] Used by permission.
†Seventy-three percent had two or more associated diseases, for an average of 2.25 diseases per patient.
‡Percentages of the group with coronary artery disease.

The other most frequent problems associated with abdominal aneurysms are coronary artery disease, previous myocardial infarction, hypertension, and diabetes. The seriousness of previous myocardial infarctions has been emphasized.[29] Therefore, the patient's cardiac status should be carefully investigated before surgery. A history of myocardial infarction or an intraventricular conduction disturbance is associated with a five-year mortality of more than 40%.[31] In patients with larger and symptomatic aneurysms, the risk of rupture exceeds the risk of coronary artery disease, and elective surgery is preferred. Coronary artery angiography is associated with a low mortality (less than 0.1%),[32] but not all patients who are to undergo aneurysmectomy can be investigated by this method. A preliminary screening test by exercise ECG may be useful because it has an accuracy of 84% for the detection of coronary artery disease, which makes it a practical screening test.

Pronounced obesity can be regarded as a severe concomitant disease when the obese patient has an abdominal aortic aneurysm. Surgery is much more difficult and more time-consuming, and the morbidity is also increased.[8]

Hypertensive patients, especially those with large aneurysms, have the worst prognosis because of the possibility of rupture,[20] which may be lethal. Therefore, these patients, even those with small aneurysms, should have their blood pressure lowered before surgery.

The value of aortography before surgery has been debated.[18] Many surgeons continue to rely on clinical evaluation as the sole guide in assessing abdominal aortic aneurysms, but there are certain advantages of preoperative aortography, such as detection of significant arterial occlusive disease in other vessels—renal, celiac, superior and inferior mesenteric iliac, and femoral arteries.[18] With the refinement of angiographic techniques, major complications of this procedure have been virtually eliminated.[18] Aortography should not be relied on to estimate the aneurysm size. It only defines the internal limits of the aneurysm or associated thrombus. In this respect, ultrasonography is clearly the method of choice for delineation of the aneurysm. It is noninvasive and remarkably accurate in defining the aneurysm size. However, it may not allow the assessment of the position of the aneurysm relative to the renal arteries or of involvement of other branch vessels in the aorta.[18]

PREOPERATIVE PREPARATION

Respiratory and renal problems are frequent causes of mortality, although cardiac disorders remain the main cause of death after the resection of abdominal aneurysm.[32] Respiratory problems usually exist before surgery. Therefore, intense respiratory therapy before the procedure may reduce the incidence of pulmonary dysfunction during the postoperative period. Atelectasis and pneumonia are the most common pulmonary complications of this type of surgery.

Renal problems usually occur during and after surgery because blood flow is compromised while the aorta is being clamped. However, the frequency of such incidents has been greatly reduced recently because of the preoperative and the intraoperative hydration of the patient and the infusion of mannitol and furosemide during surgery before aortic clamping.

Because cardiac problems are the main reason for the death of these patients, patients with heart disease and coronary artery disease should receive optimal preoperative medication. If coronary angiography is to be used in patients with high-risk coronary lesions, such as those with stenosis of 70% to 90% in the left main coronary artery (a surgically treatable condition), coronary artery bypass graft surgery should be considered before surgery on this relatively small abdominal aortic aneurysm can be done. Patients who have gone through such surgery can tolerate other noncardiac operations better than those who have not had surgery, and their postoperative myocardial infarction rate has been lower.[19]

ANESTHESIA

Premedication

Patients with abdominal aortic aneurysm who undergo elective surgery can be given premedication with any combination of narcotics or tranquilizers. As soon as the patient is brought to the operating room, ECG electrodes are attached to the patient and a blood pressure cuff is applied to each arm. Two No. 14 plastic needles are placed in the forearm or antecubital veins, with tubing attached to two 1-L bags of Ringer's lactate solution.

Monitoring

Arterial blood pressure is monitored directly by an 18-gauge Teflon catheter inserted percutaneously into a radial artery, after adequate collateral circulation has been demonstrated by clinical assessment with a modified Allen test. External (advancing the catheter through the external jugular vein with a J-wire into the superior vena cava) or internal jugular veins are used for monitoring the central venous pressure. Balloon-tipped, flow-directed catheters are useful for monitoring pulmonary wedge pressure, which reflects left atrial pressure. This type of monitoring is especially valuable for patients who have borderline cardiac function, because it is a reliable guide for fluid and blood transfusions. Otherwise, circulatory overload can occur, leading to pulmonary edema.

Monitoring the urinary output of the patient undergoing surgery for aortic aneurysm is important because renal flow is interrupted during operation. Also, renal dysfunction before surgery occurs frequently among these patients.[23]

Induction

Induction of anesthesia in patients with abdominal aortic aneurysm who undergo elective surgery is performed in a routine manner at our institution. Sodium thiopental is given intravenously in fractional doses, such as 50 to 75 mg. The myocardial depressant effects of sodium thiopental are known. Either succinylcholine (100 to 120 mg intravenously) or pancuronium (0.1 mg/kg intravenously, which requires three to four minutes to take effect) is used for intubation. Again, the patient must be completely paralyzed to prevent bucking or coughing, which may increase blood pressure. Rupture of the aneurysm, especially larger ones, in a hypertensive patient is a real danger during induction.

Maintenance

A narcotic analgesic agent, such as meperidine (Demerol) or droperidol-fentanyl (Innovar) or fentanyl, is given in fractional doses during surgery whenever it is needed. Volatile agents, such as halothane and enflurane, also can be used safely.

CROSS-CLAMPING OF AORTA

General

Halothane and enflurane can be used to control the blood pressure and the increased total peripheral resistance that occurs after the aorta is clamped.[11] Higher concentrations decrease cardiac output and peripheral resistance, therefore leading to a decrease in afterload, which in turn reduces the myocardial consumption of oxygen. This factor is important for a patient who has compromised coronary artery disease, because myocardial infarction is one of the most important causes of death during and after aortic aneurysm surgery. One study[11] showed that clamping the aorta adversely affected the cardiac contractility of patients who had an average age of 65 years. The reason for this problem was that the increase of afterload adversely affected myocardial oxygen supply-and-demand ratio, and consequently cardiac contractility worsened. Clamping time of the aorta and loss of blood also have been related to mortality. A clamping time of less than 45 minutes did not increase the mortality, but a duration greater than that had a linear relationship with increasing mortality. Also in the same study, blood loss of more than 3,000 ml greatly increased the mortality.[15]

After the aorta is cross-clamped, patients who have an acute increase of afterload leading to myocardial decompensation may require vasodilator therapy to reduce the afterload. Intravenously administered nitroprusside helps improve the hemodynamic status of the patient during cross-clamping of the aorta by reducing systemic peripheral resistance.[2, 21] Patients with chronic obstructive vascular disease (Leriche) also are not immune to hemodynamic changes during cross-clamping of the aorta. The development of collateral circulation may produce a smaller increase in systemic vascular resistance.[21] The maintenance and conduction of anesthesia should be oriented to managing any hypertensive crises and tachycardia, since these increase cardiac work and myocardial oxygen consumption and may lead to myocardial ischemia.

Declamping Hypotension During Repair

When the clamp controlling the proximal portion of the aorta is released, the systemic pressure can decrease drastically. The cause of this decrease is not known. Experimentally, interruption of the aortic flow below the renal level decreases perfusion pressure and flow distally, because of ischemia and accumulated metabolic byproducts, and causes myocardial depression, hypotension, or low-flow states.[5] Severe hypotension after declamping would have significant importance in patients with generalized arteriosclerosis and especially in those with compromised coronary arteries and carotid arteries. However, recent clinical studies have shown that declamping the aorta, with restoration of flow to the ischemic distal tissue, did not result in myocardial depression. Nevertheless, close monitoring of these patients is essential. Sequestration of fluids and acid and metabolic loads on the heart or primary myocardial factors may have a role in declamping hypotension if the left ventricle is marginally compensated.[5]

SYMPTOMATIC AND RUPTURED ABDOMINAL ANEURYSM

The first sign of a ruptured abdominal aneurysm is pain. It appears in different forms and accounts for many delayed or initially missed diagnoses. In one study, the site of the pain in ruptured aortic aneurysms was the abdomen in 54%, low back in 27%, flank in 8%, and miscellaneous sites in 11%. The variety of locations often results in admission of the patient to the urologic service for renal colic or to the orthopedic service for acute lumbar disk, causing a delay of a necessary operation.[23] It has also been reported[1] that only a small proportion of patients with ruptured abdominal aortic aneurysms received surgical treatment. Many of them died before reaching the hospital. However, if these patients with some vague back or abdominal pain had sought medical help, they might have been saved by the excision of their aneurysm before it ruptured. Their operative mortality may be as high as 64%, and even higher,[32] depending on many variables, including the patient's age, presence of other diseases, and accidents during the operation.[1] Patients who are in shock before surgery have a mortality three times that of patients who are not in shock[32] (Table 11–2).

Preoperative Preparation

Obviously the preoperative preparation of the patient should not delay the surgery. Any elevation of systolic blood pressure above 80 mm Hg may further increase the loss of blood.[26] Vasopressors are not indicated. Any procedure that provokes coughing, choking, or straining or that increases blood pressure should be avoided. Such procedures as passing a nasogastric tube or catheterizing the bladder should be delayed.

The patient is routinely prepared and draped and is ready for the incision before the induction of anesthesia. Because of the vasodilatory effects of anesthesia or any bucking or coughing during the intubation, the blood pressure in a patient with an already low blood volume may become almost nonexistent, or exsanguination may be

TABLE 11–2.—MORTALITY IN RESECTION OF RUPTURED ABDOMINAL AORTIC ANEURYSM*

	MORTALITY, %	
SOURCE	PREOPERATIVE SHOCK	NO PREOPERATIVE SHOCK
Couch, Lane, and Crane (1970)	85	43
Darling (1970)	56	10
Van Heeckeren (1970)	65	38
Yashar, Indeglia, and Yashar (1972)	70	22
Schumacher, Barnes, and King (1973)	77	8
DiGiovanni et al. (1975)	78	58
King and Evans (1975)	100	10
Hicks et al. (1975)	67	25
Sink, Myers, and James (1976)	83	48
Young, Sandberg, and Couch (1977)	89	33
Average	77	29

*From Young et al.[32] Used by permission.

increased because of more rupturing of the aneurysm.

Fortunately, bleeding freely into the intraperitoneal cavity occurs in less than 10% of patients.[26] A large percentage of hemorrhages into retroperitoneal tissues occur before operation, and this type of bleeding is easier to control. However, anterior perforation poses a much more urgent surgical problem because the retroperitoneal tamponade effect is absent.

Induction of Anesthesia

As soon as the patient is brought to the operating room, the ECG electrodes, including the V_5 chest leads, are placed. With the use of local anesthesia, two No. 14 plastic needles are inserted into the arm veins. An external or internal jugular needle is also placed while the patient is still awake. These needles are connected to strain gauges for measurements. If the patient's condition is stable (systolic blood pressure, 80 mm Hg or higher), an attempt is made to place a needle into the radial artery while the patient is waiting for induction. No attempt to raise the blood pressure is made at this time. The patient is then prepared and draped and ready for induction while the surgical team is preparing to open the chest or abdomen. The vast majority of these patients have a "full stomach," and, consequently, this factor and the precarious hemodynamic status of these patients should be considered when anesthesia is induced. After preoxygenation, a small amount of one of the nondepolarizing muscle relaxants is given (1 mg of pancuronium, 10 mg of gallamine, 3 mg of curare, or 2 mg of dimethyltubocurarine). Amnesia is induced with thiopental (100 to 200 mg) or diazepam (10 to 20 mg) intravenously, followed by 100 to 120 mg of succinylcholine to facilitate rapid tracheal intubation. Narcotic anesthetic agents, such as meperidine, fentanyl, and droperidol-fentanyl, are preferred for maintenance. After intubation, the surgical team can proceed with the incision and surgery. Obviously, preinduction preparation cannot be achieved in a patient with an actively bleeding ruptured aneurysm. Securing one or two intravenous needles, as large as possible, is all that is needed. For these patients, a dose of 60 to 80 mg of meperidine or 8 or 10 ml of fentanyl is given in increments through the intravenous lines. Sodium thiopental in 25-mg increments allows the patient to lose consciousness, and narcotics relieve the pain of the incision.

SURGICAL CONTROL OF THE BLEEDING AORTA

As soon as anesthesia is induced, the abdomen is entered. Proximal control is obtained as quickly as possible. Different methods can be used for proximal control. One method is to make an incision in the sixth intercostal space and to clamp or pinch the distal part of the thoracic aorta between the thumb and the forefinger.[26] This transthoracic approach has the advantage of being done in a matter of seconds (Fig 11–1). Second, the aorta is readily accessible for control through this route. Third, because the rupture is in the abdomen, hemorrhaging would not fill the operative field and obscure the aorta itself. Fourth, aortic clamps can be placed proximal to the aneurysm without inadvertent dam-

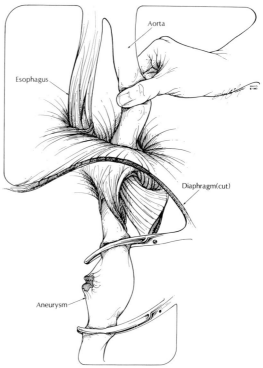

Fig 11–1.—Transthoracic approach for proximal occlusion of thoracic aorta to control bleeding. Aorta either can be cross-clamped or can be pinched between thumb and forefinger. (Modified from Stephenson and Lockhart.[26] Used by permission.)

age to the renal vessels, pancreas, or retroperitoneal structures. Finally, visual and palpatory monitoring of the status of the heart can be maintained during this critical period.[26] This transthoracic approach lends itself well to a concomitant approach through the abdomen (by a second team) to minimize supradiaphragmatic clamping time.

Once access to the abdomen is gained, several methods can be used to control the hemorrhage. Digital compression of the proximal part of the abdominal aorta is the method that is most frequently used.[26]

BLOOD TRANSFUSIONS

At this point, replacement therapy may start. The most effective replacement for hemorrhagic shock is blood that is typed and crossmatched and available in the operating room before the preparation of the patient begins.

Lactated Ringer's solution or physiologic saline solution are poor substitutes for whole blood. Although they may fill the vascular compartment, restore the blood pressure, restore the volume, and allow RBCs to reach the tissues to prevent anoxia, severe hemodilution may occur if either is used in large amounts.

Exsanguinating hemorrhages of a ruptured aortic aneurysm may require massive transfusions, causing clotting deficiencies and fibrinolysis. Heparin is the treatment of choice for fibrinolysis.[26] Old blood stored for more than 24 hours may have no platelets and may have reduced levels of factors V and VII, thus further increasing the possibility of clotting deficiencies. Fresh blood, fresh-frozen plasma, and platelets may help to correct the deficiencies. (Blood and blood component therapy are discussed in chapter 20.) One ampule (50 ml) of sodium bicarbonate for every 4 units of old blood may be administered to buffer the acidic banked blood. However, the blood gases and pH of these patients should be checked whenever it is indicated. To counteract any citrate toxicity, calcium chloride (10 ml) also is injected for every 2 or 3 units of blood given.

Giving cold blood to the patient can cause problems. The rapid administration of large quantities of cold blood may reduce the heart and body temperature. Ample evidence suggests that cardiac function is reduced when temperature is lowered. Also, temperatures as low as 30 C may irritate the myocardium, leading to ventricular fibrillation. Therefore, blood transfused should circulate through a blood-warmer.

CARDIAC ARREST

Rupture of an abdominal aortic aneurysm often is associated with cardiac arrest during surgery and is responsible for 30% to 80% of the deaths in the operating room.[26] The critical period for cardiac arrest includes induction of anesthesia, which may provoke considerable vasodilatation. Also, infusions of large quantities of cold blood can lead to reduced myocardial temperature and alterations of acid-base balance of the patient and are factors responsible for intraoperative cardiac arrest.

Cardiac arrest compounds the emergency that already exists. If it occurs during the preparation of the patient, efforts are based on life-support measures, ventilation, possibly intubation, and replacement of the lost volume of blood through infusion. A practical method of providing between 500 and 1,000 ml of blood is to elevate the legs of the patient. The left side of the chest then can be opened, and manual compression of the heart can be resumed. This maneuver also allows clamping of the thoracic aorta just above the diaphragm, thus facilitating the perfusion of the brain and myocardium. Opening the chest also allows the direct application of the defibrillator pads on the heart for defibrillation.

ACUTE AORTOVENOUS FISTULA DUE TO RUPTURE OF ABDOMINAL AORTIC ANEURYSM

A spontaneous fistula between the abdominal aorta and the inferior vena cava is rare. It probably occurs in 1% of all patients operated on for atherosclerotic aneurysms of the abdominal aorta[9] (Fig 11-2). Diagnosis may be difficult, but when fistula is suspected, confirmation is easy. Because the fistula causes severe congestive heart failure, surgery is urgently needed.

Physical findings of this syndrome frequently include a pulsatile abdominal mass in the patient before the rupture occurs. Abdominal or lower back pain associated with enlargement of the aneurysm or rupture into the vena cava (or both) may occur. Confirmation of the fistula also can be achieved by transfemoral catheterization

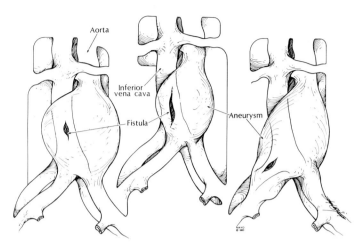

Fig 11–2.—Locations of aortocaval or aortovenous fistulas. (Modified from Johnson and Wood.[17] Used by permission.)

with a Swan-Ganz or other catheter by determining an increase in pressure in the inferior vena cava and an increase in oxygen saturation.

Compression of the inferior vena cava by a large aneurysm or a massive arteriovenous shunting (or by both) may cause extensive edema in the lower part of the body.[7]

Anesthetic Management

An aortocaval fistula produces a large increase in cardiac output, with the end result being high-output cardiac failure. Renal plasma flow decreases, causing a large increase in plasma volume as well as hemodilution.[12] Therefore, a reduction in hemoglobin level should not be considered an indication for transfusion, and such transfusion will only overload the cardiovascular system. If surgery is not urgently indicated, the use of diuretics and digitalization may improve the patient's status before surgery.

Although aortography of the patient with classic symptoms is not always needed, it can be done when the diagnosis is in doubt.[17]

Anesthetic management of these patients is not drastically different from that of patients with other types of ruptured abdominal aneurysms. The only significant difference is that the anesthesiologist should keep in mind that these patients have an increased cardiac output and a high-output cardiac failure. The operative management of aortocaval fistulas is summarized from Doty et al[9] (used by permission) as follows:

1. Monitoring of systemic arterial, right atrial, and pulmonary wedge pressures
2. Large-bore venous access in both arms
3. Minimal, careful dissection of neck of aneurysm and iliac arteries
4. Dacron graft, preclotted or low porosity
5. Heparin, intravenous to increase activated clotting time to more than 400 seconds
6. Autotransfusion of blood from aneurysm and aortocaval fistula
7. Digital control of fistula and closure by direct suture from within aorta
8. Aortic reconstruction with Dacron graft
9. Protamine sulfate to reverse heparin effect (monitor with activated clotting time)

Monitoring

Continuous monitoring of systemic arterial pressure with direct cannulation of the radial artery is mandatory. Balloon-tipped, flow-directed catheters measure pulmonary wedge pressure; this pressure reflects the left atrial pressure, which in turn makes maintenance of adequate left ventricular performance more predictable. Proper monitoring also helps in replacing the fluid and blood volume.

The purpose of surgery is obviously the closure of the aortocaval fistula, with restoration of arterial continuity. Another problem of this surgery is that a thrombus in the aneurysmal sac may enter the vena cava and cause pulmonary embolization—this should be prevented.[5]

Control of the cava by manual compression will effectively prevent pulmonary embolization during manipulation of the aortic aneurysm. This paradoxical pulmonary embolization may even cause the death of the patient.[7]

Closure of the aortocaval fistula produces dramatic relief in the high-output cardiac failure of these patients. Even during the intraoperative period, urinary output may increase and congestive heart failure will decrease promptly.

POSTOPERATIVE CARE

Usually the endotracheal tube is left in place overnight in a well-sedated patient who is artificially ventilated. Arterial blood gas levels are measured frequently to facilitate early recognition of hypoxemia. Respiratory insufficiency is a frequent event after repair of an abdominal aortic aneurysm. In one study[13] almost 18% of patients who underwent aneurysmectomy developed prolonged respiratory failure, with a high mortality (70%). Therefore, respiratory care, particularly intermittent positive-pressure breathing and ultrasonic nebulization, may reduce pulmonary problems considerably.[24]

A high rate of deaths among patients who have undergone abdominal aortic aneurysm surgery is caused by myocardial infarctions. This figure is reported to be 41%.[14] Therefore, sophisticated monitoring should continue in the intensive care unit. Arrhythmias should be promptly recognized and treated, and blood pressure fluctuations also should receive proper attention.

Renal failure is still the major contributor to morbidity. Therefore, urinary output should be monitored after operation and maintained at more than 50 ml/hour.[3] If a patient fails to have proper urinary output and renal failure is inevitable, early aggressive hemodialysis or hyperalimentation or both should be instituted to reduce the morbidity of acute renal failure. The time sequence of postoperative complications of emergency abdominal aortic aneurysmectomies from Christenson et al.[6] (used by permission) is as follows: hemorrhage (reoperation), primary circulatory insufficiency, cardiac arrhythmias (myocardial infarction), distal arterial thrombosis, renal insufficiency (uremia), posttraumatic respiratory insufficiency, pulmonary embolism, jaundice (ischemic liver cell damage), and wound rupture (wound infection).

REFERENCES

1. Armour R.H.: Survivors of ruptured abdominal aortic aneurysm: The iceberg's tip. Br. Med. J. 2:1055, 1977.
2. Attia R.R., et al.: Myocardial ischemia due to infrarenal aortic cross-clamping during aortic surgery in patients with severe coronary artery disease. Circulation 53:961, 1976.
3. Baird R.J., et al.: Abdominal aortic aneurysms: Recent experience with 210 patients. Can. Med. Assoc. J. 118:1229, 1978.
4. Bergan J.J., Yao J.S.T.: Modern management of abdominal aortic aneurysms. Surg. Clin. North Am. 54:175, 1974.
5. Bush H.L. Jr., et al.: Assessment of myocardial performance and optimal volume loading during elective abdominal aortic aneurysm resection. Arch. Surg. 112:1301, 1977.
6. Christenson J., Eklöf B., Gustafson I.: Abdominal aortic aneurysms: Should they all be resected? Br. J. Surg. 64:767, 1977.
7. Cooperman M., et al.: Spontaneous aortocaval fistula with paradoxical pulmonary embolization. Am. J. Surg. 134:647, 1977.
8. Dobell A.R.C.: Abdominal aortic aneurysms, editorial. Can. Med. Assoc. J. 118:1185, 1978.
9. Doty D.B., et al.: Aortocaval fistula associated with aneurysm of the abdominal aorta: Current management using autotransfusion techniques. Surgery 84:250, 1978.
10. Dubost C., Allary M., Oeconomos N.: Resection of an aneurysm of the abdominal aorta: Reestablishment of continuity by a preserved human arterial graft, with result after five months. Arch. Surg. 64:405, 1952.
11. Dunn E., et al.: The effect of abdominal aortic cross-clamping on myocardial function. J. Surg. Res. 22:463, 1977.
12. Epstein F.H., Ferguson T.B.: The effect of the formation of an arteriovenous fistula upon blood volume. J. Clin. Invest. 34:434, 1955.
13. Hechtman H.B., et al.: Acute pulmonary insufficiency following abdominal aortic aneurysm repair. Bibl. Anat. 15:436, 1977.
14. Hicks G.L., et al.: Surgical improvement following aortic aneurysm resection. Ann. Surg. 181:863, 1975.
15. Hildebrand H.D., Chung W.B.: Abdominal aortic aneurysmectomy: A comparative study of morbidity and mortality. Am. Surg. 37:476, 1971.
16. Interhospital Cardiovascular Surgery Group of the University of Toronto, et al.: Surgical treatment of abdominal aortic aneurysms in Toronto: A study of 1013 patients. Can. Med. Assoc. J. 107:1091, 1972.
17. Johnson J.M., Wood M.: Arteriovenous fistula

secondary to rupture of atherosclerotic abdominal aortic aneurysm: Report of five cases. *Am. J. Surg.* 136:171, 1978.
18. Kwaan J.H.M., et al.: The value of arteriography before abdominal aneurysmectomy. *Am. J. Surg.* 134:108, 1977.
19. Mahar L.J., et al.: Perioperative myocardial infarction in patients with coronary artery disease with and without aorta-coronary artery bypass grafts. *J. Thorac. Cardiovasc. Surg.* 76:533, 1978.
20. Management of abdominal aneurysm, editorial. *Br. Med. J.* 2:1106, 1977.
21. Meloche R., et al.: Haemodynamic changes due to clamping of the abdominal aorta. *Can. Anaesth. Soc. J.* 24:20, 1977.
22. Pflugfelder P., Robertson D., Cape R.D.T.: Predicting mortality after elective abdominal aortic aneurysmectomy in the elderly. *Gerontology* 23:368, 1977.
23. Scobie K., McPhail N., Hubbard C.: Early and late results of resection of abdominal aortic aneurysms. *Can. Med. Assoc. J.* 117:147, 1977.
24. Simstein N.L.: Aortic aneurysms: A five-year experience. *Milit. Med.* 143:690, 1978.
25. Sink J.D., Myers R.T., James P.M. Jr.: Ruptured abdominal aortic aneurysms: Review of 33 cases treated surgically and discussion of prognostic indicators. *Am. Surg.* 42:303, 1976.
26. Stephenson H.E. Jr., Lockhart C.G.: Treatment of the ruptured abdominal aorta. *Surg. Gynecol. Obstet.* 144:855, 1977.
27. Szilagyi D.E., Elliott J.P., Smith R.F.: Clinical fate of the patient with asymptomatic abdominal aortic aneurysm and unfit for surgical treatment. *Arch. Surg.* 104:600, 1972.
28. Szilagyi D.E., et al.: Contribution of abdominal aortic aneurysmectomy to prolongation of life. *Ann. Surg.* 164:678, 1966.
29. Tarhan S., et al.: Myocardial infarction after general anesthesia. *J.A.M.A.* 220:1451, 1972.
30. Thompson J.E., et al.: Surgical management of abdominal aortic aneurysms: Factors influencing mortality and morbidity—a 20-year experience. *Ann. Surg.* 181:654, 1975.
31. Weinberg S.L.: Natural history six years after acute myocardial infarction: Is there a low-risk group? *Chest* 69:23, 1976.
32. Young A.E., Sandberg G.W., Couch N.P.: The reduction of mortality of abdominal aortic aneurysm resection. *Am. J. Surg.* 134:585, 1977.

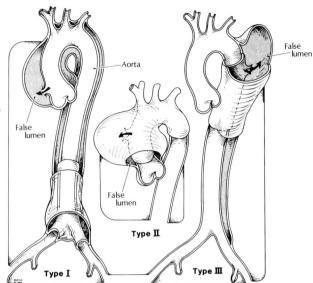

Fig 12–1.—Classification of dissecting aneurysms of aorta. **Type I,** dissection involves ascending aorta, arch, and descending aorta and extends distally. **Type II,** dissection limited to ascending aorta. **Type III,** dissection begins distal to left subclavian artery and extends distally. (Redrawn from De Bakey et al.[4])

tery. This outer layer usually has the appearance of a fusiform aneurysm, and the aortic valve is also often incompetent. This type of aneurysm is more likely to be found in Marfan syndrome.

Type III

Dissection starts in the descending thoracic aorta, most often distal to the origin of the left subclavian artery, and extends below. Sometimes, the dissection is limited to the descending thoracic aorta.

CLINICAL FEATURES

Dissecting aneurysms occur most often in patients aged between 50 and 70 years and are relatively rare in persons aged less than 40 years.[4] In spite of recent advances in operative technique and drug therapy, the mortality for these patients is still high. With medical management alone, hospital mortality varies from 14% to 67%, the highest mortality being for patients with dissection of the ascending aorta. Late mortality is reported to be as high as 55%.[15] However, De Bakey and his group[4] reported that surgery of the dissecting thoracic aneurysms of 197 patients resulted in an overall survival rate of 79%.

Symptoms produced by aneurysms of the thoracic aorta are usually the result of pressure on adjacent structures. Pressure on the trachea and bronchi often causes dyspnea and cough. There may be erosion through the ribs and sternum. Pressure on the innominate vein or superior vena cava leads to distention and edema of the neck and shoulders. The anesthetic implications of these findings are obvious. Intubation of the patient, either with a regular endotracheal tube or more often with a double-lumen tube, may be difficult and even cause rupture of the aneurysm. Such an event (rupture into the tracheobronchial tree) would be fatal. Therefore, this possibility always should be considered if a patient has blood-streaked sputum, because it is an obvious sign of leakage of the aneurysm into the trachea and bronchus.[22]

PROGNOSIS

The prognosis of patients with a thoracic aneurysm is grave, the average survival being less than one year after the onset of symptoms.[22] A study of 633 patients with saccular aneurysm of the thoracic aorta revealed that the average duration of life from the onset of symptoms was six to eight months. Patients with lesions of the ascending aorta and transverse arch had the poorest prognosis because of the location of the aneurysm and its proximity to other vital structures, such as the superior vena cava, tracheobronchial tree, and the heart itself.[8]

ANESTHESIA FOR ASCENDING AORTIC ANEURYSMS

Large fusiform or globular aneurysms of the ascending aorta tend to enlarge slowly and often cause aortic valvular insufficiency by stretching the aortic annulus without producing abnormalities of the valve leaflets themselves.[23] As the distance between the commissures is increased, the arch of each valve leaflet is lengthened and flattened. The leaflets are retracted laterally and become unable to coapt centrally.[23] Therefore, when these patients come to surgery, as an elective procedure, they may have aortic valve insufficiency. Their anesthetic management usually is not greatly different from that of patients with simple aortic valve disease in regard to induction, intubation, and monitoring. These patients have a wide pulse pressure before operation. If the diastolic pressure is low enough or nearly that of the left ventricular end-diastolic pressure, coronary flow in patients with coronary arteries that are arteriosclerotic may be reduced drastically.

The maintenance of anesthesia also is not too different from that for patients with pure valve conditions. During this stage of the surgery, these patients need a median sternotomy for exposure of the heart and ascending aorta. A large aortic aneurysm right behind the sternum may pose technical difficulties at surgery. While the sternum is being sawed, rupture of such a large aneurysm is a real danger. If we anticipate that the sternotomy may rupture the aneurysm, we use a femoral vein to femoral artery bypass technique (see chap. 8, Fig 8–6) before we attempt to open the chest. This technique provides some circulation to the vital organs.

Once the sternum is open, the aneurysm is freed. Both venae cavae then can be cannulated, and the standard vena cava to femoral artery bypass procedure can be established. In the past, the coronary arteries were cannulated and perfused, but cardioplegia for the protection of the myocardium is now the technique of choice.

The surgical technique includes cross-clamping of the aorta proximal to the innominate artery and opening of the aneurysm above the coronary cusps. Excision of the aneurysm, reconstruction of the aorta, and concentric reefing of the dilated proximal aorta at the level of the commissures produce competency of the aortic valve by allowing the leaflets to coapt normally. Although valve replacement is often indicated, it is not always needed.[23] Valve replacement can be accomplished with one of the many surgical techniques and prosthetic valves.[19] After completion of the procedure, weaning from the bypass and support of the circulation should be a routine undertaking, except that these patients are likely to have excessive blood loss through their stitches.

RESECTION AND PROSTHETIC REPLACEMENT OF ANEURYSMS OF THE AORTIC ARCH

Surgical management of the ascending or descending aorta is a relatively routine procedure,[6] but replacement of the aortic arch is still a surgical and anesthetic challenge that involves many technical problems and is infrequently undertaken. Most reports in the literature are limited to a description of very few cases.[13] However, aneurysms of the aortic arch are not rare, and the prognosis without surgery is dismal. Aneurysms of the transverse portion of the aortic arch have the poorest prognosis for life expectancy. In patients with this lesion, the average interval from the onset of symptoms until death has been reported to be 6.4 months.[8] Respiratory obstruction may lead to severe compression of the trachea and even to pneumonia, which may lead to death in 30% of the cases.[8]

There is no complete agreement among authors on the management of these patients.[1, 6, 13] The operative mortality ranges between 24.7% and 43%.[7] The management of the patient during surgery involves four critical points: (1) a technique as simple as possible should be applied; (2) cerebral protection is the most important part of the procedure; (3) the myocardium should be protected from any major insult; and (4) bleeding after the procedure is still a formidable problem, and every technical effort should be attempted to prevent or avoid it. In addition to these four considerations, damage to the CNS, secondary to the particulate or air emboli, is of major concern in aortic arch surgery. Therefore, efforts to remove air or debris from the graft and arch vessels are an important part of the procedure.

Surgery can be accomplished by different

methods: extracorporeal circulation,[13] a combination of surface cooling and deep hypothermia,[6] or temporary external shunting.[1] All have been used for the replacement of the aortic arch, and some of them are described herein just to illustrate the diversity of the methods.

Induction of Anesthesia

Large aortic aneurysms may press the trachea and cause severe respiratory failure, and the aortic arch and heart may need to be exposed by means of a median sternotomy. Attempts to accomplish this procedure may result in rupture of the aneurysm. Therefore, before induction is started, femoral vein to femoral artery bypass under local anesthesia and cardiopulmonary support to these patients may be life-saving. Once these operations are accomplished, induction with intravenously administered thiopental in fractions of 25 to 50 mg puts the patient to sleep, and pancuronium (0.1 mg/kg) facilitates the intubation. After the induction, maintenance of the patient is achieved by use of any volatile anesthetic agent or a narcotic anesthetic. During this stage, the blood pressure must be kept low enough to prevent the danger of rupture of the aneurysm. Any increase of blood pressure can be controlled by use of increased concentrations of either halothane or enflurane or by use of vasodilating agents, such as sodium nitroprusside by intravenous drip.

The patient needs to be positioned appropriately if the brachial artery is to be cannulated (supine position with arms stretched out).

Cardiopulmonary Bypass Techniques

After median sternotomy is done and the aortic arch and heart are exposed, both venae cavae or the right atrium is cannulated. The tubing that was used before for the femoral vein can be switched and connected to the right atrial cannula. The classic extracorporeal circulation circuit includes cannulation and perfusion of the femoral or iliac artery, innominate, left common carotid, and coronary arteries[13] (older concept). The technique is most complex and requires separate pumps.

A simplified method is described by Malavé and associates[13] (Fig 12–2). Cerebral perfusion catheters are brought off the main arterial line (main arterial line perfuses left femoral artery).

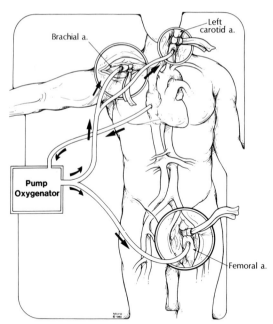

Fig 12–2.—Perfusion of right brachial artery in axilla (should perfuse right vertebral and right carotid arteries); left common carotid artery also perfused. (Redrawn from Malavé et al.[13])

The right brachial artery in the axilla is cannulated for perfusion of the right vertebral and right carotid arteries, and the left common carotid artery is cannulated separately at a point above the aortic arch with a Y-connector from the brachial artery cannulas. Also, a left ventricular sump is placed through a stab wound in the cardiac apex. The ascending aorta is then cross-clamped 3 cm above the aortic valve; and the descending aorta, brachiocephalic trunk, left carotid artery, and left subclavian are clamped if the entire aortic arch with the aneurysm is excluded from circulation.[13] The extracorporeal system is simpler to arrange (see Fig 12–2) because of the single-line cannulation of the right atrium via its appendage, and no attempt is made to control perfusion of the individual cerebral arteries by separate pumps; the cerebral blood flow regulates itself by regional vascular resistance,[13] and the left subclavian or left vertebral artery is not perfused. Use of the clamp in the proximal aorta allows coronary perfusion to continue as long as myocardial contraction remains adequate and the left ventricle has enough blood to eject. Also, some protection of the brain and myocardium is provided when the temperature of the patient decreases during bypass.[13]

Surface Cooling and Deep Hypothermia Technique

Induction and intubation are similar to those in other techniques. After they are accomplished, the patient is placed on a cooling blanket and ice bags are placed on the patient, or the patient can be immersed in a cold water bath in which the temperature is maintained at approximately 4 C by the addition of ice.[6] During surface cooling, 3 or 4 units of whole blood can be removed from the patient and replaced with Ringer's lactate solution and salt-poor albumin. When the esophageal temperature reaches 30 C, with surface cooling, the patient is positioned on the operating room table, and median sternotomy is performed, with the extension of the incision along the medial border of the left sternocleidomastoid muscle. Routine extracorporeal circulation is then performed, with inferior and superior venae cavae and common femoral artery cannulation, and core cooling starts.[6] The lungs are filled with room air, and the pulmonary artery is palpated intermittently to ensure that the left side of the heart is not distending. When the esophageal temperature reaches 12 to 15 C, the flow rate in the bypass circuit is decreased to 100 ml/minute, and the arch vessels are clamped individually. When the aortic arch is opened, an infusion catheter is placed across the aortic valve in the left ventricle, and a suction line is positioned in the ascending aorta. Saline at 4 C is then washed through the left ventricle to cool it from within during the procedure. Replacement of the aortic arch with a prosthesis is then begun. Griepp and his associates[6] reported that the average duration of cerebral ischemia with this method was 43 minutes and that the average duration of myocardial ischemia was 74 minutes. The lowest average esophageal temperature was 14 C, and the lowest average rectal temperature was 18 C.

Resection of Aneurysms of the Aortic Arch Without Cardiopulmonary Bypass or Hypothermia

Resection of aortic arch aneurysms without cardiopulmonary bypass or hypothermia is relatively new[1] and uses Tygon tubes for external temporary shunting from the ascending aorta to the femoral artery, with and without permanent bypass grafts from the ascending aorta to the ca-

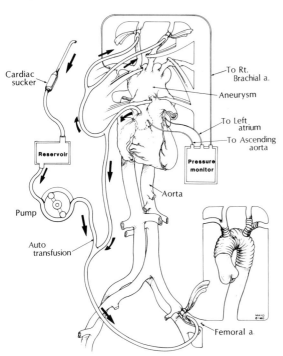

Fig 12–3.—Resection of aneurysm of arch without cardiopulmonary bypass. Cannulations during surgery. (Redrawn from Chu et al.[1])

rotid arteries. All patients receive heparin, 2 mg/kg of body weight, before external shunting.[1] Blood losses are compensated for with autotransfusion equipment. At the end of surgery, heparin is neutralized with protamine at a dose ratio of 1 to 1.5 (Fig 12–3). The overall mortality for this technique is 25%.

DISSECTING ANEURYSMS

Preoperative Assessment and Management

At presentation, these patients have a sudden onset of pain in the chest or abdomen, with increased dyspnea, loss of peripheral pulses, or a neurologic deficit. Roentgenograms of the chest may show evidence of acute edema of the lung.[24]

A patient with suspected acute dissection must be managed in an intensive care unit. Since most of the patients are hypertensive, the hypertension should be controlled as quickly as possible to prevent further dissection.[15] Arterial and central venous pressure lines are of great value for minute-to-minute monitoring.

A Swan-Ganz catheter can be introduced percutaneously into an antecubital vein to the pulmonary artery. Pulmonary capillary wedge pressure can be measured. The same catheters also can be used for cardiac output measurements. Since pulmonary capillary wedge pressure reflects left ventricular end-diastolic pressure, and if the patient with type I or II dissection has aortic valve incompetence, measurements of these pressures would give the difference between systemic diastolic pressure and left ventricular end-diastolic pressure. This evaluation helps determine the coronary artery perfusion pressure (systemic diastolic pressure minus pulmonary capillary wedge pressure) and the degree of aortic valve incompetence.

Control of Hypertension

The control of hypertension has been tried by the use of different medical regimens, such as trimethaphan, reserpine, guanethidine, and propranolol.[24] Nitroprusside intravenously administered is probably the most frequently used agent. After blood pressure is controlled, the patient's condition is stabilized and aortography can be performed. The nature and extent of the dissection and the aortic valvular incompetence and reentry point are ascertained. Also, abdominal aortography done simultaneously will reveal the status of the renal, mesenteric, and iliac vessels.[18]

To delay operation in all types of dissection is probably the current thinking in the management of aortic dissection.[15] The following tabulation, modified from Wheat[25] and used by permission, shows various treatments of dissecting aneurysm:

Drug therapy
Initial treatment for all dissecting aneurysms
Type III aneurysm, intimal tear distal to left subclavian artery
Community hospital lacking facilities for definitive aortography and an experienced cardiovascular surgical team
Patient at poor surgical risk (usually more than 50 years old)
Origin in transverse arch of aorta without extension of dissecting hematoma into ascending aorta
Site of intimal tear not identified on aortogram
False channel does not opacify
Stable chronic aneurysm, duration more than 14 days
Surgical therapy
Types I and II aneurysms, tear in ascending aorta, or ascending aorta involved by dissecting hematoma; patient reasonable surgical risk, usually less than 50 years old
Impending rupture of dissecting hematoma
Progression of dissecting hematoma
Significant aortic valve insufficiency secondary to dissecting aneurysm
Acute saccular aneurysm
Inability to relieve and control patient's pain
Inability to bring arterial pressure under control within 4 hours
Blood in pleural space or pericardium or both
Compromise or occlusion of major branch of aorta

Indications for definitive operative intervention are occlusion of the major branches of the aorta with severe ischemia, failure to control pain, and hypertension.[15] If aortic valve incompetence is present with types I and II dissections, delay of surgery may cause so much dilatation and distention of the aortic annulus that aortic valve replacement may be needed.

Medical treatment is used more often for patients with type III dissection than for patients with other types of dissection, unless the dissection progresses or vascular occlusion or rupture is imminent. With time, a saccular aneurysm forms, and these patients need resection if rupture is to be prevented.[15]

Anesthesia and Surgical Management

Type I Dissection

The anesthetic management of a type I dissection is similar to that of ascending aortic aneurysms. A median sternotomy is used for exposure. Bypass is established by cannulating the inferior and superior venae cavae and the femoral artery. Once bypass is instituted, an aortic clamp is applied to the ascending aorta proximal to the origin of the innominate artery, and the ascending aorta is transected a few centimeters above the aortic valve. If the coronary arteries are to be perfused, special catheters can be inserted into the orifices of the coronary arteries.[4] After transection of the aorta, surgery consists of obliteration of the false lumen by approximation of the inner and outer walls of the dissecting process by means of a continuous suture both proximally and distally, followed by end-to-end anastomosis of the transected aorta (Fig 12–4). In some patients, in later stages, it may be necessary to excise the diseased segment and to use a patch or tube graft.[4] (Tube graft also can be sewn inside the aortic lumen, then covered with incised segment of aorta.) These procedures can restore the normal blood flow into the aortic lumen and, by thus obliterating the false lumen, can prevent further dissection processes.

Type II Dissection

Surgical treatment of a type II dissecting aneurysm consists of resection and graft replacement of the ascending aorta. Cardiopulmonary bypass would be established, as previously described. Aortic valve insufficiency is more frequent with this type of dissection than it is with type I dissection,[4] which requires valve replacement (Fig 12–5).

Type III Dissection

A type III dissection is managed differently anesthetically, yet the surgical procedure still requires excision of the dissected portion of the aorta and replacement of the segment of the descending thoracic aorta with a graft. Because the dissecting process with this type is limited proximally to the level of the origin of the left subclavian artery, the proximal occluding clamp can be applied distally to this artery or to the common carotid artery. The distal extent of the dissecting process sometimes is limited to the de-

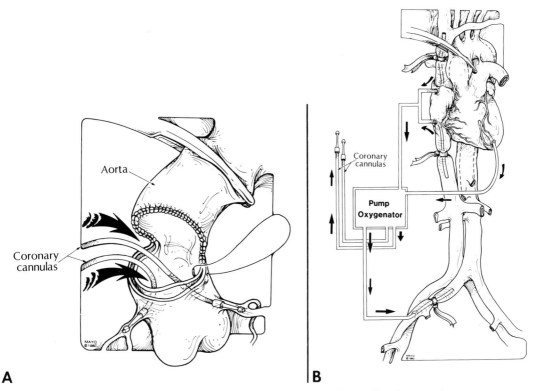

Fig 12–4.—**A,** surgical treatment of type I dissection. **B,** cardiopulmonary bypass with coronary perfusion. (Redrawn from De Bakey et al.[4])

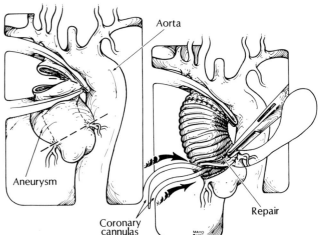

Fig 12–5.—Resection and graft replacement (with the use of cardiopulmonary bypass) in type II dissecting aneurysm. (Redrawn from De Bakey et al.[4])

scending thoracic aorta and can be completely resected.

Anesthetic Management

Patients should come to the operating room well sedated. Electrocardiographic electrodes and a blood pressure cuff are immediately attached to the right arm. The patient should have at least two large No. 14 needles attached to his forearms. Induction can be achieved in a routine manner, with intravenously administered thiopental and pancuronium. Because resection of the dissecting aneurysm is done through a left thoracotomy, the surgical field should be relatively free. A double-lumen tube (either Carlens or Robert Shaw) is used for intubation. It allows the complete elimination of lung movement on the operating side. After intubation, an arterial needle is inserted percutaneously into the right radial artery. Because the left subclavian artery could be clamped during surgery, the placement of a needle into the radial artery on this side would be useless. Catheters to measure central venous pressure also should be placed in a patient with cardiac failure. A balloon-tipped, flow-directed catheter is useful in measuring pulmonary capillary wedge pressure and will lead to more precise management of the cardiac status of the patient. The patient is positioned with the left side up, and one should have easy access to the left femoral artery if the distal portion of the aorta is to be perfused.

After the left side of the chest is opened, the upper lung can be deflated by disconnecting the left lumen of the double-lumen tube, which would allow the lung to collapse. However, this maneuver may cause severe hypoxia because blood shunts through the perfused but not ventilated upper lung. Therefore, checking the blood gases often is mandatory. If the PaO_2 is too low, the upper lung should be ventilated to improve it.

Anesthesia can be maintained with any anesthetic agent. It is most important that blood pressure be kept at preoperative levels.

After clamping the proximal and distal portions of the dissected aorta, adequate circulation can be provided to the distal level of the aortic occlusion by different methods. A left atrium to femoral artery pump bypass (Fig 12–6) can be used. The oxygenated blood is taken from the left atrium through a left atrial cannula. It is then pumped back to the femoral artery, providing perfusion to the distal aorta. However, keeping the cannula in the left atrium can cause technical difficulties, such as a tear of the atrial appendage and slippage of the cannula from the left atrium.

These difficulties led to the use of femoral vein to femoral artery partial bypass with a disposable oxygenator, which technically is more convenient. In this technique, the venous cannula must be inserted all the way up into the inferior vena cava to provide a satisfactory venous return to maintain enough flow through the oxygenator (see chap. 8, Fig 8–6).

Increasing and decreasing the pump speed in either of these techniques also increases or decreases the blood return to the heart, allowing

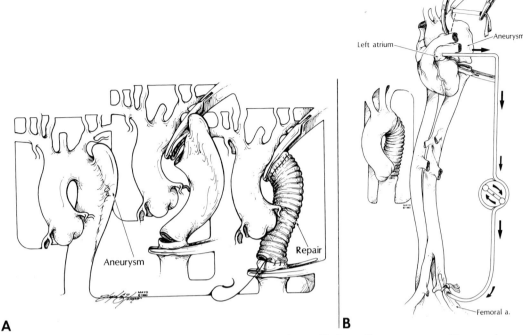

Fig 12-6.—**A,** resection and graft replacement of type III dissecting aneurysm with use of **(B)** left atrium to femoral artery pump bypass. (Redrawn from De Bakey et al.[4])

the anesthesiologist to effectively control preload. Obviously, both of these techniques require the full heparinization of the patient. However, in patients who need extensive vascular resection, systemic heparinization has been blamed for causing massive perioperative bleeding.[5]

Heparin-Coated Vascular Shunts

Generally, major operative procedures of the thoracic aorta and great vessels require the use of some type of temporary vascular bypass. Aneurysms of the descending thoracic aorta and coarctations and traumatic transections of the aorta have been managed surgically by cross-clamping the aorta with or without left heart bypass.[3] Cross-clamping of the descending aorta without rerouting the left ventricular output causes rapid overdistention of the heart and eventual failure. Left ventricular strain is even more disastrous in patients with coronary artery occlusive disease. Cerebral hypertension is also a problem with this method. To prevent these complications and to provide some perfusion distal to the clamping, shunts have been used. Reports regarding the temporary external shunts with or without heparin coating in the tube have been recently published.[3]

The use of tridodecylmethylammonium chloride (TDMAC)-heparin–coated shunts as a temporary bypass during operative procedures on the aorta and great vessels seems to be satisfactory and is a versatile method of accomplishing the two primary aims of temporary arterial bypass, as well as of avoiding the need for systemic heparinization.[5]

The TDMAC-heparin–coated polyvinyl shunt currently used for resection of a thoracic aortic aneurysm is 9 mm by 90 cm and has an indefinite shelf life for thrombus-resistant surface. A smaller shunt (7 mm by 66 cm) is also available.[5]

Placement of Vascular Shunts

After induction of the anesthesia and placement of the right radial arterial cannula and central venous pressure lines, the patient is placed in the right lateral decubitus position. After the left side of the chest is opened and access to the descending thoracic aorta is achieved, one of the three possible sites for proximal insertion of the shunt can be chosen: (1) ascending thoracic aorta, (2) transverse aorta or left subclavian artery (may be unsuitable because the disease process can extend into this region), and (3) apex of the left ventricle[5] (Fig 12-7). After insertion of the proximal shunt, a distal shunt site is selected. The site can be (1) the distal portion of the thoracic aorta, above the diaphragm, (2) the common femoral artery, or (3) the external iliac artery.[5] The distal end is inserted.

The major advantage of the TDMAC-heparin–coated shunt is that it avoids the use of systemic heparin, therefore causing less massive bleeding. Some reports have noted that the difference in bleeding in the nonheparinized patients is striking.[14]

Another method, which uses nonthrombogenic, polyurethane polyvinylgraphite–coated tubing for perfusing the lower half of the body without heparinization, is described by May et al.[14] They simply insert a nonthrombogenic cannula into the right atrium through the femoral vein and return this blood to the femoral artery with the help of a pump and perfuse the lower half of the body with mixed venous blood while the patient is ventilated with 100% oxygen. The P_{O_2} in the mixed venous blood ranges from 34 to 41 mm Hg. They did not see any adverse effects of perfusing the lower part of the body with blood with low P_{O_2}.[14]

Some resections of aneurysms of the thoracic aorta have been done without the help of any of the above techniques. With minimal dissection, normal proximal and distal aortic segments are exposed for clamping between intercostal vessels.[2] Aortic occlusion time in Crawford and associates' report[2] varied from 7 to 64 minutes. During aortic clamping, proximal blood pressure is monitored and hypertension is controlled with narcotics and halothane.[2]

Hemodynamic Effects of Aortic Clamping

The effect of aortic clamping on cardiac function in man has not been defined clearly. One recent study[11] showed that clamping of the proximal descending thoracic aorta in man is associated with a large increase in left ventricular wall stress (afterload) and deterioration in left ventricular function, which may be the result of impaired subendocardial perfusion. However, opening the shunt and decompressing the proximal aorta improve cardiac function, probably because the afterload is reduced, leading to a decrease in myocardial oxygen requirements, and because subendocardial perfusion is increased. For obvious reasons, use of a temporary shunt allows rapid decompression of the proximal aorta without the need for extracorporeal circulatory support.[11] The technique appears to provide substantial protection of the myocardium during aortic clamping, because most of the patients with aneurysms of the aorta die with heart disease either from congestive heart failure or myocardial infarction.[4]

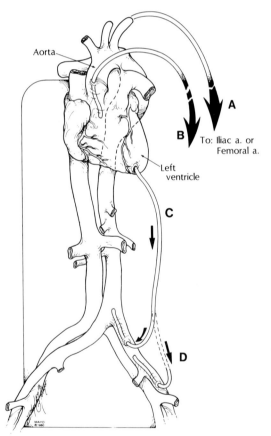

Fig 12–7.—Positions of proximal end of shunt insertions: subclavian artery **(A)**, ascending aorta **(B)**, left ventricle **(C)**, distal cannulation **(D)**. (Redrawn from Donahoo et al.[5])

Spinal Cord Damage After Procedures on the Aorta

Paraplegia is a dreaded complication of excision and graft replacement of aneurysms of the descending thoracic aorta (3% to 5%).[2] This condition can occur during operation, and the patient either does not survive or has a permanent disability afterward.[2] The same disaster also can happen during surgery of the abdominal aorta, resulting in permanent paraplegia. However, the frequency of this is low (0.25%).[20] The most important cause of paraplegia is cord ischemia from the temporary clamping of the aorta. Several methods have been devised to minimize the effects of aortic clamping. As discussed before, these techniques include hypothermia, shunts with or without heparinization, left atrium to femoral artery pump bypass, or femoral vein to femoral artery bypass with pump oxygenation. These techniques probably reduce the problems of ischemic damage to organs distal to clamping, yet paraplegia has not been eliminated by these methods.[2]

Crawford and Rubio[2] operated on 83 patients. In the first 38, various shunts were applied, and in the last 45 patients no shunts were used. One patient in the no-shunt group became paraplegic, compared with three patients in the shunt group. Because shunting does not prevent paraplegia, other factors probably are more important: hypotension, removal of long segments of the aorta, and removal of the aortic segments from which collateral circulation to the spinal cord had not had time to develop.[2]

Blood Supply of the Spinal Cord

The arterial blood supply of the spinal cord in man is segmental (Fig 12–8).[17] Three main arteries traverse the length of the cord: a single anterior spinal artery and two posterior spinal arteries. Preoperatively, the exact anatomy of the anterior spinal artery cannot be determined in a particular patient. As many segmental arteries as possible should be preserved during the aortic resection, either by limited resection of the aorta or by careful reattachment of the major intercostal or lumbar arteries to the graft when major thoracic aortic resection is performed.[17]

Postoperative Hemorrhage

Immediate postoperative hemorrhage is a frequent complication of major reconstruction of thoracic aneurysms. Hemorrhage at the suture line is frequent and can easily exsanguinate the patient. Hemodilution, hypothermia, and long cardiopulmonary bypass time greatly alter the coagulation system. Therefore, blood components should be available for immediate administration as soon as cardiopulmonary bypass is discontinued and protamine sulfate has been administered. Blood component therapy is discussed in chapter 20. Repeated tests for coagulation factors are essential, and component therapy should be guided by the results of these tests.

TRAUMATIC RUPTURED THORACIC AORTA

General Remarks

Transection of the thoracic aorta secondary to blunt trauma is a life-threatening condition that requires early diagnosis and treatment. Rupture of the aorta with nonpenetrating trauma is now accepted as a clinical entity.[21] Approximately 60% of deaths after high-speed deceleration accidents are associated with aortic trauma. Tears of the aorta are located in the ascending aorta (23%), aortic arch (8%), descending aorta (12.7%, isthmus not included), abdominal aorta (4.7%), and multiple areas (6%). The most frequent area of rupture (45%) is the aortic isthmus.[16] Ruptures other than the isthmus are usually fatal because of massive exsanguination. Tears at the isthmus may become stabilized by adventitia and pleura. The patient may survive until medical treatment is available.[21]

Therefore, the diagnosis of these injuries in the emergency room should be based on a high degree of suspicion and physical findings. The most important diagnostic tool is the posteroanterior chest roentgenogram. It may reveal widened mediastinum, blurring of the aortic knob, tracheal deviation, and depression of the left main-stem bronchus. Aortography provides a definite diagnosis and is necessary to guide the optimal surgical approach. In our institution, we use retrograde femoral aortography. Aortography should include both the thoracic and abdominal segments of the aorta, because multiple aortic injuries may exist simultaneously.

Although these injuries occur mostly in young healthy adults,[9] the mortality for these patients who undergo surgery is still high (20%). The surgical mortality for patients with ruptured arteriosclerotic aneurysms is 50%.

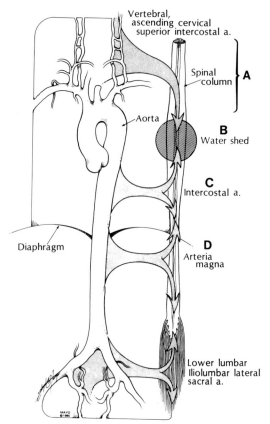

Fig 12–8.—Arterial supply of spinal cord. **A,** cervical and upper thoracic cord supplied by radicular branches of vertebral, ascending cervical, and superior intercostal arteries. **B,** watershed. **C,** midthoracic cord supplied from a single intercostal artery. **D,** thoracolumbar region supplied by a large vessel near diaphragm, and cauda equina supplied from lower lumbar, iliolumbar, and lateral sacral arteries. (Redrawn from Pasternak et al.[17])

Induction and Maintenance of Anesthesia

Anesthetic management of these patients is not substantially different from that of patients with ruptured or dissected arteriosclerotic thoracic aneurysms. Induction and maintenance of anesthesia in these patients have been discussed previously in detail. There is no agreement on the use of a shunt or of an atrial-femoral pump or oxygenator after the aorta is cross-clamped during repair. All methods have been used with equal success.[2] Simple aortic cross-clamping also has been tried, but it has the theoretical disadvantages of left heart overload with upper extremity hypertension and ischemia of the lower body, causing visceral organ damage and spinal cord ischemia. Yet, the method avoids the use of systemic heparinization (such heparinization being associated with high mortality and morbidity[21] because it may cause excessive bleeding in patients with multiple injuries, which is common among these patients).

Another method of avoiding total heparinization is to use a TDMAC-heparin–coated cannula, which is nonthrombogenic. One end of the shunt is inserted into the aortic lumen above the cross-clamp, and the other end is inserted into the distal aortic lumen. The distal delivery of blood, driven by proximal aortic pressure, prevents an increase in afterload and hypertension caused by cross-clamping of the aorta. However, paraplegia still can occur with this method (3% to 5%).[2, 10] If reconstruction of the descending aorta is attempted with simple cross-clamping, no more than 30 minutes of cross-clamping should be used.[21] Hypertension of the upper extremities can be controlled with the use of a vasodilator drug, such as sodium nitroprusside.

REFERENCES

1. Chu S.-H., et al.: Resection of aneurysm of the aortic arch without cardiopulmonary bypass. *J. Thorac. Cardiovasc. Surg.* 74:928, 1977.
2. Crawford E.S., Rubio P.A.: Reappraisal of adjuncts to avoid ischemia in the treatment of aneurysms of descending thoracic aorta. *J. Thorac. Cardiovasc. Surg.* 66:693, 1973.
3. Cukingnan R.A., Fee H.J., Carey J.S.: Repair of lesions of the descending thoracic aorta with the TDMAC-heparin shunt. *J. Thorac. Cardiovasc. Surg.* 75:227, 1978.
4. De Bakey M.E., et al.: Surgical management of dissecting aneurysms of the aorta. *J. Thorac. Cardiovasc. Surg.* 49:130, 1965.
5. Donahoo J.S., Brawley R.K., Gott V.L.: The heparin-coated vascular shunt for thoracic aortic and great vessel procedures: A ten-year experience. *Ann. Thorac. Surg.* 23:507, 1977.
6. Griepp R.B., et al.: Prosthetic replacement of the aortic arch. *J. Thorac. Cardiovasc. Surg.* 70:1051, 1975.
7. Inoue T., et al.: Surgical treatment of the aortic aneurysm. *Jpn. J. Surg.* 8:86, 1978.
8. Kampmeier R.H.: Saccular aneurysm of the thoracic aorta: A clinical study of 633 cases. *Ann. Intern. Med.* 12:624, 1938.
9. Katz S.: Traumatic rupture of the thoracic aorta. *J. Maine Med. Assoc.* 68:304, 1977.

CEREBRAL BLOOD FLOW.—The classic technique for measuring cerebral blood flow has been described by Kety and Schmidt.[16] Nitrous oxide is breathed to equilibration, and samples from the carotid artery and jugular vein are used to quantitate flow by appropriate integration procedures. In clinical practice and the clinical research laboratory, the cerebral blood flow is usually measured by radioisotopes, external counting devices, and computer integrative functions.[18]

The clinical use of measurements of cerebral blood flow during carotid endarterectomy can provide useful information and at the same time remain relatively uncomplicated, although the tests are expensive. Our system uses ^{133}Xe as the radioisotope, a single sodium iodide scintillation detector, and a small computer with a digital readout.[28] The detector is mounted on a Zeiss operating microscope stand and is positioned over the hand and face area of the motor strip before the operation is begun. With the external carotid artery occluded, 200 μCi of ^{133}Xe in 0.4 ml of isotonic saline are rapidly injected through a 27-gauge needle into the internal carotid artery. As the β particles penetrate the skull and reach the detector, the light energy in the crystal is electrically converted to counts per minute. The computer calculates the cerebral blood flow from the initial slope of the washout curve (Fig 13–1), and the digital readout shows the rate of cerebral blood flow within one minute after injection.

The nasal plethysmograph is a small, light-emitting diode device that can be inserted into the nose to measure pulsations in the nasal circulation. Theoretically, the anterior ethmoidal artery pulsations might be directly related to the pulsations in the distal internal carotid artery during carotid artery occlusion. We studied 19 patients undergoing carotid endarterectomy with simultaneous EEG monitoring and cerebral blood flow determinations by ^{133}Xe washout. When comparing the percent change in pulse height from the nasal plethysmograph with the percent change in cerebral blood flow, there was little correlation between the two. Besides failing to estimate reductions in cerebral blood flow, the nasal plethysmograph failed to identify patients with critically low cerebral blood flows producing EEG changes of ischemia. We believe that this lack of correlation is due to the rich arterial anastomotic network of the face and nose.

STUMP PRESSURE MEASUREMENT.—The arterial blood pressure in the distal end of the occluded carotid artery can be easily determined by standard direct arterial pressure measurement systems. This back pressure from the cephalad portion of the carotid artery has been called the internal carotid artery "stump" pressure. Numerous attempts have been made to correlate stump pressure with the need for a shunt during carotid artery surgery. However, pressure measurement cannot be expected to correlate accurately with flow in any situation that involves a variable resistance. Anesthetics can and do effect changes in cerebral vascular resistance.

A correlation of stump pressure, regional cerebral blood flow, and the EEG has been noted

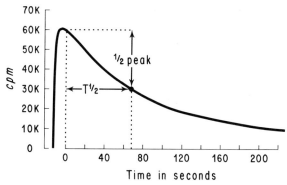

Fig 13–1.—Typical cerebral blood flow curve after intra-arterial injection of xenon 133 into internal carotid artery. Cerebral blood flow is determined by dividing 3,600 by the time in seconds for curve to fall to one half its peak value. Cerebral blood flow = 3,600/65 = 55.5 ml/100 gm/minute. Kilocounts (1,000 counts, K). (From Sundt et al.[26] Used by permission.)

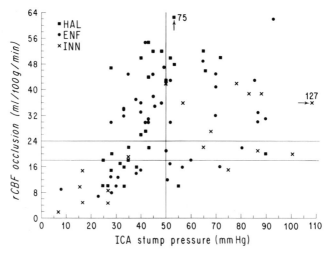

Fig 13-2.—Scattergram of regional cerebral blood flow *(rCBF)* during occlusion plotted against internal carotid artery *(ICA)* stump pressures. Vertical line represents stump pressure of 50 mm Hg (considered the critical level). Two horizontal lines represent critical flow level (rCBF≤18 ml/100 gm/minute) and marginal zone (rCBF 28 to 24 ml/100 gm/minute). Halothane *(HAL)*, enflurane *(ENF)*, Innovar (droperidol-fentanyl) *(INN)*.

in patients undergoing carotid endarterectomy[19] (Fig 13-2). Of 35 patients with stump pressures of >50 mm Hg, 7 had low regional cerebral blood flow of less than 18 ml/100 gm/minute. Four of the 7 patients had EEG changes of ischemia, and 3 did not. However, an internal carotid artery shunt was placed in all 7 patients before waiting for EEG changes to occur. Thus, about 4% of the patients with stump pressures greater than 50 mm Hg in that study still needed a shunt (Fig 13-3). These patients with "missed shunts" might be expected to have a poor surgical outcome without a shunt. However, 28% of the patients with stump pressures less than 50 mm Hg would be subjected to a needless shunt and to the risk of embolic complications even though their regional cerebral blood flow was adequate (>18 ml/100 gm/minute). Thus, stump pressure does not always correlate positively with regional cerebral blood flow and EEG signs of ischemia. These data indicate that if a stump pressure of 60 mm Hg

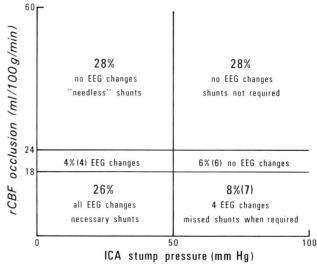

Fig 13-3.—Modification and interpretation of data in Figure 13-2 to correlate regional cerebral blood flow *(rCBF)*, internal carotid artery *(ICA)* stump pressure, EEG, and "need" for ICA shunt.

were used as a guide for shunt placement, more "needless" shunts would be placed and only three "missed" shunts would have occurred (none of which had EEG changes during the time required to place the shunt).

INTRAOPERATIVE EEG.—The use of continuous EEG recordings during carotid artery surgery has aided in the detection of cerebral ischemic episodes during carotid artery occlusion. A 16-channel EEG can be used, with recording beginning before the induction of anesthesia and extending through the emergence. During anesthesia, two basic patterns can be seen: a symmetric pattern, and an asymmetric pattern with a persistent delta focus from a previous neurologic deficit.[26] A pattern of sustained rhythmic activity of 10 to 24 Hz is sought by using light levels of inhalation anesthesia. Slower activity of 2 to 6 Hz appears as anesthesia is deepened.

Major focal EEG changes occur in 15% to 20% of the patients undergoing carotid endarterectomy.[8, 26] The severity of the changes closely parallels the relative reduction in cerebral blood flow. In patients with very low values for regional cerebral blood flow, the EEG changes are more severe and of more rapid onset. The EEG changes are consistent. Faster background frequencies are first replaced by higher-amplitude Θ components and then by lower-amplitude Δ components. In extreme situations, the residual EEG activity is reduced to low-voltage irregular Δ activity with total absence of faster background components. The changes are usually unilateral and occur in nearly all patients with a regional cerebral blood flow less than 18 ml/100 gm/minute. After placement of a shunt, the focal EEG changes resolve in from two to seven minutes (Fig 13–4). Persistent EEG changes due to emboli during surgery also can occur.

Intraoperative EEG monitoring not only involves complicated equipment but also requires highly skilled personnel to interpret the recordings. Because of this, such monitoring has not gained wide acceptance in the operating room. Modern electronics can provide EEG data in various processed forms. The compressed spectrum analysis and cerebral function monitor (CFM) are examples. A processed EEG signal, which can simplify identification of a pattern indicative of cerebral ischemia, may be a useful operating room monitor during carotid endarterectomy.

The CFM is a one-channel EEG filter-processor (Fig 13–5). The efficacy of this device in detecting hemispheric cerebral ischemia during carotid artery occlusion was compared with that

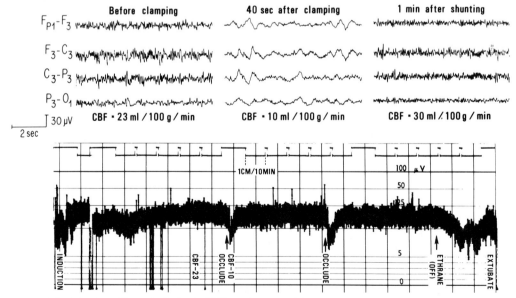

Fig 13–4.—Changes in both EEG and cerebral function monitor with low regional cerebral blood flow (CBF) during left carotid artery occlusion. (From Cucchiara et al.[8] Used by permission.)

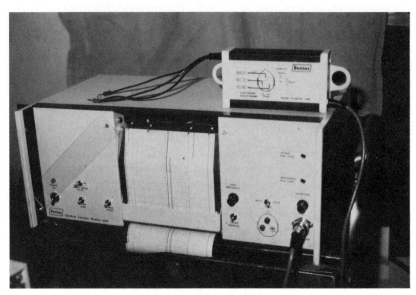

Fig 13-5.—Cerebral function monitor manufactured by Devices Limited, 501 George St., New Brunswick, NJ 08903.

of the standard 16-channel EEG in a study of ^{133}Xe washout determinations of regional cerebral blood flow in a series of 70 patients undergoing carotid endarterectomy.[8] Bilateral lead placement was ineffective in detecting ischemic changes in 15 patients. Unilateral lead placement over the hemisphere supplied by the diseased carotid artery greatly improved the unit's sensitivity in 55 patients. With both CFM recording electrodes over the affected hemisphere, neither the EEG nor the CFM changed in 44 of 55 patients (Table 13-2). In 11 patients, EEG changes and measurements of regional cerebral blood flow indicated cerebral ischemia during carotid artery clamping; the CFM baseline decreased in 9 of the 11. The 2 patients in whom the CFM did not change had only a loss of higher frequency waves (10 to 15 Hz) from the standard 16-channel EEG. The values for regional cerebral blood flow were 7 and 15 ml/100 gm/min in these patients.

Some changes in CFM tracing during changing anesthetic depth were similar to those obtained during hemispheric ischemia. Maintenance of a steady level of anesthesia during carotid artery occlusion was necessary to clearly interpret the CFM tracing. The following conclusions were drawn: (1) Bilateral symmetric application of the CFM leads was inadequate for detecting hemispheric cerebral ischemia during carotid endarterectomy. (2) The CFM with unilateral lead placement was not as sensitive as the combination of the 16-channel EEG and regional cerebral blood flow measurement in the detection of cerebral ischemia. (The CFM, however, did identify cerebral ischemia in those patients in whom obvious EEG changes occurred, but it was inadequate to detect subtle EEG changes of ischemia.) (3) Changes in the CFM tracing due to changing anesthetic depth can resemble very closely those seen with cerebral ischemia during carotid artery clamping (thus, anesthetic level must be steady during this part of the operation). (4) A diagnosis of hemispheric ischemia in the setting of this clinical situation could be made from the CFM tracing *only* at carotid artery occlusion.

"CRITICAL" HUMAN CEREBRAL BLOOD FLOW

The tolerance of human nervous tissue to ischemia is difficult to study. From such attempts, however, has evolved the concept of "critical" cerebral blood flow in man. The critical cerebral blood flow is that flow below which cerebral ischemia occurs. The brain can tolerate considerable reduction in cerebral blood flow

TABLE 13–2.—EEG AND CEREBRAL FUNCTION MONITOR (CFM) CHANGES AT CAROTID ARTERY OCCLUSION IN ELECTIVE CAROTID ENDARTERECTOMY*

OCCLUSION CHANGES	NO. OF PATIENTS	REGIONAL CEREBRAL BLOOD FLOW <18 ML/100 GM/ MIN
In both EEG and CFM	9	9
In EEG without CFM changes	2	2
In neither EEG nor CFM	44	3
Total	55	14

*Internal carotid artery shunt used in all patients with regional cerebral blood flow less than 18 ml/100 gm/minute.

without metabolic or functional disturbance. Even a very low cerebral blood flow, one that produces functional neurologic deficit, can be tolerated for short periods, with subsequent return of function. Because there is no surgical technique for carotid endarterectomy that does not require temporary occlusion of the carotid artery, patients undergoing this procedure are candidates for evaluation of cerebral blood flow during this period. Ultimately, determination of this critical flow depends on the ability to detect critical regional metabolic states in the brain.

The EEG has been used as an indirect measure of reduced regional supply of cerebral oxygen. With the use of the EEG in patients undergoing carotid artery clamping, significant information about critical flow levels has been obtained.[2, 8, 19, 27] Some patients can tolerate a reduction of cerebral blood flow to below 30 ml/100 gm/minute for 20 minutes. A critical flow of 20 ml/100 gm/minute during nitrous oxide–halothane anesthesia with normocarbia has been tolerated.[2] Below this cerebral blood flow, EEG changes of ischemia occur within 5 to 10 minutes, as reported by Boysen et al.[2] Regional cerebral blood flow above 24 ml/100 gm/minute did not result in EEG changes, but flow reductions to less than 18 ml/100 gm/minute were associated with EEG changes of ischemia in more than 100 patients undergoing carotid endarterectomy. Flows between 18 and 24 ml/100 gm/minute were variably adequate.[27] Thus, a critical cerebral blood flow level of approximately 20 ml/100 gm/minute in man is an experimentally supported figure, at least during inhalation anesthesia and normocarbia.

ANESTHETIC TECHNIQUE

Agents

Inhalation

HALOTHANE.—The halogenated hydrocarbons have evolved as the most useful inhalation agents. Halothane has gained wide acceptance as a rapidly acting, well-tolerated inhalation anesthetic. It is both a cerebral vasodilator and a bronchodilator. Halothane has been proved to be useful in providing light levels of anesthesia for the patient undergoing carotid endarterectomy without undue myocardial depression and without reducing the readability of the EEG monitoring systems. Halothane has been implicated in the entity of halothane-associated hepatitis, but the risk to a patient undergoing carotid endarterectomy of developing halothane-associated hepatitis is extremely small. Halothane, placed in the proper perspective, is a suitable agent for carotid artery surgery, especially because it is a cerebral vasodilator.

ENFLURANE.—As one of the newer halogenated inhalation anesthetics, enflurane has proved to be useful, safe, and versatile. It has the desirable property of cerebral vasodilation. Under certain clinical circumstances, enflurane can be a convulsant. Dogs anesthetized with deep enflurane anesthesia under hypocarbic conditions demonstrate spiked patterns on their EEG and, with an auditory stimulus, can demonstrate grand mal seizure activity. This seizure activity is identical in motor activity and effects on cerebral blood flow and metabolic rate for oxygen to that produced by pentylenetetrazol.[20] Such spike activity under deep enflurane anesthesia with hypocarbia has been demonstrated in human beings.[22] Abnormal EEGs may be noted weeks after the anesthetic in patients who have had a seizure while under enflurane anesthesia.[4]

An examination of the EEGs of more than 200 patients undergoing carotid endarterectomy under light levels of enflurane anesthesia with normocarbia has revealed no episodes of spike activity during the anesthesia. The EEG data on patients before, during, and after carotid artery surgery (Table 13–3) did not show a significant difference in postoperative worsening of the EEG after enflurane anesthesia as compared with halothane or droperidol-fentanyl (Innovar) anesthesia (see Table 13–3). Thus, the risk of seizures during light enflurane anesthesia with normocarbia probably is extremely small, as is the risk of abnormal encephalographic changes after light levels of enflurane anesthesia.

Intravenous

Intravenously administered anesthetics generally are cerebral vasoconstrictors and have variable effects on the cerebral metabolic rate for oxygen.

THIOPENTAL.—Even though sodium thiopental is a cerebral vasoconstrictor and can reduce cerebral blood flow to half its control value, it is also an extremely effective drug in reducing cerebral metabolic rate for oxygen.[7] The decrease in cerebral blood flow and metabolic rate for oxygen are concomitant and do not appear to jeopardize the patient who has limited cerebral circulation. In fact, sodium thiopental is a cerebral protective agent in some situations of cerebral ischemia. Therefore, it is a logical and useful intravenous induction agent for a patient undergoing carotid endarterectomy.

DROPERIDOL-FENTANYL.—The cerebral vasoconstrictive effects of droperidol-fentanyl result in higher stump pressures, with correspondingly low cerebral blood flow values[19] (Fig 13–6). This finding indicates that the cerebrovascular resistance is increased by the drug. It reduces the cerebral metabolic rate for oxygen but only by 10% to 15%.[12] Droperidol-fentanyl is thus a potent cerebral vasoconstrictor that produces only a mild reduction in the cerebral metabolic rate for oxygen. This evidence of cerebral vasoconstrictive effects provides our primary reasoning for not using this agent in carotid artery surgery.

KETAMINE.—Although cerebral blood flow is increased during ketamine anesthesia, the cerebral metabolic rate for oxygen is also increased.[9] Because the metabolic rate might be increased in a localized area of the brain beyond the ability of the vasculature to supply that part of the brain with increased blood flow, ketamine might be expected to aggravate a cerebral ischemic episode. While the blood pressure is well maintained during anesthesia with ketamine, emergence from ketamine anesthesia does not always allow proper neurologic evaluation of the patient immediately after completion of the surgery.

Muscle Relaxants

Intubation

Either depolarizing or nondepolarizing muscle relaxants can be used for intubation of the patient undergoing carotid endarterectomy. Care must be exercised in the use of succinylcholine in the hemiplegic patient because of the possibility of producing hyperkalemia and subsequent cardiac arrest.[6] Pancuronium bromide at a dose of 0.1 to 0.15 mg/kg is a useful nondepolarizing muscle relaxant for intubation. Pulse rate increases after the intravenous administration of pancuronium, and a normal sinus tachycardia may be converted to atrial flutter requiring digitalization and treatment with propranolol. For the EEG to be used as a monitoring device, the anesthetic level must be light to achieve the appropriate tracing. This effect requires the use of a maintenance muscle relaxant to ensure a quiet surgical field. Our choice is pancuronium; however, in special situations of labile hypertension, d-tubocurare or metocurine may be useful substitutes.

Anesthetic Depth

Because the blood pressure should be maintained at normal preoperative levels and because EEG recording is conducted, light levels of inhalation anesthesia are preferred. We prefer use of normocarbia during general anesthesia for carotid endarterectomy because of the prin-

TABLE 13–3.—EEG FINDINGS ASSOCIATED WITH VARIOUS ANESTHETIC AGENTS BEFORE, DURING, AND AFTER CAROTID ENDARTERECTOMY*

EEG	DROPERIDOL-FENTANYL		HALOTHANE		ENFLURANE		TOTAL
	NO.	CHANGE	NO.	CHANGE	NO.	CHANGE	
Unchanged preop to postop	15	...	26	...	42	...	83
Changed preop to postop	3	Dys I to Asym I Dys I to normal Dys II to Asym I	3	Normal to Dys III† Normal to Dys II Dys I to Dys III‡	1	Normal to Dys II	7
Total	18		29		43		90

*Abbreviations are as follows: Dys, dysrhythmia; Asym, asymmetry.
†Clinical stroke.
‡After emergency reoperation.

ciple that the patient can maintain cerebral blood flow at normocarbia while awake, and therefore he will not be compromised by normocarbia while asleep. Hypocarbia has been advocated by some for carotid artery surgery in the hope that the normal cerebrovasculature would constrict in response to the reduced PCO_2 and would shunt more flow to the ischemic area. Hypercarbia has been advocated in the hope of increasing cerebral blood flow to the entire brain, although it has been realized recently that this increase may reduce the flow to a specific ischemic area. Studies on cerebral blood flow in man at varying PCO_2 values have indicated that the flow response of an ischemic area of brain to altered PCO_2 cannot be predicted accurately in the individual patient.

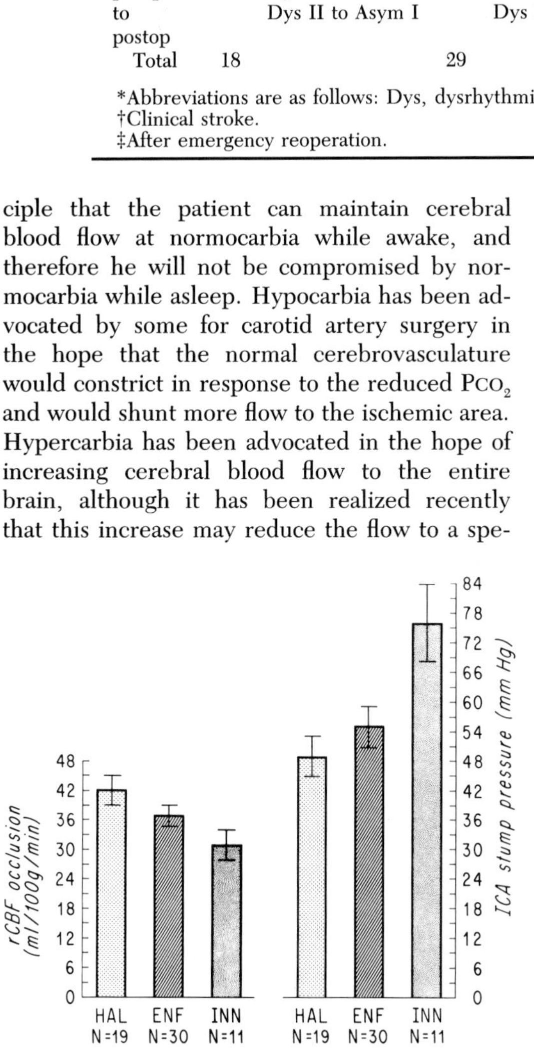

The lowest preoperative pressure at which the patient is asymptomatic should be the lower limit of acceptable pressure during surgery. In general, the blood pressure is maintained at least at the preoperative minimum, and in the presence of low cerebral blood flow during occlusion, the blood pressure may be increased 20% with the use of phenylephrine. Hypovolemia must be avoided. Therefore, early transfusion with blood or colloid in the patient undergoing carotid endarterectomy is important. These patients may have reduced blood volumes from being bedridden or from hypertension, even though their hematocrit and hemoglobin levels may be adequate. The lack of appropriate transfusion during surgery may result in hypovolemia and acute hypotension during the immediate postoperative period.

Fig 13–6.—Inverse relationships of occlusion regional cerebral blood flow (rCBF) and stump pressure with halothane (HAL), enflurane (ENF), and droperidol-fentanyl (Innovar [INN]) in patients with rCBF values more than 18 ml/100 gm/minute. (From McKay et al.[19] Used by permission.)

RECOMMENDATIONS

Our preferred anesthetic technique for carotid endarterectomy includes light levels of inhalation anesthesia, normocarbia, and the use of a maintenance muscle relaxant. Other techniques have been advocated by others.[11, 14, 23] In our experience the most sensitive system for monitoring the CNS in regard to focal cerebral ischemia has been a 16-channel EEG and determinations of regional cerebral blood flow. This system is generally not widely available in the operating theater. A monitoring system composed of measurements of stump pressure and an EEG processor (for example, the CFM) appears to be a commercial monitoring system that could be expected to provide reliable sensitivity to cerebral ischemic episodes but with somewhat more limited selectivity. Since such a system of cerebral monitoring is still moderately elaborate, the surgeon and anesthesiologist may decide to forego a cerebral monitoring system in an attempt to provide pharmacologic protection to the brain if ischemia occurs during carotid artery occlusion. In this situation the use of sodium thiopental as a cerebral protective agent probably would help decrease the morbidity from cerebral ischemia during a limited period of carotid artery occlusion. A dose of thiopental sufficient to produce burst suppression should be ideal in this regard; however, such a dose might produce unacceptable hypotension. Clinically, a "sleep" dose of thiopental might be used just before carotid crossclamping.

Advances in anesthetic and surgical management of patients undergoing carotid endarterectomy can be expected to be made in the field of improved monitoring of the CNS during the procedure and in the field of cerebral pharmacologic protection.

REFERENCES

1. Allen E.V.: Thromboangiitis obliterans: Methods of diagnosis of chronic occlusive arterial lesions distal to the wrist with illustrative cases. Am. J. Med. Sci. 178:237, 1929.
2. Boysen G., et al.: On the critical lower level of cerebral blood flow in man with particular reference to carotid surgery, editorial. Circulation 49:1023, 1974.
3. Browne T.R. III, Poskanzer D.C.: Treatment of strokes. N. Engl. J. Med. 281:594, 1969.
4. Burchiel K.J., et al.: Relationship of pre- and postanesthetic EEG abnormalities to enflurane-induced seizure activity. Anesth. Analg. 56:509, 1977.
5. Cervantes F.D., Schneiderman L.J.: Anticoagulants in cerebrovascular disease: A critical review of studies. Arch. Intern. Med. 135:875, 1975.
6. Cooperman L.H., Strobel G.E. Jr., Kennell E.M.: Massive hyperkalemia after administration of succinylcholine. Anesthesiology 32:161, 1970.
7. Cucchiara R.F., Michenfelder J.D.: The effect of interruption of the reticular activating system on metabolism in canine cerebral hemispheres before and after thiopental. Anesthesiology 39:3, 1973.
8. Cucchiara R.F., et al.: An electroencephalographic filter-processor as an indicator of cerebral ischemia during carotid endarterectomy. Anesthesiology 51:77, 1979.
9. Dawson B., Michenfelder J.D., Theye R.A.: Effects of ketamine on canine cerebral blood flow and metabolism: Modification by prior administration of thiopental. Anesth. Analg. 50:443, 1971.
10. Easton J.D., Sherman D.G.: Stroke and mortality rate in carotid endarterectomy: 228 consecutive operations. Stroke 8:565, 1977.
11. Fitch W.: Anaesthesia for carotid artery surgery. Br. J. Anaesth. 48:791, 1976.
12. Fitch W., et al.: The influence of neuroleptanalgesic drugs on cerebrospinal fluid pressure. Br. J. Anaesth. 41:800, 1969.
13. Frank G.: Comparison of anticoagulation and surgical treatments of TIA: A review and consolidation of recent natural history and treatment studies. Stroke 2:369, 1971.
14. Geevarghese K.P., Patel T.C.: Anesthesia and surgical treatment of cerebrovascular insufficiency. Int. Anesthesiol. Clin. 15:57, Fall, 1977.
15. Kaplan J.A., King S.B. III: The precordial electrocardiographic lead (V_5) in patients who have coronary-artery disease. Anesthesiology 45:570, 1976.
16. Kety S.S., Schmidt C.F.: The effects of altered arterial tensions of carbon dioxide and oxygen on cerebral blood flow and cerebral oxygen consumption of normal young men. J. Clin. Invest. 27:484, 1948.
17. Larson C.P. Jr., et al.: Jugular venous oxygen saturation as an index of adequacy of cerebral oxygenation. Surgery 62:31, 1967.
18. Lassen N.A.: Control of cerebral circulation in health and disease. Circ. Res. 34:749, 1974.
19. McKay R.D., et al.: Internal carotid artery stump pressure and cerebral blood flow during carotid endarterectomy: Modification by halothane, enflurane, and Innovar. Anesthesiology 45:390, 1976.
20. Michenfelder J.D., Cucchiara R.F.: Canine cerebral oxygen consumption during enflurane anesthesia and its modification during induced seizures. Anesthesiology 40:575, 1974.
21. Millikan C.H.: Anticoagulant or surgical treatment of cerebral ischemia, in Ingelfinger F.J., et al. (eds.): Controversy in Internal Medicine: II. Philadelphia, W.B. Saunders Co., 1974, p. 787.
22. Rosén I., Söderberg M.: Electroencephalo-

graphic activity in children under enflurane anesthesia. *Acta Anaesthesiol. Scand.* 19:361, 1975.
23. Smith A.L., Wollman H.: Cerebral blood flow and metabolism: Effects of anesthetic drugs and techniques. *Anesthesiology* 36:378, 1972.
24. Sublett J.W., Seidenberg A.B., Hobson R.W., II: Internal carotid artery stump pressures during regional anesthesia. *Anesthesiology* 41:505, 1974.
25. Sundt T.M. Jr., Sandok B.A., Whisnant J.P.: Carotid endarterectomy: Complications and preoperative assessment of risk. *Mayo Clin. Proc.* 50:301, 1975.
26. Sundt T.M. Jr., et al.: Monitoring techniques for carotid endarterectomy. *Clin. Neurosurg.* 22:199, 1975.
27. Waltz A.G., Sundt T.M. Jr., Michenfelder J.D.: Cerebral blood flow during carotid endarterectomy. *Circulation* 45:1091, 1972.
28. Waltz A.G., Wanek A.R., Anderson R.E.: Comparison of analytic methods for calculation of cerebral blood flow after intracarotid injection of ^{133}Xe. *J. Nucl. Med.* 13:66, 1972.

14 / Myocardial Preservation

GLENN A. FROMME
ROGER D. WHITE

ISCHEMIC HEART DISEASE is the most frequent cause of morbidity and mortality in the United States. Each year, more than 600,000 persons die of complications of ischemic heart disease and more than 1 million new myocardial infarctions occur. Because complications of myocardial infarction, such as arrhythmias and congestive heart failure, appear to be related to the size of the infarct, it is important to safeguard as large a mass of viable myocardium as is possible. This holds true for the patient undergoing cardiac surgery, as well as for the patient suffering an acute infarction. The former group of patients presents the more complex problem because of the severity of the insult that occurs during operations on such a vital structure. This chapter reviews the metabolic changes that occur in the heart with ischemia, examines some of the various interventions that protect the myocardium during acute ischemia, and discusses the techniques involved in protecting the myocardium during operations on the heart.

MYOCARDIAL CHANGES OCCURRING WITH ISCHEMIA

Myocardial preservation is fundamentally a matter of supply versus demand. If myocardial oxygen demands are not met by the oxygen supply, anaerobic metabolism, ischemia, and infarction occur. Myocardial oxygen demand is determined by heart rate, preload, afterload, and the inotropic state, whereas oxygen supply is determined by oxygen saturation, Po_2, hemoglobin concentration, and regional coronary blood flow. Changes in any of these factors can shift the ratio of supply versus demand either favorably or adversely and, in the marginally compensated situation, may make the difference between normal metabolism and ischemia.

With ischemia, various metabolic and functional changes occur. First, myocardial oxygen supply is rapidly depleted. Myocardial oxygen supply is totally expended in approximately 8 seconds as tissue Po_2 decreases below 5 mm Hg.[24] Then, there is a brief burst of accelerated glycolysis, which decreases quickly to well below control levels. Adenosine triphosphate and phosphocreatine levels rapidly decrease. Because anaerobic metabolism ensues, lactic acid accumulates, and the resulting intracellular acidosis serves to further depress glycolysis by interfering with several key enzymes in the glycolytic pathway. Fatty acid oxidation, which supplies the heart with most of its energy in the normal state, is also impaired because of reduction in the activity of carnitine palmityl coenzyme A[48]—a mitochondrial enzyme that is important in fatty acid oxidation.

This process occurs quickly after the onset of ischemia. After about 15 minutes, levels of adenosine triphosphate are decreased to 60% of their preischemic levels, and phosphocreatine levels, which are essential for the transfer of a phosphoryl group to adenosine diphosphate for the regeneration of adenosine triphosphate, are reduced to between 5% and 10% of preischemic levels.[26] With reperfusion after 15 minutes of ischemia, there are rapid increases in phosphocreatine levels to 150% of normal, and a more gradual return of adenosine triphosphate and glycogen levels to normal. These changes correspond closely with the return of normal conduction and contractility. However, with more extended periods of ischemia and greater decrease in high-energy phosphate levels, the return to normal levels during reperfusion becomes increasingly prolonged. These metabolic changes correlate closely with decreased functional recovery.[15]

INTERVENTIONS AFFECTING MYOCARDIAL PRESERVATION

Interventions Increasing Ischemia

Because ischemia results from oxygen demands that are unsatisfied by oxygen supply, any intervention that increases oxygen demand or decreases oxygen supply is detrimental. Myocardial oxygen demands, and therefore ischemic damage, are increased by inotropic drugs, primarily isoproterenol, by digitalis in the nonfailing heart, by all other catecholamines, and by hypertension and hyperthermia. Also, anemia, hypoxemia, and decreased myocardial perfusion increase ischemic injury by hampering the delivery of oxygen.

In global ischemia, isoproterenol causes rapid deterioration.[29] In regional ischemia, however, the effects vary. In severely ischemic areas, function deteriorates, whereas moderately ischemic and normal areas show functional improvement by increasing blood supply in these areas. However, infarct size has been shown to increase with isoproterenol use in dogs with experimental coronary artery occlusion.[29] Digitalis increases oxygen consumption only in the nonfailing heart. In the failing heart, it improves myocardial performance and decreases ventricular chamber size, which reduces ventricular wall tension (afterload) and therefore decreases oxygen consumption.

Coronary artery perfusion can decrease in various ways. The most common is from gradual narrowing of a coronary artery from coronary atherosclerosis. Because coronary artery perfusion is dependent on systemic diastolic pressure, during hypotensive conditions a seemingly insignificant coronary lesion could also result in regional ischemia.

Various drugs cause coronary vasodilatation that, under conditions of regional ischemia, may shunt blood away from the ischemic region. This shunting occurs because arteries in the ischemic region are already maximally dilated, owing to metabolic factors, and the increased flow therefore is diverted to the normal areas of myocardium, resulting in an actual decrease in flow to the ischemic region. Nitroprusside is one of these drugs and has been shown experimentally to increase infarct size.[6]

Interventions Decreasing Ischemia

Many factors favorably affect the amount of ischemic injury. Basically, these interventions either increase oxygen supply or decrease demand. Some of the factors, whose efficacies are unproved, are considered to be effective by increasing available substrate for anaerobic metabolism, thus preserving high-energy compounds, or by protecting against destruction of cells. A list of interventions that decrease myocardial ischemia (modified from Hillis and Braunwald[19]) is as follows:

By decreasing oxygen demands
    Adrenergic blockade
    Digitalis in the failing heart
    Afterload reduction
By increasing oxygen supply
    Increase arterial oxygenation
        Correcting anemia
        Increasing P_{O_2}
    Increase coronary perfusion
        Adrenergic stimulation
        Intra-aortic balloon counterpulsation
        Pharmacologic agents that increase regional coronary flow (heparin, nitroglycerin, mannitol, hyaluronidase), dipyridamole
By increasing substrate utilization
    Glucose, glucose–insulin–potassium chloride, adenosine triphosphate, phosphocreatine
By protecting against cellular destruction
    Steroids
    Cobra venom factor
    Aprotinin

Interventions Decreasing Oxygen Demands

In patients with ischemic heart disease, perfusion to the ischemic region is relatively fixed. Therefore, the most effective way to change the supply-demand relationship favorably is to decrease oxygen demands. This change is achieved by the use of β-adrenergic blockade. Propranolol decreases both the rate and the contractile state and has been shown to decrease the size of the infarct in experimental coronary arterial occlusion in dogs[29, 37] and to decrease infarct size, the determination being based on ST-segment mapping in man.[13] As mentioned previously, digitalis in the failing heart decreases the demand for oxygen by increasing the efficiency of the heart and decreases the extent of ischemic injury.[44]

Reduction in afterload is not a clear-cut issue. The reduction of systemic blood pressure in hypertensive patients who suffer an acute infarction decreases infarct size.[40] Afterload reduction also improves left ventricular hemodynamics, even in patients with severe pump failure, during an acute myocardial infarction.[5] However, in animal experiments, hypertension has been shown to be beneficial in reducing ischemic injury in the nonfailing heart, whereas hypotension induced by hemorrhage increases myocardial damage.[29] In the failing heart, blood pressure elevation above normal increases infarct size.[44] The effect of raising or lowering blood pressure in acute infarction seems to be highly dependent on the inotropic state.

Reducing excessively elevated arterial pressure in acute infarction decreases oxygen demand and affects the balance favorably. Nitroglycerin and nitroprusside, two drugs used clinically to reduce blood pressure, have opposite effects on myocardial ischemia.[6] Nitroglycerin decreases infarct size in experimental coronary occlusion, whereas nitroprusside increases infarct size. This opposite effect indicates a difference in their effects on coronary blood flow—nitroglycerin appears to increase flow to the ischemic zone, whereas nitroprusside appears to decrease it. Therefore, nitroglycerin appears to be a more favorable drug for reducing afterload in acute infarction because it not only decreases afterload but also increases perfusion.

Agents Increasing Oxygen Supply

Inhalation of increased FIO_2 decreases the infarct size in dogs[33] and man[27] because of the increased availability of oxygen to the ischemic tissue.

The use of α-adrenergic stimulating agents, such as phenylephrine and methoxamine, is also controversial. Hypertension in the presence of acute infarction is a two-edged sword. The increase in oxygen consumption secondary to increased afterload increases the oxygen debt. However, the increase in diastolic pressure and the subsequent increase in coronary perfusion pressure may be beneficial, and the reflex bradycardia helps decrease oxygen demands also. The amount of benefit derived from these agents depends on numerous factors, such as degree of hypertension reached, ability of the ischemic region to respond to the increased coronary perfusion pressure, and the inotropic state of the myocardium.

Intra-aortic balloon counterpulsation is occasionally used in patients with acute myocardial infarction and cardiogenic shock. Its benefits are the reduction of afterload and the diastolic augmentation of systemic blood pressure, thus increasing coronary perfusion pressure. In dogs and in man, balloon counterpulsation has been shown to decrease ischemic injury in acute myocardial infarction.[31]

Various pharmacologic agents favorably affect the size of the infarct, presumably by improving coronary collateral blood flow. Heparin,[39] probably because of its anticoagulant effect in reducing thrombosis, improves collateral flow and reduces ischemic injury in acute myocardial infarction. Dipyridamole is a potent coronary vasodilator and reduces platelet adhesiveness and thus may be helpful in patients with ischemia.[18] Studies proving any benefit in acute infarction, however, remain to be done.

Mannitol, by its hyperosmolar properties, presumably reduces cell swelling, thus improving collateral blood flow. It improves the function of ischemic regions and decreases the extent of ischemia.[36, 45, 47]

Hyaluronidase limits the extent of ischemic injury and infarction in experimental coronary occlusion,[32] presumably by improving collateral blood flow to the ischemic region.

Agents Increasing Substrate Utilization

Because glucose is the primary source of energy during ischemia, it seems likely that increasing the amount of this substrate available might be beneficial. Weissler et al.[46] showed that infusion of glucose during anoxia improves myocardial performance during anoxia and allows for a more rapid return of myocardial function after a return to an aerobic environment. Maroko et al.[30] demonstrated a reduction in infarct size with infusion of glucose solutions and glucose–insulin–potassium chloride solutions. Levitsky et al.[25] demonstrated better preservation of adenosine triphosphate levels with the infusion of creatine in experimental coronary occlusion.

Agents Protecting Against Myocardial Cell Degradation

The value of the remaining agents has been proved less conclusively. They generally are considered to be helpful because of their effects on the mechanisms that produce cell destruction.

Corticosteroids have been advocated for use during ischemia because of their effect of decreasing cellular edema and thereby increasing regional coronary perfusion. Results in laboratory animals have been promising, but in clinical trials with steroids, conflicting results have been reported.

Aprotinin and cobra venom factor are inhibitors of the kallikrein and complement systems, respectively. Their use in myocardial protection is based on decreasing the inflammatory response to ischemia and thus the interstitial edema and proteolytic activity they initiate. They have been shown to limit infarct size in experimental animals.[8, 28]

Many of these compounds have yet to survive clinical trials, and their clinical use has not been established. However, the possibility that metabolic, hemodynamic, and pharmacologic intervention, even up to six hours after the onset of myocardial ischemia, can affect the amount of myocardium suffering damage cannot be denied. Results so far have been promising, and further work should improve our understanding and clinical management of myocardial ischemia.

EFFORTS AT PROTECTING THE HEART DURING CARDIAC SURGERY

The basic principles of protecting the heart from ischemia during cardiac surgery are the same as those during acute myocardial infarction. Supply versus demand is still the basic concept; however, differences exist because the heart is frequently excluded from the circulation by cardiopulmonary bypass and the coronary circulation often needs to be interrupted for varying periods. These changes cause much larger swings in the balance of supply versus demand than is usually seen in other clinical situations.

Because patients undergoing cardiac operations have previous cardiac disease, occasionally with pump failure and limited cardiac reserve, protection of as much of their remaining myocardium as possible is mandatory. Therefore, various methods have been devised for myocardial preservation during cardiac surgery: intermittent cross-clamping, direct coronary perfusion, hypothermia, and cardioplegia. These are most important when interruption of the coronary circulation for long periods is necessary, such as during aortic valve surgery, coronary artery bypass, and complex congenital repairs. Each of these methods is based on increasing the oxygen supply or decreasing the oxygen demand, and each has advantages and disadvantages.

Intermittent Cross-Clamping With Periods of Reperfusion

This technique has been popular since the early days of cardiac surgery and has the following advantages and disadvantages:

Advantages
  Relatively quiet and bloodless operative field
  Simple—small risk of introducing coronary air emboli
  Reperfusion period theoretically allows high-energy compounds to return toward normal values and metabolic waste products to be eliminated
Disadvantages
  Increases bypass time because of waiting during reperfusion
  Generally results in long periods of ventricular fibrillation, with resultant increased myocardial oxygen consumption during ischemia
  Initiation of ischemic arrest results in release of endogenous catecholamines, with increased myocardial oxygen consumption and decreased tolerance to ischemia

Interruption of coronary flow results in ischemic arrest, usually in 8 to 15 minutes.[14] However, because permanent damage results with longer periods of arrest, the technique of 15 minutes of arrest, followed by 3 to 5 minutes of reperfusion, has been used. The reperfusion period allows the partial regeneration of high-energy metabolites and permits the washout of metabolic end products.

Numerous clinical trials, based on mortality, morbidity, and need for inotropic agents after operation, support the efficacy of this technique, and the technique has been the mainstay of cardiac surgery for many years. However, several experimental studies have shown significant depression of contractility[9, 15, 26] and increased intraoperative myocardial infarction rate[1] with this technique.

With the use of metabolic measurements and contractility studies to compare intermittent versus continuous ischemia, Levitsky et al.[26] studied this technique in dogs. They found no significant difference in the decrease in adenosine triphosphate levels between intermittent reperfusion and continuous ischemia (Fig 14–1) and significantly better preservation of adenosine triphosphate levels with hypothermia and potassium chloride–arrested hearts. They found that, although adenosine triphosphate levels increased slightly during the 5-minute reperfusion period, the increase was insignificant; during the subsequent period of ischemia, the level decreased promptly to the same value as in the group with continuous ischemia. Levels of phosphocreatine increased dramatically during the 5-minute reperfusion but decreased during the subsequent period of ischemia to levels that were no different from those for the group with continuous ischemia. They also found significant (greater than 50%) postischemic depression of maximal rate of pressure change in the left ventricle (dp/dt) in both groups, the one with continuous ischemia and the other with intermittent reperfusion. However, there was no significant difference between the two groups.

Theoretically, intermittent reperfusion may have some detrimental characteristics, because contractile activity is regenerated during the reperfusion periods and continues for 5 to 7 minutes after each cross-clamping. This process increases myocardial oxygen consumption and hastens degradation of high-energy compounds. These results seem to indicate that the detrimental effects cancel out the possible benefits of reperfusion.

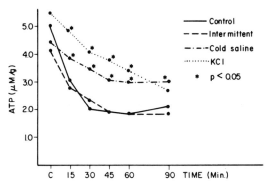

Fig 14–1.—Comparison of levels of adenosine triphosphate (ATP) by different myocardial preservation techniques. No significant difference is seen between continuous ischemia and intermittent reperfusion. Significant difference in maintenance of ATP levels is seen with hypothermia and potassium chloride-arrested hearts. (From Levitsky et al.[26] Used by permission.)

Direct Coronary Perfusion

Direct coronary perfusion was introduced in 1958 and, before the revival of cardioplegia, was the technique of choice for operations requiring open aortotomy. It entails placing two separate coronary perfusion lines from the bypass machine directly into the coronary arteries. Its main advantage is that it maintains myocardial oxygenation and therefore decreases the total ischemia time. The disadvantages are primarily technical problems; early bifurcation of the left main coronary artery can result in nonperfusion of a segment of myocardium, and damage to the ostia of the coronary arteries themselves can occur, sometimes necessitating coronary artery bypass grafting. The introduction of platelet thrombi and coronary air emboli can occur, as can myocardial damage secondary to increased perfusion pressure. The inconvenience of the cannula frequently dislodging during the operation is a time-consuming problem that has made an alternate method desirable. The technique is also of little value in coronary artery bypass graft surgery, which requires a relatively bloodless field. However, when properly conducted, this procedure should result in adequate myocardial protection.

Hypothermia

Hypothermia is based on decreasing myocardial oxygen consumption and thus greater tolerance to ischemia. Greenberg et al.[14] showed that myocardial oxygen consumption decreases proportionally with temperature. They found that, even though the heart becomes mechanically and electrically arrested at 16 C, the oxygen consumption continues to decrease in a linear fashion, even below this temperature (Fig 14–2). Oxygen consumption in the nonworking canine heart has an upper value at normothermia of about 3.2 ml/100 gm/minute. In the intact working heart, the oxygen consumption is 9.5 to 24 ml/100 gm/minute, which indicates that cardiopulmonary bypass alone, eliminating afterload, decreases the myocardial oxygen consumption at least threefold. This favorably affects the balance of oxygen supply and demand.

Several studies have reported superior protection with significantly better postarrest function with hypothermia, as well as better preservation of myocardial adenosine triphosphate and

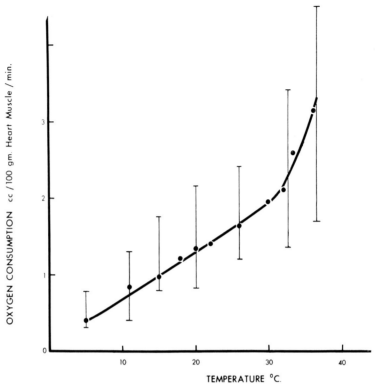

Fig 14–2.—Myocardial oxygen consumption as a function of temperature. (From Greenberg et al.[14] Used by permission.)

phosphocreatine levels.[14, 15, 42] Generally, myocardial temperature is kept between 10 and 20 C, by either perfusion with cold blood or topical hypothermia or both.

Chemically Induced Cardioplegia

In 1883, Ringer[38] studied the effects of various blood constituents on the heart. He found that calcium increases contractility of the heart and eventually leads to tetanus of cardiac muscle, whereas potassium has the opposite effect, decreasing contractions and eventually stopping cardiac activity. In 1929, Hooker[21] suggested the use of potassium chloride solutions to stop the heart during ventricular fibrillation. He suggested calcium chloride as an antidote in restarting the heart, and he showed in animals that this method was effective in converting electrical shock–induced ventricular fibrillation.

Until the introduction of extracorporeal circulation, this information was not of much clinical usefulness. However, in the early days of cardiac surgery, the concept of being able to stop the heart and then restart it after the operation seemed like a good method to provide ideal surgical conditions and still protect the myocardium from ischemic insult by decreasing and almost eliminating its demand for oxygen.

Because myocardial oxygen consumption is rate- and rhythm-dependent, chemically induced cardiac standstill should result in minimal oxygen consumption and superb myocardial protection. Myocardial oxygen consumption varies with rhythm[11] (Table 14–1). Oxygen consumption nearly doubles with ventricular fibrillation and is reduced to about one fourth with arrest, and coronary vascular resistance decreases during arrest because the myocardium is flaccid.

In 1955, Melrose et al.[34] followed up Ringer's and Hooker's work with the original set of experiments suggesting that potassium arrest be used in cardiac surgery. They did three sets of experiments using potassium citrate as the arresting agent. In their initial experiments, 25 to 100 mg of potassium citrate (potassium, 245 to

TABLE 14–1.—CORONARY ARTERIOVENOUS OXYGEN DIFFERENCE AND VASCULAR RESISTANCE WITH VARIOUS RHYTHMS*

EXPERIMENTAL GROUP	RANGE	AVERAGE
Oxygen difference, vol/dl		
Control	1.60–5.91	3.62
Pacing	1.20–5.92	3.78
Fibrillation	3.81–9.85	6.22
Arrest	0.68–1.38	0.92
Vascular resistance, mm Hg/ml/min		
Control	0.50–0.90	0.73
Pacing	0.30–1.10	0.60
Fibrillation	0.40–0.95	0.52
Arrest	0.36–0.65	0.48

*From Gay.[11] Used by permission.

980 mEq/L) resulted in persistent ventricular fibrillation and poor ventricular function; they attributed this effect to calcium chloride and epinephrine, which had been used during the recovery phase.

In the second set of experiments, they used 1 to 5 mg of potassium citrate (potassium, 10 to 50 mEq/L) and found that with 10 mEq/L atrial activity that was just barely perceptible remained, whereas 50 mEq/L resulted in the complete absence of electrical activity. They avoided the use of inotropic drugs during the recovery phase in this group and found consistent recovery of electrical activity and nearly complete recovery of force, even after 45 minutes of arrest. They also found that, when solutions containing more than 50 mEq of potassium per liter were used, there was a longer interval between reperfusion and the recovery of electrical activity and force.

In the third set of experiments, they used 2 ml of 25% potassium citrate diluted to 20 ml with blood (250 mEq of potassium per liter) (same as in the first set of experiments). They again avoided the use of inotropic drugs and found good electrical activity, but they did not make any evaluation of functional recovery.

These experiments showed that 10 to 50 mEq of potassium chloride could induce temporary cardiac arrest, which was nearly completely reversible even after 45 minutes. This result was perceived to be a method of achieving excellent surgical conditions, as well as superb myocardial preservation. Unfortunately, the results were interpreted as suggesting that 250 mEq of potassium or more be used, and in numerous animal experiments and clinical trials, persistent ventricular fibrillation, focal myocardial necrosis, and depressed left ventricular function were seen with potassium-induced arrest.[17, 35, 42, 43] As a result, the technique was abandoned.

In the early 1970s, interest in potassium-induced arrest was revived. Gay and Ebert in 1973,[11, 12] using an iso-osmotic solution of potassium chloride with 12 to 15 mEq of potassium per liter, found only mild depression of left ventricular function curves in animals undergoing 60 minutes of potassium-induced arrest at normothermia; after 60 minutes of normothermic ischemic arrest, none of the control hearts recovered enough for function curves to be obtained (Fig 14–3). After 48 hours, they examined microscopically the hearts arrested with potassium chloride and found only mild interstitial edema.

The reason for the poor results was believed to be elevated levels of potassium (250 mEq or ten times the amount needed to induce arrest) and the increased osmolarity (greater than 400 mOsm with Melrose's solution). Both of these factors increase the microscopic damage to the myocardium and result in depressed left ventricular function.[42] It was determined that 10 to 50 mEq of potassium per liter was the safe range for cardioplegia.[42]

Since that time, numerous studies have shown superior protection of left ventricular

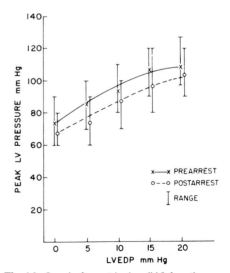

Fig 14–3.—Left ventricular *(LV)* function curves inscribed before and 30 minutes after a 60-minute period of normothermic cardiac ischemia in potassium chloride-arrested hearts. (From Gay.[11] Used by permission.)

pass, sites of distal graft anastomosis are found and marked by dissecting the epicardial fat from these segments of the vessel, because the presence of a clear cardioplegic solution in the coronary artery will make later recognition of the sites difficult. Once the sites for anastomosis are located, the aorta is cross-clamped and the cardioplegic solution is infused through a needle inserted proximal to the aortic cross-clamp. Blanching of the myocardium and then arrest of the heart in diastole occurs. If all distal graft anastomoses are done before the proximal ones, infusion of additional cardioplegic solution is repeated after each distal anastomosis. However, if each graft is completed as an individual step, then the solution is reinfused before the distal anastomosis of the next graft is begun.

Volume of Infusion

Generally, the volume of cardioplegic solution is estimated according to the body surface area and is given at a rate of 150 ml/minute/sq m for two minutes.[7] This volume also can be calculated on the basis of the weight of the patient: 10 ml/kg for adults; 15 ml/kg for children between 10 and 20 kg; and 20 ml/kg for children less than 10 kg. These volumes are not absolute values. They serve only as a guide for safe administration, without excessive pressure in the

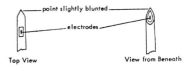

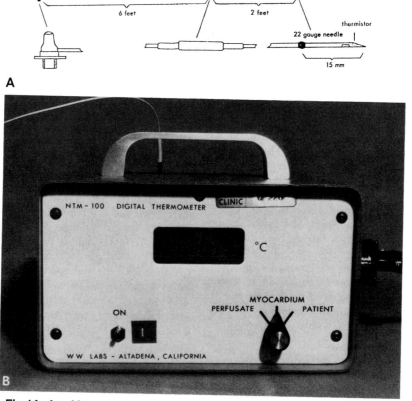

Fig 14–4.—Myocardial temperature monitoring system. **A,** needle probes. **B,** digital thermometer (Milton Webster Laboratories, Altadena, Calif.)

lines. The actual volume is dictated by the effects of solution on the heart, measurements of temperature of the myocardium, and cessation of electromechanical activity of the heart.

Temperature

At the completion of infusion, the temperature of the myocardium should be less than 20 C and usually reaches between 12 and 15 C and is maintained at approximately 20 C. The myocardial temperature is measured with a temperature needle probe and monitored (Fig 14–4).

During cardiac ischemia, measures such as the external cooling of the heart by bathing it with cold saline placed in the pericardial sac and the reduction of the temperature of perfusate in the heart-lung machine to the range of 22 to 25 C can reduce the temperature gradient between the myocardium and its surroundings. This reduction helps to maintain the desired hypothermia[7] and also allows reducing the total body perfusion to between 1.0 and 1.5 L/minute/sq m without significant risk.

Such low body and perfusate temperatures are frequently required for patients with complex cyanotic congenital conditions because of the need for better surgical exposure. However, patients with simple congenital conditions or acquired heart disease can be managed with higher temperatures because they often do not require a reduction in perfusion.

During closure of the aortotomy in patients with aortic valve replacement (perfusate temperature usually is returned to normal during this stage), a short period (three to five minutes) of coronary perfusion with the perfusate temperature momentarily lowered to between 25 and 30 C may be useful to flush the cardioplegic solution from the coronary system, and this short, cold perfusion may further provide myocardial protection for the duration of the aortotomy closure.[7]

REFERENCES

1. Adappa M.G., et al.: Cold hyperkalemic cardiac arrest versus intermittent aortic cross-clamping and topical hypothermia for coronary bypass surgery. *J. Thorac. Cardiovasc. Surg.* 75:171, 1978.
2. Behrendt D.M., Jochim K.E.: Effect of temperature of cardioplegic solution. *J. Thorac. Cardiovasc. Surg.* 76:353, 1978.
3. Bixler T.J., et al.: Effects of procaine-induced cardioplegia on myocardial ischemia, myocardial edema, and postarrest ventricular function: A comparison with potassium-induced cardioplegia and hypothermia. *J. Thorac. Cardiovasc. Surg.* 75:886, 1978.
4. Bretschneider H.J., et al.: Myocardial resistance and tolerance to ischemia: Physiological and biochemical basis. *J. Cardiovasc. Surg.* 16:241, 1975.
5. Chatterjee K., et al.: Hemodynamic and metabolic responses to vasodilator therapy in acute myocardial infarction. *Circulation* 48:1183, 1973.
6. Chiariello M., et al.: Comparison between the effects of nitroprusside and nitroglycerin on ischemic injury during acute myocardial infarction. *Circulation* 54:766, 1976.
7. Devloo R.A.: Personal communication.
8. Diaz P.E., Maroko P.R.: The effects of aprotinin on myocardial ischemic injury following experimental coronary artery occlusion, abstracted. *Clin. Res.* 23:180A, 1975.
9. Ebert P.A., et al.: Experimental comparison of methods for protecting the heart during aortic occlusion. *Ann. Surg.* 155:25, 1962.
10. Engelman R.M., et al.: Myocardial reperfusion, a cause of ischemic injury during cardiopulmonary bypass. *Surgery* 80:266, 1976.
11. Gay W.A. Jr.: Potassium-induced cardioplegia. *Ann. Thorac. Surg.* 20:95, 1975.
12. Gay W.A. Jr., Ebert P.A.: Functional, metabolic, and morphologic effects of potassium-induced cardioplegia. *Surgery* 74:284, 1973.
13. Gold H.K., Leinbach R.C., Maroko P.R.: Propranolol-induced reduction of signs of ischemic injury during acute myocardial infarction. *Am. J. Cardiol.* 38:689, 1976.
14. Greenberg J.J., Edmunds L.H. Jr., Brown R.B.: Myocardial metabolism and postarrest function in the cold and chemically arrested heart. *Surgery* 48:31, 1960.
15. Hearse D.J., Stewart D.A., Braimbridge M.V.: Hypothermic arrest and potassium arrest: Metabolic and myocardial protection during elective cardiac arrest. *Circ. Res.* 36:481, 1975.
16. Hearse D.J., Stewart D.A., Braimbridge M.V.: Myocardial protection during ischemic cardiac arrest: The importance of magnesium in cardioplegic infusates. *J. Thorac. Cardiovasc. Surg.* 75:877, 1978.
17. Helmsworth J.A., et al.: Myocardial injury associated with asystole induced with potassium citrate. *Ann. Surg.* 149:200, 1959.
18. Hickey P.A.: Prevention of intraoperative myocardial injury by pretreatment with pharmacological agents. *Ann. Thorac. Surg.* 20:101, 1975.

19. Hillis L.D., Braunwald E.: Myocardial ischemia. N. Engl. J. Med. 296:971, 1034, and 1093, 1977.
20. Holland C.E. Jr., Olson R.E.: Prevention of hypothermia of paradoxical calcium necrosis in cardiac muscle. J. Mol. Cell. Cardiol. 7:917, 1975.
21. Hooker D.R.: On the recovery of the heart in electric shock. Am. J. Physiol. 91:305, 1929.
22. Jynge P., et al.: Protection of the ischemic myocardium: Ultrastructural, enzymatic, and functional assessment of the efficacy of various cardioplegic infusates. J. Thorac. Cardiovasc. Surg. 76:2, 1978.
23. Kirsch U., Rodewald G., Kalmár P.: Induced ischemic arrest: Clinical experience with cardioplegia in open-heart surgery. J. Thorac. Cardiovasc. Surg. 63:121, 1972.
24. Kübler W., Spieckermann P.G.: Regulation of glycolysis in the ischemic and the anoxic myocardium. J. Mol. Cell. Cardiol. 1:351, 1970.
25. Levitsky S., Feinberg H.: Protection of the myocardium with high-energy solutions. Ann. Thorac. Surg. 20:86, 1975.
26. Levitsky S., et al.: Does intermittent coronary perfusion offer greater myocardial protection than continuous aortic cross-clamping? Surgery 82:51, 1977.
27. Madias J.E., Madias N.E., Hood W.B. Jr.: Precordial ST-segment mapping: 2. Effects of oxygen inhalation on ischemic injury in patients with acute myocardial infarction. Circulation 53:411, 1976.
28. Maroko P.R., Carpenter C.B.: Reduction in infarct size following acute coronary occlusion by the administration of cobra venom factor, abstracted. Clin. Res. 22:289A, 1974.
29. Maroko P.R., et al.: Factors influencing infarct size following experimental coronary artery occlusions. Circulation 43:67, 1971.
30. Maroko P.R., et al.: Effect of glucose-insulin-potassium infusion on myocardial infarction following experimental coronary artery occlusion. Circulation 45:1160, 1972.
31. Maroko P.R., et al.: Effects of intraaortic balloon counterpulsation on the severity of myocardial ischemic injury following acute coronary occlusion: Counterpulsation and myocardial injury. Circulation 45:1150, 1972.
32. Maroko P.R., et al.: Reduction by hyaluronidase of myocardial necrosis following coronary artery occlusion. Circulation 46:430, 1972.
33. Maroko P.R., et al.: Reduction of infarct size by oxygen inhalation following acute coronary occlusion. Circulation 52:360, 1975.
34. Melrose D.G., et al.: Cited by Gay and Ebert.[12]
35. Nunn D.D., et al.: A comparative study of aortic occlusion alone and of potassium citrate arrest during cardiopulmonary bypass. Surgery 45:848, 1959.
36. Powell W.J. Jr., et al.: The protective effect of hyperosmotic mannitol in myocardial ischemia and necrosis. Circulation 54:603, 1976.
37. Reimer K.A., Rasmussen M.M., Jennings R.B.: Reduction by propranolol of myocardial necrosis following temporary coronary artery occlusion in dogs. Circ. Res. 33:353, 1973.
38. Ringer S.: A further contribution regarding the influence of different constituents of the blood on the contraction of the heart. J. Physiol. 4:29, 1883.
39. Saliba M.J. Jr., Covell J.W., Bloor C.M.: Effects of heparin in large doses on the extent of myocardial ischemia after acute coronary occlusion in the dog. Am. J. Cardiol. 37:599, 1976.
40. Shell W.E., Sobel B.E.: Protection of jeopardized ischemic myocardium by reduction of ventricular afterload. N. Engl. J. Med. 291:481, 1974.
41. Tyers G.F.O.: Metabolic arrest of the ischemic heart. Ann. Thorac. Surg. 20:91, 1975.
42. Tyers G.F.O., et al.: The mechanism of myocardial damage following potassium citrate (Melrose) cardioplegia. Surgery 78:45, 1975.
43. Waldhausen J.A., et al.: Left ventricular function following elective cardiac arrest. J. Thorac. Cardiovasc. Surg. 39:799, 1960.
44. Watanabe T., et al.: Effects of increased arterial pressure and positive inotropic agents on the severity of myocardial ischemia in the acutely depressed heart. Am. J. Cardiol. 30:371, 1972.
45. Weisfeldt M.L., et al.: Effect of mannitol on the performance of the isolated canine heart after fibrillatory arrest. J. Thorac. Cardiovasc. Surg. 66:290, 1973.
46. Weissler A.M., et al.: Role of anaerobic metabolism in the preservation of functional capacity and structure of anoxic myocardium. J. Clin. Invest. 47:403, 1968.
47. Willerson J.T., et al.: Improvement in myocardial function and coronary blood flow in ischemic myocardium after mannitol. J. Clin. Invest. 51:2989, 1972.
48. Wood J.M., et al.: Effect of chronic myocardial ischemia on the activity of carnitine palmityl-coenzyme A transferase of isolated canine heart mitochondria. Circ. Res. 32:340, 1973.
49. Zimmerman A.N.E., et al.: Morphological changes of heart muscle caused by successive perfusion with calcium-free and calcium-containing solutions (calcium paradox). Cardiovasc. Res. 1:201, 1967.

15 / Protection of the Brain from Ischemic and Embolic Phenomena

ROY F. CUCCHIARA
CARL R. NOBACK
RONALD J. FAUST

Cerebral pathophysiologic changes produced during cardiopulmonary bypass are examined in observations of the final result—patient neurologic function. The need to repair cardiac defects has always been balanced against the risk of surgery, a part of which has been cerebral risk. Physical, technical, and pharmacologic techniques to protect the brain during ischemic and embolic episodes hold the key to another step in improving the safety of cardiopulmonary bypass.

CEREBRAL ISCHEMIA

There has been a renewed interest in modifying, reducing, and preventing irreversible loss of neurologic function after a cerebral ischemic episode. Permanent loss of neurologic function can be expected when cell death occurs during or immediately after the period of cerebral ischemia. A return of neurologic function implies that the responsible neurons were not irreversibly damaged during the ischemic episode or that their role was assumed by other neurons not irreversibly damaged.

Cellular Ischemia

Although ischemia or hypoxia (or both) can damage the neurons of the CNS beyond repair, the mechanism of such damage at a cellular level is still the subject of considerable study. The level of adenosine triphosphate in the brain decreases rapidly during the first five minutes of anoxia but changes only slowly during the next four minutes.[30] In this circumstance of anoxia (nitrogen inhalation), there was no difference in the rate of depletion of adenosine triphosphate in dogs treated with thiopental or untreated, although the EEGs showed longer activity in the treated dogs. With hypotension and normal oxygenation, thiopental-treated dogs showed a slower depletion of adenosine triphosphate, and EEG activity was sustained in both groups.[30]

Attention has been focused on the bilipid layer of the cell membrane as a possible site of structural cell damage during hypoxia. Such damage might be due to lipid peroxidation by the formation of free radicals during hypoxia.[14]

Animal Studies

Because considerable differences exist between experimental models of cerebral ischemia, reasonable groupings can be made into models of complete or global cerebral ischemia and incomplete or focal cerebral ischemia. Global ischemia may be complete if no oxygen is delivered to the brain (anoxia) or incomplete if some flow, however small, continues to the brain (hypoxia). Regional ischemia may be complete to a specific area of brain, but because perfusion may continue to some areas around the ischemic zone owing to overlapping circulation, regional cerebral ischemia is usually incomplete. Anoxia is complete deprivation of oxygen supply to the brain, independent of flow (which usually ceases). Hypoxia is incomplete deprivation, independent of flow (which usually persists). Cardiac arrest produces complete global ischemia, whereas hypotension produces incomplete global ischemia. There is still some technical inconsistency in the terminology used in models of cerebral ischemia. In a more exact sense, complete global ischemia means that no blood flow to the brain is present. In anoxia, oxygen is not delivered to the brain, and a situation analogous to, but not identical to, complete global ischemia is produced because flow can continue for a short period without oxygen delivery.

Global Complete Cerebral Ischemia (Animal Models)

The task of producing an animal model of global ischemia in which there is survival with severe neurologic damage is difficult. Large variability in collateral cerebral circulation exists in different species. The vertebral vessels are protected from compression by the bony spinal column. Extracranial-intracranial collateral pathways may exist. Occlusion of carotid and vertebral arteries does not reliably produce global ischemia.[12]

The comparison of neurologic damage with ischemia time probably produces an S-shaped curve. No permanent neurologic damage is produced up to a given time of global ischemia. A relatively shorter ischemic period from that point could be expected to produce a steep increase in animals with permanent damage. From the end of that period, another plateau would be reached at which all the animals would be so severely damaged as not to survive. Thus, a model of global cerebral ischemia should be able to reproducibly place animals on the steep portion of such a curve so as to produce serious neurologic injury without death. Because such a curve would be steep, small variations in intensity of insult might produce striking changes in results.

Global ischemia can be produced by elevating intracranial pressures to pressures exceeding blood pressure. However, such elevations in intracranial pressure usually preclude survival of the animal.[28] Clearly, global cerebral ischemia can be produced by total circulatory arrest, as occurs in ventricular fibrillation, but again too few animals can be resuscitated.[36]

Global ischemia can be produced by aortic occlusion in dogs. Goldstein et al.[16] reported some survivors and an improved neurologic outcome after such an insult in animals treated with pentobarbital.

With the use of the same experimental preparation, Steen et al.[41] were unable to verify these results and found no difference between pentobarbital-treated and untreated dogs. Most dogs tolerated 8 minutes of aortic occlusion without neurologic sequelae, but sustained severe deficits or death after 10 minutes of occlusion.

The application of a high-pressure neck tourniquet and systemic arterial hypotension has recently been used in a monkey model of global cerebral ischemia.[4] Thiopental improved neurologic recovery and increased survival after 16 minutes of neck compression and hypotension. That report was accompanied by an editorial that pointed out several difficulties with the experimental design and data interpretation in the work.[34] Global anoxic injury was not mitigated by thiopental in dogs asphyxiated and subjected to cardiopulmonary resuscitation.[37]

Regional Cerebral Ischemia (Primate Models)

While a cerebral protective effect of barbiturates in global ischemia remains less than clearly demonstrated, such an effect in regional cerebral ischemia has considerable experimental support. In a baboon model of occlusion of the middle cerebral artery, consistent cerebral infarction was produced. Neurologic status was clearly better, and the infarct was smaller when 90 mg of pentobarbital per kilogram was administered intravenously, when comparisons were made to a control group given 1.2% halothane.[23] Similar results were found, although indicating a more limited effect of barbiturates, in monkeys anesthetized with ketamine who had occlusion of the middle cerebral artery by focal injection of silicone cylinders.[31] The effect of barbiturates and intensive care in reducing infarct size and improving neurologic outcome has been studied.[29] Java monkeys with permanent surgical occlusion of the middle cerebral artery were treated with pentobarbital and given 48 hours of intensive care. The monkeys that did not receive pentobarbital had severe neurologic deficits and large infarcts, and several died. The monkeys given barbiturates and intensive care had statistically smaller deficits and infarcts, and none died.

Primate model studies thus point to a clearly protective effect of barbiturates on the brain in the circumstance of regional cerebral ischemia.

NEUROLOGIC SEQUELAE OF CARDIOPULMONARY BYPASS

The incidence and severity of neurologic complications after cardiopulmonary bypass have been assessed since the early days of open-heart surgery. Physiologic changes in the EEG during anesthesia and open-heart surgery were correlated early with neurologic outcome.[45] Postcardiotomy delirium was recognized early by clinicians and examined from several approaches.[3, 25, 35] Animal studies directed at the quantitation of cerebral blood flow and metabolism during cardiopulmonary bypass became progressively more sophisticated.[5] Neuropathologic correlations among intraoperative course, neurologic outcome, and cerebral autopsy specimens sought to help define the causes of brain damage after cardiopulmonary bypass.[6] Improvements in anesthetic, surgical, and cardiopulmonary bypass techniques and the application of technical advances in filter technology have steadily reduced the incidence and severity of neurologic dysfunction after open-heart surgery.[19]

Some factors associated with brain dysfunction are advanced age, severity of preoperative and postoperative illness, and time on cardiopulmonary bypass.[19] Pump-generated microemboli can be related to a reduction in cerebral blood flow; filtration can significantly reduce this change in flow.[5] Intensive care seems to have a role for some patients with postbypass delirium.[3] However, intraoperative hypotension or embolism or both are probably the most important current causes for compromise in cerebral function after bypass. The correlation between intraoperative hypotension and postoperative neurologic sequelae has been suggested in pathologic studies.[46] Diffuse neuronal degeneration was the most frequent pathologic manifestation of the encephalopathic syndrome after operation, while focal cerebral necrosis (suggesting emboli) was most often associated with postoperative motor changes.[48] In one study, hemiplegia could be accounted for by cerebral emboli, whereas "gnostic disorders" could not.[15]

Protection of the brain from emboli during cardiopulmonary bypass has continued to improve. The limit of hypotension that can be tolerated during cardiopulmonary bypass without neurologic sequelae is not precisely defined. For example, in one study, one patient sustained 8 minutes of cerebral perfusion pressure below 20 mm Hg, and 15 more minutes between 20 and 40 mm Hg, with no deficit even though the EEG was "flat" for the last 4 minutes of the most severe hypotension, whereas another patient suffered a recurrence of hemiparesis from a prior cerebrovascular accident after only moderate hypotension (cerebral perfusion pressure 40 mm Hg).[42] Thus, high systemic flow alone cannot be considered adequate for cerebral perfusion—cerebral perfusion pressure also must be very important, especially in the older patient. What level of cerebral perfusion pressure on cardiopulmonary bypass is adequate in order to reliably prevent irreversible cerebral ischemia? Reliable data on human beings are lacking; the answer is not known. In our practice, vasopressors are used to maintain a cerebral perfusion pressure of at least 50 mm Hg in middle-aged and older patients.

After an unavoidable hypotensive episode, what blood pressure level should be sought? The importance of the cerebral "no-reflow" phenomenon after hypotension during cardiopulmonary bypass in human beings is not well defined. Considerable work suggests that the conditions associated with cardiopulmonary bypass and cerebral ischemia can contribute to the no-reflow phenomenon.[1, 8, 17, 18] These findings suggest that a higher cerebral perfusion pressure should be sought after a hypotensive episode. Stockard et al.[42] suggested that low reperfusion pressures and the no-reflow phenomenon may have had an important role in the irreversibility of the hypotension-induced EEG changes in some patients in their study.

EMBOLIC PHENOMENA DURING CARDIOPULMONARY BYPASS

Neurologic and psychiatric damage has been noted in as many as two thirds of patients after cardiopulmonary bypass.[20] The relationship of this damage to embolic phenomena is largely circumstantial; however, deleterious effects of air and gaseous emboli entering the systemic or cerebral circulation are well established. Methods are available for protection against the development of emboli, whether particulate or gaseous, during cardiopulmonary bypass.

Several potential sources of microemboli exist. These include formation of microaggregates of the patient's endogenous platelets and leukocytes; cellular aggregation and generation of gaseous microemboli by the oxygenator; the return of large amounts of fats, solids, and activated platelets through the cardiotomy suction system; infusion during the initial phase of cardiopulmonary bypass of particles retained in the oxygenator in the manufacturing process; and exogenous sources of emboli, such as transfused blood and intravenous solutions.

Organ Involvement by Emboli During Cardiopulmonary Bypass

The microcirculation of the brain was shown by Brierley[7] to be particularly susceptible to the effects of inadequate blood flow and air embolism. Williams et al.[47] showed that visual symptoms arising in the occipital cortex of patients who had undergone cardiopulmonary bypass probably were due to migrating thrombi or emboli. Brennan et al.[5] demonstrated that the depression in cerebral blood flow and cerebral metabolic rate was correlated with the titer of microparticles in the bypass system and could be avoided by the use of filters. Evidence suggesting pulmonary damage from particulate microembolization includes deposition of platelet-fibrin aggregates, margination of leukocytes, endothelial swelling, interstitial edema, leukocyte infiltration, perivascular damage, and alveolar structural damage.[21] These findings are nonspecific, but the constellation of them may result in significant functional pulmonary impairment. Histologic studies of other organs downstream from the arterial inflow line have revealed entrapped emboli. Using emboli of ^{51}Cr-labeled platelets and surface gamma-scintillation counters, Hicks and Edmunds[20] showed an increase of 50% in background levels of liver and spleen activity during the first hour of bypass, thus indicating that platelet-aggregate emboli formed during extracorporeal circulation are at least temporarily sequestered in the liver and spleen. Such a histologic method does not even detect gaseous emboli or those that may transiently occlude the microcirculation.

Quantifying Emboli Produced During Cardiopulmonary Bypass

Ultrasonic devices using the Doppler principle may detect gaseous emboli, but these are effectively limited to detecting particles greater than 100 μm in diameter.[20] The use of this method has established that gas-interface (bubble) oxygenators produce myriads of gaseous microemboli, whereas membrane oxygenators produce few such emboli.[20]

Swank et al.[43] devised the screen-filtration pressure test, which measures the pressure required to maintain a constant rate of blood flow through a filter with a pore size of 20 μm. Peak pressure increases reflect the volume of particulate matter filtered; however, this method does not identify size, number, or composition of particles detected. The model-T Coulter counter used by Solis and Gibbs[38] similarly identifies the particle size and number as well as volume of the filtered material, but not its composition.

Dutton et al.[13] demonstrated that emboli 50 to 500 μm in diameter were produced by both membrane and bubble oxygenators. The emboli consisted of platelets (some of which were disrupted) and a few leukocytes (Fig 15–1). Platelet-aggregate emboli formed at the rate of 0.5 to 1 embolus per milliliter of filtrate. Particles greater than 50 μm in diameter were removed by a nylon filter of 40-μm pore size. Such a filter, however, may produce smaller emboli. Dutton et al. also showed that a filter of 27-μm

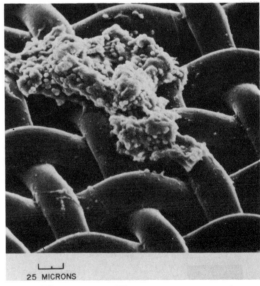

Fig 15–1.—Scanning electron micrograph of platelet-aggregate emboli recovered from patient perfused with gas-interface oxygenator. Scattered platelets and leukocytes adhere to surrounding nylon strands. (From Hicks and Edmunds.[20] Used by permission.)

pore size removed particles greater than 50 μm in diameter, but not those less than 50 μm in diameter. This finding suggests that the filter may produce smaller microemboli by fragmentation of emboli less than 50 μm in diameter.

Large numbers of microemboli have been demonstrated during the initial portion of perfusion and are seen to decrease with time.[11] The introduction of an arterial line filter when the numbers of emboli are at their greatest, as determined by ultrasonic techniques, decreased the number of circulating particles. Removal of the filter at a later time increased the number of particles detected (Fig 15–2). The embolus count also was increased by the introduction of nitrogen, the use of cardiotomy suction, and tapping or hitting of the extracorporeal device.[10] The influence of the arterial line filter in removing microspheres of 100-μm diameter is shown in Figure 15–3.

These emboli are composed primarily of intact and disrupted platelets and leukocytes.

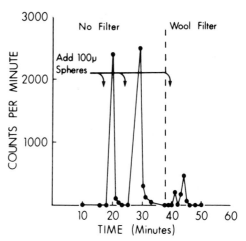

Fig 15–3.—Epoxy resin microspheres (100 μm) injected into oxygenator and microemboli counts were recorded. Influence of arterial line filter is shown. (From Clark et al.[11] Used by permission.)

Platelet emboli may form by contact of activated platelets or by dislodgement of surface-bound aggregates. The mechanism of aggregate formation involves the surface activation of factor XII (Hageman factor), the kallikrein-kininogen system, and adenosine diphosphate. A thin film of protein is deposited when blood contacts a foreign surface, and platelets begin to adhere to it. Shortly thereafter, platelet counts in both bubble and membrane oxygenators decrease to between 15% and 60%[20, 21] of the preperfusion levels. This decrease is greater than that expected from hemodilution alone.

Solis et al.[40] showed that, after 30 minutes of cardiopulmonary bypass, the volume of both platelets and aggregates decreased but that a greater percentage of platelets aggregated, thus suggesting that platelet reactivity to adenosine diphosphate may have increased. This finding also indicates that the reduction of platelet aggregation seen during cardiopulmonary bypass is due to thrombocytopenia rather than to decreased platelet reactivity. No change was seen in mean platelet size before and 30 minutes after the institution of cardiopulmonary bypass. This result is significant because younger platelets, which are functionally more active than older platelets, are larger than older ones. The lack of change in mean platelet size suggests that the rate of removal of the larger and smaller platelets was the same.[40]

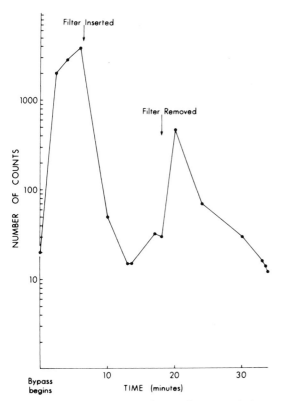

Fig 15–2.—Microemboli counting rate during initial stage of perfusion in dog. Influence of arterial line filter is shown. (From Clark et al.[11] Used by permission.)

Hill et al.[21] showed that arterial inflow line filtration with Dacron-wool filters during normothermic bypass "virtually eliminates nonfat emboli, reduces overall mortality, and improves the postoperative clinical picture." Hill et al. also studied arterial inflow line filtration during hypothermic bypass. With filtration, the microembolus count is typically high during the early phase of perfusion and decreases with time. During continued perfusion, the microembolus count is relatively stable until the onset of rewarming, when Clark et al.[11] showed significant increases in the embolus formation rate. In addition, perfusion times in excess of three hours increase the incidence of CNS abnormalities, low cardiac output, high pulmonary vascular resistance, and hepatic and renal dysfunction.[10] Hissen et al.[22] found that the group with Dacron-wool filters on the arterial inflow line had a significant decrease in postoperative neurologic damage when compared to the group without such filters.

Cardiopulmonary Bypass Devices and Embolus Formation

The type of oxygenator also can affect embolus formation. A gradient of microemboli developed on passage of blood through a bubble oxygenator but not through a membrane oxygenator.[39] The volume of aggregates was significantly greater with bubble oxygenation, thus indicating a relative reduction of particulate microembolization with membrane oxygenation (Fig 15–4). Bubble oxygenators produce gaseous emboli, which may decrease cerebral metabolism[5] and which can be eliminated by an arterial line filter of 40-μm pore size.[20] In further studies on the formation of gaseous microemboli, Katoh and Yoshida[24] found that, with a blood-gas interface, the rate of microemboli formation increased with the speed of agitation. Without the interface, and with the same rate of agitation, the screen-filtration pressure did not change, thus indicating a lack of microembolus formation. Two conclusions were reached: (1) the blood-gas interface is essential for microembolus formation and (2) blood turbulence contributes little to microembolus formation. Thus, membrane oxygenators, in which the blood is separated from the gas by a gas-permeable membrane, are more suitable than bubble oxygenators for prolonged cardiopulmonary bypass.

The cardiotomy suction return may contribute

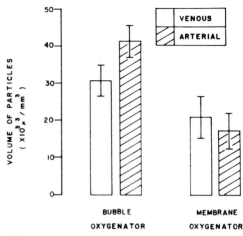

Fig 15–4.—Particulate microembolization during extracorporeal oxygenation. Volume of particles 18 to 80 μm in diameter (mean ± SE) in venous and arterial blood during first ten minutes on cardiopulmonary bypass with bubble (N = 35) and membrane (N = 19) oxygenation. (From Solis et al.[39] Used by permission.)

significant amounts of fats and solids, including activated platelets and cellular fragments, to the oxygenator reservoir. Osborn et al.[32] began a controlled clinical study to evaluate the effectiveness of Dacron-wool filtration of the cardiotomy suction return, but they soon abandoned the control group because of an "overwhelming conviction" that the group with the filter suffered fewer postoperative complications. Solis et al.[39] showed, with both oxygenators, an increased volume of microemboli in cardiotomy-return blood compared with arterial blood, thus emphasizing the need for an effective cardiotomy-return filtration system, regardless of the type of oxygenator used. Dacron-wool filtration of the cardiotomy suction return, similar to arterial inflow-line filtration, is effective, as is filtration with a filter of three separate elements of polyurethane foam containing progressively smaller pores (diameter 150 to 27 μm) placed between the coronary suction line and the cardiotomy reservoir.[44]

With respect to embolic complications of oxygenator systems, most attention has been directed to the production of gaseous emboli by the system and the effect of filtration on the removal of platelet-aggregate emboli. Another significant consideration was elucidated by Reed et al.,[33] namely, that of particulate contamination of the various bubble oxygenators in use. Particulate matter washed from bubble oxygenators by priming solutions included fibers (86%), plastic chips (10%), and particles of an undetermined nature (4%). A wide variation in particulate contamination among the oxygenators was found (Table 15–1). Since the introduction of a filter with a pore size of 5 μm between the arterial and venous lines during pump priming procedures at the Texas Heart Institute,[33] the incidence of neurologic deficits after cardiopulmonary bypass has decreased from 14.3% to 10.7%.

Filtration and choice of oxygenator system or brand can have a significant effect on the size and incidence of microemboli. A filter with a pore size of 20 to 40 μm may be included on the arterial inflow line. Cardiotomy suction return should pass through a similar filter. Additionally, a 5-μm filter placed between the arterial and venous lines may be beneficial. A membrane oxygenator results in less particulate and gaseous emboli than does a bubble oxygenator.

Air Embolism

In addition to the embolic problems, another form of gaseous embolus must be considered—air embolus (Fig 15–5). The possible problems associated with air embolism were first discussed by Carrel[9] in 1914, and further elucidation of the consequences of air entering the systemic or cerebral circulation during the ensuing years leaves no doubt as to the seriousness of the problem. Several sources of air embolism exist, including generation of bubbles by the oxygenator system used, retention of air in the left ventricle after cardiotomy closure, entrance of air to the systemic circulation through interatrial

TABLE 15–1.—COUNTS* OF FOREIGN-BODY PARTICLES IN VARIOUS BUBBLE OXYGENATORS†

OXYGENATOR	MEAN	RANGE
Bentley Q 100	130,046	10,530–480,100
Harvey H200	39,598	20,702–66,773
Harvey H200B	7,912	927–25,458
Galen Optiflo	5,719	987–30,125
Rygg	23,730	1,974–115,893
Travenol 6 LF	1,429	239–4,248
Travenol 2 LF	845	299–2,812

*Ten of each model.
†From Reed et al.[33] Used by permission.

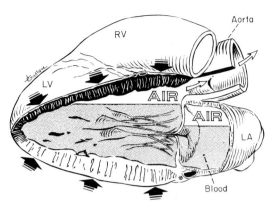

Fig 15–5.—Mechanism of air embolism. If mitral valve is competent and left ventricle *(LV)* contracts, blood and air would be ejected to unclamped aorta, and air would enter systemic circulation. Right ventricle *(RV)*, left atrium *(LA)*. (From McGoon D.C.: Technics of open heart surgery for congenital heart disease. *Curr. Probl. Surg.*, April 1968, p. 1. Used by permission.)

or interventricular defects, or introduction of air into the left ventricle through needle holes or the vent insertion site. Oxygen bubbles may form when supersaturated cold blood from the oxygenator is warmed on entering the patient.[27]

Air embolism may affect the heart itself. With the patient supine, the ostium of the right coronary artery is at the highest point of the aortic root, which increases the chance of air embolism to the right coronary artery. Cardiac effects of air embolism may be manifested by poor right ventricular contractility, arrhythmias, ST-segment elevation on the ECG, and higher pressures in the right atrium than the left atrium.[44] Trapped air in the left atrium also creates the danger of air embolism, especially if the blood level is decreased below the septal opening by suction during closure of an atrial septal defect.

Many methods have been described to prevent or minimize air embolism. Among these are induction of elective ventricular fibrillation or the use of cardioplegia to bring the heart to a standstill during open cardiotomy, cross-clamping the aorta before incision of the right atrium, venting the heart (especially the apex), needle aspiration of the aortic root or cardiac chambers, filling the cardiac chambers with blood or saline and then compressing them, the use of the Trendelenburg position, and aortic cross-clamping for three or four beats to allow coronary artery flushing.[2]

Air embolism occurs most commonly at the termination of cardiopulmonary bypass and after defibrillation.[26] Patients undergoing aortic valve replacement are most likely to suffer air embolism.[26] Efforts to remove air from the left side of the heart are best made before the termination of bypass. The heart should be elevated, and the left atrial appendage invaginated, with the left ventricular vent open to expel entrapped air. Increasing airway pressure by use of either the anesthesia bag or the ventilator, concurrent with the invagination and compression, forces blood from the pulmonary veins into the left atrium and ventricle. The air trapped can then be expelled through the left ventricular vent. Air bubbles also can be removed by an aortic root vent.[11, 44] Elevation, invagination, and compression may be repeated as necessary.

Air emboli may be detected by clinical signs or by the use of Doppler monitoring. Intraoperatively, Doppler flow studies may provide a means of detecting continued showers of air emboli or the entrance of new bubbles, which may otherwise go unnoticed.[26] If a Doppler device is used, with the probe secured on the right brachiocephalic artery, air emboli may be detected into the postbypass period. Lemole and Pinder[27] observed the liberation of air bubbles up to 20 minutes after the termination of bypass and decannulation.

Air embolism to the coronary arteries may be minimized if the aortic cross-clamp is slowly released after three or four beats and the proximal right coronary artery is gently pinched. This maneuver allows blood to fill the proximal aorta from below, forcing any air trapped in the aortic root through an aortic root vent. Although Lawrence et al.[26] found that the use of an aortic vent button or needle did not seem to eliminate intravascular air embolism sufficiently to warrant its continued use, the experience at our institution differs. We have found that a thumbtack needle vent connected to the suction line is useful for preventing air embolism (Fig 15–6). There is a slit along the length of the shaft of the needle vent that allows continuous suction of accumulated foam and air bubbles when the needle vent is placed in the ascending aorta.[44]

Lemole and Pinder[27] described a technique of partial occlusion of the ascending aorta with a clamp applied before the termination of bypass (Fig 15–7). This method creates a cupula in the aortic flow, into which a needle vent is placed.

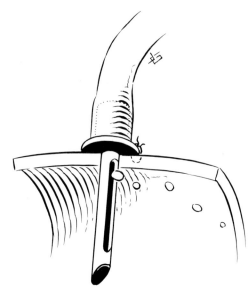

Fig 15–6.—Thumbtack needle vent placed in ascending aorta and connected to suction line can evacuate foam and air bubbles continually. (From McGoon D.C.: Technics of open-heart surgery for congenital heart disease. *Curr. Probl. Surg.*, April 1968, p. 1. Used by permission.)

Air bubbles in the aortic stream then rise and escape through the needle vent. They stated that the critical reduction of the lumen is three fourths of the arterial cross-section; thus, adequate flow continues despite a significant luminal compromise.

The effectiveness of the major techniques to

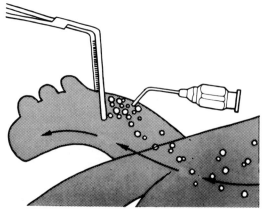

Fig 15–7.—Schematic view showing cupula filling with air bubbles that will be released by needle vent. (From Lemole and Pinder.[27] Used by permission.)

reduce air embolism—apical ventricular venting, aortic root venting, and cardiac chamber compression after chamber filling—was evaluated with Doppler flow studies by Lawrence et al.[26] They found that approximately two thirds of the patients undergoing cardiopulmonary bypass had no detectable bubbles. Air emboli were detected in only 8% of patients undergoing coronary artery bypass grafting procedures. None of the maneuvers was totally effective in preventing air embolism when used alone or in combination; however, repetition of the triad of venting, filling, and compressing the cardiac chambers provided an effective mechanism for removing trapped air.

Embolic phenomena present a significant problem to the patient undergoing cardiopulmonary bypass. Particulate emboli, regardless of their source, can be removed by filters appropriately placed in the bypass circuit. The choice of oxygenator may significantly affect the production of gaseous microemboli, with the membrane oxygenator producing less particulate and gaseous emboli. Air embolism remains a significant potential problem, which is minimized by the use of such maneuvers as elevating and compressing the heart, cardiac chamber venting, and aortic root venting. Thus, no single panacea exists for the problem of embolic phenomena. The team's attention must be focused on several areas at once, and attention to detail will reduce intraoperative embolic complications.

REFERENCES

1. Ames A. III, et al.: Cerebral ischemia: II. The no-reflow phenomenon. *Am. J. Pathol.* 52:437, 1968.
2. Balderman S.C., Bates R.J., Anagnostopoulos C.E.: Cardiac valve replacement: Improved survival related to air exclusion and myocardial protection. *I.M.J.* 151:113, 1977.
3. Blachy P.H., Starr A.: Post-cardiotomy delirium. *Am. J. Psychiatry* 121:371, 1964.
4. Bleyaert A.L., et al.: Thiopental amelioration of brain damage after global ischemia in monkeys. *Anesthesiology* 49:390, 1978.
5. Brennan R.W., Patterson R.H. Jr., Kessler J.: Cerebral blood flow and metabolism during cardiopulmonary bypass: Evidence of microembolic encephalopathy. *Neurology* 21:665, 1971.
6. Brierley J.B.: Neuropathological findings and patients dying after open-heart surgery. *Thorax* 18:291, 1963.
7. Brierley J.B.: Brain damage complicating open-heart surgery: A neuropathological study of 46 patients. *Proc. R. Soc. Med.* 60:858, 1967.
8. Cantu R.C., et al.: Hypotension: A major factor limiting recovery from cerebral ischemia. *J. Surg. Res.* 9:525, 1969.
9. Carrel A.: Experimental operations on the orifices of the heart. *Ann. Surg.* 60:1, 1914.
10. Clark R.E., Dietz D.R., Miller J.G.: Quantification of microemboli in extracorporeal circulation systems. *Surg. Forum* 25:139, 1974.
11. Clark R.E., Dietz D.R., Miller J.G.: Continuous detection of microemboli during cardiopulmonary bypass in animals and man. *Circulation* 54(suppl. 3):74, 1976.
12. Donald D.E., White R.J.: Temporary bilateral occlusion of the common carotid and vertebral arteries in the monkey at normal body temperature. *Neurology* 11:836, 1961.
13. Dutton R.C., et al.: Platelet aggregate emboli produced in patients during cardiopulmonary bypass with membrane and bubble oxygenators and blood filters. *J. Thorac. Cardiovasc. Surg.* 67:258, 1974.
14. Flamm E.S., et al.: Possible molecular mechanisms of barbiturate-mediated protection in regional cerebral ischemia. *Acta Neurol. Scand. Suppl.* 64:150, 1977.
15. Gilman S.: Cerebral disorders after open-heart operations. *N. Engl. J. Med.* 272:489, 1965.
16. Goldstein A. Jr., Wells B.A., Keats A.S.: Increased tolerance to cerebral anoxia by pentobarbital. *Arch. Int. Pharmacodyn. Ther.* 161:138, 1966.
17. Hekmatpanah J.: Cerebral circulation and perfusion in experimental increased intracranial pressure. *J. Neurosurg.* 32:21, 1970.
18. Hekmatpanah J.: Cerebral blood flow dynamics in hypotension and cardiac arrest. *Neurology* 23:174, 1973.
19. Heller S.S., et al.: Psychiatric complications of open-heart surgery: A re-examination. *N. Engl. J. Med.* 283:1015, 1970.
20. Hicks R.E., Edmunds L.H. Jr: Microembolus production and blood filtration during extracorporeal perfusion, in Zapol W.M., Qvist J. (eds.): *Artificial Lungs for Acute Respiratory Failure: Theory and Practice*. New York, Academic Press, 1976.
21. Hill D.G., et al.: Protection from lung damage by blood filtration during deep hypothermia in puppies. *J. Thorac. Cardiovasc. Surg.* 70:133, 1975.
22. Hissen W., et al.: Effect of Dacron wool filtration in microembolism in extracorporeal circulation. *Bull. Soc. Int. Chir.* 33:290, 1974.
23. Hoff J.T., et al.: Barbiturate protection from cerebral infarction in primates. *Stroke* 6:28, 1975.

24. Katoh S., Yoshida F.: Physical factors affecting microembolus formation in extracorporeal circulation. *Ann. Biomed. Eng.* 4:60, 1976.
25. Kornfeld D.S., Zimberg S., Malm J.R.: Psychiatric complications of open-heart surgery. *N. Engl. J. Med.* 273:287, 1965.
26. Lawrence G.H., McKay H.A., Sherensky R.T.: Effective measures in the prevention of intraoperative aeroembolus. *J. Thorac. Cardiovasc. Surg.* 62:731, 1971.
27. Lemole G.M., Pinder G.C.: A method of preventing air embolus in open-heart surgery. *J. Thorac. Cardiovasc. Surg.* 71:557, 1976.
28. Marshall L.F., et al.: Experimental cerebral oligemia and ischemia produced by intracranial hypertension. *J. Neurosurg.* 43:308, 1975.
29. Michenfelder J.D., Milde J.H., Sundt T.M. Jr.: Cerebral protection by barbiturate anesthesia: Use after middle cerebral artery occlusion in Java monkeys. *Arch. Neurol.* 33:345, 1976.
30. Michenfelder J.D., Theye R.A.: Cerebral protection by thiopental during hypoxia. *Anesthesiology* 39:510, 1973.
31. Moseley J.I., Laurent J.P., Molinari G.F.: Barbiturate attenuation of the clinical course and pathologic lesions in a primate stroke model. *Neurology* 25:870, 1975.
32. Osborn J.J., et al.: Clinical use of a Dacron wool filter during perfusion for open-heart surgery. *J. Thorac. Cardiovasc. Surg.* 60:575, 1970.
33. Reed C.C., et al.: Particulate matter in bubble oxygenators. *J. Thorac. Cardiovasc. Surg.* 68:971, 1974.
34. Rockoff M.A., Shapiro H.M.: Barbiturates following cardiac arrest: Possible benefit or Pandora's box, editorial. *Anesthesiology* 49:385, 1978.
35. Sachdev N.S., et al.: Relationship between postcardiotomy delirium, clinical neurological changes, and EEG abnormalities. *J. Thorac. Cardiovasc. Surg.* 54:557, 1967.
36. Safar P., Stezoski W., Nemoto E.M.: Amelioration of brain damage after 12 minutes' cardiac arrest in dogs. *Arch. Neurol.* 33:91, 1976.
37. Snyder B.D., et al.: Failure of thiopental to modify global anoxic injury. *Stroke* 10:135, 1979.
38. Solis R.T., Gibbs M.B.: Filtration of the microaggregates in stored blood. *Transfusion* 12:245, 1972.
39. Solis R.T., et al.: Cardiopulmonary bypass: Microembolization and platelet aggregation. *Circulation* 52:103, 1975.
40. Solis R.T., et al.: Platelet aggregation: Effects of cardiopulmonary bypass. *Chest* 67:558, 1975.
41. Steen P.A., Milde J.H., Michenfelder J.D.: No barbiturate protection in a dog model of complete cerebral ischemia. *Ann. Neurol.* 5:343, 1979.
42. Stockard J.J., et al.: Hypotension-induced changes in cerebral function during cardiac surgery. *Stroke* 5:730, 1974.
43. Swank R.L., Roth J.G., Jansen J.: Screen filtration pressure method and adhesiveness and aggregation of blood cells. *J. Appl. Physiol.* 19:340, 1964.
44. Tarhan S, White R.D., Moffitt E.A.: Anesthesia and postoperative care for cardiac operations. *Ann. Thorac. Surg.* 23:173, 1977.
45. Theye R.A., Patrick R.T., Kirklin J.W.: The electro-encephalogram in patients undergoing open intracardiac operations with the aid of extracorporeal circulation. *J. Thorac. Surg.* 34:709, 1957.
46. Tufo H.M., Ostfeld A.M., Shekelle R.: Central nervous system dysfunction following open-heart surgery. *J.A.M.A.* 212:1333, 1970.
47. Williams I.M., Merrillees N.C.R., Robinson P.M.: Microembolism and the visual system: II. The consequence of emboli in the microcirculation of nervous tissue, especially that comprizing the visual system. *Proc. Aust. Assoc. Neurol.* 12:179, 1975.
48. Witoszka M.M., et al.: Electroencephalographic changes and cerebral complications in open-heart surgery. *J. Thorac. Cardiovasc. Surg.* 66:855, 1973.

16 / Renal Function and Cardiovascular Anesthesia

JOSEPH M. MESSICK, JR.
DAVID M. WILSON
ROY F. CUCCHIARA

RENAL DYSFUNCTION after cardiopulmonary bypass is not uncommon and may be a serious complication. The reported incidence of acute renal failure varies from 2% to 15%, while that of less severe renal dysfunction ranges from 26% to 39%.[4, 39, 40] Mortality ranges from 30% to 38% in mild dysfunction up to 70% in severe dysfunction,[39] and the rates for patients requiring dialysis are especially high.[5] Renal failure after cardiac surgery reportedly occurs less frequently in children than in adults.[5] One study reported an incidence of 8% in infants less than 1 year of age.

A number of factors associated with cardiovascular surgery may contribute to renal dysfunction, and the detection of impending renal problems and the application of possible corrective measures are important. Because a review of renal physiology, the effects of anesthesia and surgery on renal function,[3, 14, 16, 22, 28, 59] and the general management of acute renal failure is beyond the scope of this chapter, only those aspects of renal function that are appropriate to cardiovascular surgery will be discussed.

RENAL FUNCTION

Major functions of the kidneys are as follows[18]: (1) regulation of water balance, electrolyte balance, and acid-base balance; (2) excretion of metabolic waste products; (3) detoxification and elimination of toxins; (4) blood pressure regulation (renin-angiotensin system and prostaglandins); (5) erythropoietic principle; and (6) vitamin D activation (1,25-dihydroxycholecalciferol production). The kidney must filter if it is to function and must be perfused if it is to filter.

The kidneys screen the circulating intravascular fluid compartment at high flow rates to regulate the body fluids and their constituents and to excrete the end products of body metabolism.[18] The kidneys receive 20% to 25% of the cardiac output, although they comprise only approximately 0.5% of the total body weight.[12, 18] Greater appreciation of the high renal blood flow rate may be realized if one considers that, during a 24-hour period, the total blood volume circulates through the kidneys approximately 300 times (or 180 L/day).[19] As a result of this high renal blood flow, most renal tissue is maintained at a relatively high Po_2, delivery of oxygen and other substrates normally is not perfusion-limited, the arteriovenous oxygen extraction is small (approximately 14%), and renal tissue Pco_2 is relatively independent of renal tissue metabolic rate and remains within a relatively narrow range.[12, 18]

Approximately 20% of renal plasma flow filters passively through the glomerular capillary walls to form a filtrate closely resembling an ultrafiltrate of plasma.[6, 7] This passive fluid movement occurs because the hydraulic pressure difference across the glomerular capillary membrane (glomerular capillary hydrostatic pressure minus the hydrostatic pressure in Bowman's space) is greater than the colloid osmotic pressure difference (effective glomerular capillary colloid osmotic pressure minus the effective colloid osmotic pressure of Bowman's space).[6, 7] Under normal conditions, the effective colloid osmotic pressure in Bowman's space is zero, the glomerular capillary hydrostatic pressure approximates 45 mm Hg, and the hydrostatic pressure in Bowman's space approximates 10 mm

Hg.[6,7,19,51] Thus, the difference in glomerular transmembrane hydraulic pressure favoring filtration is approximately 35 mm Hg, whereas the plasma oncotic pressure opposing filtration approximates 27 mm Hg.[6,7,19] Although the plasma oncotic pressure increases (because of the formation of protein-free glomerular ultrafiltrate) as blood travels from the afferent to the efferent end of the glomerular capillary network, in man the net ultrafiltration pressure probably always favors filtration in normal situations.[6,7,30,31,43] Thus, since the entire glomerular capillary network normally is used for filtration, an increase in renal plasma flow per se will not increase glomerular filtration rate. In this sense, glomerular filtration rate is relatively independent of renal blood flow per se.[31,43]

Renal oxygen consumption rate is relatively high, comprising approximately 7% of the total-body oxygen consumption rate.[12] This high oxygen consumption rate is consistent with the high work load of the kidney. Most of this work is internal, related to various tubular transport mechanisms,[12] unlike the external work performed by some other organs such as the heart. A significant portion of renal oxygen consumption rate is directly related to the rate of sodium reabsorption.[12,60] In turn, the sodium load that the kidneys must process is related to the glomerular filtration rate, which is related to renal blood flow. This factor emphasizes a peculiarity between the blood flow and the oxygen consumption rate in the kidney compared with that of other organs. In most organs, alterations in metabolism lead to changes in tissue blood flow, whereas in the kidney, blood flow regulates oxygen consumption.[60] Although transport involved in reabsorption of the filtered sodium load is a primary determinant of renal oxygen consumption, the "basal" renal oxygen consumption required for other renal functions is significant and is variously estimated at from 3% to 18% of the total renal oxygen consumption.[12]

Autoregulation

If renal function changed with the changes in blood pressure and cardiac output that occur in various activities during a day, this would be a great disadvantage. Fortunately, the kidney has the ability to autoregulate both renal blood flow and glomerular filtration rate. Autoregulation refers to the ability of the kidney to maintain renal blood flow and glomerular filtration rate relatively constant as renal perfusion pressure (which approximates mean arterial pressure) varies. Autoregulation is accomplished by changing the renal vascular resistance as perfusion pressure changes. The limits of autoregulation of renal blood flow are renal perfusion pressures of approximately 75 to 180 mm Hg.[38] Glomerular filtration rate is autoregulated at slightly higher pressures than is renal blood flow.[38] The primary site of autoregulation appears to be the renal afferent arteriole.[38] Autoregulation of renal blood flow involves primarily the 90% of the total renal blood flow that perfuses the renal cortex; medullary blood flow tends to be related directly to systemic blood flow.[18]

Although various mechanisms have been proposed for renal autoregulation, agreement has not been reached. Currently, the primary mechanisms proposed for autoregulation of renal blood flow are (1) the *myogenic hypothesis* (smooth muscle cells intrinsically can contract when they are stretched; hence, afferent arterioles could contract in response to an increase in renal perfusion pressure),[18,31] and (2) the *macula densa hypothesis*, in which autoregulation functions primarily to maintain a normal glomerular filtration rate and hence a normal sodium load. The renin-angiotensin system is a presumed mediator in the macula densa hypothesis.[18,38] Major hypotheses for autoregulation of glomerular filtration rate are the *myogenic hypothesis*, the *macula densa feedback hypothesis*, a *prostaglandin hypothesis*, and a *metabolic mechanism*.[31] Although there is considerable controversy over the role of the macula densa in the autoregulation of glomerular filtration rate, this hypothesis and the current myogenic hypothesis probably have the greatest support, with prostaglandins involved as modifying factors and in the intrarenal distribution of renal blood flow.

Extrinsic Regulation of Renal Blood Flow

The sympathetic nervous system and certain hormones (for example, vasopressin, angiotensin, serotonin) also influence renal blood flow, as do pharmacologic agents, such as anesthetics and sedatives.[18] Although most of these factors primarily affect the afferent arteriole, the sympathetic nervous system also influences intrarenal distribution of flow.[18]

RENIN-ANGIOTENSIN-ALDOSTERONE SYSTEM

The renin-angiotensin-aldosterone system is involved in the regulation of renal blood flow and glomerular filtration rate, of body fluid volume and composition, and of blood pressure.

Renin, a proteolytic enzyme synthesized and stored in specialized granular epithelial cells (juxtaglomerular cells), initiates the formation of a series of active peptides, angiotensins I, II, and III, by converting the tetradecapeptide α-globulin (synthesized primarily in the liver) into a decapeptide, angiotensin I.[11, 23, 42, 44] Angiotensin I, in turn, is cleaved by several aminopeptidases and by converting enzyme, which splits off two terminal amino acids to form the vasoactive octapeptide angiotensin II.[11, 15, 44] Converting enzyme is present in various tissues but is present in the lung in sufficiently high concentration to convert nearly all the angiotensin I entering the pulmonary circulation into angiotensin II during a single pass through the lung.[45, 61] Angiotensin II is removed from the circulation by hydrolysis by tissue peptidases. One product, angiotensin III, may be a primary stimulus to aldosterone secretion. (Angiotensin II may stimulate aldosterone secretion also.[23, 44])

Angiotensin II influences blood pressure directly and indirectly.[41] It is a vasoconstrictor of arteriolar smooth muscle.[11, 15, 41] Indirectly, angiotensin II influences blood pressure via the CNS, the sympathetic nervous system, the adrenal medulla, the heart, and possibly systemic veins.[41] Different vascular beds, and different portions of the same vascular bed, vary in their response to angiotensin II.[15] The splanchnic, hepatic, renal, and cutaneous beds appear to be the most sensitive.[15] The pulmonary vascular bed seems to be relatively resistant.[15] Renal vascular response to angiotensin II is inversely related to plasma renin activity, blunted by sodium depletion (acute or chronic), and enhanced by acute sodium loading or chronic high-sodium diets and desoxycorticosterone acetate.[41]

Control of renal renin release involves three groups of mechanisms:[15]

(1) two intrarenal receptors, the renal vascular receptor [in the renal afferent arteriole] and the macula densa; (2) the renal sympathetic nerves . . . ; and (3) several humoral agents including epinephrine, norepinephrine, sodium and potassium ions, angiotensin II, and antidiuretic hormone.

In general, (1) renal renin release is stimulated by factors that decrease renal afferent arteriolar wall tension, (2) (the current view is that) decreased sodium or chloride load at the macula densa stimulates renin release, (3) increased sympathoadrenal activity stimulates renin release via an intrarenal β-adrenergic receptor, (4) changes in plasma sodium or potassium concentrations produce inverse changes in renin release, and (5) renin release is inhibited by angiotensins I and II and by antidiuretic hormone.[15, 44]

To recapitulate briefly, two important physiologic actions of angiotensin II are its vasoconstrictor effect, including the renal vasculature, and its stimulation of aldosterone secretion.[26] With regard to regulation of renal renin release, the renal vascular baroreceptor mechanism probably is dominant within the autoregulatory range, while the macula densa mechanism achieves increasing importance at perfusion pressures below this range.[15]

Anesthesia can alter the renin-angiotensin-aldosterone axis at the site of renin release and at the site of aldosterone synthesis.[46] Blood pressure during anesthesia may become angiotensin-dependent, especially in instances of sodium depletion.[36, 46] Miller et al.[37] suggested that blood pressure support becomes more angiotensin-dependent during anesthesia with agents that depress the sympathetic nervous system but is not significantly angiotensin-dependent when anesthetic agents that stimulate the sympathetic nervous system are used. Plasma renin activity has been reported to increase threefold during surgery, particularly when fluid intake is low,[53] and to remain elevated 3½-fold during surgery involving cardiopulmonary bypass.[46] Increased renin levels may have contributed to elevated levels of aldosterone, sodium retention, and potassium losses seen in these patients.[46, 53] Taylor et al.[62] reported a large (threefold) increase in plasma angiotensin II levels above prebypass levels in ten patients undergoing normothermic, nonpulsatile bypass. Angiotensin II levels remained at these high levels for approximately two hours postoperatively, returned toward normal at approximately four hours postoperatively, and persisted at low levels for 24 hours. The elevation in angiotensin II levels was significantly greater than that occurring during or after closed mitral valvulotomy in six other patients. The authors suggested that the renin-angiotensin system is a significant factor in early postbypass peripheral vasoconstriction and hypertension and may contribute to the low-output syndrome.

Defining hypertension as a "persistent systolic blood pressure greater than or equal to 160 mm Hg and/or diastolic pressure greater than or equal to 90 mm Hg despite increased anesthesia intraoperatively or treatment of pain and anxiety postoperatively," Roberts et al.[52] noted that increased plasma catecholamine and renin levels were associated with the perioperative hypertension seen in 48% of their 100 patients undergoing coronary artery bypass graft operations. The hypertension was characterized primarily by an increased systemic vascular resistance and could be treated effectively by sodium nitroprusside.

Plasma renin activity increased above surgical levels after release of the aortic cross-clamping in 21 patients undergoing major surgery of the abdominal aorta.[20] The authors suggested that the contributing factors may be decreased renal blood flow during aortic cross-clamping (even with infrarenal clamp placement), hypotension when the clamp is released, loss of blood, and visceral retraction.

Rocchini et al.[55] reported that hypertension after resection of coarctation of the aorta may be initiated by the sympathetic nervous system and maintained, at least partially, by the renin-angiotensin system.

ANTIDIURETIC HORMONE

A major factor in the ability of the kidneys to concentrate urine and conserve body water is antidiuretic hormone (arginine vasopressin). Antidiuretic hormone is synthesized in the hypothalamic supraoptic and paraventricular nuclei, packaged in secretory granules, and transported by axon flow primarily to either the posterior lobe of the pituitary gland (main pathway) or the median eminence (second pathway).[66]

The major physiologic stimuli for vasopressin release are an increase in plasma osmolality and a depletion of blood volume.[24, 32]

Under normal conditions, plasma osmolality is the principal regulator of secretion of antidiuretic hormone.[32] A sensitive osmoreceptor located near the thirst center in the anterior hypothalamus stimulates an increase in plasma antidiuretic hormone of 0.34 pg/ml for each unit increase in plasma osmolality above the threshold level.[54] This effect means that a change of 1% (2.9 mOsm/kg) in plasma osmolality would cause a change of approximately 1 pg/ml in plasma antidiuretic hormone.[54] Another sensitive mechanism, the urine concentrating mechanism, correlates directly with the plasma concentration of antidiuretic hormone, so that urine osmolality increases 250 mOsm/kg (average) for each unit increment in plasma antidiuretic hormone above threshold.[54] The combination of these two sensitive mechanisms results in a system in which small changes in plasma osmolality are transformed rapidly into relatively large changes in urine osmolality and flow.[54] For example, a change of 1 mOsm/kg in plasma osmolality normally leads to a change of about 95 mOsm/kg in urine osmolality, nearly a hundredfold gain.[54]

Volume depletion as a stimulus for vasopressin secretion is distinct from hypertonicity[24] and presumably is mediated by baroreceptors in the left atrium, the great pulmonary veins, the aortic arch, the carotid sinus, and the right subclavian artery.[24, 32] The baroreceptors seemingly are stretch receptors that respond to change in tension in the receptor wall, rather than to a change in the actual volume of blood present. A decrease in wall tension causes a decrease in afferent impulses (which travel via the glossopharyngeal and vagus nerves and the aortic nerves), which in turn results in an increase in vasopressin secretion.[32] An increase in wall tension increases afferent activity, which decreases vasopressin secretion. A decrease in effective blood volume of more than 8% to 10%, independent of change in renal hemodynamics or plasma osmolality, results in a large increase in vasopressin secretion,[24, 32] while a decrease greater than 25% produces up to a 25- to 50-fold increase in the rate of vasopressin secretion. In high concentrations, vasopressin appears to act as a pressor agent, as well as an antidiuretic agent,[24, 32] and is one of the most potent endogenous vasoconstrictors in man (direct action on vascular smooth muscle).[13, 47] (Maximal antidiuretic effect is seen at plasma vasopressin concentrations of less than 20 pg/ml.[47]) Thus, at very high concentrations, the pressor action of vasopressin may be advantageous to the patient and may be more responsible for changes in urine flow (due to hemodynamic changes) than for its antidiuretic effect on the collecting duct cells in the kidney. High doses of vasopressin, in the pharmacologic range, decrease renal plasma flow and glomerular filtration rate, with decreases in renal plasma flow being greater.[65]

Philbin and co-authors[47–49] found some of the highest levels of antidiuretic hormone reported in man in patients undergoing surgery and cardiopulmonary bypass. The antidiuretic hormone levels, well above those required for the antidiuretic action of the hormone, did not occur with anesthesia alone, but rather increased after surgery began. These authors suggested that the unphysiologic state of cardiopulmonary bypass, with loss of pulsatile flow and large decrease in left atrial pressure, initiates an endogenous attempt to achieve pressor action of the hormone and that the maximal secretion of antidiuretic hormone in response to the stress of bypass overrides the usual osmotic control of vasopressin secretion.

Vasopressin travels via the systemic circulation to its major receptors in the kidney, where it binds with specific receptors in the serosal basal membrane of cells in the collecting ducts and late segments of the distal convoluted tubule. Through a series of steps involving cyclic adenosine monophosphate, water permeability of the luminal membrane of these cells is increased, permitting water to be drawn from the tubular lumen by the medullary interstitial osmotic gradient maintained by the countercurrent mechanism.[17, 24, 30]

DIURETICS

Loop Diuretics

The "loop diuretics" (those that work in the loop of Henle), primarily furosemide and ethacrynic acid, are bound to plasma proteins, which limits their filtration at the glomerulus. They are secreted into the proximal tubular fluid by the transport system that secretes p-aminohippuric acid, and they inhibit active chloride transport in the thick portion of the ascending limb of Henle's loop.[8, 9, 21, 57] These drugs increase renal sodium and chloride excretion. Renal potassium secretion is stimulated by the increased fluid and sodium delivery to the distal tubule, with potassium excretion increasing to two to five times the predrug level.[8] (For a description of regulation of potassium secretion, see Giebisch.[21]) The decrease in glomerular filtration rate associated with these drugs appears to be related primarily to a decrease in extracellular fluid volume.[57] Intravenous furosemide or ethacrynic acid has its onset of action within five minutes and its peak effect in 15 to 20 minutes.[8] Most of the sodium excretion is completed within one to three hours. Ethacrynic acid and furosemide have a steep dose-response curve and can produce diuresis even in the presence of severe volume depletion, metabolic alkalosis, or severe hyponatremia, if the kidneys are functioning.[50] Thus, improper use of these diuretics may produce serious complications and may result in death.[50] The main adverse effects of these drugs, volume depletion and metabolic abnormalities, result from their improper and excessive use.[50]

Excessive intravascular volume depletion, the most frequent complication, can result in orthostatic hypotension or shock, which may be complicated by hypokalemia and may result in death. The hemodynamic effects result from reduction in left ventricular preload, owing primarily to the depleted intravascular volume. Furosemide also directly decreases venous tone, increasing venous capacitance. The diuresis may cause little change in heart rate or cardiac index if preexisting left ventricular pressure was high but may result in a decrease in stroke volume and cardiac index, with a compensatory increase in heart rate, if preexisting left ventricular filling pressure was normal or low. In this regard, caution should be exercised when interpreting left atrial pressure as an index of left ventricular filling pressure in patients with obstruction to left ventricular filling (for example, mitral stenosis, constrictive pericarditis, or pericardial tamponade). Volume depletion also may result in inadequate perfusion of the brain, bowel, or extremities.

Metabolic abnormalities include hypokalemia, hyponatremia, metabolic alkalosis, or hyperuricemia. Hypokalemia is especially dangerous in patients receiving digitalis and having a propensity for ventricular dysrhythmias. Hyponatremia occurs more frequently in edematous patients, in whom it may be present even though the total-body sodium value is increased. Recall also that acute diuresis may result in sodium depletion from the walls of blood vessels, which may contribute to hypotension.

Osmotic Diuretics

Osmotic diuretics, such as mannitol, work predominantly in the proximal tubule, where they decrease water reabsorption and hence sodium reabsorption. This action results in an increased intraluminal fluid flow rate and delivery of an increased sodium load to the distal tubule. This combination increases potassium secretion in the distal tubule, and the increased flow rate also decreases the effectiveness of the countercurrent mechanism.[21, 29] Osmotic diuretics have been used for both prophylaxis and treatment of acute renal failure. The proposed benefits, together with some less enthusiastic aspects of their use in acute renal failure, are discussed in the following section on acute renal failure.

ACUTE RENAL FAILURE

"Acute renal failure" is a term frequently used in descriptions of renal dysfunction associated with cardiovascular surgery. What is acute renal failure? The following discussion from the medical and physiology literature concerns acute renal failure in general and is not oriented toward postoperative cardiovascular patients per se.

Acute renal failure has been defined as a rapid decrease in renal function characterized by rapidly progressive oliguria and azotemia.[35] Oliguria implies a urinary volume that is inadequate for the excretion of waste products without a change in body fluids and is influenced by diet.[35] For practical purposes, oliguria can be defined as urinary output of less than 400 ml/day (<20 ml/hour).[35] Although oliguria usually is a characteristic feature of acute renal failure, a milder nonoliguric form can occur in 5% to 30% of patients.

The terms "acute renal failure" (a clinical description) and "acute tubular necrosis" (a histo-

TABLE 16–1.—Major Causes of Acute Renal Failure*

CLASSIFICATION	EXAMPLES
A. Postrenal failure	
1. Obstruction	Calculi, neoplasms of bladder and pelvic organs, prostatism, surgical accidents, ureteral instrumentation
2. Rupture of bladder	. . .
B. Prerenal failure	
1. Hypovolemia	Skin losses (sweating, burns)
	Gastrointestinal losses (diarrhea, vomiting)
	Renal losses (diuretics, osmotic diuresis in diabetes mellitus)
	Hemorrhage
	Sequestration (burns, peritonitis)
2. Cardiovascular failure	
a. Myocardial failure	Infarction, tamponade, dysrhythmias
b. Vascular pooling	Sepsis, septic abortion, anaphylaxis, extreme acidosis
C. Acute tubular necrosis	
1. Postischemic	All conditions causing prerenal failure (see classification B above)
2. Heme pigments	
a. Intravascular hemolysis	Transfusion reactions, hemolysis due to toxins or immunologic damage, malaria
b. Rhabdomyolysis and myoglobinuria	Trauma, muscle disease, prolonged coma, seizures, heat stroke, severe exercise
3. Nephrotoxins	. . .
4. Pregnancy-related	Toxic abortifacients, septic abortion, uterine hemorrhage
D. Other renal diseases	
1. Glomerulitis	Poststreptococcal, lupus erythematosus
2. Vasculitis	Periarteritis, hypersensitivity angiitis
3. Malignant nephrosclerosis	. . .
4. Acute diffuse pyelonephritis, papillary necrosis	. . .
5. Severe hypercalcemia	. . .
6. Intratubular precipitation	Myeloma, urates after cytotoxic drugs, sulfonamides
7. Hepatorenal syndrome	. . .
8. Pregnancy-related	Eclampsia, postpartum renal failure
E. Vascular obstruction	
1. Arterial	Thrombosis, embolism, aneurysm
2. Venous	Thrombosis, vena caval obstruction, diffuse small vein thrombosis in amyloidosis

*From Levinsky and Alexander.[35] Used by permission.

logic description) frequently are used interchangeably. However, the incidence of histologic acute tubular necrosis in patients with acute renal failure may be only 10% to 20%,[56] and acute tubular necrosis is one class of acute renal failure[35] (Table 16–1).

Major causes of acute renal failure as classified by Levinsky and Alexander[35] are listed in Table 16–1. This chapter will focus on factors that may result in acute renal failure (prerenal failure and acute tubular necrosis), although the diagnosis of acute renal failure might not become clear until the postoperative period. In general, acute tubular necrosis accounts for approximately 75% of all cases of acute renal failure.[35] Probably the most frequent causes of acute renal failure and acute tubular necrosis are prolonged prerenal azotemia and renal ischemia, respectively.[34, 35, 56]

Prerenal Failure

Cardiac failure, volume depletion, and peripheral vasodilatation are the principal causes of renal hypoperfusion and prerenal azotemia.[56] At this stage of prerenal failure, restoration of cardiac output or adequate blood volume will restore adequate renal function.[35] If renal insufficiency progresses, however, it reaches an irreversible stage at which prerenal failure becomes acute tubular necrosis.[35] "Clinical experience indicates that there is great variation in both the duration and the severity of circulatory insufficiency needed to precipitate acute tubular necrosis."[35] Similarly,

noteworthy renal ischemia can occur in normotensive man during modest reductions of cardiac output. Thus, it should not be surprising that minor episodes of circulatory insufficiency may trigger acute renal failure in man, even if there has been no prior hypotension or shock.[34]

Factors that predispose to acute renal failure include advanced age, hypovolemia, decreased cardiac output, and exposure to nephrotoxins. Both the incidence of and the mortality from acute renal failure are higher in the elderly.[56] Contributing factors include the known deterioration in renal function with increasing age and the greater likelihood that the patient will be taking medications that have renal effects for other systemic pathophysiologic conditions. Examples of such medications include prostaglandin synthesis inhibitors (for example, indomethacin) for arthritis or diuretics for hypertension.

A progressive decline in total renal blood flow and in glomerular filtration rate occurs with advancing age at a rate of approximately 10% per decade.[58] Contributing factors may include a decrease in cortical perfusion; greater age-related atrophy in the cortex than in the medulla; and the predilection of associated vascular lesions for small arteries rather than arterioles, resulting in a distribution that favors simultaneous filtration pressure reduction in numerous glomeruli.[27] Although glomerular filtration rate declines, the decline in renal plasma flow is greater, so the calculated filtration fraction increases.[27] Explanations offered for this phenomenon have included an increase in postglomerular resistance or preferential obliteration of the outer cortical nephrons, which normally have higher renal plasma flow and lower glomerular filtration rate than inner cortical nephrons.[27] Although not without problems, creatinine clearance (C_{Cr}) often is used as an indicator of glomerular filtration rate. Two formulas for estimating expected "normal" creatinine clearance in milliliters per minute are:

$$C_{Cr} = 1.33\,[0.64\ \text{age (yr)}] \pm 30\ \text{ml/minute}^{58}$$

and

$$C_{Cr} = \frac{140 - \text{age (yr)}}{\text{serum creatinine (mg/dl)}}\ (\text{males})$$
$$= \text{above formula} \times 0.9\ (\text{females})^{64}$$

Because a creatinine clearance of 100 ml/minute or more is considered to be adequate, the number obtained with the second equation also represents the patient's percentage of normal renal function.[64] Some consider a glomerular filtration rate greater than 50 ml/minute to indicate adequate renal function with respect to filtration.[27]

Cardiac Failure

Decreased cardiac output can cause renal hypoperfusion. If cardiac failure is the cause, the resulting elevated left atrial pressure may provide some early renal protection because of the reflex decrease in renal sympathetic tone it causes.[56] In cardiac failure, renal blood flow decreases approximately in proportion to the decrease in cardiac output. Decreased renal perfusion results in increased renin release and formation of angiotensin II.[10, 63] Angiotensin II causes vasoconstriction and stimulates the release of aldosterone from the adrenal cortex.[63]

Aldosterone stimulates sodium reabsorption from the tubular lumen.[63] The decrease in cardiac output causes a decrease in arterial distending pressure, which also elicits systemic compensatory mechanisms.[10] One such mechanism is an increase in sympathetic tone, including an increase in arteriolar vasoconstriction, which contributes to a decrease in renal blood flow.[10] Increased sympathetic and renin-angiotensin activity are believed to be the primary mediators of renal vasoconstriction in cardiac failure.[10] In addition to a decrease in total renal blood flow, some workers believe that there is a preferential decrease in flow to the outer renal cortex, with a shift in flow toward the inner cortical and juxtamedullary nephrons. Schrier[56] has noted that, "for a given decrement in blood pressure, the degree of renal ischemia is less during cardiac failure (increase in left atrial pressure) than it is during hemorrhage (decrease in left atrial pressure)."

In mild heart failure, the glomerular filtration rate declines, but not to the extent that the renal blood flow does.[10] Therefore, the calculated filtration fraction increases. Greater efferent than afferent vasoconstriction is the mechanism believed to be responsible.[10] Such differential vasoconstriction tends to maintain glomerular capillary hydrostatic pressure, promoting filtration while simultaneously decreasing the hydrostatic pressure in the capillaries. The increased plasma oncotic pressure in the peritubular capillaries (secondary to the increased filtration fraction), together with the decreased hydrostatic pressure, would promote return of fluid in the filtrate from the tubular lumen into the peritubular capillaries. Increased tubular reabsorption of sodium chloride and water occurs in patients with congestive heart failure, although there is no consensus of opinion on the precise renal tubular location(s) where this occurs.[10] Physical forces, the renin-angiotensin-aldosterone axis, and the intrarenal effects of the sympathetic nervous system, the renin-angiotensin-aldosterone system, the kinin-kininogen system, and renal prostaglandins may be involved.[10]

Reduction in the sodium and water content of the body is important in the therapy of heart failure.[63] Decrease in intake and promotion of excretion of sodium and water are necessary.[63] An increase in cardiac output and renal perfusion, which may involve use of cardiotonic drugs, will help promote excretion.[63] Avoidance of cardiac depressants is desirable.

In therapy, one must consider primarily increasing cardiac function to reverse the factors set in motion. Concurrently, one must be aware that a decreased plasma volume will not allow the reversal of renal sodium retention and poor perfusion. Thus, with renal insufficiency in the presence of cardiac failure, cardiac function should not be improved at the expense of a normal plasma volume.

Acute Tubular Necrosis

Conditions that cause prerenal failure can also cause acute tubular necrosis (see Table 16–1). Two other causes of acute tubular necrosis are the heme pigments (hemoglobin, myoglobin) and nephrotoxins.

A discussion of nephrotoxins is beyond the scope of this chapter. We should note, however, that the aminoglycoside antibiotics (amikacin, gentamicin, kanamycin, neomycin, streptomycin, and tobramycin) can be nephrotoxic.[56] This nephrotoxicity seems to be related to cortical tissue-binding, which in turn is related to the number of free amino groups.[56] The half-life of these drugs in the serum is approximately 30 minutes; their half-life in renal tissue is approximately 109 hours.[56] Radiographic dyes may be toxic in patients with mild renal insufficiency, prerenal insufficiency, or diabetes. If the time interval between angiography and surgery is less than 48 hours, this complication may not be recognized before surgery.

Of the heme pigments, myoglobinuria may cause acute renal failure more often than hemoglobinuria.[56] Examples of clinical settings in which myoglobinuria may occur include muscle damage, viral infections, hypokalemia, alcoholism, drug abuse, and acute hypophosphatemia.[56] Purified hemoglobin is not nephrotoxic.[35] Infusion of hemoglobin alone does not elicit a reproducible model of acute renal failure. The toxic or vasoconstrictive elements that produce the renal failure associated with hemoglobinuria appear to come from RBC membranes or stroma or from muscle.[35, 56] Volume depletion may contribute also.[56] "Intravascular hemolysis of any type may precipitate acute tubular necrosis."[35]

Factors to be considered in the differential diagnosis of prerenal failure versus acute tubular necrosis are summarized in Table 16–2.

TABLE 16-2—URINARY INDICES OF ACUTE RENAL FAILURE

	PRERENAL	ACUTE OLIGURIC	ACUTE TUBULAR NECROSIS
Urine sodium (random sample),* mEq/L	Usually <10†; <20*	>40*	≥25 in oliguric; no consistent elevation in nonoliguric†
Urine osmolality, mOsm/kg of water	Usually >500*	<350*	. . .
U/P‡ osmolality	High†	. . .	Usually ≤1:1†
U/P urea nitrogen	>20:1†; >8:1*	<3*	Usually ≤3:1; rarely >10:1†
U/P creatinine	Usually >40:1*†; rarely <10:1†	<20*	Usually <10:1†
Renal failure index* $\frac{U_{Na}}{(U/P)_{Cr}}$	<1*	>1*	. . .
Fractional excretion of filtered sodium, % $\frac{(U/P)_{Na}}{(U/P)_{Cr}} \times 100$	<1*	>1*	. . .

*Data from Schrier.[56]
†Data from Levinsky and Alexander.[35]
‡Urine-plasma ratio.

The pathophysiology of nonspecific acute renal failure (ignoring specific causes such as glomerulonephritis, vascular disease, and so forth) is multifactorial.[34, 56] Two major points of view have emerged as to the principal cause of acute renal failure: tubular necrosis, with tubular luminal obstruction by cell debris and proteinaceous casts and "back-leak" of filtrate through the damaged tubular epithelium; and vasoconstriction with "persistent self-perpetuating renal ischemia."[54] Renal vasoconstriction persists during acute renal failure, with reduction of total renal blood flow to between one fourth and one half of normal, and pronounced diminution in the outer cortical flow as determined by inert-gas washout curves.[34] In most patients with acute renal failure, plasma renin activity increases during failure and decreases to normal with return of adequate renal function; this is compatible with persistent vasoconstriction.[34] That renal vasoconstriction is not the whole answer is evidenced by other data, such as the observation that infusion of known vasodilators (for example, acetylcholine, prostaglandins) into the renal artery of patients with acute renal failure produces large increases in renal blood flow, but oliguria persists.[34] Decreased glomerular filtration rate, back-leak of filtrate, and obstruction of tubular lumen may contribute to the persistent oliguria.[35] We have referred to back-leak and tubular obstruction previously. One explanation for decreased glomerular filtration rate is persistent afferent arteriolar constriction concomitant with efferent arteriolar dilatation[56]; this combination would lower the glomerular capillary hydrostatic pressure.

Thus, both vascular mechanisms and tubular mechanisms are important in the pathogenesis of acute renal failure and are probably interdependent.[34, 56] Levinsky and Alexander[35] have summarized a proposed scheme (Fig 16–1). The relative contributions of the various pathogenetic factors in acute renal failure probably vary with the cause, severity, and duration of the initial insult and the failure.[34, 56]

Prevention is the key.

Acute tubular necrosis usually occurs in predictable clinical settings; anticipation is the key to prevention. Postischemic acute tubular necrosis may be prevented by prompt and adequate replacement of fluid and blood losses in surgical, burned, or traumatized patients.[35]

The use of mannitol or other potent diuretics for either prophylaxis or treatment is controversial. Proposed benefits include decreased reabsorption of filtrate (decreasing the danger of tubular obstruction) or decreased renal vaso-

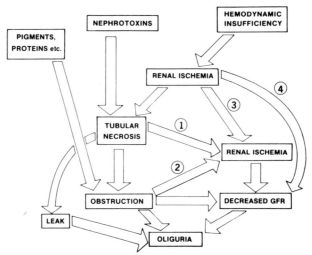

Fig 16-1.—Tubular factors are grouped on left and vascular factors on right. *Unnumbered arrows* indicate well-established relationships. Current hypotheses for which some experimental evidence is available are indicated by the *numbered arrows*: (1) tubular cell damage may alter concentration of salt at macula densa, thereby stimulating renin-angiotensin; (2) obstruction of nephron may cause vasoconstriction of afferent arteriole of attached glomerulus (through unknown mechanisms); (3) vascular mechanisms (deficiency of renal vasodilators; vascular swelling; unknown) may cause self-perpetuating ischemia after initial hemodynamic insult; and (4) ischemia may damage glomerular filtration apparatus, thereby directly decreasing filtration (GFR). (From Levinsky.[34] Used by permission.)

dilatation (particularly of the afferent arterioles) or both.[35] In addition, mannitol might (1) shrink swollen capillary endothelium, with reversal of the "no-reflow" phenomenon, (2) decrease renin secretion by some mechanism not clearly defined, and/or (3) exert some nonspecific beneficial effects, perhaps involving extracellular fluid volume expansion or reduced blood viscosity.[35]

Despite a voluminous literature, it is difficult to determine whether mannitol and loop diuretics prevent acute tubular necrosis in man, because there are no controlled studies. The theory that mannitol prevents acute renal failure in high-risk surgery is supported by clinical testimonials and uncontrolled trials in open-heart, complicated biliary, and major vascular surgery. . . .

Even more attractive and less well substantiated than the view that mannitol or diuretics prevent acute renal failure is the concept that they will reverse early or incipient acute tubular necrosis.[35 (p. 816)]

Implicit in the last quotation is the knowledge that increased urine flow does not necessarily indicate improved renal function. Having briefly reviewed both sides of the controversy, Levinsky and Alexander[35] summarized their own clinical impressions. It seems reasonable to use mannitol (preferably) or furosemide, together with intravenous fluids, to maintain urine output in patients with severe trauma (particularly muscle injury), transfusion reaction, or rapid intravascular hemolysis. In patients undergoing surgical procedures in whom the risk of acute tubular necrosis is high (for example, cardiac surgery, aortic surgery), adding 25 to 50 gm of mannitol per day to the intravenous fluids on the day of surgery and for one to two days after surgery may be beneficial. Of greater importance, however, is what Levinsky and Alexander term "meticulous management of overall fluid balance to avoid volume deficits."[35] Noting that their results using mannitol or furosemide in "incipient" acute tubular necrosis have been "disappointing," they nevertheless agree that a single dose of mannitol or furosemide may be worth trying. They caution, however, that if 25 gm of mannitol or 200 to 400 mg of furosemide is not effective, the use of higher doses probably is unwise.[35] Mannitol or furosemide should not be used to differentiate prerenal failure from acute tubular necrosis.[35]

Preoperative fluid balance may be even more important than postoperative fluid balance, avoiding severe volume depletion, which stimulates antidiuretic hormone and the renin-angiotensin system. In high-risk renal patients, this balance may be accomplished by infusing intravenous fluids containing saline or mannitol (or both) to avoid overnight dehydration.

RENAL DYSFUNCTION ASSOCIATED WITH CARDIAC SURGERY

Abel et al.[1] conducted a prospective study of 500 consecutive patients who survived 24 hours or longer after closed or open cardiac surgical procedures (503 operations, 94.2% involving cardiopulmonary bypass). "Morphine anesthesia," moderate hemodilution, and hypothermia, with Ringer's lactate prime and bubble oxygenation, were usual in patients undergoing open procedures. Diuretics were not used routinely, and there was no specific protocol for treating incipient or established renal failure. Oliguria in the operating room usually was treated initially with mannitol infusion and occasionally with small doses of furosemide. Maintenance of cardiac output was the major thrust of the management of oliguria, including during the postoperative period. Hemoglobinuria was not a significant problem in the patients in their study, and there was no specific protocol for its treatment. The degree of hemoglobinuria did not correlate well with the subsequent development of renal failure. Abel et al. concluded, "Therefore, we do not support the suggestion of others that 'prophylactic' mannitol therapy in high-risk patients is indicated because of the possibility that the drug will promote a diuresis of hemoglobinuric urine."[1] A presumptive diagnosis of acute tubular necrosis was made when fixed oliguria or anuria occurred that was unresponsive to increased cardiac output, increased left atrial pressure, intravenous infusion of 50 gm of mannitol, and a single intravenous bolus of 100 to 200 mg of furosemide. The diagnosis was considered confirmed by the finding of hyposthenuric urine and a high urine sodium excretion.

Either moderate or severe acute renal failure occurred in 35 patients, and mild prerenal azotemia developed in an additional 102 patients in the Abel study.[1] The overall mortality was 6.8%, but the mortality was significantly higher in patients with greater renal dysfunction. The factors that correlated significantly with the incidence of acute renal failure listed in the following are considered to be positive risk factors[1]: (1) degree of preoperative renal dysfunction ("By all methods of statistical comparison, the degree of preoperative renal dysfunction statistically predicted the onset of renal failure in the postoperative period . . ." [p. 326]); (2) degree of hemodynamic impairment; (3) history of chronic renal disease; (4) duration of operation; (5) duration of aortic cross-clamping; (6) age; (7) mean blood pressure in operating room just before transfer to intensive care unit; (8) requirement for intra-aortic balloon pump to wean from bypass (35 patients; class III or IV disease developed in ten); and (9) furosemide use, classes III and IV versus I and II.

Abel et al. also listed the following factors that did not correlate significantly with the incidence of acute renal failure: (1) history of possible intake of nephrotoxins preoperatively; (2) diabetes mellitus; (3) hypertension; (4) arteriosclerotic peripheral vascular disease; (5) cerebrovascular accident (old); (6) chronic obstructive pulmonary disease; (7) anesthetic agent (halothane, methoxyflurane, morphine, droperidol-fentanyl, or diazepam); (8 to 11) degree of hypothermia, mean blood pressure, lowest blood pressure, and mean perfusion flow rates during cardiopulmonary bypass; (12) urine output during operation; (13) occurrence of hemoglobinuria after open-heart procedures; and (14) mannitol use.

The patient classification used by Abel et al. is given in Table 16–3. In their study, the mortality for established acute renal failure was extremely high (88.8%), and there were no survivors among those who required dialysis.[1] All 15 dialysis patients were in class IV. As the authors pointed out, the high mortality in classes III and IV were due primarily to multiple organ failure secondary to inadequate cardiac output, and in only 2 of the 35 deaths was acute renal failure considered to be the direct cause of death, most of the deaths being due to sepsis or to cardiac or respiratory dysfunction. The incidence of acute renal failure after closed-heart procedures was low and was similar to that for general surgical patients.

Abel et al. pointed out that (1) the correlation between the duration of cardiopulmonary bypass and the incidence of acute renal failure was compatible with previous reports of a decrease

TABLE 16-3.—PATIENT CLASSIFICATION IN ACUTE RENAL FAILURE*

	COMMENT
Class I	Normal renal function Serum creatinine not >1.5 mg/dl No dialysis
Class II	Mild azotemia Serum creatinine not >2.5 mg/dl No dialysis
Class III	Mild renal failure Serum creatinine not >5.0 mg/dl No dialysis
Class IV	Severe acute renal failure (mostly acute tubular necrosis) Serum creatinine >5.0 mg/dl or dialysis required

*Data from Abel et al.[1]

in renal blood flow with time during cardiopulmonary bypass; (2) the lack of statistical correlation between acute renal failure and perfusion flow rates or hypotension during cardiopulmonary bypass in this study differed from previous retrospective studies; (3) their study did not support a "protective" effect of mannitol or furosemide, but it also did not incriminate them as etiologic factors in the development of acute renal failure; (4) the study suggested that the use of furosemide may not be justified to augment urine volume alone during the perioperative period; (5) age, preoperative renal failure, and preoperative hemodynamic impairment have in common decreased glomerular filtration rate; and (6) blood urea nitrogen and serum creatinine levels appear to be better predictors of acute renal failure than urinary volume during the first postoperative week.

FREE-WATER CLEARANCE

Early diagnosis of renal insufficiency is not easy. Fractional excretion of sodium, the ratio of urine osmolality to plasma osmolality, and osmolar clearance are helpful in diagnosing renal insufficiency. These parameters are less reliable in patients with increased osmotic load, altered sodium intake, and elevated levels of antidiuretic hormone, as after bypass. Free-water clearance has been reported to be a sensitive and reliable early indicator of acute renal insufficiency or acute renal failure in this setting.[2, 25, 33] It represents renal excretion of water over and above that water required for excretion of the solute load the kidneys are obligated to process (hence, solute-"free" water). It is an indicator of renal concentrative ability and is calculated as the difference between urinary output and osmolar clearance[2, 33]:

$$C_{H_2O} = U_v - C_{osm}$$

where C_{H_2O} is the free-water clearance in milliliters per hour, U_v is the urine volume in milliliters per hour, and C_{osm} is the osmolar clearance calculated as follows:

$$C_{osm} = (U_{osm} \times U_v)/P_{osm}$$

where U_{osm} is urine osmolality in milliosmoles per kilogram and P_{osm} is the plasma osmolality in milliosmoles per kilogram.

Free-water clearance in this setting normally is negative, with a range of -25 to -100 ml/hour, but it becomes less negative or even positive in renal failure.[2, 25, 33]

Baek et al.,[2] studying sequential changes in renal function in 38 postoperative patients in intensive care units, proposed that free-water clearance values near zero be used as criteria for the early diagnosis of acute renal failure. They had diagnosed acute renal failure by standard clinical and laboratory criteria (oliguria, low urinary specific gravity, urine sodium excretion greater than 40 mEq/L, and increasing creatinine and blood urea nitrogen levels), paying particular attention to osmolar and free-water clearances. Free-water clearances near zero were found one to three days before the standard clinical and laboratory criteria indicated acute renal failure.

Heimann et al.[25] studied 40 consecutive patients undergoing cardiopulmonary bypass with a hyperosmolar prime (mean osmolality 450 mOsm/kg). (Neither perfusion pressure during bypass nor the anesthetic agents and technique were described.) Postoperative renal dysfunction (defined as a blood urea nitrogen value >50 mg/dl) occurred in 23% of the patients, with a higher incidence in diabetic than in nondiabetic patients. Free-water clearance was significantly less negative in the renal dysfunction group after one hour of bypass, remained so for the duration of the study (to 18 hours after bypass), and was a more reliable indicator of renal dysfunction than was urine osmolality, osmolar clearance, or urinary sodium excretion.

Defining postoperative acute renal insufficiency as an increase of 100% in serum creatinine concentration or an increase of 400% in blood urea nitrogen levels over preoperative values, Landes et al.[33] found this complication in five of 59 adult patients (8.5% incidence) undergoing nonpulsatile cardiopulmonary bypass involving hemodilution with Ringer's lactate 16 ml/kg and mannitol 0.5 gm/kg. Free-water clearance values were equal to or more positive than −8 ml/hour in the renal dysfunction group but were −20 ml/hour or less in the patients without renal dysfunction. These authors, noting that early recognition of impending renal insufficiency is important, concluded that free-water clearance is a more consistent indicator than is duration of bypass, hemolysis, perfusion, or urine output during bypass.

Unfortunately, the thesis has not been tested as to whether earlier recognition and treatment of acute renal failure in this way will improve morbidity or mortality. (It is possible that the renal dysfunction is irreversible at this point, and thus loop diuretics or mannitol will neither help nor hinder.)

REFERENCES

1. Abel R.M., et al.: Etiology, incidence, and prognosis of renal failure following cardiac operations: Results of a prospective analysis of 500 consecutive patients. *J. Thorac. Cardiovasc. Surg.* 71:323, 1976.
2. Baek S.M., Brown R.S., Shoemaker W.C.: Early prediction of acute renal failure and recovery: I. Sequential measurements of free water clearance. *Ann. Surg.* 177:253, 1973.
3. Bastron R.D., Deutsch S.: *Anesthesia and the Kidney*. New York, Grune & Stratton, 1976.
4. Bevan D.R., et al.: Fluid-loading and cardiopulmonary bypass: A study of renal function. *Anesthesia* 28:631, 1973.
5. Bourgeois B.F., et al.: Effects of cardiac surgery on renal function in children. *J. Thorac. Cardiovasc. Surg.* 77:283, 1979.
6. Brenner B.M., Baylis C., Deen W.M.: Transport of molecules across renal glomerular capillaries. *Physiol. Rev.* 56:502, 1976.
7. Brenner B.M., Humes H.D.: Mechanics of glomerular ultrafiltration. *N. Engl. J. Med.* 297:148, 1977.
8. Burg M.B.: Mechanisms of action of diuretic drugs, in Brenner B.M., Rector F.C. Jr. (eds.): *The Kidney*. Philadelphia, W.B. Saunders Co., 1976, vol. 1, p. 737.
9. Burg M.B.: Renal chloride transport and diuretics, editorial. *Circulation* 53:587, 1976.
10. Cannon P.J.: The kidney in heart failure. *N. Engl. J. Med.* 296:26, 1977.
11. Chonko A.M., Stein J.H., Ferris T.F.: Renin and the kidney. *Nephron* 15:279, 1975.
12. Cohen J.J., Kamm D.E.: Renal metabolism: Relation to renal function, in Brenner B.M., Rector F.C., Jr. (eds.): *The Kidney*. Philadelphia, W.B. Saunders Co., 1976, vol. 1, p. 126.
13. Corliss R.J., et al.: Systemic and coronary hemodynamic effects of vasopressin. *Am. J. Med. Sci.* 256:293, 1968.
14. Cousins M.J., Mazze R.I.: Anaesthesia, surgery and renal function: Immediate and delayed effects. *Anaesth. Intensive Care* 1:355, 1973.
15. Davis J.O., Freeman R.H.: Mechanisms regulating renin release. *Physiol. Rev.* 56:1, 1976.
16. Deutsch S.: Effects of anesthetics on the kidney. *Surg. Clin. North Am.* 55:775, 1975.
17. Dousa T.P., Valtin H.: Cellular actions of vasopressin in the mammalian kidney. *Kidney Int.* 10:46, 1976.
18. Frohnert P.P.: Renal blood flow, in Knox F.G. (ed.): *Textbook of Renal Pathophysiology*. Hagerstown, Md., Harper & Row, 1978, p. 43.
19. Frohnert P.P.: Glomerular filtration, in Knox F.G. (ed.): *Textbook of Renal Pathophysiology*. Hagerstown, Md., Harper & Row, 1978, p. 49.
20. Gal T.J., Cooperman L.H., Berkowitz H.D.: Plasma renin activity in patients undergoing surgery of the abdominal aorta. *Ann. Surg.* 179:65, 1974.
21. Giebisch G.: Effects of diuretics on renal transport of potassium. *Methods Pharmacol.* 4A:121, 1976.
22. Granberg P.-O., Wåhlin Å.: The effect of enflurane (Ethrane[R]) on the renal function with special reference to tubular rejection of sodium. *Acta Anaesthesiol. Scand.* 17:41, 1973.
23. Haber E.: The role of renin in normal and pathological cardiovascular homeostasis. *Circulation* 54:849, 1976.
24. Hays R.M.: Antidiuretic hormone. *N. Engl. J. Med.* 295:659, 1976.
25. Heimann T., et al.: Urinary osmolal changes in renal dysfunction following open-heart operations. *Ann. Thorac. Surg.* 22:44, 1976.
26. Hollenberg N.K., et al.: Reciprocal influence of salt intake on adrenal glomerulosa and renal vascular responses to angiotensin II in normal man. *J. Clin. Invest.* 54:34, 1974.
27. Hollenberg N.K., et al.: Senescence and the renal vasculature in normal man. *Circ. Res.* 34:309, 1974.
28. Jensen B.H., et al.: Glomerular filtration rate during enflurane anaesthesia. *Acta Anaesthesiol. Scand.* 22:13, 1978.

29. Knox F., Tucker R.: Personal communication.
30. Knox F.G., Ott C.E.: Filtration pressure disequilibrium in the dog glomerulus, in Giovannetti S., Bonomini V., D'Amico G. (eds.): *Sixth International Congress of Nephrology.* Basel, Switzerland, S Karger AG, 1976, p. 216.
31. Knox F.G., et al.: Regulation of glomerular filtration and proximal tubule reabsorption. *Circ. Res.* 36(suppl. 1):107, 1975.
32. Kurtzman N.A., Boonjarern S.: Physiology of antidiuretic hormone and the interrelationship between the hormone and the kidney. *Nephron* 15:167, 1975.
33. Landes R.G., et al.: Free-water clearance and the early recognition of acute renal insufficiency after cardiopulmonary bypass. *Ann. Thorac. Surg.* 22:41, 1976.
34. Levinsky N.G.: Pathophysiology of acute renal failure. *N. Engl. J. Med.* 296:1453, 1977.
35. Levinsky N.G., Alexander E.A.: Acute renal failure, in Brenner B.M., Rector F.C. Jr. (eds.): *The Kidney.* Philadelphia, W.B. Saunders Co., 1976, vol. 2, p. 806.
36. Miller E.D. Jr., Ackerly J.A., Peach M.J.: Blood pressure support during general anesthesia in a renin-dependent state in the rat. *Anesthesiology* 48:404, 1978.
37. Miller E.D. Jr., Longnecker D.E., Peach M.J.: The regulatory function of the renin-angiotensin system during general anesthesia. *Anesthesiology* 48:399, 1978.
38. Navar L.G.: Renal autoregulation: Perspectives from whole kidney and single nephron studies. *Am. J. Physiol.* 234:F357, 1978.
39. Nuutinen L., Hollmén A.: Cardiopulmonary bypass time and renal function. *Ann. Chir. Gynaecol.* 65:191, 1976.
40. Nuutinen L.S.: The effect of nitrous oxide on renal function in open heart surgery. *Ann. Chir. Gynaecol.* 65:200, 1976.
41. Oliver J.A., Cannon P.J.: The effect of altered sodium balance upon renal vascular reactivity to angiotensin II and norepinephrine in the dog. *J. Clin. Invest.* 61:610, 1978.
42. Oparil S., Haber E.: The renin-angiotensin system. *N. Engl. J. Med.* 291:389; 446, 1974.
43. Ott C.E., et al.: Determinants of glomerular filtration rate in the dog. *Am. J. Physiol.* 231:235, 1976.
44. Peach M.J.: Renin-angiotensin system: Biochemistry and mechanisms of action. *Physiol. Rev.* 57:313, 1977.
45. Peart W.S.: Renin-angiotensin system. *N. Engl. J. Med.* 292:302, 1975.
46. Pettinger W.A.: Anesthetics and the renin-angiotensin-aldosterone axis. *Anesthesiology* 48:393, 1978.
47. Philbin D.M., Coggins C.H.: Plasma antidiuretic hormone levels in cardiac surgical patients during morphine and halothane anesthesia. *Anesthesiology* 49:95, 1978.
48. Philbin D.M., et al.: Radioimmunoassay of antidiuretic hormone during morphine anaesthesia. *Can. Anaesth. Soc. J.* 23:290, 1976.
49. Philbin D.M., et al.: Antidiuretic hormone levels during cardiopulmonary bypass. *J. Thorac. Cardiovasc. Surg.* 73:145, 1977.
50. Plumb V.J., James T.N.: Clinical hazards of powerful diuretics: Furosemide and ethacrynic acid. *Mod. Concepts Cardiovasc. Dis.* 47:91, 1978.
51. Renkin E.M., Gilmore J.P.: Glomerular filtration, in Orloff J., Berliner R.W., Geiger S.R. (eds.): *Handbook of Physiology.* Section 8: *Renal Physiology.* Washington, D.C., American Physiological Society, 1973, p. 185.
52. Roberts A.J., et al.: Systemic hypertension associated with coronary artery bypass surgery: Predisposing factors, hemodynamic characteristics, humoral profile, and treatment. *J. Thorac. Cardiovasc. Surg.* 74:846, 1977.
53. Robertson D., Michelakis A.M.: Effect of anesthesia and surgery on plasma renin activity in man. *J. Clin. Endocrinol. Metab.* 34:831, 1972.
54. Robertson G.L., Shelton R.L., Athar S.: The osmoregulation of vasopressin. *Kidney Int.* 10:25, 1976.
55. Rocchini A.P., et al.: Pathogenesis of paradoxical hypertension after coarctation resection. *Circulation* 54:382, 1976.
56. Schrier R.W.: Acute renal failure. *Kidney Int.* 15:205, 1979.
57. Seely J.F., Dirks J.H.: Site of action of diuretic drugs. *Kidney Int.* 11:1, 1977.
58. Slack T.K., Wilson D.M.: Normal renal function: C_{In} and C_{PAH} in healthy donors before and after nephrectomy. *Mayo Clin. Proc.* 51:296, 1976.
59. Stanley T.H., et al.: The effects of high dose morphine and morphine plus nitrous oxide on urinary output in man. *Can. Anaesth. Soc. J.* 21:379, 1974.
60. Stein J.H.: The renal circulation, in Brenner B.M., Rector F.C. Jr. (eds.): *The Kidney.* Philadelphia, W.B. Saunders Co., 1976, vol. 1, p. 215.
61. Strong C.G.: The renin-angiotensin-aldosterone system, in Knox F.G. (ed.): *Textbook of Renal Pathophysiology.* Hagerstown, Md., Harper & Row, 1978, p. 173.
62. Taylor K.M., et al.: Hypertension and the renin-angiotensin system following open-heart surgery. *J. Thorac. Cardiovasc. Surg.* 74:840, 1977.

References

63. Tucker R.M.: Mechanism of edema formation, in Knox F.G. (ed.): *Textbook of Renal Pathophysiology*. Hagerstown, Md., Harper & Row, 1978, p. 199.
64. Van Scoy R.E., Wilson W.R.: Antimicrobial agents in patients with renal insufficiency. *Mayo Clin. Proc.* 52:704, 1977.
65. Wesson L.G. Jr.: *Physiology of the Human Kidney*. New York, Grune & Stratton, 1969.
66. Zimmerman E.A., Robinson A.G.: Hypothalamic neurons secreting vasopressin and neurophysin. *Kidney Int.* 10:12, 1976.

17 / Mechanisms, Diagnosis, and Treatment of Cardiac Arrhythmias

ROGER D. WHITE

SINCE there are numerous, and frequently easily recognized, explanations for cardiac arrhythmias in patients undergoing anesthesia and operation, this chapter will focus on the electrophysiologic mechanisms underlying the genesis and perpetuation of arrhythmias and how these mechanisms can be altered by pharmacologic or electrical interventions. That hypoxia, hypercapnia, electrolyte derangements, and too light or too deep an anesthetic state can produce cardiac arrhythmias is well known to every anesthesiologist. Perhaps less well appreciated and understood are the electrophysiologic derangements responsible for the rhythm disorder and also the presumed mechanisms of action of several antiarrhythmic drugs. The understanding of such pharmacologic actions has undergone considerable alteration for some of the drugs as a result of recent studies of drug action in diseased, rather than normal, cardiac tissue.

NORMAL MECHANISMS OF IMPULSE FORMATION AND CONDUCTION

Regardless of the site of origin of an abnormal rhythm, rhythm disorders can be caused by disturbances in impulse formation or impulse conduction or a combination of the two.[14] To more fully understand these disturbances, a brief review of normal impulse formation and conduction is necessary.

Action potentials recorded from different sites within the heart have different configurations (Fig 17–1). Sinoatrial pacemaker cells normally generate the spontaneous activity that ultimately depolarizes all of the cardiac cells sequentially. Pacemaker cells in the sinoatrial node possess the intrinsic property, automaticity, of spontaneous phase 4 depolarization. Since these cells are innervated by the autonomic nervous system, the rate at which they depolarize and discharge spontaneously is influenced by the relative tone of the sympathetic and parasympathetic nervous systems.

Sinoatrial impulses are rapidly conveyed along specialized atrial conducting tracts (internodal tracts), permitting simultaneous atrial muscle depolarization and propagation of the impulse to the atrioventricular junction[43] (Fig 17–2). Here, the advancing wave front encounters a functionally important conduction delay effected by virtue of the action potential characteristics of cells in the atrioventricular junction. Atrioventricular nodal cells in the junction generate action potentials rather similar to those in the sinoatrial node in that the resting potential is considerably less negative than that found in other portions of the conducting system (-60 mV as opposed to -85 to -90 mV), and the rate of increase of the upstroke and the amplitude (phase 0) are reduced.[12] These latter two action potential characteristics, which are normal findings in the sinoatrial and atrioventricular nodes, are related to a reduced conduction velocity of the advancing wave front. The functional importance of this property in cells of the atrioventricular node is apparent in that it provides a means of assuring atrial and ventricular contractile synchrony. Such action potentials, with reduced resting voltages and relatively slow rates of increase of phase 0 and reduced phase 0 amplitude, are known as slow-response action potentials.[12] More discussion will follow about how such action potentials, when generated in diseased cardiac tissue, can be causes of and contribute to the perpetuation of cardiac arrhythmias.

The advancing wave front, having passed

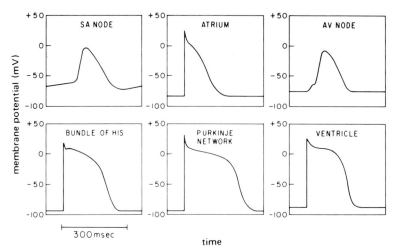

Fig 17-1.—Action potential configurations in different regions of the mammalian heart. (From Katz A.M.: *Physiology of the Heart.* New York, Raven Press, 1977. Used by permission.)

through the atrioventricular junction, enters the three fascicles of the ventricular conducting system (see Fig 17-2) and is conducted to the ramifying terminal portions of the fascicles, Purkinje's fibers, from which the impulse is then conveyed into the ventricular muscle.

Because action potentials of Purkinje's fibers have such an apparently crucial role in ventricular arrhythmias, closer analysis of such action potentials is needed. The configuration of a normal Purkinje fiber potential and the most important currents that seem to be responsible for the various phases of the action potential are depicted in Figure 17-3. Note, in contrast to the sinoatrial and atrioventricular nodal potentials, the high (-90 mV) resting potential, the very steep rate of increase of phase 0 and total amplitude, and the prominent sustained plateau (phase 2) before the period of rapid repolarization (phase 3) and return to resting potential (beginning of phase 4).[19, 21] Rapid depolarization (phase 0) is due to a sudden and explosive increase in membrane sodium permeability that permits a dense, inward sodium current to rapidly carry the interior of the cell to a positive charge.[20] This rapid sodium current, responsible for the steepness of the slope of phase 0, relates to the very rapid conduction velocity in Purkinje's fibers of approximately 2 m/second. When the membrane voltage approaches about -50 mV, another current, carried by both sodium and calcium ions, is activated.[20, 46] This current has much slower kinetics and is known as the slow inward current.[12, 49] It is this slow, inward, positive current that is believed to be primarily responsible for the sustained plateau (phase 2) of the action potential and that also, by virtue of the inward flow of calcium ions and triggered release of calcium ions from the sarcoplasmic reticulum, accounts for the intricate coupling of action potential excitation with the ventricular muscle response—tension generation and fiber shortening (excitation-contraction coupling).[49] Inactivation of this slow inward current permits an outward potassium current to rapidly repolarize the cell (phase 3) and return it to its resting potential. Action potentials recorded from ventricular muscle resemble closely those generated by Purkinje's fibers. These types of action potentials, with high resting voltages, steep phase 0 slopes, and high amplitudes, are called "fast response action potentials" and are found in cells conducting the impulse at a rapid conduction velocity.[47]

ABNORMAL MECHANISMS

As was stated earlier, cardiac arrhythmias can be conceived as being the consequence of disturbances in impulse formation or conduction, or both acting simultaneously. Some of these possibilities will be illustrated and discussed in this section.

Alterations in the slope of phase 4 depolarization or in the threshold potential at which rapid (phase 0) depolarization begins can cause

Abnormal Mechanisms 343

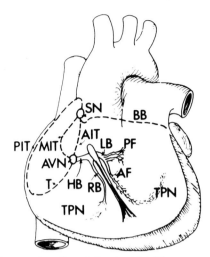

Fig 17-2.—Specialized atrial fibers connecting sinus node *(SN)* and atrioventricular node *(AVN)* form three noninsulated tracts: the anterior, middle, and posterior internodal tracts *(AIT, MIT,* and *PIT)*. Bachmann's bundle *(BB)*, a branch of the anterior internodal tract, crosses atrial roof to left appendage. Atrioventricular node, which lies close to coronary sinus ostium, is connected to main bundle of His *(HB)*. The latter gives rise to left bundle branch *(LB)*, with its segmental anterior and posterior fascicles *(AF* and *PF)*, and right bundle branch *(RB)*. Resulting trifascicular system includes terminal Purkinje's network *(TPN)*, which conducts impulse to ventricular muscle. (From Childers R.: Classification of cardiac dysrhythmias. *Med. Clin. North Am.* 60:3, 1976. Used by permission.)

changes in automaticity. For example, sympathetic discharge will steepen the slope of phase 4 in sinoatrial pacemaker cells and so accelerate the rate of discharge, causing sinus tachycardia. Conversely, parasympathetic discharge will depress the phase 4 slope and slow the rate at which threshold is attained, thus slowing the heart rate.

When the slope of phase 4 depolarization is steepened in Purkinje's fibers (for example, by administration of catecholamines), such fibers can discharge "prematurely" and thus generate ventricular ectopic depolarizations. Such a focus of enhanced automaticity in the ventricles can account for isolated ventricular ectopic depolarizations, salvos of ventricular ectopic depolarizations, or sustained runs of ventricular tachycardia. Such enhanced automaticity is an example of arrhythmia generation secondary to disturbances in impulse formation.

As was already pointed out, two of the most critical determinants of conduction velocity are the maximal rate of increase in the action potential voltage during phase 0 depolarization (maximal dV/dt of phase 0) and the magnitude of the depolarization, that is, the amplitude of phase 0. Furthermore, the level of resting membrane potential itself at the moment of cell excitation is a determinant of the rate of increase of phase 0; therefore, if the resting potential of a cardiac fiber is reduced (less negative—for example, from −90 mV to −65 mV), the maximal rate of increase of phase 0 will be reduced, and conduction velocity in the cardiac fiber also will be reduced accordingly.[46]

Many clinically applicable factors alter conduction velocity in cardiac fibers. The most intensively studied area in laboratory investigation has been the effects of acute ischemia and infarction on the electrical activity of both Purkinje's fibers and ventricular muscle.[39, 46, 47] Because these findings have such clinical relevance, particularly with the increasing frequency of coronary artery bypass operation in patients with ischemic heart disease, it is necessary to understand how ischemia can be the mechanism for the onset and perpetuation of arrhythmias with life-threatening potential. Such

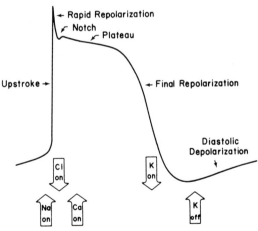

Fig 17-3.—Diagrammatic representation of cardiac action potential, emphasizing characteristics of Purkinje's fiber action potential. Ionic events related to each phase are discussed in text. *Arrows* below diagram refer to approximate time when indicated ion is influencing membrane potential. They point in direction of effect on membrane potential: upward for depolarization and downward for repolarization. (From Fozzard and Gibbons.[21] Used by permission.)

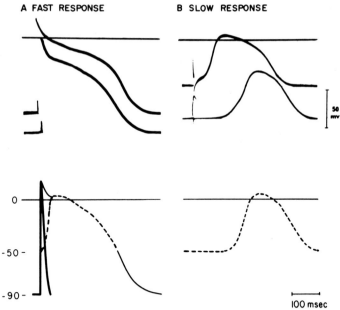

Fig 17-4.—Comparison of fast and slow responses. Panel A *(top)* shows two transmembrane action potentials recorded from different cells in bundle of canine Purkinje's fibers (fast fibers) perfused with normal Tyrode's solution (K^+ = 4 mmol). Reference line 0 is for top action potential only. Microelectrodes are located 15 mm apart at either end of unbranched bundle, and Purkinje's fiber bundle is stimulated at one end. Action potentials shown in panel A are examples of fast response. Panel B *(top)* shows transmembrane action potentials recorded from same two cells while Purkinje's fiber bundle is being perfused with Tyrode's solution containing high K^+ (16 mmol) and epinephrine levels. Stimulation of Purkinje's fiber bundle now results in slow response action potentials. Diagrams at bottom of each panel indicate relative time course of Na^+ *(dark trace)* and Ca^{++} *(dashed trace)* currents. (From Wit and Friedman.[47] Used by permission.)

ischemia-provoked arrhythmias are likely to be secondary to acute alterations in membrane potential, leading to sudden depression of conduction velocity and even conduction block. These conditions set the stage for reentry of wave fronts and sustained arrhythmias.

These complex events can be summarized as follows. Acutely ischemic cardiac cells are unable to maintain their normal intracellular ion concentrations. In particular, potassium ions leak from the ischemic cells, and sodium ions accumulate intracellularly. The loss of potassium ions into the surrounding extracellular fluid elevates the potassium concentration outside the cell, which brings about a reduction in the level of resting membrane potential. A reduction in membrane potential, for example, from −90 mV to −60 mV, profoundly impairs the fast inward sodium current responsible for the rapid rate of increase of phase 0, resulting in a reduced upstroke velocity and amplitude and therefore a reduced conduction velocity. Indeed, the fast inward current can be completely inactivated by high extracellular potassium concentrations, with membrane potentials reduced to between −50 mV and −40 mV.[46, 47] The slow inward current carried by both sodium and calcium, however, remains functional at such low levels of membrane potential, particularly when locally released catecholamines are present, as is probably the case in acutely ischemic areas (Fig 17–4). Thus, Purkinje's fibers in ischemic zones may be converted from fast response to slow response action potential fibers, with the characteristics discussed previously, and with depressed conduction velocity as the consequence.[46, 47] This process can be schematically illustrated as a form of reentry (Fig 17–5).

In this case, a main bundle (MB) of Purkinje's fibers bifurcates into branches A and B before

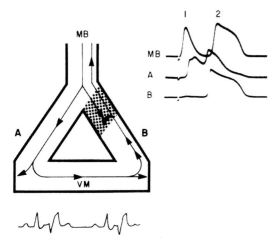

Fig 17–5.—Sequence of activation of a loop of Purkinje's fiber bundles *(A and B)* and ventricular muscle *(VM)* during reentry. Region of unidirectional conduction block is indicated by darkly shaded area in branch *B*. Conduction cannot occur through this area in the antegrade direction (from *B* to *VM*), but only in the retrograde direction (from *VM* to *B*). Slow conduction is present throughout loop. At right, action potentials recorded from a similar anatomic arrangement of canine Purkinje's fibers are shown. Conduction in the loop was depressed, with elevated K$^+$ and catecholamine levels. Action potentials in top trace were recorded from main bundle leading into loop *(MB)*. Action potential in middle trace was recorded from branch *A* and action potential in the bottom trace from branch *B*. Action potential 1 in *MB* results from antegrade propagation in this bundle, the response in trace *A* was elicited as the impulse conducted through branch *A*, and the action potential in *B* occurred as it propagated retrograde in this branch. Action potential 2 in *MB* is the retrogradely conducting reentrant impulse. At the bottom of the figure is shown a possible ECG pattern that may result from this type of reentry. (From Wit et al.[48] Used by permission.)

terminating on a length of ventricular muscle (VM).[48] There is a region of acute ischemia and therefore profound depression of conduction properties in branch B, indicated by the stippled zone. The advancing wave front, shown by the arrows, enters branch A and is conducted through this branch into the muscle. In branch B, the wave front is blocked in the depressed zone (unidirectional block). The impulse entering ventricular muscle from branch A depolarizes the muscle and then enters branch B. In this retrograde conduction, the impulse can penetrate the depressed area at a severely reduced conduction velocity and finally emerge and reenter the now recovered tissue proximally. An ECG pattern that might be a result of such reentry is shown as ventricular bigeminy. The pattern could as easily be one of sustained ventricular tachycardia and finally ventricular fibrillation, depending on the precise timing of the reentry wave front and its ability to fractionate into daughter wavelets, the latter event inevitably terminating in ventricular fibrillation. Conduction in ischemic zones is highly complex, with numerous potential reentrant pathways, functionally dissociated areas, and areas of localized ventricular fibrillation.[15] However, the likelihood that reentrant mechanisms are responsible for ventricular arrhythmias in ischemic and infarcted hearts is well established.

Another way of illustrating the phenomenon of reentry is shown in Figure 17–6. These drawings are examples of arrhythmia generation and perpetuation as a consequence of acute disturbances in impulse conduction. Ischemia need not be the only mechanism for reentry. Any (even slight) variations in conduction velocity or refractoriness could permit a wave front to establish reentry. For example, paroxysms of supraventricular tachycardia can be initiated and sustained by reentry within the atrioventricular node (Fig 17–7). It is proposed that the atrioventricular node is longitudinally dissociated into two functional pathways, α and β.[24] The sinus impulse traverses the faster conducting β pathway to depolarize the His-Purkinje system and ventricles. Simultaneous conduction of the impulse down the α pathway is slower, reaching the bundle of His slightly after the impulse traversing the β pathway. An atrial premature depolarization will be blocked in the β pathway with its longer refractoriness (despite its more rapid conduction) but will proceed slowly through the α pathway, which has a shorter refractory period. If conduction in the α pathway is sufficiently slow, the previously refractory β pathway will have recovered and will conduct the impulse retrogradely, producing atrial depolarization (an atrial echo). If the α pathway recovers its excitability, it will permit the returning impulse from the β pathway to reenter, and supraventricular tachycardia will be established using this atrioventricular nodal reentrant cir-

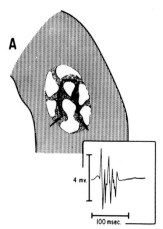
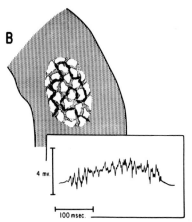

Fig 17–6.—Suggested mechanism of complex desynchronization and slow propagation. In this schematic figure, the white areas represent severely depressed (unexcitable) myocardium. *Stippled areas* represent less severely depressed, nonhomogeneously excitable myocardium. The area of *wavy lines* represents normally excited myocardium in the absolute refractory period. In **A**, more coarsely distributed nonhomogeneity results in fewer spikes of larger amplitude and shorter duration of activity than in **B**. In **B**, more finely distributed nonhomogeneity of depressed excitability results in more complex and effectively longer pathways. Greater degree of asynchronous excitation in **B** results in a larger number of spikes of smaller amplitude and a greatly prolonged duration of the circuitous activity confined to this region. Activity is confined by the absolute refractory state of surrounding myocardium that has previously been excited by normally propagated wave front through this region. In this example there is interplay between duration of persistent desynchronized activity and duration of the recovery period of surrounding myocardium, a factor that determines whether or not reentrant preventricular contractions are generated. (From Boineau J.P., Cox J.L.: Slow ventricular activation in acute myocardial infarction: A source of re-entrant premature ventricular contractions. *Circulation* 48:702, 1973. Used by permission of the American Heart Association.)

cuit. A delicate balance of conduction and refractoriness is necessary to both initiate and sustain such a reentrant tachycardia.

To spontaneous impulse formation (automaticity) and alterations in conduction (reentry) must be added a third probable source of cardiac rhythm disturbances, triggered activity.[13] This recently described phenomenon is distinguished from spontaneous or automatic activity in that a triggerable focus becomes rhythmically active if driven only at a critical rate or by a critically timed premature impulse. Such triggered activity seems dependent on afterpotentials (early or delayed after-depolarization, early after-hyperpolarization). An example of such triggered activity arising from afterpotentials is shown in Figure 17–8. Triggered activity of this type might be still another cause of paroxysmal tachycardia of atrial or ventricular origin. Triggerable fibers have been identified in the coronary sinus that can drive the entire atrium and may sustain a paroxysm of supraventricular tachycardia. While much remains to be learned about the role of such triggered activity as a cause of cardiac arrhythmias, enough is already known to justify inclusion of this mechanism in a review of electrophysiologic derangements as sources of cardiac arrhythmias.

DIAGNOSIS AND TREATMENT

One of the most serious and sometimes disastrous errors committed in the management of cardiac arrhythmias is that of treating the ECG findings and rhythm rather than the patient and the underlying problem. This factor cannot be overemphasized, especially in the patient under anesthesia, in whom ventilation and its effects,[2] electrolyte derangements,[17] hypotension or hypertension, and the depth of the anesthetic state itself all may be the only, the primary, or at least a contributory explanation for the rhythm

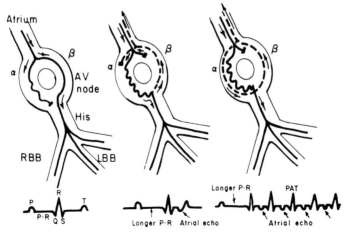

Fig 17–7.—Mechanism of atrioventricular nodal reentrant tachycardia. Each part of figure is shown as atrium, atrioventricular node (which is divided into α and β pathway), bundle of His, and bundle branches. *Left,* sinus rhythm is present and mechanism of resulting QRS is shown. *Center,* response of atrioventricular node to single atrial premature beat with single atrial echo is depicted. *Right,* initiation of supraventricular tachycardia with atrial premature beat is shown. Paroxysmal atrial tachycardia *(PAT),* right bundle branch *(RBB),* left bundle branch *(LBB).* (From Josephson and Kastor.[24] Used by permission.)

disorder. The assumption is that the anesthesiologist is thoroughly aware of this possibility and has ruled out (or corrected) these problems and that the patient and his rhythm disorder require pharmacologic treatment. Only representative problems requiring treatment and the proposed mechanisms of drug action, where appropriate, will be considered herein.

Supraventricular Arrhythmias

Sinus or Junctional Bradycardia

In general, sinus or junctional bradycardia requires treatment only if it is hemodynamically significant (hypotension and low cardiac outpute, measured or clinically evident) or if it is accompanied by electrical "instability" in the form of frequent ventricular ectopic depolarizations, which may, at least in some instances, be precursors of more serious ventricular arrhythmias.[44] Atropine in increments of 0.4 to 0.5 mg is usually effective; however, if the bradycardia has not been corrected after a total dose of 2.0 mg has been given incrementally at intervals of four to five minutes, isoproterenol can be used. One milligram of isoproterenol in 250 ml of 5% dextrose in water provides 4 μg/ml. The infusion can be started in the adult at 2 μg/min and titrated until the desired response is obtained. The deleterious effect of undue increases in heart rate (and myocardial oxygen requirements) in patients with coronary artery disease must be clearly understood when embarking on cardioaccelerator therapy in such patients.[29] Worsened ischemia or even acute infarction can be provoked if the rate is accelerated excessively.[38] Here again, the anesthesiologist must seek out the explanation for the bradycardia. In the operating room, after bypass and with the chest still open, temporary myocardial wires can be placed and the rate can be ideally controlled if bradycardia is a persistent problem.

Sinus Tachycardia

Sinus tachycardia demands a thorough assessment as to cause. Management of the cause almost always constitutes management of the arrhythmia. However, especially in hyperdynamic patients undergoing coronary artery surgery, such increases in heart rate are most easily and rapidly controlled by the use of 0.25 to 0.50 mg of propranolol or 5.0 mg of edrophonium; the latter drug can be given again in four to five minutes, using as much as 15 to 20 mg if it is needed. In this setting the high myocardial oxygen requirement imposed by the tachycardia

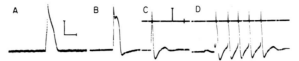

Fig 17–8.—Action potentials obtained from canine Purkinje's fiber exposed to sodium-free, calcium-rich solution. Action potential in **A** shows no afterpotentials; that in **B** shows only an early after-hyperpolarization. In **C**, early after-hyperpolarization is followed by a delayed after-depolarization. In **D**, single stimulus applied to a quiescent fiber evokes a driven action potential, followed by four nondriven action potentials that arise from delayed after-depolarizations of the sort seen at the end of the record. Calibrations: the horizontal calibration in **A** represents 1 second for **A** and 2 seconds for **B**; the vertical calibration in **A** represents 20 mV for **A** and **B**. The calibrations in **C** represent 20 mV and 2 seconds for **C** and **D**. (From Cranefield.[13] Used by permission.)

justifies and, indeed, necessitates prompt, even though etiologically nonspecific, treatment.[33]

Atrial Flutter

Generally, atrial flutter (Fig 17–9) is secondary to a circus movement of excitation within the atrium (a form of reentry) (Fig 17–10). The atrial rate is typically 250 to 350 beats per minute, with sawtooth undulations of the baseline called "F waves." Conduction into the ventricles is usually at a constant rate, for example, 2:1 or 3:1, though it may be variable. In 2:1 conduction, with a flutter rate of 300 per minute, the ventricular rate will be regular at 150 beats per minute (see Fig 17–9). Atrial flutter may become life-threatening if the rate of ventricular response produces an acute decrease in cardiac output and precipitous hypotension. The tachycardia also may stress the relationship of myocardial oxygen supply and demand and provoke acute myocardial ischemia and further intensify the low cardiac output and hypotension. This occurrence is especially likely in patients with coronary artery disease, and this potential complication of tachyarrhythmias of any type must be considered in such patients.

Atrial flutter is usually sensitive to direct-current cardioversion at low energies, for example, 25 joules, and this treatment should be the choice when the arrhythmia has precipitated acute hypotension. If cardioversion cannot be used, rapid digitalization can be effected. In the adult who has not previously received digitalis, 0.5 mg of digoxin can be given, followed by 0.25 mg in two to four hours. A total digitalizing dose of 0.9 mg/sq m of body surface area given in increments in this manner usually will control the ventricular rate, even if the flutter is not terminated. In addition, propranolol in increments of 0.25 mg can be added to the digoxin treatment in doses up to about 3.0 mg during a 20- to 30-minute period, if necessary. While congestive cardiac failure is considered a contraindication to propranolol therapy, it is possible for the rapid tachyarrhythmia to precipitate acute cardiac failure and therefore justify combined digoxin-propranolol therapy.

Atrial Fibrillation

Unlike atrial flutter, atrial fibrillation (Fig 17–11) is usually a chronic disorder, for which oral digitalis preparations have been prescribed. It too is likely to be secondary to a circus movement of excitation within the atria. If it is of acute onset, or if, because of previous withdrawal of digitalis in preparation for cardiac op-

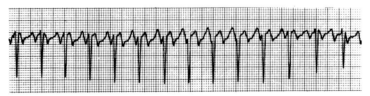

Fig 17–9.—Atrial flutter with 2:1 conduction. (From *A Manual for Instructors of Advanced Cardiac Life Support.* Dallas, American Heart Association, 1977. Used by permission.)

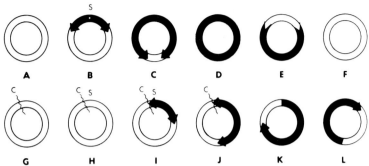

Fig 17–10.—Role of unidirectional block in establishing circus movement. Application of stimulus to ring of excitable tissue *(unshaded area)* in absence of block *(B)* initiates impulse *(shaded area)* that depolarizes entire ring *(D)*. Mutual cancellation of impulses moving in opposite directions *(C)* allows tissue to repolarize completely *(E* and *F)*. However, if unidirectional block is established by temporary clamping of tissue *(C* in *H–J)*, impulse propagated in clockwise direction can continue to travel around the ring *(K* and *L)*, thereby establishing circus movement. (From Silber E.N., Katz L.N.: *Heart Disease.* New York, Macmillan Publishing Co., 1975. Used by permission.)

eration, the ventricular rate is very rapid, the fast ventricular rate may necessitate prompt treatment in the operating room. Treatment principles follow the guidelines for management of atrial flutter. If synchronized cardioversion is used, higher energies, for example, 100 joules or higher, are usually required to terminate atrial fibrillation as opposed to atrial flutter.

Paroxysmal Supraventricular Tachycardia

Paroxysmal supraventricular tachycardia (Fig 17–12) embraces a group of arrhythmias with similar ECG features. As was described earlier, reentrant mechanisms probably generate most of these arrhythmias, which include such types as atrioventricular nodal reentrant tachycardia, sinus nodal reentrant tachycardia, and bypass tract reentrant tachycardia, as in the Wolff-Parkinson-White syndrome.[9, 41] In addition, supraventricular tachycardia may result from abnormal automaticity in atrial tissues. Here, triggered activity associated with afterpotentials, discussed earlier, may be a cause of such tachycardias of atrial origin.

On a surface ECG, it is difficult to identify the precise origin of these tachycardias, except to say that they arise above the bifurcation of the bundle of His. Therefore, the term "paroxysmal supraventricular tachycardia" applies to this group, regardless of the exact site and mechanism of origin.[24] The rhythm is characteristically regular, with rates of 160 to 200 beats per minute, although they may be as low as 100 or as high as 250 beats per minute. They are identified as supraventricular in origin because the QRS complexes are of normal duration ("narrow complex tachycardias"). However, when preexistent bundle-branch block or aberrant conduction is present, then it may be difficult or even impossible to identify with certainty the rhythm as supraventricular in origin. Aberrant conduction, usually with a right bundle-branch block configuration, is not infrequent when the ventricular rate is extremely rapid.[34, 50] In such instances, if hemodynamic deterioration has ensued, treatment must be instituted in spite of lack of confident differentiation of supraventricular from ventricular origin. The following plan of treatment can be instituted as a gen-

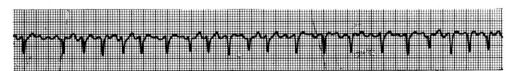

Fig 17–11.—Atrial fibrillation. (From *A Manual for Instructors of Advanced Cardiac Life Support.* Dallas, American Heart Association, 1977. Used by permission.)

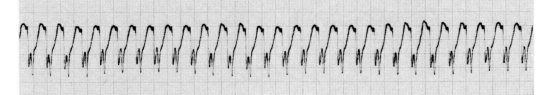

Fig 17–12.—Paroxysmal atrial tachycardia in patient with known Wolff-Parkinson-White syndrome. Ventricular rate, 220 beats per minute. Hemodynamic deterioration necessitated immediate direct-current cardioversion. (From White R.D.: Drugs in cardiac supportive care. *Anesth. Analg.* 55:633, 1976. Used by permission.)

eral approach applicable to most paroxysms of supraventricular tachycardia, regardless of the exact site and mechanism of origin.[40, 42]

Carotid sinus pressure, through its reflex vagal stimulation, can be tried first. Other vagotonic manipulations can be tried, such as the use of edrophonium in 5.0-mg increments, digoxin in doses as discussed previously, or α-adrenergic agents, such as phenylephrine (2.0 mg) or methoxamine (5.0 mg). The last two drugs can be given again if necessary; the pressure, heart rate, and drug effect should be observed. Propranolol in increments of 0.25 to 0.50 mg up to 3.0 to 4.0 mg also may slow or terminate the arrhythmia by prolonging atrioventricular nodal conduction and refractoriness. Procainamide in increments of 50 mg every three to four minutes, up to about 500 to 700 mg, also may be effective, especially if the tachycardia is using an accessory pathway for reentry, as in the Wolff-Parkinson-White syndrome. In this situation, procainamide slows conduction and prolongs refractoriness in the accessory pathway, thereby interrupting conduction in this limb of the reentrant circuit.[35] Also, lidocaine in a bolus of 1.0 mg/kg and repeated every five minutes, up to about 300 mg, in the adult can be tried in this setting, since it may block conduction in the bypass tract and slow the ventricular response by favoring conduction through the more refractory atrioventricular node.[25]

Here again, as with atrial flutter and atrial fibrillation, synchronized cardioversion can be used to terminate the tachycardia and is nearly always effective with energies as low as 25 joules.[37] In those infrequent instances when drug or electrical (or both) therapy has failed to attain or maintain rate control or arrhythmia conversion, pacing via placement of a temporary transvenous electrode may be required. The pacing-induced depolarization wave front terminates the arrhythmia by penetrating the atrioventricular node and colliding with the circulating wave front, thereby extinguishing the reentrant circuit.

Atrioventricular Block

First-Degree Atrioventricular Block

First-degree atrioventricular block can be defined as a PR interval of 210 ms or greater, without failure of atrial impulses to capture the ventricles.[36] Such block usually reflects excessive vagal effects or direct effects of drugs on the atrioventricular junction (in the latter instance, that of digitalis in particular). It also may accompany acute myocardial infarction, usually of the inferior wall. While treatment is unnecessary, sudden appearance of first-degree block justifies identification of the cause and observation for progression to a higher degree of block.

Second-Degree Atrioventricular Block

Second-degree atrioventricular block is characterized by a failure of some, but not all, supraventricular impulses to cross the atrioventricular junction. In Mobitz type I second-degree block (Wenckebach's phenomenon), there is a progressive prolongation of the PR interval, leading finally to a dropped beat[36] (Fig 17–13). The cycle is then resumed. An additional characteristic of this entity is that, prior to the dropped beat, the PR interval increases by decreasing increments, so that the incremental increase in the PR interval can be seen to decrease prior to the dropped beat. The PR intervals therefore become shorter prior to the dropped beat. This form of block is almost always supra-Hisian, that is, within the atrioventricular junction, and is

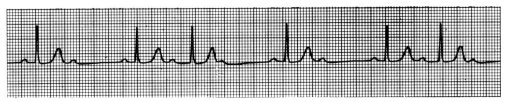

Fig 17–13.—Second-degree atrioventricular block, type I (Wenckebach). (From *A Manual for Instructors of Advanced Cardiac Life Support.* Dallas, American Heart Association, 1977. Used by permission.)

seen with acute infarction involving the inferior wall with ischemia and edema in the region of the atrioventricular junction.[26, 36] Treatment is usually not required unless the ventricular rate is very slow, in which case atropine in doses discussed for the treatment of sinus bradycardia can be tried.[1] This form of block generally does not progress to complete heart block, but if it should, an escape pacemaker with a rate of more than 40 beats per minute and located in the bundle of His will usually provide adequate hemodynamics. If necessary, isoproterenol can be given to improve atrioventricular conduction or to accelerate the rate of the escape pacemaker.

A different situation is present when the second-degree block is characterized by intermittently dropped beats without prior progressive lengthening of the PR interval (Fig 17–14). This form of block, known as Mobitz type II, is usually caused by infra-Hisian conduction system disease, and QRS widening, reflecting such disturbance, is often present.[27] This condition may progress suddenly and unpredictably to complete heart block, and because of the infra-Hisian site, the escape pacemaker is usually idioventricular in location, with resulting very slow rates (<30 beats per minute) that are associated with low cardiac output and hypotension. While temporizing treatment can be initiated with atropine or isoproterenol (or both), Mobitz type II block is generally considered a clear indication for placement of a temporary transvenous pacemaker. Indeed, the degree of block may increase with atropine when the site of block is in the His-Purkinje system (infra-Hisian),[1] probably because, while the sinus rate and atrioventricular nodal conduction are enhanced, increasing the frequency of impulse passage to infra-Hisian tissues, there is no improvement by atropine in conduction within the His-Purkinje system. This system thus becomes increasingly refractory.

Third-Degree (Complete) Atrioventricular Block

When there is complete interruption of all conduction between atria and ventricles, complete heart block is present. The P waves and QRS complexes on the ECG bear no constant relationship to each other. The site of the pacemaker that controls the ventricles can be inferred from the configuration of the QRS complex. When the pacemaker resides in the atrioventricular junction, the QRS complex is narrow in the absence of other conduction abnormalities.[26] This feature is true in most instances of congenital complete heart block, in which the QRS complexes are normal and ventricular rates are only slightly slower than normal. However, with the pacemaker idioventricular in location, as is usually true in acquired complete heart block, the QRS complex is wide

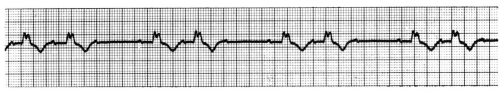

Fig 17–14.—Second-degree atrioventricular block, type II. (From *A Manual for Instructors of Advanced Cardiac Life Support.* Dallas, American Heart Association, 1977. Used by permission.)

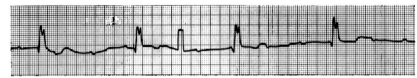

Fig 17–15.—Third-degree atrioventricular block. (From *A Manual for Instructors of Advanced Cardiac Life Support.* Dallas, American Heart Association, 1977. Used by permission.)

and bizarre and the rate is slow, for example, 35 to 40 beats per minute (Fig 17–15).

The definitive treatment for complete heart block is pacing. Here again, however, an adequate rate and hemodynamic stability can be temporarily maintained by the use of atropine or isoproterenol (or both). If the pacemaker is situated in the ventricles, with wide QRS complexes on the ECG, isoproterenol is much more likely to be effective in temporary acceleration of the ventricular rate than is atropine, but ventricular tachyarrhythmias and disproportionate increases in myocardial oxygen requirement may be consequences of too rapid an infusion of isoproterenol.

Ventricular Arrhythmias

Because these arrhythmias are seen frequently in patients undergoing cardiac operations and often require treatment with drugs, as well as the usual manipulations accompanying onset of arrhythmias in anesthetized patients, a more detailed consideration of drug action will be included herein.

Ventricular Ectopic Beats

There are numerous possible causes of ectopic depolarizations of ventricular origin occurring in patients under anesthesia. Obvious possibilities

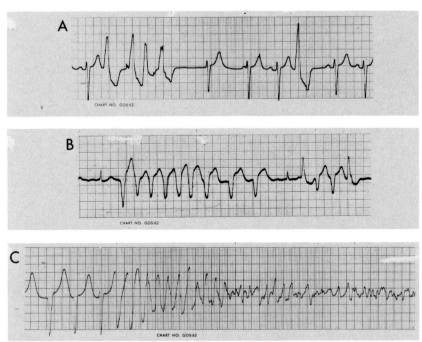

Fig 17–16.—**A,** ventricular ectopy, with run of four successive ventricular ectopic beats on left, followed by junctional escape beat. **B,** burst of ventricular tachycardia. **C,** brief burst of ventricular tachycardia initiated by close-coupled ventricular ectopic beats (fourth beat from left) with rapid degeneration into ventricular fibrillation. (From White R.D.: Drugs in cardiac supportive care. *Anesth. Analg.* 55:633, 1976. Used by permission.)

include blood-gas abnormalities, electrolyte imbalances (especially hypokalemia), a light anesthetic state with accompanying sympathetic discharge (as may occur during laryngoscopy and intubation), and direct or indirect effects of anesthetic drugs themselves. In open-cardiac surgery, manipulation of the heart often provokes isolated salvos of ventricular ectopic beats. Treatment is always first directed toward the provocation; when it is identified and corrected, specific antiarrhythmic drug treatment is infrequently required.

In patients with coronary artery disease, ventricular arrhythmias may develop as a consequence of an acute imbalance between myocardial oxygen supply and demand, with acute myocardial ischemia the cause of such ectopic activity. The electrophysiologic mechanisms underlying such rhythm disturbances already have been discussed. Here again, the primary and immediate thrust of management must be to restore, as rapidly as possible, the balance between supply and demand. For example, if frequent ventricular ectopic beats appear and persist during and after intubation, especially with accompanying hypertension and ST-segment depression, rapid deepening of anesthesia may be all that is required for correction. If an ischemic focus continues to discharge ventricular premature depolarizations, treatment with antiarrhythmic drugs is usually necessary. Traditionally accepted indications for prompt suppression of ventricular ectopic beats include those that are occurring frequently (>5 beats per minute), are multiform in configuration, are closely coupled, and are occurring in salvos of two or more in succession.[44] These patterns are generally accepted as carrying malignant potential, with a propensity to rapid degeneration into ventricular tachycardia or ventricular fibrillation (Fig 17–16).

Lidocaine remains the drug of choice for treatment of ventricular arrhythmias.[6, 10] In ischemic zones, lidocaine may further slow conduction in already depressed areas and so terminate reentrant excitation [16, 30–32] (Fig 17–17). In other circumstances, lidocaine may actually improve conduction velocity and thus terminate reentrant mechanisms by eliminating unidirectional block.[5] The dose is 1 mg/kg as an intravenous bolus, repeated in three to five minutes if needed, and, if necessary, a continuous infusion

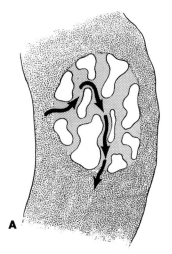 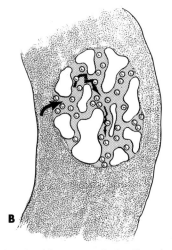

Fig 17–17.—Schematic depiction of conduction through ischemic-infarcted intramural zone of ventricular muscle. *White areas* are islands of inexcitable, severely depressed tissue. *Dotted areas* within ischemic zone are still excitable, though also depressed, and conduct wave front at reduced conduction velocities. Ischemic zone is surrounded by normal muscle indicated by the *wavy lines*. **A,** wave front propagates through depressed area at reduced conduction velocity but is able to sustain itself and emerge to reenter surrounding normal myocardium. **B,** after lidocaine administration, lidocaine-induced further depression of conduction velocity impairs advance of wave front to extent that it is blocked and unable to reenter normal surrounding muscle. Reentrant dysrhythmias sustained via such pathways of depressed conduction would then be terminated.

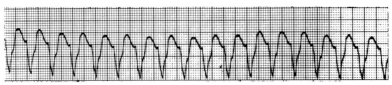

Fig 17–18.—Ventricular tachycardia. (From *A Manual for Instructors of Advanced Cardiac Life Support.* Dallas, American Heart Association, 1977. Used by permission.)

at 30 to 50 μg/kg/minute is begun to sustain the blood level of lidocaine in a range sufficient to suppress discharge from the ectopic focus.[44, 45]

If lidocaine is ineffective, procainamide can be used. It both depresses phase 4 depolarization in Purkinje's fibers and prolongs conduction velocity, the latter effect probably contributory to termination of reentrant excitation.[28] It is given intravenously in increments of 25 to 50 mg/minute, until the ectopy is suppressed or until 700 to 1,000 mg has been given.[22, 45] The arterial pressure must be constantly observed for hypotension, and the ECG should be monitored for QRS widening or PR or QT interval lengthening. The latter are evidence of toxicity and necessitate terminating the use of the drug. Given at the above rate of administration, procainamide may be safely given and will often effectively suppress ventricular ectopy.[22]

The β-adrenergic blocker propranolol, given intravenously in increments of 0.25 mg up to about 3.0 mg, is also an effective antiarrhythmic agent, especially if sympathetic overactivity is likely to be contributing to the ectopic discharge. Ventricular tachycardia (Fig 17–18) can be treated with any of the previously mentioned drugs.[34] Sustained ventricular tachycardia is best treated by synchronized cardioversion. If treatment is externally applied, energies as low as 25 to 50 joules are usually effective. After termination of ventricular tachycardia by cardioversion, drug therapy (for example, with lidocaine as a bolus or infusion) should be begun immediately to prevent recurrence. In the meantime, the probable cause should be identified and corrected if possible. It is usually difficult to be certain that a wide QRS-complex tachycardia is ventricular in origin.[18] Notwithstanding this fact, such a tachycardia, usually in the range of 150 to 180 beats per minute, sudden in onset and sustained, should be assumed to be ventricular in origin and so treated according to these guidelines.

Ventricular Fibrillation

Ventricular fibrillation is best treated by immediate direct-current defibrillation with externally applied energies of 200 to 320 joules.[11] If there is delay in defibrillation, a single precordial thump can be applied (also in ventricular tachycardia). If this does not remove the ventricular fibrillation, cardiopulmonary resuscitation must be instituted while preparations for defibrillation are made. In cardiac operating rooms, a defibrillator should always be immediately available and ready for use. As in ventricular tachycardia, drug therapy should be begun after defibrillation, preferably with lidocaine, to prevent recurrence.[44]

When either ventricular tachycardia or ventricular fibrillation is unresponsive to this therapeutic approach or recurs after transient removal, bretylium tosylate may be effective.[3, 23] It can be given intravenously as a 5 mg/kg bolus. If ventricular tachycardia or ventricular fibrillation persists with continued standard treatment, including cardiopulmonary resuscitation, a second bolus of 10 mg/kg can be given and repeated in 15 to 30 minutes, to a maximum of 30 mg/kg. Its pharmacologic properties appear to be different from those of other antiarrhythmic agents.[4] It possesses adrenergic blocking properties, in addition to its antiarrhythmic action, and may cause hypotension by this mechanism.[8] Its action in terminating ventricular arrhythmias in ischemic events may be related to its property of reducing the disparity in action potential duration and refractory period between normal and infarcted regions, thus eliminating conditions conducive to reentrant excitation.[7]

REFERENCES

1. Akhtar M., et al.: Electrophysiologic effects of atropine on atrioventricular conduction studied by His bundle electrogram. *Am. J. Cardiol.* 33:333, 1974.

2. Ayres S.M., Grace W.J.: Inappropriate ventilation and hypoxemia as causes of cardiac arrhythmias: The control of arrhythmias without antiarrhythmic drugs. Am. J. Med. 46:495, 1969.
3. Bernstein J.G., Koch-Weser J.: Effectiveness of bretylium tosylate against refractory ventricular arrhythmias. Circulation 45:1024, 1972.
4. Bigger J.T. Jr., Jaffe C.C.: The effect of bretylium tosylate on the electrophysiologic properties of ventricular muscle and Purkinje fibers. Am. J. Cardiol. 27:82, 1971.
5. Bigger J.T. Jr., Mandel W.J.: Effect of lidocaine on the electrophysiological properties of ventricular muscle and Purkinje fibers. J. Clin. Invest. 49:63, 1970.
6. Borer J.S., et al.: Beneficial effect of lidocaine on ventricular electrical stability and spontaneous ventricular fibrillation during experimental myocardial infarction. Am. J. Cardiol. 37:860, 1976.
7. Cardinal R., Sasyniuk B.I.: Electrophysiological effects of bretylium tosylate on subendocardial Purkinje fibers from infarcted canine hearts. J. Pharmacol. Exp. Ther. 204:159, 1978.
8. Chatterjee K., et al.: Cardiovascular effects of bretylium tosylate in acute myocardial infarction. J.A.M.A. 223:757, 1973.
9. Chung E.K.: Tachyarrhythmias in Wolff-Parkinson-White syndrome: Antiarrhythmic drug therapy. J.A.M.A. 237:376, 1977.
10. Collinsworth K.A., Kalman S.M., Harrison D.C.: The clinical pharmacology of lidocaine as an antiarrhythmic drug. Circulation 50:1217, 1974.
11. Cranefield P.F.: Ventricular fibrillation. N. Engl. J. Med. 289:732, 1973.
12. Cranefield P.F.: *The Conduction of the Cardiac Impulse: The Slow Response and Cardiac Arrhythmias*. Mount Kisco, N.Y., Futura Publishing Co., 1975, pp. 135–137.
13. Cranefield P.F.: Action potentials, afterpotentials, and arrhythmias. Circ. Res. 41:415, 1977.
14. Cranefield P.F., Wit A.L., Hoffman B.F.: Genesis of cardiac arrhythmias. Circulation 47:190, 1973.
15. El-Sherif N., et al.: Re-entrant ventricular arrhythmias in the late myocardial infarction period: 1. Conduction characteristics in the infarction zone. Circulation 55:686, 1977.
16. El-Sherif N., et al.: Re-entrant ventricular arrhythmias in the late myocardial infarction period: 4. Mechanism of action of lidocaine. Circulation 56:395, 1977.
17. Fisch C.: Relation of electrolyte disturbances to cardiac arrhythmias. Circulation 47:408, 1973.
18. Fisch C., Noble R.J.: Ventricular tachycardia, editorial. Am. Heart J. 89:551, 1975.
19. Fozzard H.A.: Cardiac contractility, in Vassalle M. (ed.): *Cardiac Physiology for the Clinician*. New York, Academic Press, 1976.
20. Fozzard H.A.: Cardiac muscle: Excitability and passive electrical properties. Prog. Cardiovasc. Dis. 19:343, 1977.
21. Fozzard H.A., Gibbons W.R.: Action potential and contraction of heart muscle. Am. J. Cardiol. 31:182, 1973.
22. Giardina E.-G.V., Heissenbuttel R.H., Bigger J.T. Jr.: Intermittent intravenous procaine amide to treat ventricular arrhythmias: Correlation of plasma concentration with effect on arrhythmia, electrocardiogram, and blood pressure. Ann. Intern. Med. 78:183, 1973.
23. Holder D.A., et al.: Experience with bretylium tosylate by a hospital cardiac arrest team. Circulation 55:541, 1977.
24. Josephson M.E., Kastor J.A.: Supraventricular tachycardia: Mechanisms and management. Ann. Intern. Med. 87:346, 1977.
25. Josephson M.E., Kastor J.A., Kitchen J.G. III: Lidocaine in Wolff-Parkinson-White syndrome with atrial fibrillation. Ann. Intern. Med. 84:44, 1976.
26. Kastor J.A.: Atrioventricular block. N. Engl. J. Med. 292:462, 1975.
27. Kastor J.A.: Atrioventricular block. N. Engl. J. Med. 292:572, 1975.
28. Kastor J.A., et al.: Human ventricular refractoriness: II. Effects of procainamide. Circulation 56:462, 1977.
29. Knoebel S.B., et al.: Atropine-induced cardioacceleration and myocardial blood flow in subjects with and without coronary artery disease. Am. J. Cardiol. 33:327, 1974.
30. Kupersmith J.: Antiarrhythmic drugs: Changing concepts, editorial. Am. J. Cardiol. 38:119, 1976.
31. Kupersmith J., Antman E.M., Hoffman B.F.: In vivo electrophysiological effects of lidocaine in canine acute myocardial infarction. Circ. Res. 36:84, 1975.
32. Lazzara R., et al.: Effects of lidocaine on hypoxic and ischemic cardiac cells. Am. J. Cardiol. 41:872, 1978.
33. Loeb H.S., et al.: Effects of pharmacologically-induced hypertension on myocardial ischemia and coronary hemodynamics in patients with fixed coronary obstruction. Circulation 57:41, 1978.
34. Lown B., Temte J.V., Arter W.J.: Ventricular tachyarrhythmias: Clinical aspects. Circulation 47:1364, 1973.

35. Mandel W.J., et al.: The Wolff-Parkinson-White syndrome: Pharmacologic effects of procaine amide. *Am. Heart J.* 90:744, 1975.
36. Merideth J., Pruitt R.D.: Disturbances in cardiac conduction and their management. *Circulation* 47:1098, 1973.
37. Resnekov L.: Theory and practice of electroversion of cardiac dysrhythmias. *Med. Clin. North Am.* 60:325, 1976.
38. Richman S.: Adverse effect of atropine during myocardial infarction: Enhancement of ischemia following intravenously administered atropine. *J.A.M.A.* 228:1414, 1974.
39. Russell D.C., Oliver M.F., Wojtczak J.: Combined electrophysiological technique for assessment of the cellular basis of early ventricular arrhythmias: Experiments in dogs. *Lancet* 2:686, 1977.
40. Ticzon A.R., Whalen R.W.: Refractory supraventricular tachycardias. *Circulation* 47:642, 1973.
41. Tonkin A.M., Gallagher J.J., Wallace A.G.: Tachyarrhythmias in Wolff-Parkinson-White syndrome: Treatment and prevention. *J.A.M.A.* 235:947, 1976.
42. Warner H.: Therapy of common arrhythmias. *Med. Clin. North Am.* 58:995, 1974.
43. Watanabe Y., Dreifus L.S.: Factors controlling impulse transmission with special reference to A-V conduction. *Am. Heart J.* 89:790, 1975.
44. White R.D.: Essential drugs in emergency cardiac care, in *Advanced Cardiac Life Support*. Dallas, American Heart Association, 1975, p. 1.
45. Winkle R.A., Glantz S.A., Harrison D.C.: Pharmacologic therapy of ventricular arrhythmias. *Am. J. Cardiol.* 36:629, 1975.
46. Wit A.L., Bigger J.T. Jr.: Possible electrophysiological mechanisms for lethal arrhythmias accompanying myocardial ischemia and infarction. *Circulation* 52(suppl. 3):96, 1975.
47. Wit A.L., Friedman P.L.: Basis for ventricular arrhythmias accompanying myocardial infarction: Alterations in electrical activity of ventricular muscle and Purkinje fibers after coronary artery occlusion. *Arch. Intern. Med.* 135:459, 1975.
48. Wit A.L., Rosen M.R., Hoffman B.F.: Electrophysiology and pharmacology of cardiac arrhythmias: II. Relationship of normal and abnormal electrical activity of cardiac fibers to the genesis of arrhythmias: B. Re-entry: Section I. *Am. Heart J.* 88:664, 1974.
49. Zipes D.P., Besch H.R. Jr., Watanabe A.M.: Role of the slow current in cardiac electrophysiology, editorial. *Circulation* 51:761, 1975.
50. Zipes D.P., Fisch C.: Supraventricular arrhythmia with abnormal QRS complex. *Arch. Intern. Med.* 129:993, 1972.

18 / Support of the Circulation During and After Cardiac Operation

GLENN A. FROMME
ROGER D. WHITE

THE FUNCTIONS of the circulatory system are the distribution of oxygen and nutrients to metabolically active tissues and the removal of waste products and carbon dioxide. Certain tissues, primarily the brain, heart, and kidney, cannot tolerate poor perfusion or hypoxia for long before severe and sometimes irreversible pathologic sequelae develop, and therefore diagnosis and correction of the cause of low cardiac output must be enacted promptly. In ischemic heart disease, a low cardiac output can result in decreased coronary perfusion, which results in further ischemia, depression of myocardial function, lower cardiac output, and further decreased coronary perfusion and ischemia. Such a vicious cycle can be fatal unless certain interventions are instituted promptly to interrupt these events.

The purpose of this chapter is to review the management of low cardiac output, with specific reference to the cardiac surgical patient. Presented first is a discussion of some basic considerations in normal cardiac function and the compensatory mechanisms that occur when cardiac output decreases.

TERMINOLOGY

Low cardiac output, cardiac failure, and shock are terms that are sometimes used interchangeably and often loosely. All three can be defined as "inadequate perfusion to meet the needs of the tissues." However, certain types of shock, such as that due to sepsis or sympathetic block, actually may have an increased cardiac output. Cardiac failure also can occur with high cardiac output in conditions such as thyrotoxicosis, in which the metabolic rate of the tissues is so high that even a supernormal circulation is inadequate. In the severe stages of these conditions, the cardiac output begins to decrease, and this event can further confuse the situation. Usually, these conditions can be diagnosed on clinical bases, aided by monitoring of filling pressures and measurement of cardiac output.

This discussion will be limited to those situations in which the origin of the circulatory failure is actually in the pumping action of the heart. This failure can be due to intrinsic myocardial disease, ischemia, valvular dysfunction, dysrhythmias, and pericardial disease, either inhibiting myocardial function or decreasing venous return, as well as other causes of decreased venous return, such as hypovolemia and venous obstruction. Since the treatment depends on the cause, prompt diagnosis is the key to proper management.

The two cardinal features of cardiac failure are decreased cardiac output and increased filling pressures. All the signs and symptoms are secondary to these two physiologic changes, which are the basis for the division into forward failure and backward failure. Forward failure refers to all the signs of low cardiac output: (1) cool, clammy skin; (2) weak, thready pulse; (3) confusion, disorientation, restlessness; and (4) oliguria. The blood pressure may be low, high, or normal at this point, depending on the systemic vascular resistance. Backward failure refers to the signs of increased venous pressure: (1) pulmonary congestion, manifested by dyspnea and cyanosis, (2) ankle edema, and (3) hepatic dysfunction due to passive congestion.

In normal as well as in pathologic conditions, the performance of the heart is governed by four primary determinants: (1) preload, (2) afterload, (3) inotropic state, and (4) heart rate.

PRIMARY DETERMINANTS OF CARDIAC PERFORMANCE

Preload

The effect of preload on myocardial performance is the basis of Starling's law or the Frank-Starling phenomenon. This law basically states that the force of contraction of a muscle fiber is dependent on the initial fiber length.[7] In the isometric muscle preparation, this relationship is shown in the length-tension curve (Fig 18–1). In the intact heart, the end-diastolic wall tension represents preload and ultimately determines sarcomere length and the force of contraction. The end-diastolic wall tension is related to ventricular end-diastolic volume and pressure (Fig 18–2). However, end-diastolic wall tension, end-diastolic volume, and end-diastolic pressure cannot be considered synonymous. Since the last two can be measured clinically, they can be used as an estimation of preload, although other than for acute directional changes, their relationship to actual preload is unreliable.[7]

The question of whether a descending limb of Starling's curve exists is unresolved. In the isovolumetric perfused preparation of the dog heart, ventricular end-diastolic pressures as high as 60 mm Hg resulted in no decline in left ventricular systolic pressures, and left ventricular end-diastolic pressures as high as 100 mm Hg resulted in a decline in left ventricular systolic pressure of only 7.5%.[48] It has been postulated that the apparent descending limb observed in whole-heart preparations is actually related to an increase in afterload, which has been shown to occur with volume loading.[42]

Afterload

Afterload is the tension in the ventricular wall during systole and is dependent on end-diastolic radius, systemic vascular resistance, and ventricular wall thickness. Changes in ventricular wall tension have an inverse relationship with stroke volume if preload is held constant (Fig 18–3). However, with the intact circulation and a normal heart, increases in afterload result in maintenance of stroke volume due to a compensatory increase in left ventricular end-diastolic volume. In the diseased heart, stroke volume tends to decrease with an increase in afterload.[55] The reciprocal is also true—that is, decrease in afterload results in increase in stroke volume and augmentation of cardiac output in the failing heart.

Inotropic State

The inotropic state is a function of the intrinsic ability of the heart to develop a force of contraction independent of preload and afterload. Since changes in contractile state also occur with changes in preload and afterload, to assess the actual intrinsic inotropic state, these variables must be held constant. One way to assess these changes is to compare some indicator of left ventricular function such as stroke volume, stroke

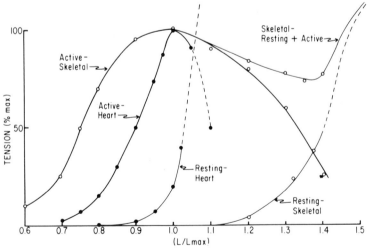

Fig 18–1.—Relationship between initial fiber length and actively developed isometric tension, both expressed as function of maximum. (From Braunwald et al.[7] Used by permission.)

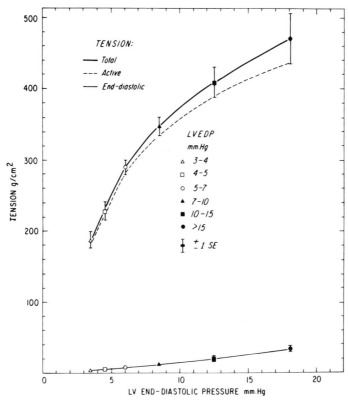

Fig 18–2.—Relationship between left ventricular end-diastolic pressure *(LVEDP)* and calculated peak tension in single induced isovolumetric beats in the intact, sedated dog. (From Taylor R.R., et al.: A quantitative analysis of left ventricular myocardial function in the intact, sedated dog. *Circ. Res.* 21:99, 1967. Used by permission of the American Heart Association.)

work, or rate of pressure change in the ventricle (dp/dt) over a whole range of preloads while holding afterload and heart rate constant (Fig 18–4). This ventricular function curve shows a series of Frank-Starling curves at different contractile states. Displacement upward and to the left represents an increased contractile state; displacement downward and to the right indicates a depressed contractile state.

The maximal velocity of shortening at zero afterload (V_{max}) is another method of measuring inotropic state, but it is of limited usefulness in the clinical situation. Inotropic state is affected by catecholamines, cardiac glycosides, anesthetics, anoxia, acidosis, and various other conditions and pharmacologic agents.

Heart Rate

Heart rate is the fourth determinant of myocardial performance. Increased heart rate over the physiologic range results in a small increase in inotropic state.[7] However, because of reflex changes in venous return, cardiac output is affected minimally. In the depressed heart, as well as during general anesthesia, these effects may be more significant. If venous return is increased appropriately, increased heart rate can result in increased cardiac output, as occurs with exercise. Inordinately fast rates, which decrease time for diastolic filling, and very slow rates, which cannot be compensated for by maximal increase in stroke volume, can decrease cardiac output.

PHYSIOLOGIC CHANGES WITH DECREASE IN CARDIAC OUTPUT

As cardiac performance decreases, two compensatory mechanisms maintain cardiac output: (1) the Frank-Starling mechanism and (2) increased release of catecholamines.

The Frank-Starling mechanism, as previously discussed, maintains cardiac output by increas-

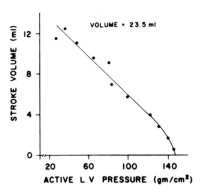

Fig 18-3.—Inverse relationship between stroke volume and left ventricular systolic pressure *(active LV pressure)* in isotonically contracting left ventricle of dog. Left ventricular end-diastolic volume was held constant. (From Burns J.W., Covell J.W., Ross J. Jr.: Mechanics of isotonic left ventricular contractions. *Am. J. Physiol.* 224:725, 1973. Used by permission.)

ing preload or end-diastolic volume. As ventricular function declines, ejection fraction decreases and more blood is left in the ventricle at end-systole. After diastolic filling occurs, a greater end-diastolic volume is achieved, which can serve to maintain cardiac output despite decreased function only to a certain point. As cardiac function continues to deteriorate, end-diastolic volume increases further and signs of venous congestion with dyspnea and cyanosis develop.

The second compensatory mechanism is release of catecholamines. As heart failure progresses and cardiac output decreases, release of catecholamines from cardiac adrenergic nerves and the adrenal medulla is increased. This change augments the contractile state and increases blood pressure by means of arterial vasoconstriction, but it also increases total peripheral vascular resistance and afterload. Under neuronal control, there is also redistribution of flow with increasing heart failure, so that delivery of oxygen to vital structures, such as brain and kidneys, is maintained at the expense of visceral and splanchnic flow.

As long as these mechanisms continue to work, the heart failure remains compensated. However, they are of limited effectiveness, and as heart failure progresses, compensation eventually fails. At this point, the patient has elevated venous pressure, low cardiac output, increased total peripheral vascular resistance, and often some depletion of myocardial catecholamines.

The management of this symptom complex is the topic of this chapter.

INTRAOPERATIVE HYPOTENSION

Intraoperatively, there are three primary causes of hypotension: (1) anesthetic overdose, (2) hypovolemia, and (3) pump failure.

All anesthetic agents have the potential for cardiovascular depression. This is due to direct myocardial depression, which occurs with most

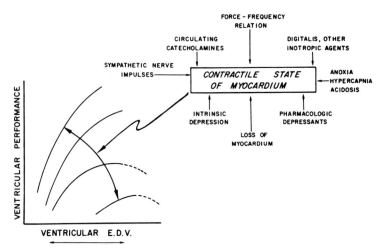

Fig 18-4.—Schematic ventricular function curves showing displacement of the curve with changes in contractile state; end-diastolic volume *(E.D.V.)* (From Braunwald et al.[7] Used by permission.)

anesthetic drugs, and, with some agents, vasodilatation with decrease in preload. Because many cardiac surgical patients have limited cardiac reserve, even a small amount of myocardial depression may not be tolerated. Also, the adrenergic stimulation that maintains blood pressure in compensated heart failure may be overcome easily by agents that cause vasodilatation, such as morphine, resulting in a decrease in blood pressure. With such an occurrence, immediate diagnosis and treatment must be instituted. If vascular dilatation is the cause, as reflected in a low central venous pressure or left atrial pressure, the rapid administration of fluid or blood may be necessary until acceptable hemodynamics are reestablished. The concentration of inhalation agents, including nitrous oxide, may need to be decreased; or their use may need to be withdrawn in some circumstances.

If these two maneuvers fail to restore blood pressure to acceptable levels and cardiopulmonary bypass cannot be established within a few minutes, the use of a short-acting inotropic or pressor agent may be indicated. The decision whether to treat should be aimed at the protection of vital structures. If coronary and cerebral perfusion is inadequate, myocardial or cerebral damage may occur before institution of bypass. Assessment of whether perfusion of these structures is adequate must be done on the basis of systolic and diastolic blood pressure, ECG changes, and previous history of hypertension, coronary artery disease, and cerebrovascular disease.

With coronary artery disease, the use of inotropic or pressor agents is a two-edged sword. Myocardial oxygen utilization is a balance between supply and demand. Increased oxygen demand and decreased oxygen supply can both result in ischemia. If diastolic blood pressure is decreased, coronary perfusion may be decreased also. However, treating decreased blood pressure with either an inotropic agent or a pressor agent that increases afterload will increase myocardial oxygen demands.

When the benefits are deemed to outweigh the risks of treatment in this situation, there are numerous drugs from which to choose. Generally, a single-bolus agent of rapid onset and short duration of action is preferable for this purpose, because cardiopulmonary bypass will be established shortly and the agent or agents chosen may or may not be needed after emergence from bypass.

AGENTS USED TO TREAT INTRAOPERATIVE HYPOTENSION

Calcium

Calcium is an important element in excitation-contraction coupling. It is a potent inotropic substance,[19, 28] and increased extracellular concentration of calcium ion generally leads to parallel increases in three parameters: (1) the amount of adenosine triphosphate consumed by the contractile system, (2) the magnitude of mechanical tension developed, and (3) the uptake of oxygen related to the contractile force generated.[17] Actually, the positive inotropic action of cardiac glycosides and β-adrenergic agents is related to increased availability of calcium to the contractile system.[16, 38] And the oxygen-saving action and myocardial protection with agents such as verapamil are due to calcium antagonistic action.[16] Calcium also has a constrictor effect on vascular smooth muscle and can increase coronary vascular resistance, as well as systemic vascular resistance.[17] It is used intravenously as an inotropic agent and is the first-line agent used for hypotension before cardiopulmonary bypass.

Three calcium salts are available, but only calcium chloride has shown consistent increases in plasma levels of ionized calcium[70] and is the preparation that we use exclusively. A bolus of 5 to 10 mg of 10% calcium chloride per kilogram injected intravenously usually produces a clinically significant increase in arterial pressure. Untoward effects at this dosage are infrequent, although severe bradycardia and cardiac standstill have been described with rapid injection. Calcium salts potentiate the effects of digitalis, and therefore caution must be exercised when using calcium preparations in digitalized patients. Calcium chloride is also a useful agent for profound cardiovascular collapse in the form of electromechanical dissociation or asystole.

Sympathomimetic Drugs

Another group of drugs useful for hypotension are the sympathomimetic agents (Table 18–1). These agents act in two ways: (1) by β-adrenergic action on the heart, increasing the inotropic state (central); and (2) by α-adrenergic stimulation on the peripheral vasculature, resulting in vasoconstriction (peripheral). β-Adrenergic stimulation of the peripheral vessels results in vasodilatation,

TABLE 18-1.—Sympathomimetic Agents Used as Inotropes and Vasopressors

AGENT	HEART* α	HEART* β₁	PERIPHERAL* α	PERIPHERAL* β₂	DIRECT ACTIVITY	INDIRECT ACTIVITY	BLOOD PRESSURE†	HEART RATE†	CARDIAC OUTPUT†	SYSTEMIC VASCULAR RESISTANCE†	MYOCARDIAL OXYGEN CONSUMPTION†
Epinephrine	+	++++	++++	+++	Yes	No	++	+	++	−,+	++
Norepinephrine	+++	++++	++++	0,+	Yes	No	+++	−	0,−	++	++
Isoproterenol	0	++++	0	++++	Yes	No	−	+++	++	− −	++
Metaraminal	0	0,+	++	0,+	Yes	Yes	++	− −	0,−	++	+
Phenylephrine	+	0	++	0	Yes	No	+	−	−	+	+
Methoxamine	0	0,−	++	0	Yes	No	++	− −	− −	++	+
Mephentermine	0	+++	++	+	Yes	Yes	+	+	+	0,+	+
Ephedrine	0	+++	++	++	Yes	Yes	+	+	+	±	+

*Key: 0, no activity at receptor; +, mild activity at receptor; ++, moderate activity at receptor; +++, strong activity at receptor; ++++, very strong activity at receptor; and −, mild antagonistic activity at receptor.
†Key: +, mild increase; ++, moderate increase; +++, marked increase; 0, no change; −, mild decrease; − −, moderate decrease; ±, negligible change.

which may not be a desired response in this setting of acute hypotension. Agents in this class act in two ways: by direct α- or β-adrenergic action of the drugs themselves and by indirect action of secondarily released neurotransmitter substances, primarily norepinephrine. The prototype drugs are the naturally occurring catecholamines: epinephrine, norepinephrine, and isoproterenol.

Epinephrine[20, 24, 37, 53, 58, 68, 69] has very potent β-adrenergic effects on the heart and increases both rate and force of contraction. Its vascular effects are the result of action on both α- and β-adrenergic receptors in the peripheral vasculature. With very low doses, β-adrenergic effects predominate, but as dosage increases, α-adrenergic activity becomes more pronounced. The net result is increased cardiac output, increased blood pressure, and decreased total peripheral vascular resistance, although increased peripheral vascular resistance occurs with high doses. There also is decreased flow to skin, viscera, and renal vascular beds and increased myocardial oxygen demand.[68] The increase in myocardial oxygen demand is undesirable, and ischemia can result. However, if hypotension has decreased coronary perfusion significantly, the increased diastolic pressure may increase coronary perfusion and therefore improve the myocardial oxygen supply-demand ratio. Epinephrine is seldom used as a bolus for acute hypotension in the operating room but is frequently used for profound cardiovascular collapse and cardiac arrest. Side effects are ventricular arrhythmias, myocardial ischemia, and cerebral hemorrhage. It is more commonly used, in cardiac surgical patients, as an intravenous infusion.

Isoproterenol* is the prototype of pure β-stimulating agents. It has a potent β₁-adrenergic action on the heart, increasing rate and contractile state, and a potent β₂-adrenergic activity on peripheral receptors, with vasodilatation and decreased peripheral vascular resistance. Because blood pressure either remains stable or decreases, the drug is seldom useful as a bolus for acute hypotension in the operating room, unless hypotension is due to bradycardia that is unresponsive to atropine. Isoproterenol is also useful as an intravenous infusion.

Norepinephrine[20, 24, 37, 53, 58, 68, 69] exerts a predominance of α-adrenergic activity on peripheral vascular receptors, with resultant vasoconstriction, including venoconstriction, which increases venous return. Norepinephrine also has β₁-adrenergic activity on the heart, which increases contractile state and heart rate. However, when the drug is given in vivo, reflex vagal stimulation occurs, owing to the intense vasoconstriction, and usually results in a net decrease in heart rate. Thus, norepinephrine increases blood pressure and peripheral vascular resistance, decreases heart rate, and either does not affect or decreases cardiac output due to increased afterload. Myocardial oxygen demand is

*References 20, 24, 37, 53, 58, 62, 64, 65, and 68.

again increased and the balance of supply versus demand is altered, the net effect being the summation of four factors: (1) increased inotropic state and (2) increased afterload, both of which increase oxygen demand, (3) decreased heart rate, which decreases oxygen demand, and (4) increased diastolic pressure, which increases coronary perfusion and thus increases oxygen supply. The end result depends on the initial conditions: blood pressure, peripheral vascular resistance, and preload and the ability to increase coronary flow to meet demands, as well as the preinjection state of the myocardium. Norepinephrine is not clinically used for hypotension of short duration in the operating room but is used occasionally in intravenous infusions, although it has several undesirable properties: (1) as previously stated, the intense vasoconstriction increases afterload and may actually decrease cardiac output, (2) flow is reduced to mesenteric and renal vascular beds, (3) ventricular arrhythmias are common, (4) the increased venous return, together with the increased afterload, may be too much for the failing left ventricle to tolerate, and pulmonary edema may be precipitated, and (5) tissue sloughing and necrosis are seen frequently, even without extravasation.

The drugs commonly used to treat brief periods of hypotension in the operating room are all sympathomimetic agents that lack the catechol nucleus. They have properties similar to those of the parent compounds but are generally less potent and have less serious side effects. They can be subdivided into predominantly α-adrenergic agents (metaraminol, methoxamine, and phenylephrine) and mixed α- and β-adrenergic agents (mephentermine and ephedrine).

The three α-stimulating agents act in a similar manner. All three have potent α-adrenergic activity, similar to (although much less potent than) norepinephrine. They have little (metaraminol) or no (methoxamine and phenylephrine) β_2-adrenergic activity on the peripheral vasculature.[58]

Their effects on the heart vary. Metaraminol has a small β_1-adrenergic effect, whereas phenylephrine has no β_1-adrenergic activity but has a positive inotropic effect on the heart that is mediated by α-adrenergic receptors within the heart and is blocked by phentolamine.[58] Actually, some of the positive inotropic action of epinephrine is apparently mediated by α-adrenergic receptors and is blocked by α-adrenergic blocking agents.[25] Methoxamine has a negative inotropic effect mediated by reflex vagal activity.[58]

Phenylephrine and methoxamine are purely direct acting, as is norepinephrine. Metaraminol has both direct and indirect actions. The cardiovascular effects of all three agents are increased blood pressure, increased peripheral vascular resistance, increased venous return, increased myocardial oxygen demand, and decreased cardiac output due to increased afterload and reflex bradycardia.

Mephentermine and ephedrine both have direct and indirect properties, predominantly cardiac.[58,69] They both stimulate β_1-adrenergic myocardial receptors and increase both the strength and the rate of contraction. They both have mixed α- and β-adrenergic effects on the peripheral vasculature, with slight α-adrenergic predominance; mephentermine has a relatively greater effect on resistance vessels, and ephedrine has a greater effect on capacitance vessels.[58] The net effect of both of these agents is increased blood pressure, increased cardiac output, increased myocardial oxygen demand, slight increase in heart rate, and little change or slight increase in peripheral vascular resistance.

How aggressively to treat brief episodes of hypotension in the operating room, especially in cardiac patients, and which agent to use are unresolved issues. Hypotension, especially diastolic hypotension, can lead to decreased coronary perfusion and myocardial ischemia. However, all the agents that have been discussed increase myocardial oxygen demands, which may have an adverse effect on a patient with coronary artery disease. The ideal approach is the avoidance of hypotension by the prudent use of minimally depressant anesthetic techniques in patients with limited cardiac reserves. It may be advisable to insert an intra-aortic balloon under local anesthesia in certain patients with marginal hemodynamics before operation or to have femoral-femoral partial bypass established as standby under local anesthesia before the induction of general anesthesia.

When hypotension occurs before bypass, the use of all depressant anesthetic agents is decreased or withdrawn. When this is ineffective, calcium chloride, 5 to 10 mg/kg, is the agent of choice, with rapid institution of cardiopulmonary bypass if possible. If hypotension is refrac-

TABLE 18-2.—Catecholamines Used as Intravenous Infusions for Inotropic Support

AGENT	INOTROPIC STRENGTH*	HEART RATE*	BLOOD PRESSURE*	α†	β₁†	β₂†	NOREPINEPHRINE RELEASE*	MESENTERIC FLOW*	RENAL FLOW*
Dopamine (µg/kg/min)									
<2	+	0,+	0,−	0	+	+	Yes	+	+
2–10	++	0,+	−,0,+	0	++	0,+	Yes	++	++
>10	+++	+	+	++	+++	0	Yes	−	−
Dobutamine	++	0,+	0,+	+	++	±	No	±	±
Epinephrine									
Low dose	++	+	−	+	++	+++	No	−	−
High dose	+++	++	++	+++	+++	++	No	−	−−
Isoproterenol	+++	+++	−	0	+++	+++	No	+	+
Norepinephrine	+++	−	+++	++++	+++	0	No	−−	−−

*Key: −−−, marked decrease; −−, moderate decrease; −, mild decrease; 0, no change; ±, negligible change; +, mild increase; ++, moderate increase; and +++, marked increase.
†Key: +, mild activity; ++, moderate activity; +++, strong activity; ++++, very strong activity; 0, no activity; and 0,+, minimal activity.

tory to calcium, such drugs as ephedrine and mephentermine are the best second-line agents because of their predominant cardiac effects and their lesser effects on the peripheral vasculature. These agents are infrequently needed when the anesthetic depth and hemodynamic responses are closely monitored, and attempts at avoiding the situations where they are needed are recommended. The use of α-stimulating agents is limited to treating hypotension due to supraventricular tachycardias, although these arrhythmias may be better managed by cardioversion (see chap. 17).

EMERGENCE FROM BYPASS

Emergence from bypass is a critical time for the cardiac patient, and low cardiac output may become manifest at this time. Depressant anesthetic agents are usually withdrawn five to ten minutes before the termination of bypass. Bypass is terminated by clamping the venous return line and transfusing through the arterial cannula until satisfactory hemodynamics are obtained. Usually a left atrial pressure of 10 to 15 mm Hg is sufficient. However, overtransfusion up to left atrial pressures as high as 20 mm Hg is sometimes done to allow for continued bleeding and vasodilatation. If hemodynamics are unsatisfactory despite adequate filling pressure, further assessment is necessary. Calcium chloride, 5 to 10 mg/kg, can be given intravenously if volume is adequate and arterial pressure is low. (Hypocalcemia can occur after bypass secondary to hemodilution[13] and citrate binding, and injection of calcium may be all that is necessary to restore hemodynamics.) To attenuate these effects on levels of calcium, calcium chloride is always added to the priming solution. If inadequate hemodynamics persist, the patient can be returned to bypass while the cause of left ventricular dysfunction is evaluated.

Mechanical problems, such as residual ventricular septal defect or residual gradient across a valve, should be searched for and evaluated, preferably while the patient is off bypass, if hemodynamics will allow, but compromised hemodynamics should not be accepted for long. If such problems exist, further repair may be required. Coronary air emboli can occur and may be manifested by ST-segment changes. Putting the patient back on bypass and perfusing the coronary arteries will decrease the work load of the heart while allowing time for air to pass through the coronary circulation. Once these problems have been ruled out or resolved, if poor hemodynamics persist, left ventricular dysfunction is the cause, usually secondary to poor preoperative left ventricular function or ischemic insult during bypass, or both. Often the metabolic and functional changes that occur with either cardioplegia or intermittent perfusion and hypothermia can take 30 minutes or longer to even approach normal.[40, 63] Sometimes keeping the patient on bypass for a short period, allowing the heart to beat with no work load, can be helpful.

SKELETAL MUSCLE FLOW*	CORONARY FLOW*	ARRHYTHMOGENICITY*	MYOCARDIAL OXYGEN CONSUMPTION*	VENOCONSTRICTION*	PULMONARY VASCULAR RESISTANCE*	SYSTEMIC VASCULAR RESISTANCE*
+	0, +	+	+	+	−	− −
0, −	0, +	+ +	+ +	+ +	−	−
−	0, +	+ + +	+ + +	+ + +	+	+
±	0, +	0, +	+ +	+ +	0, −	0, −
+ +	+	+	+ +	+	0, +	− −
−	+	+ + +	+ + +	+ +	0, +	−
+ + +	+	+ + +	+ + +	+ +	−, 0, +	− − −
− −	+	+ +	+ + +	+ + +	+	+ +

INOTROPIC SUPPORT DURING EMERGENCE FROM BYPASS

During emergence from bypass, most patients who need support have low cardiac output, tachycardia, and increased peripheral vascular resistance, although normal and decreased peripheral vascular resistance may occur as well.[1] The ideal agent for this purpose would be one that increases the contractile state, reduces peripheral resistance to normal, does not increase heart rate, and does not increase myocardial oxygen demand. Naturally, this ideal agent does not exist. Several inotropic agents, though not ideal, are used for treating low cardiac output (Table 18–2). Epinephrine, isoproterenol, dopamine, and dobutamine all share the common property of increasing contractile state, and each has different effects on heart rate and rhythm and on the peripheral vessels.

Epinephrine

Epinephrine[20, 24, 37, 53, 58, 68, 69] is a naturally occurring catecholamine that possesses both α- and β-adrenergic effects. As an intravenous infusion, epinephrine, when used in small doses up to 0.30 µg/kg/minute, increases cardiac output and heart rate and decreases peripheral vascular resistance.[20] Epinephrine increases coronary flow and skeletal muscle flow but markedly decreases renal blood flow, even at very low doses. At higher doses, α-adrenergic effects predominate in most vascular beds and peripheral vascular resistance may actually increase. With these doses, blood pressure increases, and this may increase coronary flow. However, myocardial oxygen demand is also increased.[68] In other words, epinephrine increases blood pressure and cardiac output at the expense of increasing myocardial oxygen demand and jeopardizing renal blood flow. It also increases ventricular ectopy, and arrhythmias are commonly seen.

Isoproterenol

Isoproterenol* has only β-adrenergic effects and is a more powerful inotropic drug than epinephrine.[58] Isoproterenol acts only on β_2-adrenergic receptors on the peripheral vessels, and although it increases flow to all vascular beds, including the renal circulation, it preferentially increases flow to skeletal muscle beds because of the greater number of β-adrenergic receptors at those sites. Peripheral vascular resistance is decreased, which may be accompanied by a decline in arterial diastolic pressure and therefore by decreased coronary perfusion. Isoproterenol also decreases pulmonary vascular resistance[2] and causes tachycardia and ventricular arrhythmias to a greater degree than does epinephrine. The greatest usefulness of isoproterenol is in patients with low cardiac output, bradycardia, and very high peripheral vascular resistance. (Initial dose rate 0.02 to 0.1 µg/kg/minute; adjust rate to response.)

*References 20, 24, 37, 53, 58, 62, 64, 65, 68, and 69.

Dopamine

Dopamine* is a naturally occurring catecholamine and was first synthesized in 1910. However, not until the mid-1960s were its cardiovascular effects thoroughly studied. Dopamine has several advantages over epinephrine and isoproterenol. First, dopamine has greater inotropic than chronotropic activity on cardiac β_1-adrenergic receptors, so that, for equal increases in contractile state, dopamine has much less effect on heart rate. Dopamine is also associated with less ventricular ectopic activity than is either epinephrine or isoproterenol. Its action on the heart is partially direct and partially indirect by stimulating the release of norepinephrine. Action on peripheral receptors is complex, but it possesses some desirable properties. First of all, dopamine has mixed α- and β-adrenergic activities, with β-adrenergic activity predominating at relatively low-dose ranges (<10 μg/kg/minute). It also exhibits a unique vasodilating activity in the renal and mesenteric vascular beds that is not mediated by α- or β-adrenergic receptors. This effect has been called "dopaminergic." Dopaminergic vasodilatation occurs at all dosage ranges, until α-adrenergic activity begins to predominate (>10 μg/kg/minute), increasing the resistance in the peripheral vascular bed. This dopaminergic-mediated dilatation is not blocked by α- or β-adrenergic blocking agents but can be specifically blocked by dopaminergic blocking agents, such as the butyrophenones[71] and phenothiazines.[23] Since these receptors predominate in the renal and mesenteric vascular beds and do not appear to be significantly present in skeletal muscle beds, flow is preferentially diverted toward renal and mesenteric beds rather than toward skeletal muscle, as long as the dosage range is kept below 10 μg/kg/minute.

According to Schuelke et al.,[56] dopamine also causes dopaminergic-mediated dilatation of coronary arteries, but this can be detected only after α- and β-adrenergic blockade.

Thus, dopamine at low doses increases contractile state, with minimal increase in heart rate and ectopy. It causes decreased total peripheral resistance while diverting flow to renal and mesenteric beds. At higher dosages, α-adrenergic effects predominate, and the actions of dopamine then are similar to those of epinephrine, with decreased renal blood flow and increased peripheral resistance. Like all other catecholamines except norepinephrine, dopamine has little or no effect on cerebral vessels, with cerebral blood flow being more sensitive to changes in blood pressure and P_{CO_2}.

Dobutamine

Dobutamine† is a synthetic catecholamine that was developed by modifying the chemical structure of isoproterenol so that certain desirable properties, such as positive inotropy, were retained while undesirable actions, such as chronotropy, arrhythmogenicity, and strong peripheral vascular activity, were minimized.[66] The resulting compound was one of 16 modifications of dopamine that were developed.

Dobutamine retains strong β_1-adrenergic activity, although none of the compounds studied has the inotropic potency of isoproterenol. However, the chronotropic activity compared with that of isoproterenol is reduced fourfold, and in this respect is comparable to that of dopamine.

Dobutamine has less effect on automaticity, resulting in less ectopic activity compared with norepinephrine, isoproterenol, or dopamine.[64, 66] An advantage of dobutamine over dopamine is that all of dobutamine's activity is direct, whereas dopamine's activity is in part dependent on the release of norepinephrine. This factor is important in the patient whose myocardial catecholamine stores are depleted.

The structure of dobutamine was modified in such a way as to reduce α- and β_2-adrenergic activity, and thus dobutamine has little effect on the peripheral vasculature. It causes only a modest increase in blood pressure and decreases peripheral vascular resistance less than does either isoproterenol or dopamine. Dobutamine does not stimulate dopaminergic receptors and therefore does not produce the direct increase in renal blood flow that is seen with dopamine. (Initial rate of infusion 2 to 5 μg/kg/minute; maximal rate 20 μg/kg/minute.)

Comparisons Among Catecholamines

Clinical studies have supported the use of all four of these agents during emergence from cardiopulmonary bypass. Recent studies have

---

*References 12, 15, 20-24, 30, 32, 37, 41, 44, 46, 51, 53, 54, 56, 62, 68, 69, and 71.

†References 4, 22, 24, 32, 41, 45, 59, and 64-68.

shown certain advantages of dopamine and dobutamine. Tinker et al.[64] found greater increase in cardiac index, less increase in heart rate, and fewer arrhythmias with dobutamine than with isoproterenol. Steen et al.,[59] in a later study, compared the effects of epinephrine (0.04 µg/kg/minute), dopamine (5, 10, and 15 µg/kg/minute), and dobutamine (5, 10, and 15 µg/kg/minute) for emergence from bypass. They found consistent increases in cardiac index with all three agents, greatest with dopamine; a moderate increase in mean arterial pressure (20% to 30%) with all three agents; a small increase in heart rate (7% to 13%), with no major difference among the three agents in this regard; and no major difference in arrhythmogenicity. They described four patients given dobutamine and one given dopamine who did not respond with increased cardiac index but who did respond to the other drug. All patients treated with epinephrine responded with increased cardiac index.

These studies suggest that, despite the theoretical and experimental evidence showing advantages for dopamine and dobutamine, epinephrine seems to be an equally adequate agent, at least as far as emergence from bypass is concerned. These three agents probably are superior to isoproterenol for this purpose.[64] The long-term effects of possibly compromising renal flow with epinephrine during emergence from bypass, however, are not certain.

Stephenson et al.[61] compared dopamine and epinephrine during the immediate postoperative period and found significantly increased urinary flow with dopamine. They also found a greater incidence of tachycardia with dopamine than with epinephrine, for a comparable increase in cardiac index. This finding is in disagreement with most studies.

With all of these agents, changes in cardiac index correlate poorly with changes in blood pressure; in certain situations significant increase in cardiac index occurs despite little change or decrease in blood pressure, and in other situations elevation of blood pressure occurs with no change or with a decrease in cardiac index. Thus, the importance of monitoring cardiac output seems evident. Monitoring cardiac output and calculating vascular resistances aid in the selection of an inotrope that properly fits the situation. With high systemic vascular resistance and low cardiac index, dopamine or even isoproterenol may be preferable to dobutamine or epinephrine. There also are certain situations on emergence from bypass in which the cardiac index is high and the systemic vascular resistance is low, and as a result blood pressure is low. This situation sometimes occurs after aortic valve replacement.[1] Treatment with an inotropic agent, especially isoproterenol, is unphysiologic. Treatment with an α-adrenergic agent, such as phenylephrine, is much more physiologically sound and probably is the best choice.

Data from clinical studies suggest that dopamine and dobutamine are the most effective first-line agents for inotropic support during emergence from bypass, with substitution of the other agent if the first is unsatisfactory. Epinephrine would be the third choice, although substitution of a pharmacologic regimen that would preserve renal blood flow should be instituted as soon as possible during the postoperative period. Isoproterenol should be reserved for patients in whom an increase in heart rate would be advantageous or in whom a large decrease in systemic vascular resistance, as well as increased cardiac index, is needed. The tachycardia and arrhythmogenicity with isoproterenol may still require substitution of another agent. α-Adrenergic agents should be reserved for the specific situation in which cardiac index is normal or increased and systemic vascular resistance is low.

Because all of the previously described catecholamines have properties that differ from each other, when used in combination they may result in advantages to certain patients. Talley et al.[62] described two patients who had a significantly greater increase in cardiac index with isoproterenol than with dopamine, but who had a significantly greater increase in urinary output with dopamine. Combined therapy resulted in greater increased cardiac index and urinary output than with either drug alone. Filner et al.[15] described four patients who had a more favorable response to dopamine and isoproterenol in combination than to either drug alone and three other patients who responded better to a combination of dopamine plus other agents. Holzer et al.[30] reported two cases in which isoproterenol and dopamine resulted in better hemodynamics than either drug alone and two cases in which dopamine and epinephrine or dopamine and norepinephrine proved to be superior.

These studies indicate that the individual advantages of each drug, such as a greater decrease in systemic vascular resistance with isoproterenol, greater vasoconstriction with epinephrine, and augmentation of urinary flow with dopamine, may be enhanced to give an overall improvement in hemodynamics.

MECHANICAL SUPPORT: INTRA-AORTIC BALLOON PUMP

Another means of support during emergence from bypass is the intra-aortic balloon pump* (see chap. 19). This device is inserted through a femoral artery into the descending aorta. Inflations of the balloon are triggered by the R wave of the ECG, so that inflation occurs during diastole to augment coronary perfusion and deflation occurs during systole to decrease afterload and increase cardiac output.

Actually, three types of mechanical support in cardiogenic shock have been described. In 1961, Clauss et al.[10] described the concept of counterpulsation. Counterpulsation was achieved by mechanically withdrawing blood from the femoral arteries during systole and reinjecting it during diastole. Reduction of afterload and increase in coronary blood flow could be demonstrated, but problems with hemolysis and synchronization led to its abandonment.

In 1962, Moulopoulos et al.[49] devised the prototype intra-aortic balloon, which after various modifications developed into the present-day intra-aortic balloon pump.

The third device is the external counterpulsator, which was described by Dennis et al.[14] in 1963. This device entails use of a half-body pressure suit or some type of external sleeve on the lower extremities that inflates during diastole and deflates during systole. These actually have produced changes similar to those produced by the intra-aortic balloon pump, although to a much lesser degree.

The only device actually in use at this time clinically is the intra-aortic balloon pump. With initiation of counterpulsation, there is an immediate decrease in peak systolic pressure and an increase in mean diastolic pressure. Actually, the entire arterial pressure tracing is altered such that peak systolic pressure is slightly reduced, and as the balloon is inflated at about the position of the dicrotic notch, arterial pressure increases to a peak that decreases markedly just before the next systole (Fig 18–5). Documented increases in cardiac index have been shown, as well as decreased pulmonary capillary wedge pressure, increased coronary blood flow, and decreased myocardial oxygen consumption.

The two primary indications for use of the intra-aortic balloon pump are myocardial infarction shock and emergence from cardiopulmonary bypass. Studies have shown increased survival with[33] and without[27] surgery when the intra-aortic balloon pump is used in myocardial infarction shock. Numerous clinical studies have reported the use of the intra-aortic balloon pump for successful emergence from bypass in patients who were unable to be weaned from bypass despite inotropic support.[31]

Intra-aortic balloon counterpulsation is also used during the postoperative period for treatment of low cardiac output by itself and in conjunction with inotropic support. Holzer et al.[30] reported the use of dopamine in conjunction with intra-aortic balloon counterpulsation and achieved more satisfactory results than with norepinephrine or isoproterenol. Dopamine seems to be particularly well suited for additional support with the intra-aortic balloon because of its effect on renal blood flow, which may be compromised by intra-aortic balloon counterpulsation.

POSTOPERATIVE LOW CARDIAC OUTPUT

Low cardiac output is also encountered during the immediate postoperative period. The principles of management are similar to those used for emergence from bypass, but there are a few subtle differences. The major difference is that the support is of longer duration, and as a result long-term preservation of organ function, such as of the kidney, is of more significance. Also, the conditions are more stable; minute-to-minute changes are not seen as frequently as they are in the operating room; and weaning from support is a longer and slower process. Aside from these differences, principles of management are similar and management during the postoperative period is basically an extension of support initiated in the operating room.

The principles of management are based on the four primary determinants of myocardial

---

*References 10, 14, 27, 31, 33, 34, 36, 39, 49, and 50.

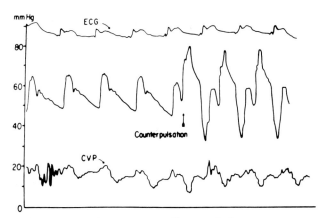

Fig 18–5.—Changes in arterial pulse contour with initiation of intra-aortic balloon counterpulsation; central venous pressure *(CVP)*. (From Mueller.[50] Used by permission.)

performance discussed earlier in this chapter: heart rate, preload, afterload, and inotropic state.

Controlling Heart Rate

As mentioned previously, heart rate changes within the physiologic range have relatively minor effects on cardiac output, and therefore only significant bradycardias and tachycardias outside the physiologic range benefit significantly from treatment (see chap. 17). Optimal heart rate actually covers a large range; however, heart rate is probably the most important determinant of myocardial oxygen demand, and thus rapid heart rates, even if hemodynamically insignificant, should be avoided if possible.

Optimizing Preload

The preload should be made optimal if the best cardiac output is to be obtained. As mentioned previously, increasing preload increases cardiac output up to a certain point. This point varies from person to person and in the same person from time to time. Because left atrial pressure is only an estimation of left ventricular preload and the correct end point is unknown, the best way to make the preload optimal is by observing the corresponding changes in cardiac output that are associated with elevations in left atrial pressure. If elevation of left atrial pressure results in no change or a decrease in cardiac index or signs of "backward failure," optimal preload has been exceeded, and further increases would be of no benefit or even detrimental.

Low output that persists after optimal preload has been achieved is cardiogenic shock, by definition, and can result from various causes. A sudden deterioration in left ventricular function is suggestive of an acute problem, such as tamponade, myocardial ischemia or infarction, or pulmonary embolism. Diagnosis and differentiation among these three may be difficult after operations on the heart, yet delay in diagnosis and treatment may be fatal. Once an acute process has been ruled out, two treatment modalities remain: (1) inotropic or mechanical support and (2) afterload reduction.

Inotropic Support

The specific agents for inotropic support have been discussed previously in connection with emergence from bypass, as has intra-aortic balloon counterpulsation. The theoretical considerations during the postoperative period are much the same as those during emergence from bypass; however, the thinking has changed considerably during the past decade, with more aggressive monitoring and careful attention being paid to the physiologic changes that occur with low output cardiac failure. This change has caused a shift from treating the low cardiac output with inotropic agents to treating the increased systemic vascular resistance with afterload reducers.

Afterload Reduction

As was mentioned previously, as the left ventricle starts to fail and cardiac output decreases,

TABLE 18–3.—Spectrum of Vasodilators Used for the Treatment of Heart Failure*

AGENT	PREDOMINANT SITE OF ACTION	MODE OF ADMINISTRATION	DURATION OF ACTION
Phentolamine	Arterial	Continuous intravenous	Minutes
		Oral	Hours
Phenoxybenzamine	Arterial	Oral	Hours
Hydralazine	Arterial	Oral, IV, IM	Hours
Minoxidil	Arterial	Oral	Hours
Nitroprusside	Arterial and venous	Continuous intravenous	Minutes
Trimethaphan	Venous and arterial	Continuous intravenous	Minutes
Prazosin	Arterial and venous	Oral	Hours
Nitroglycerin	Venous	Intravenous or sublingual	Minutes
		Ointment	Hours
Isosorbide dinitrate	Venous	Sublingual, oral	Minutes–hours

*From Braunwald.[6] Used by permission.

neural and humoral factors cause a reflex increase in systemic vascular resistance. This increase in afterload may cause further deterioration in left ventricular function. Treatment of left ventricular dysfunction by reducing afterload is based on the contention that at least part of the reflex increase in vascular resistance is inappropriate and its correction will result in hemodynamic improvement. This effect has been shown to be true, and several agents are of benefit in acute and chronic heart failure. The major differences among these agents are their differential effects on resistance versus capacitance vessels (Table 18–3).

Sodium Nitroprusside

Sodium nitroprusside* is the most thoroughly studied and widely used agent for reducing afterload in low-output states. Nitroprusside acts by the direct relaxation of arteriolar and venular smooth muscle,[52] thus decreasing both preload and afterload. Administration to patients with low cardiac output generally produces decreased systemic vascular resistance, increased cardiac output, and little or no decrease in blood pressure. In postoperative cardiac patients with elevated mean arterial pressure before the administration of nitroprusside, Bixler et al.[5] found a decrease in mean arterial pressure, whereas in those with initially low mean arterial pressure,

*References 5, 6, 8, 11, 18, 26, 35, 43, 47, 52, and 57.

they noted similar changes in systemic vascular resistance and cardiac output but little or no change in blood pressure.

The effect on cardiac output actually depends on the function of the left ventricle before the administration of the drug. Patients with normal cardiac output and systemic vascular resistance before the administration of sodium nitroprusside will not have an increased cardiac output and may actually have a decrease because of the decrease in preload. Maintaining preload with volume infusion may be necessary. Nitroprusside also decreases pulmonary vascular resistance and may dilate reflexly constricted pulmonary arterioles, resulting in increased intrapulmonic shunt and decreased Po_2.[8]

Reflex tachycardia is a common problem in patients with normal cardiac index during nitroprusside infusion for induced hypotension. However, patients receiving nitroprusside for afterload reduction and low cardiac output often have little change or even a decrease in heart rate, presumably because of the improvement in stroke volume and cardiac output.[45]

The effect of nitroprusside on renal function depends on the response of the cardiac output. With increase in cardiac output, renal blood flow and urinary output usually increase, whereas with acute reduction in mean arterial pressure, renal blood flow and urinary output may decrease. The dosage of nitroprusside needed for afterload reduction varies from 10 to 800 µg/minute.[57]

Trimethaphan

Trimethaphan is a short-acting ganglionic blocking agent that, like nitroprusside, has effects on both venous and arterial vessels, and for many years has been used for hypertensive crises and induction of hypotension. An advantage when the drug is used in this setting is that ganglionic blockade prevents reflex tachycardia. The effects of trimethaphan actually are predominantly on the capacitance vessels, and thus preload is decreased more than afterload.[11] Because of varying and unstable response, it is not commonly used for reduction of afterload in heart failure.

Prazosin

Prazosin is a quinazoline derivative that causes arteriolar and venular dilatation and therefore, like nitroprusside, decreases preload and afterload. In a study by Mehta et al.,[43] hemodynamic changes found with oral prazosin (4 mg) were similar to those found with 20 to 200 μg/minute of sodium nitroprusside, although the changes with prazosin were quantitatively slightly less. Prazosin exerts its beneficial effects in one to six hours after oral administration and is most useful in the management of chronic cardiac failure.

Other Agents That Reduce Afterload

There are several agents that act almost exclusively on the arterial side, including hydralazine and the α-adrenergic blocking agents phentolamine and phenoxybenzamine. Phentolamine decreases systemic vascular resistance and markedly increases cardiac output when infused at 0.2 to 2 mg/minute.[11] Filling pressure generally decreases, but only minimally, the decrease being due to improved cardiac output. However, the drug is expensive, and its lack of advantages over nitroprusside limits its clinical usefulness.

Hydralazine acts almost exclusively on arteriolar smooth muscle and consequently decreases systemic vascular resistance and increases cardiac output in patients with cardiac failure.[6] Again, a small reduction in left atrial pressure is seen because of the improvement in cardiac performance. An advantage of hydralazine is that, like prazosin, it can be given orally and thus may be useful in the management of chronic cardiac failure. A disadvantage of these agents that act only on the resistance vessels is that they affect preload only minimally, and therefore symptoms of backward failure may be relatively unaltered.

Nitrates

The last group of vasodilators includes the nitrates, which act almost exclusively on capacitance vessels and therefore decrease preload with little or no effect on afterload. Nitroglycerin given intravenously, sublingually, or orally has a profound effect on right- and left-sided filling pressures and also decreases pulmonary artery pressures (see chap. 8). However, the systemic vascular resistance is minimally changed, and therefore cardiac output remains unchanged or may even decrease if the decrease in preload is significant.[47] If preload is maintained, then cardiac output may increase because of the smaller effect on the resistance vessels, causing a slight decrease in systemic vascular resistance. The other nitrate preparations have similar effects, with the only differences being the route of administration and the duration of action.

Treatment of Low Cardiac Output With Vasodilators

Vasodilator treatment of low-output cardiac failure has proved to be beneficial in numerous clinical trials and has become the first-line treatment in many situations in which inotropic support used to be the treatment of choice. There has been a change toward treating the patient's compensatory response (increased systemic vascular resistance) and away from treating the pump failure. Greater knowledge of the physiologic derangements involved and more thorough monitoring, including that of cardiac output and vascular resistance, have permitted more precise application of drug therapy to specific clinical entities.

Nitroprusside is the agent most frequently chosen when afterload reduction is indicated. It has two advantages over other vasodilators: (1) reduction of both preload and afterload, which is beneficial to most patients with low-output failure, and (2) rapid onset and termination of effect for minute-to-minute control.

Vasodilators Versus Inotropes

Patients with low-output cardiac failure generally have decreased cardiac output, increased systemic vascular resistance, and increased preload. Nitroprusside and the inotropic drugs all act to return these measures toward normal, but by attacking opposite ends of the problem. The decision whether to treat with inotropes or afterload reducers must be guided by physiologic changes and patient response.

Nitroprusside offers (1) reduction in afterload, (2) less tachycardia and arrhythmogenicity than with epinephrine, isoproterenol, and perhaps dopamine and dobutamine,[45] and (3) an increase in cardiac output with probably less increase in myocardial oxygen demand, although the effects of nitroprusside on the myocardial oxygen supply-demand ratio are complex.[9] The possible disadvantages are (1) too great a reduction in diastolic blood pressure, compromising coronary flow, (2) unsatisfactory increase in cardiac output, and (3) cyanide toxicity.

In comparing the hemodynamic response of nitroprusside and dobutamine in patients with low-output cardiac failure, Mikulic et al.[45] found similar increases in cardiac index and greater reduction in systemic vascular resistance and pulmonary artery wedge pressure with nitroprusside, but a reduction in mean and diastolic arterial pressures as well. Dobutamine caused little change or an increase in mean arterial pressure, but less reduction in pulmonary wedge pressure and systemic vascular resistance. Berkowitz et al.[4] found similar hemodynamic changes when they compared the two agents, but in seven of 19 patients, they observed increases in cardiac index that were too small to permit comparison with dobutamine.

These findings support both afterload reduction and inotropic support as being efficacious in low-output cardiac failure and suggest an advantage of nitroprusside when increased systemic vascular resistance dominates the physiologic changes and an advantage of dobutamine if a decrease in arterial pressure could be deleterious. However, individual patient response exists, and patients with low mean arterial pressure before institution of nitroprusside often have an insignificant decrease in mean arterial pressure. This factor suggests that a trial period with nitroprusside under careful observation may be the best way to evaluate its effectiveness.

Because these two groups of agents cause similar hemodynamic changes by different mechanisms, combined therapy may be more beneficial than either agent alone. Experimental studies have shown that dopamine and phentolamine act synergistically, with greater increased cardiac output and renal blood flow when infused simultaneously.[3] Clinical trials show a greater increase in cardiac index and a greater reduction in pulmonary wedge pressure and systemic and pulmonary vascular resistance with nitroprusside in combination with either dobutamine or dopamine.[4,46,60]

Digitalis

No discussion of circulatory support would be complete without some mention of digitalis.[24,29] Digitalis preparations have been used in the treatment of cardiac failure since the 19th century and still hold a prestigious place in the treatment of chronic congestive heart failure. Several factors have limited the use of digitalis in the management of acute cardiac failure: (1) onset of action, even with the most rapidly acting preparation, is five to ten minutes; (2) due to the long half-life, control is difficult; (3) the therapeutic index is low, and therefore toxic manifestations are common; (4) consistent increase in cardiac index, especially in ischemic heart disease, is sometimes not seen[29]; (5) the increase in contractile state is not as impressive as that seen with catecholamines; and (6) like all agents that increase the contractile state, it can increase myocardial oxygen demand and therefore can increase ischemia.

Digoxin, the most commonly used preparation, is still frequently used for the chronic management of all types of cardiac failure. The hemodynamic effects seen with digoxin vary in the failing and the nonfailing heart. In the nonfailing heart, digoxin increases inotropic state, increases venous tone, and increases total peripheral vascular resistance. The increased impedance to ventricular ejection nullifies the increased inotropic state, and the net effect on cardiac index is no change. There is, however, an increase in myocardial oxygen consumption. In the failing heart, with reflex peripheral vasoconstriction already present, the increase in myocardial performance reduces the reflex vasoconstriction and results in a net decrease in total peripheral vascular resistance, and therefore cardiac output increases. Because of decreased afterload and improved myocardial efficiency, myocardial oxygen consumption decreases. When digoxin is administered intravenously, its onset of action is between 15 and 30 minutes, with peak effect at one to five hours. (Digitalizing dose 0.9 mg/sq m of body surface; initially one half of the estimated total dose intravenously, then one fourth or one eighth added intravenously 1 to 2 hours until desired effect is obtained or adverse effects appear.) The major use of digitalis preparations is for the chronic management of congestive heart failure, and they remain the most commonly used drugs for this purpose.

CONCLUSIONS

The proper management of low cardiac output demands knowledge of physiologic changes in the four primary determinants of myocardial performance. Various degrees of decreased cardiac output, increased systemic vascular resistance, and increased filling pressures occur with low-output cardiac failure. Treatment involving preload and afterload reduction, inotropic support, and mechanical support is guided by the physiologic changes that are needed to best improve the clinical situation. Various combinations of inotropic drugs with or without vasodilators often achieve a more optimal effect than either alone. Although observed physiologic changes are a guide to therapy, considerable variation among patients exists, and the individual patient response to various combinations should dictate the proper therapy.

REFERENCES

1. Arkin D.B., Saidman L.J., Benumof J.L.: Case history number 98: Hypotension following cardiopulmonary bypass. *Anesth. Analg.* 56:720, 1977.
2. Aviado D.M. Jr., Schmidt C.F.: Effects of sympathomimetic drugs on pulmonary circulation: With special reference to a new pulmonary vasodilator. *J. Pharmacol. Exp. Ther.* 120:512, 1957.
3. Bagwell E.E., Daniell H.B., Freeman B.F.: Influence of phentolamine on the cardiovascular effects of dopamine in experimental cardiogenic shock. *Arch. Int. Pharmacodyn. Ther.* 208:197, 1974.
4. Berkowitz C., et al.: Comparative responses to dobutamine and nitroprusside in patients with chronic low output cardiac failure. *Circulation* 56:918, 1977.
5. Bixler T.J., et al.: Improved myocardial performance in postoperative cardiac surgical patients with sodium nitroprusside. *Ann. Thorac. Surg.* 25:444, 1978.
6. Braunwald E.: Vasodilator therapy—a physiologic approach to the treatment of heart failure, editorial. *N. Engl. J. Med.* 297:331, 1977.
7. Braunwald E., Ross J. Jr., Sonnenblick E.H.: *Mechanisms of Contraction of the Normal and Failing Heart*, ed. 2. Boston, Little, Brown & Co., 1976.
8. Brodie T.S., et al.: Effect of nitroprusside on arterial oxygenation, intrapulmonic shunts and oxygen delivery, abstracted. *Am. J. Cardiol.* 37:123, 1976.
9. Chiariello M., et al.: Comparison between the effects of nitroprusside and nitroglycerin on ischemic injury during acute myocardial infarction. *Circulation* 54:766, 1976.
10. Clauss R.H., et al.: Assisted circulation: I. The arterial counterpulsator. *J. Thorac. Cardiovasc. Surg.* 41:447, 1961.
11. Cohn J.N., Franciosa J.A.: Drug therapy: Vasodilator therapy of cardiac failure. *N. Engl. J. Med.* 297:27 and 254, 1977.
12. Costello D.L., Mueller H.S., Ayres S.M.: Dopamine in the treatment of low cardiac output state: Comparison with isoproterenol and L-norepinephrine, abstracted. *Clin. Res.* 22:678A, 1974.
13. Das J.B., et al.: Changes in serum ionic calcium during cardiopulmonary bypass with hemodilution. *J. Thorac. Cardiovasc. Surg.* 62:449, 1971.
14. Dennis C., et al.: Studies on external counterpulsation as a potential measure for acute left heart failure. *Trans. Am. Soc. Artif. Intern. Organs* 9:186, 1963.
15. Filner B., Karliner J.S., Daily P.O.: Favorable influence of dopamine on left ventricular performance in patients refractory to discontinuation of cardiopulmonary bypass. *Circ. Shock* 4:223, 1977.
16. Fleckenstein A.: Specific inhibitors and promoters of calcium action in the excitation-contraction coupling of heart muscle and their role in the prevention or production of myocardial lesions, in Harris P., Opie L. (eds.): *Calcium and the Heart*. New York, Academic Press, 1971, p. 135.
17. Fleckenstein A.: Specific pharmacology of calcium in myocardium, cardiac pacemakers, and vascular smooth muscle. *Annu. Rev. Pharmacol. Toxicol.* 17:149, 1977.
18. Franciosa J.A., Cohn J.N.: Hemodynamic effects of oral ephedrine given alone or combined with nitroprusside infusion in patients

with severe left ventricular failure. *Am. J. Cardiol.* 43:79, 1979.
19. Gilmore J.P., et al.: Influence of calcium on myocardial potassium balance, oxygen consumption, and performance. *Am. Heart J.* 75:215, 1968.
20. Goldberg L.I.: Use of sympathomimetic amines in heart failure. *Am. J. Cardiol.* 22:177, 1968.
21. Goldberg L.I.: Cardiovascular and renal actions of dopamine: Potential clinical applications. *Pharmacol. Rev.* 24:1, 1972.
22. Goldberg L.I., Hsieh Y.-Y., Resnekov L.: Newer catecholamines for treatment of heart failure and shock: An update on dopamine and a first look at dobutamine. *Prog. Cardiovasc. Dis.* 19:327, 1977.
23. Goldberg L.I., Yeh B.K.: Attenuation of dopamine-induced renal vasodilation in the dog by phenothiazines. *Eur. J. Pharmacol.* 15:36, 1971.
24. Goodman L.S., Gilman A.: *The Pharmacological Basis of Therapeutics*, ed. 5. New York, Macmillan Publishing Co., 1975.
25. Govier W.C.: Myocardial *alpha* adrenergic receptors and their role in the production of a positive inotropic effect by sympathomimetic agents. *J. Pharmacol. Exp. Ther.* 159:82, 1968.
26. Guiha N.H., et al.: Treatment of refractory heart failure with infusion of nitroprusside. *N. Engl. J. Med.* 291:587, 1974.
27. Hagemeijer F., et al.: Effectiveness of intraortic balloon pumping without cardiac surgery for patients with severe heart failure secondary to a recent myocardial infarction. *Am. J. Cardiol.* 40:951, 1977.
28. Harrison D.C., Nelson D.: The effects of calcium on isometric tension in isolated heart muscle during coupled pacing. *Am. Heart J.* 74:663, 1967.
29. Hodges M., et al.: Effects of intravenously administered digoxin on mild left ventricular failure in acute myocardial infarction in man. *Am. J. Cardiol.* 29:749, 1972.
30. Holzer J., et al.: Effectiveness of dopamine in patients with cardiogenic shock. *Am. J. Cardiol.* 32:79, 1973.
31. Housman L.B., et al.: Counterpulsation for intraoperative cardiogenic shock: Successful use of intra-aortic balloon. *J.A.M.A.* 224:1131, 1973.
32. Jewitt D., Jennings K., Jackson P.G.: Efficacy of new inotropic drugs in clinical coronary heart failure. *Am. J. Med.* 65:197, 1978.
33. Johnson S.A., et al.: Treatment of cardiogenic shock in myocardial infarction by intraaortic balloon counterpulsation and surgery. *Am. J. Med.* 62:687, 1977.
34. Kantrowitz A.: The development of mechanical assistance to the failing human heart. *Med. Instrum.* 10:224, 1976.
35. Kötter V., et al.: Comparison of haemodynamic effects of phentolamine, sodium nitroprusside, and glyceryl trinitrate in acute myocardial infarction. *Br. Heart J.* 39:1196, 1977.
36. Kuhn L.A.: Current status of diastolic augmentation for circulatory support. *Am. Heart J.* 81:281, 1971.
37. Lappas D.G., Powell W.M.J. Jr., Daggett W.M.: Cardiac dysfunction in the perioperative period: Pathophysiology, diagnosis, and treatment. *Anesthesiology* 47:117, 1977.
38. Lee K.S., Klaus W.: The subcellular basis for the mechanism of inotropic action of cardiac glycosides. *Pharmacol. Rev.* 23:193, 1971.
39. Lefemine A.A., et al.: Results and complications of intraaortic balloon pumping in surgical and medical patients. *Am. J. Cardiol.* 40:416, 1977.
40. Levitsky S., et al.: Does intermittent coronary perfusion offer greater myocardial protection than continuous aortic cross-clamping? *Surgery* 82:51, 1977.
41. Loeb H.S., Bredakis J., Gunnar R.M.: Superiority of dobutamine over dopamine for augmentation of cardiac output in patients with chronic low output cardiac failure. *Circulation* 55:375, 1977.
42. MacGregor D.C., et al.: Relations between afterload, stroke volume, and descending limb of Starling's curve. *Am. J. Physiol.* 227:884, 1974.
43. Mehta J., et al.: Comparative hemodynamic effects of intravenous nitroprusside and oral prazosin in refractory heart failure. *Am. J. Cardiol.* 41:925, 1978.
44. Merin G., et al.: The hemodynamic effects of dopamine following cardiopulmonary bypass. *Ann. Thorac. Surg.* 23:361, 1977.
45. Mikulic E., Cohn J.N., Franciosa J.A.: Comparative hemodynamic effects of inotropic and vasodilator drugs in severe heart failure. *Circulation* 56:528, 1977.
46. Miller R.R., et al.: Combined dopamine and nitroprusside therapy in congestive heart failure: Greater augmentation of cardiac performance by addition of inotropic stimulation to afterload reduction. *Circulation* 55:881, 1977.
47. Miller R.R., et al.: Pharmacological mechanisms for left ventricular unloading in clinical congestive heart failure: Differential effects of nitroprusside, phentolamine, and nitroglycerin

on cardiac function and peripheral circulation. *Circ. Res.* 39:127, 1976.
48. Monroe R.G., et al.: Left ventricular performance at high end-diastolic pressures in isolated, perfused dog hearts. *Circ. Res.* 26:85, 1970.
49. Moulopoulos S.D., Topaz S., Kolff W.J.: Diastolic balloon pumping (with carbon dioxide) in the aorta: A mechanical assistance to the failing circulation. *Am. Heart J.* 63:669, 1962.
50. Mueller H.: Are intra-aortic balloon pumping and external counterpulsation effective in the treatment of cardiogenic shock? *Cardiovasc. Clin.* 8:87, 1977.
51. Mueller H.S., Evans R., Ayres S.M.: Effect of dopamine on hemodynamics and myocardial metabolism in shock following acute myocardial infarction in man. *Circulation* 57:361, 1978.
52. Palmer R.F., Lasseter K.C.: Sodium nitroprusside. *N. Engl. J. Med.* 292:294, 1975.
53. Rosenblum R.: Physiologic basis for the therapeutic use of catecholamines. *Am. Heart J.* 87:527, 1974.
54. Rosenblum R., Frieden J.: Intravenous dopamine in the treatment of myocardial dysfunction after open-heart surgery. *Am. Heart J.* 83:743, 1972.
55. Ross J. Jr., Braunwald E.: The study of left ventricular function in man by increasing resistance to ventricular ejection with angiotensin. *Circulation* 29:739, 1964.
56. Schuelke D.M., et al.: Coronary vasodilatation produced by dopamine after adrenergic blockade. *J. Pharmacol. Exp. Ther.* 176:320, 1971.
57. Shah P.K.: Ventricular unloading in the management of heart disease: Role of vasodilators. *Am. Heart J.* 93:256 and 403, 1977.
58. Smith N.T., Corbascio A.N.: The use and misuse of pressor agents. *Anesthesiology* 33:58, 1970.
59. Steen P.A., et al.: Efficacy of dopamine, dobutamine, and epinephrine during emergence from cardiopulmonary bypass in man. *Circulation* 57:378, 1978.
60. Stemple D.R., Kleiman J.H., Harrison D.C.: Combined nitroprusside-dopamine therapy in severe chronic congestive heart failure: Dose-related hemodynamic advantages over single drug infusions. *Am. J. Cardiol.* 42:267, 1978.
61. Stephenson L.W., Blackstone E.H., Kouchoukos N.T.: Dopamine vs. epinephrine in patients following cardiac surgery: randomized study. *Surg. Forum* 27:272, 1976.
62. Talley R.C., et al.: A hemodynamic comparison of dopamine and isoproterenol in patients in shock. *Circulation* 39:361, 1969.
63. Tarhan S., White R.D., Moffitt E.A.: Anesthesia and postoperative care for cardiac operations. *Ann. Thorac. Surg.* 23:173, 1977.
64. Tinker J.H., et al.: Dobutamine for inotropic support during emergence from cardiopulmonary bypass. *Anesthesiology* 44:281, 1976.
65. Tuttle R.R.: The inotropic and chronotropic effects of dobutamine and isoproterenol on cat atria and papillary muscles at different temperatures, abstracted. *Fed. Proc.* 33:503, 1974.
66. Tuttle R.R., Mills J.: Dobutamine: Development of a new catecholamine to selectively increase cardiac contractility. *Circ. Res.* 36:185, 1975.
67. Tuttle R.R., et al.: Dobutamine: Containment of myocardial infarction size by a new inotropic agent, abstracted. *Circulation* 48 (suppl. 4):132, 1973.
68. Vasu M.A., et al.: Myocardial oxygen consumption: effects of epinephrine, isoproterenol, dopamine, norepinephrine, and dobutamine. *Am. J. Physiol.* 235:H237, 1978.
69. Weil M.H., Shubin H., Carlson R.: Treatment of circulatory shock: Use of sympathomimetic and related vasoactive agents. *J.A.M.A.* 231:1280, 1975.
70. White R.D., et al.: Plasma ionic calcium levels following injection of chloride, gluconate, and gluceptate salts of calcium. *J. Thorac. Cardiovasc. Surg.* 71:609, 1976.
71. Yeh B.K., McNay J.L., Goldberg L.I.: Attenuation of dopamine renal and mesenteric vasodilation by haloperidol: Evidence for a specific dopamine receptor. *J. Pharmacol. Exp. Ther.* 168:303, 1969.

19 / Intra-aortic Balloon Counterpulsation

SAIT TARHAN
RONALD J. FAUST

COUNTERPULSATION (the intra-aortic balloon pump is based on the same principle) was first recommended by Harken[7] in 1958. His proposal was to remove the blood via the femoral route during ventricular systole and then to reinfuse the same blood rapidly during diastole to increase coronary perfusion pressure.[1] The same action also would decrease left ventricular work while increasing coronary blood flow. However, such difficulties as excessive hemolysis, need for bilateral femoral arteriotomies, and lack of evidence of increased coronary blood flow in the hypotensive state with counterpulsation via the femoral route made the technique impractical.[1] Different methods to create the same effect were tried by other investigators.

One idea[13] was to use a single-chambered intra-aortic balloon inserted and placed in the descending thoracic aorta and providing the same benefit as would counterpulsation. The balloon was inflated in diastole, beginning with closure of the aortic valve, and deflated rapidly at the onset of ventricular systole. Inflation would displace the intra-aortic blood toward the coronary arteries, resulting in an increase of coronary pressure and flow; collapse of the balloon would decrease the impedance to left ventricular ejection and afterload. In turn, this would decrease the left ventricular work.[3] The first clinical application of single-chambered intra-aortic balloon pulsation was achieved successfully in 1968.[10] Since then, the balloon has been modified, dual- and triple-segmented versions have been introduced, its indications have expanded, and the method has become most important in the treatment of refractory left ventricular failure.

CARDIOGENIC SHOCK

The indications for intra-aortic balloon counterpulsation are changing and expanding rapidly, yet its main use is still for cardiogenic shock, whether due to acute myocardial infarction or to postcardiotomy myocardial failure. A list of indications for the procedure, from Curtis et al.[4] and used by permission, is as follows: (1) preinfarction angina; (2) complications of myocardial infarction (persistent angina, progressing infarct, and pump failure, particularly when mechanical defects such as ventricular septal defect, mitral regurgitation, and ventricular aneurysm are present); (3) aid in weaning from cardiopulmonary bypass; (4) postcardiotomy low output; and (5) miscellaneous (low-output sepsis and myocardium-suppressing drug overdose).

Cardiogenic shock secondary to acute myocardial infarction has been a discouraging entity, yet use of intra-aortic balloon pumping has provided new hope for these patients.

Cardiogenic shock is a result of loss of functioning left ventricular myocardium beyond that needed to support essential circulation. If shock is not treated early, a dangerous cycle ensues (Fig 19–1). Systemic hypotension and acidosis decrease coronary blood flow, leading to myocardial hypoxia and arrhythmias, and further impair myocardial performance, causing additional necrosis in the tissue adjacent to the initial infarction.[5] Mortality is close to 100% in spite of the use of catecholamines, diuretics, and respiratory assistance. Any therapy that increases myocardial oxygen demand without increasing oxygen supply may increase the myocardial dysfunction and necrosis.[11] However, intra-aortic balloon counterpulsation can break the vicious cycle by decreasing left ventricular work and oxygen demand.[15]

Patients with cardiogenic shock should receive intervention as soon as possible. Intra-aortic balloon counterpulsation applied within eight hours of the initiation of chest pain and shock gives the best results.[2] Changes in clinical out-

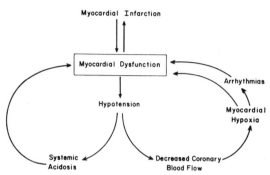

Fig 19–1.—Self-perpetuating cycles in cardiogenic shock. (From Dunkman et al.[5] Used by permission.)

look for the patient, such as clearance of obtundation, a sense of well-being, and a response to diuretics, are usually observed within one to two hours of intra-aortic balloon counterpulsation.

These patients should be treated according to a program such as supportive therapy, which should be applied at first for about one hour[1]; the program should include medications for pain, acidosis, and cardiac failure (Table 19–1). Hypoxia should be treated by providing oxygen by mask. A central venous catheter should be inserted for central venous pressure, or a Swan-Ganz catheter should be placed to monitor pulmonary capillary wedge pressure. If central venous pressure is less than 15 cm H_2O or if pulmonary capillary wedge pressure measured with a Swan-Ganz catheter is less than 18 mm Hg, the patient may need a volume infusion.[1] Inotropic agents, such as dopamine, can be used in doses of 5 to 15 μg/kg/minute. However, some recent studies have indicated that dopamine in doses sufficient to increase peripheral perfusion and arterial blood pressure in patients with cardiogenic shock after acute myocardial infarction greatly increases myocardial oxygen consumption and leads to the deterioration of myocardial metabolism. It has been concluded that dopamine is potentially harmful to acute ischemic myocardium.[14]

Inotropic agents and vasopressors act by increasing the inotropic state of the myocardium or cardiac afterload. In each of these conditions, the myocardial oxygen requirements increase when total oxygen availability and delivery is decreased. Therefore, once cardiogenic shock is diagnosed, an intra-aortic balloon should be used as early as is possible, because it decreases myocardial oxygen requirements and utilization[8] by decreasing the systolic blood pressure. This decrease reduces left ventricular work and lowers myocardial oxygen requirements. Diastolic blood pressure is also increased during counterpulsation, resulting in an increased coronary blood flow and greater oxygen availability.[8] A more favorable oxygen supply and demand improves coronary blood flow to the ischemic areas of the myocardium, and counterpulsation also may open coronary collateral vessels.[9] Another study demonstrated that the early institution of intra-aortic balloon counterpulsation decreases the size of the potential myocardial infarction after coronary occlusion.[12]

Our current policy is for patients with refractory shock after myocardial infarction to receive intra-aortic balloon counterpulsation, after which coronary arteriography or left ventriculography (or both) can be done on an emergency

TABLE 19–1.—SEQUENCE OF SUPPORTIVE THERAPY IN CARDIOGENIC SHOCK*†

Step 1	Initial treatment comprises (1) standard supportive treatment for 1 hr, (2) digitalis, and (3) volume addition (trial of dextrose-water or dextrose-water with albumin).
Step 2	Perform cardiac output studies if (1) systolic pressure is less than 80 mm Hg (or less than 100 mm Hg in formerly hypertensive patient) and (2) urinary excretion is less than 20 ml/hr.
Step 3	Administer positive inotropic agent therapy with 5 to 15 μg of dopamine per kilogram per minute while cardiac studies are being done.

Continue treatment if any two of the following result: (1) low output improves; (2) cardiac index is 2.2 L/min/sq m or more; (3) central venous pressure decreases 3 cm H_2O; (4) pulmonary capillary wedge pressure decreases 3 mm Hg; (5) systolic pressure is greater than 80 mm Hg or is 10 mm Hg above basal level; (6) urinary output is more than 20 ml/hr.

Start intra-aortic balloon pulsation if any two of the following result: (1) low output persists; (2) cardiac index is 2.0 L/min/sq m or less; (3) systolic pressure is less than 80 mm Hg (or less than 100 mm Hg in formerly hypertensive patient); and (4) urinary output is less than 20 ml/hr.

*Low cardiac output syndrome; systolic pressure less than 80 mm Hg or pressure less than 100 mm Hg in formerly hypertensive patient; urinary output less than 20 ml/hr.
†Modified from Bregman.[1]

basis. If the patient does not sustain a satisfactory response to intra-aortic balloon counterpulsation and a correctable disorder has been defined, immediate surgical intervention should be considered. Despite the high risk of surgery in this group, this aggressive therapy has resulted in improved survival rates.[4] If clinical improvement is satisfactory with intra-aortic balloon counterpulsation and the patient can be weaned from intra-aortic balloon counterpulsation, surgery can be delayed for six weeks.

POSTCARDIOTOMY CARDIOGENIC SHOCK

The rationale and methods used in the previous section can be applied in postcardiotomy myocardial failure, with the assumption that the temporary depression of left ventricular function or the myocardial injury from perioperative ischemia or infarction is reversible. Effective assistance to the myocardium may result in the ultimate recovery of the heart.

Intra-aortic balloon counterpulsation is needed most often for patients who cannot be weaned from cardiopulmonary bypass. These patients cannot maintain circulatory stability (systolic pressure greater than 60 mm Hg) when cardiopulmonary bypass is terminated, despite intensive treatment with conventional methods (vasopressors or inotropic agents). However, some patients can sustain a reasonable blood pressure with the help of vasopressor agents during the emergence from bypass; yet, despite the contin-

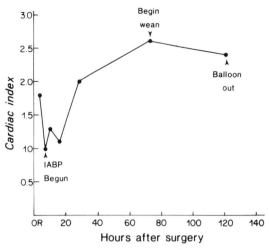

Fig 19–2.—Changes of cardiac index in patient during postoperative period and effects of intra-aortic balloon pulsation *(IABP)* on hemodynamics. (From Curtis et al.[4] Used by permission.)

ued use of these agents, the cardiac index of these patients decreases gradually during the period after bypass. They also need intra-aortic balloon counterpulsation. A cardiac index profile of a patient in need of counterpulsation is shown in Figure 19–2. In that patient, intra-aortic balloon counterpulsation was instituted six hours after operation, and the patient experienced immediate improvement in hemodynamics and did not need inotropic agents.[4]

Some patients require prolonged intra-aortic

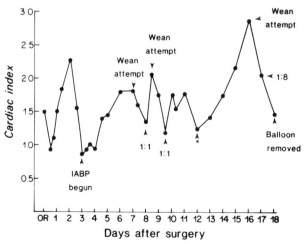

Fig 19–3.—Prolonged application of intra-aortic balloon pulsation *(IABP)* in patient during postoperative period. Cardiac output taken after episode of ventricular tachycardia terminated by cardioversion and prolonged resuscitation. (From Curtis et al.[4] Used by permission.)

balloon assist. An illustrative example of such a patient (Fig 19–3) shows that the patient's cardiac index decreased from 1.5 to 0.92 during the early postoperative hours but responded favorably to a combination of cardiotonic agents. However, the hemodynamics again deteriorated on the second postoperative day, and intra-aortic balloon pulsation was needed. Several attempts to wean the patient from circulatory assist were not successful. Finally, the balloon was removed after 15 days of assisting, and the patient survived a stormy course of hospitalization after removal of intra-aortic balloon counterpulsation.[4]

TECHNIQUE AND EQUIPMENT

Placement of Intra-aortic Balloon

The placement of the intra-aortic balloon in a patient with cardiogenic shock after cardiac surgery is relatively easy. These patients are already heparinized and maintained on cardiopulmonary bypass during the insertion of the balloon. A Dacron or Teflon graft is sutured end-to-side to the isolated common femoral artery, and the balloon is inserted into the thoracic aorta through this site (Figs 19–4,A and B).

The position of the balloon in the descending thoracic aorta can be verified by direct palpation, and the tip of the balloon catheter is placed just distal to the origin of the left subclavian artery (Fig 19–4,C). After counterpulsation is initiated, cardiopulmonary bypass is discontinued and heparin can be neutralized by the use of protamine sulfate. The incisions then are closed and the patient can be transported to the cardiac surgical intensive care unit, while receiving continuous intra-aortic balloon assistance.

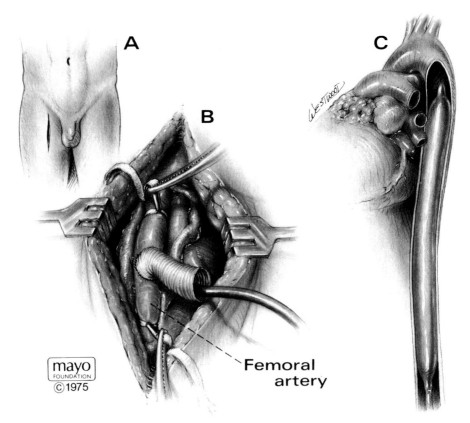

Fig 19–4.—A, location of incision to secure common femoral artery for intra-aortic balloon pulsation. **B,** suture of Dacron graft to femoral artery. **C,** placement of balloon into descending thoracic aorta.

Intra-aortic Balloon Counterpulsation in Pediatric Patients

In smaller children, intra-aortic balloon counterpulsation can be accomplished by insertion of the balloon via the ascending aorta.[4] Such a procedure is facilitated by the availability of 12- and 4-ml balloons. However, a more extensive trial of intra-aortic balloon pulsation in pediatric patients with postoperative low cardiac output or in those who cannot be weaned from cardiopulmonary bypass is needed to confirm its feasibility in these patients.[4]

Intra-aortic Balloon Counterpulsation Equipment

The Avcothane-51 balloon has good blood compatibility, which minimizes the danger of clot formation on the surface of the balloon and therefore makes intra-aortic balloon pumping possible without the need for systemic anticoagulation.[6] This feature is important for the use of intra-aortic balloon counterpulsation during the immediate postoperative period, because it permits a satisfactory hemostasis without the need for continuous systemic anticoagulation. The AVCO IABP Model 7 console (Fig 19–5,A) and, more recently, the AVCO IABP Model 10 (both developed by AVCO Corporation and manufactured for Roche Medical Electronics Division, Cranbury, NJ 08512) with internal portable power supply make the transport of the patient from the operating room to the cardiac surgical intensive care unit possible while the patient is receiving circulatory assistance.

Intra-aortic Balloon

The three-segment nonocclusive design eliminates the trapping of blood around the balloon; such trapping may strain the aortic wall and impair effective pumping. The balloon is 25.4 cm long, and the total length of the catheter is 91.4 cm (Fig 19–6). The usual sizes are 20, 30, and 40 ml (14 mm, 16 mm, and 18 mm in diameter), mounted on 12 F, 14 F, and 14 F catheters, respectively. A 12-ml balloon on a 9 F catheter and a 4.5-ml balloon on an 8 F catheter also are available.[4] Balloon size is selected on the basis of the total-body surface area and the size of the femoral artery after dissection of the artery.

AVCO Intra-aortic Balloon Pump Console

The console houses all electronic and pneumatic controls (see Fig 19–5). The balloon is in-

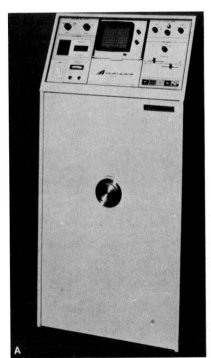

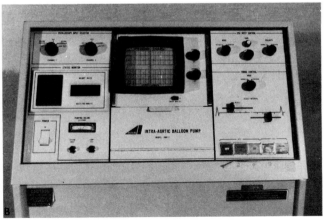

Fig 19–5.—AVCO IABP-7. **A,** console; **B,** front panel with controls.

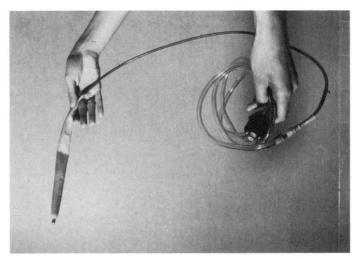

Fig 19-6.—Three-segment nonocclusive intra-aortic balloon.

flated with helium because helium is light and inert and has a low viscosity. Gas movement is rapid, and inflation and deflation require little time. Therefore, helium provides longer periods of full inflation and more efficient pumping and pumping rates. Inflation and deflation of the balloon are synchronized within the console circuitry with regard to the QRS complex.

BALLOON MANAGEMENT

Because the action of intra-aortic balloon counterpulsation is regulated with the patient's ECG, good-quality tracings are necessary.

R Wave

The largest positive spike of the ECG is sensed by the console and is interpreted as an R wave, which then synchronizes the balloon motion accordingly. To trigger the motion, the positive spike (R wave) has to be between 0.5 and 1.5 V on the ECG oscilloscope, which is located on the console's front panel (see Fig 19-5,B). This voltage can be calculated by adding the positive spike to the downstroke below the isoelectric baseline (total QR upstroke, Fig 19-7). Therefore, the amplitude of the R wave should be made maximal, and all other waves and artifacts should be reduced. Also any interference should be eliminated.

The ECG lead that shows the highest R wave can be used for this purpose. If necessary, the electrodes can be duplicated to provide the dedicated lead for the intra-aortic balloon pulsation.

If the lead amplitude is inadequate, either the sensitivity on the monitor can be increased or different leads with high enough amplitude can be selected.

Other Waves and Artifacts

If the other segments of the ECG show an increase of their voltage, such as T wave, ST upstroke, or atrial pacing, the console will sense it and trigger the motion (Fig 19-8). Adequate voltage of both the R wave and the other ECG segments would be sensed and would trigger intra-aortic balloon counterpulsation (double-triggering). However, if one of the other segments (other than the R wave) of the ECG has a high enough voltage, the motion would be triggered and pronounced asynergy would be produced between the cardiac and the balloon action. In turn, this would reduce the efficiency of pumping. For example, a T wave of more than 1.5 V with an R wave of less than 1.5 V would cause only the T wave to be sensed.[6]

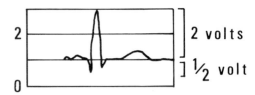

Fig 19-7.—Calculation of voltage of positive spike. (From Ford and Weintraub.[6] Used by permission.)

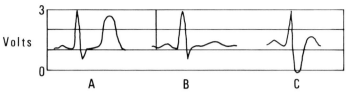

Fig 19–8.—Other ECG waves and artifacts may trigger intra-aortic balloon pulsation. Each one of these tracings can cause double-triggering. *A*, hyperacute T wave. *B*, atrial pace spike. *C*, pronounced ST upstroke.

Pacing Spike and Double-Triggering

Because of its proximity to the R wave, a ventricular pacing spike does not significantly disrupt timing.[6] However, an atrial pacing spike can be a problem. Yet, such a spike can be reduced by reversing the polarity of the spike either by changing the connections or by adjusting the voltage of the pacemaker. Other moves, such as reducing the gain control on the balloon console, switching to another lead, or repositioning the electrodes, also can help. If interference persists in spite of these measures, a second generator can be used transiently to trigger the balloon.[6]

Interference From Other Waves on the ECG

Interference from other waves can be reduced by changing to a different lead or by reversing the polarity of the cardiogram on the console. The upstroke of the R wave and the ST segment would be sensed and would cause double-triggering (Fig 19–9,A). However, only one upstroke would remain and be sensed by the console if a different lead is used or polarity is reversed[6] (Fig 19–9,B).

If the slope of a wave is too gradual, it may not be sensed by the console even if the voltage of the wave is adequate (Fig 19–10).

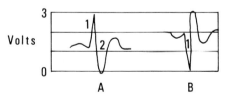

Fig 19–9.—*A*, upstroke of R wave *(1)* and deep ST segment *(2)* would be sensed and would trigger intra-aortic balloon pulsation motion. *B*, reverse polarity would provide only one upstroke.

Balloon Timing

The correct synchronization of the cardiac action with the balloon action is one of the most important parts in the timing adjustments, which can be accomplished by inflation and deflation markers. Before the insertion of the balloon, the ECG can be used as a timing guide. A positive inflation marker is superimposed on the T wave. A negative deflation marker is positioned within the PR interval; yet once the balloon is inserted and operational, the timing adjustments can be made with an arterial trace.[6]

Timing Landmarks

A dicrotic notch represents aortic valve closure. The balloon should inflate immediately after closure of the valve (Fig 19–11). If the timing is taken from peripheral arterial traces, the waveform is delayed and aortic valve closure occurs centrally, before it shows itself as a dicrotic notch on the peripheral arterial tracing. Also, the retrograde transmission of the balloon pressure pulse to the aortic root is delayed.[6]

Adjustment of the Inflation Marker

The inflation marker can be moved to the right, which would indicate that the curve of the diastolic augmentation of the balloon (Fig 19–12, No. 4) is moving to the right, away from the patient's own systolic curve; the two curves become completely separated and a dicrotic notch becomes visible between them.

If the inflation marker is moved to the left, the dicrotic notch will disappear (Fig 19–13, No. 2) and the area of the notch will take the shape of the U wave configuration.[6] This change would signify that the augmentation curve is exactly at the level of the dicrotic notch. If the curve is taken from the radial trace, the inflation time for the balloon would occur 50 ms before

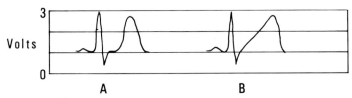

Fig 19–10.—*A,* balloon and console would sense both R wave and T wave, and double-triggering would ensue. *B,* T wave would not be sensed because of its gradual slope.

the notch (delay of the appearance of the notch in the peripheral arterial trace). If it continues to move leftward, the notch area will assume a sharp V wave, indicating that the balloon inflation has reached a proper point. As the timing improves, the peak (Fig 19–14, No. 4) also will increase.

Adjustment of the Deflation Marker

First, the timing landmarks, such as systolic peak and diastolic low (see Fig 19–11, No. 1 and 3), are determined with the balloon off. Then the balloon is turned on at the 1:2 setting. This permits comparison of the systolic and diastolic levels while the balloon is on and off[6] (Fig 19–15). The deflation marker then is moved more slowly to the right, which would decrease the depth of the end-diastolic dip after balloon augmentation (Fig 19–16, No. 6). The marker is moved to the right until the end-diastolic dip is equal to or 10 to 15 mm below the level of the patient's diastolic pressure without assistance (Fig 19–16, No. 6 and 3). The height of the systolic peak (the one after the balloon augmentation) (see Fig 19–15, No. 5) declines relative to the systolic peak, unaffected by the preceding balloon action (see Fig 19–15, No. 1). Once the adjustment of the deflation marker accomplishes the above waveforms, no more changes are necessary. The maximal reduction of the height of the systolic peak (see Fig 19–15, No. 5) demonstrates the unloading effect of the balloon.[6]

Weaning From Intra-aortic Balloon Counterpulsation

After hemodynamic variables are stabilized and the inotropic agent requirements are decreased, an attempt at reducing the circulatory assist can be made. The ratio of the number of balloon inflations to the number of the patient's heartbeats can be reduced from 1:1 to 1:2, then to 1:4, and finally to 1:8. This reduction can be accomplished by switching the indicator to the selected ratio by turning the knob under the scope on the front panel of the console. While the ratio is being reduced, the patient should be under constant care for signs of deterioration, such as low blood pressure, increasing pulmonary capillary wedge and left atrial pressures, diminished urinary output, clouding of the sensorium, ST-segment changes on the ECG, angina, or changes in heart rate and rhythm. If these signs appear, circulatory assist should continue until a new trial at weaning is attempted.

When the patient can maintain an adequate blood pressure for 12 hours at an assist ratio of 1:8, then the balloon can be removed using local anesthesia. The range of success of weaning the patient from cardiopulmonary bypass with intra-aortic balloon counterpulsation varies among institutions from 22% to 85%, with an average of 58%.[1] Therefore, its value in clinical situations is apparent. Also important is that, if the patient

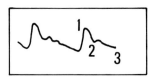

Fig 19–11.—Arterial pressure trace (balloon off). Dicrotic notch *(2)* represents aortic valve closure. Note systolic peak (without balloon effect) *(1)* and diastolic low *(3).*

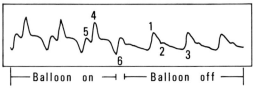

Fig 19–12.—Arterial pressure tracing (balloon on 1:1 and balloon off). Note diastolic peak *(4)* balloon augmentation and systolic peak *(1),* dicrotic notch *(2),* diastolic low *(3),* diastolic peak *(4),* systolic peak *(5),* and end-diastolic dip *(6).*

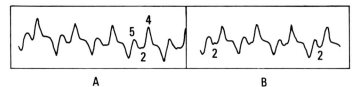

Fig 19-13.—*A*, exposure of dicrotic notch with movement of inflation marker to right on front panel of console. *B*, disappearance of dicrotic notch with movement of inflation marker to left. Note dicrotic notch *(2)*, diastolic peak *(4)*, and systolic peak *(5)*.

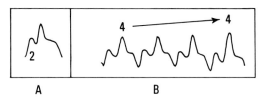

Fig 19-14.—*A*, note V wave configuration *(2)*. *B*, rise of peak *(4)*.

is successfully weaned from cardiopulmonary bypass with the aid of intra-aortic balloon counterpulsation, a large percentage will be hospital survivors (59% of the patients in three studies).[4]

COMPLICATIONS OF INTRA-AORTIC BALLOON COUNTERPULSATION

Complications involve variable vascular insufficiency in the catheterized limb after removal of the balloon, dissection of the aorta by the balloon catheter during its introduction, findings of small emboli at autopsy, and a moderate reduction in the platelet count during pumping.[5] One study noted a decrease of 50% in platelet count during the first 60 hours of pumping, compared with the level before intra-aortic balloon counterpulsation.[5] Serum hemoglobin levels also were elevated modestly (average, 23 mg/dl), but renal damage did not occur with this degree of hemoglobinemia.[5] In a study of 34 patients at our institution,[4] nine were found to have complications: four had arterial insufficiency that did not require surgery and one each had arterial insufficiency of the extremity that hosted the catheter (necessitating amputation at the knee), embolus to the opposite extremity, deep vein thrombosis, groin infection, and groin hematoma. These patients were treated expectantly with removal of the balloon electively after hemodynamic stability had been obtained.

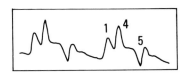

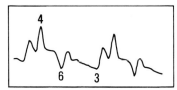

Fig 19-15 (top).—Systole without preceding balloon effect *(1)*, systole *(5)* affected by preceding balloon action *(4)*.

Fig 19-16 (bottom).—Diastole without preceding balloon effect *(3)*. Diastole *(6)* affected by preceding balloon action *(4)*.

REFERENCES

1. Bregman D.: Dual-chambered intra-aortic balloon counterpulsation, in Ionescu M.I., Wooler G.H. (eds.): *Current Techniques in Extracorporeal Circulation.* London, Butterworth & Co., 1976, p. 408.
2. Buckley M.J., et al.: Hemodynamic evaluation of intra-aortic balloon pumping in man. *Circulation* 41 (suppl. 2):130, 1970.
3. Corday E., et al.: Physiologic principles in the application of circulatory assist for the failing heart: Intraaortic balloon circulatory assist and venoarterial phased partial bypass. *Am. J. Cardiol.* 26:595, 1970.
4. Curtis J.J., et al.: Intra-aortic balloon assist: Initial Mayo Clinic experience and current concepts. *Mayo Clin. Proc.* 52:723, 1977.
5. Dunkman W.B., et al.: Clinical and hemodynamic results of intraaortic balloon pumping and surgery for cardiogenic shock. *Circulation* 46:465, 1972.
6. Ford P.J., Weintraub R.M.: *Intra-aortic Balloon Pumping Manual,* ed. 2. Boston, Beth Israel Hospital, 1975.
7. Harken D.E.: Cited by Bregman.[1]
8. Housman L.B., et al.: Counterpulsation for intraoperative cardiogenic shock: Successful use

of intra-aortic balloon. *J.A.M.A.* 224:1131, 1973.
9. Jacobey J.A., et al.: A new therapeutic approach to acute coronary occlusion: II. Opening dormant coronary collateral channels by counterpulsation. *Am. J. Cardiol.* 11:218, 1963.
10. Kantrowitz A., et al.: Initial clinical experience with intraaortic balloon pumping in cardiogenic shock. *J.A.M.A.* 203:113, 1968.
11. Maroko P.R., et al.: Factors influencing infarct size following experimental coronary artery occlusions. *Circulation* 43:67, 1971.
12. Maroko P.R., et al.: Effects of intraaortic balloon counterpulsation on the severity of myocardial ischemic injury following acute coronary occlusion: Counterpulsation and myocardial injury. *Circulation* 45:1150, 1972.
13. Moulopoulos S.D., Topaz S.R., Kolff W.J.: Extracorporeal assistance to the circulation and intraaortic balloon pumping. *Trans. Am. Soc. Artif. Intern. Organs* 8:85, 1962.
14. Mueller H.S., Evans R., Ayres S.M.: Effect of dopamine on hemodynamics and myocardial metabolism in shock following acute myocardial infarction in man. *Circulation* 57:361, 1978.
15. Soroff H.S., et al.: Assisted circulation: II. Effects of counterpulsation on left ventricular oxygen consumption and hemodynamics. *Circulation* 27:722, 1963.

20 / Blood and Cardiovascular Anesthesia

RONALD J. FAUST
ROY F. CUCCHIARA
JOSEPH M. MESSICK, JR.

IN ANESTHESIA for cardiac surgery, far more blood than halothane or any other drug will be used. The proper use of blood and blood components is necessary for the success of most cardiac surgical procedures, and the misuse of blood can produce a disastrous outcome in almost any procedure. Thus, most practicing anesthesiologists should have a thorough understanding of the clinical use of blood products and certain aspects of hematology.

HEMATOLOGY OF THE RED BLOOD CELL

The nonnucleated red blood cell (RBC) circulates in the body continually for four months while maintaining its function, size, plasticity, and shape.

In adults, RBCs are normally produced in the marrow of the vertebrae, ribs, sternum, pelvis, scapulae, skull, and proximal humerus and femur. In the fetus and in certain disease states, they are produced in many other sites, most importantly the liver, spleen, and lymph nodes. Certain primitive stem cells can differentiate into various types of cells found in the circulation (erythrocytes, neutrophils, monocytes, eosinophils, lymphocytes, and platelets), and differentiation of these stem cells is controlled by erythropoietin, a hormone secreted primarily by the kidney. The production of this hormone is affected by hypoxemia, anemia, and many stimuli. In the marrow, the hormone is believed to activate certain genes that are essential to synthesis of hemoglobin, in addition to causing proliferation of the RBC precursors. The maturation of the RBC involves a progression through the stages of proerythroblast, normoblast, and reticulocyte as the cell nucleus disappears and the hemoglobin content increases. Maturation of the RBC in the marrow takes only three to seven days, and under normal conditions, a reticulocyte will remain in the marrow two to three days more before it is released into the circulation.

The life span of the erythrocyte, as measured by many techniques, is approximately 120 days. After loss of its nucleus, mitochondria, and ribosomes, the RBC can no longer synthesize proteins. Hence, the activity of some of its enzymes is gradually lost, and it eventually becomes nonviable and is destroyed in the reticuloendothelial system. Also called the "mononuclear phagocyte system," the reticuloendothelial system includes tissues in the spleen, liver, kidney, lymph nodes, and bone marrow. Most (80% to 90%) of RBC destruction occurs extravascularly in the spleen and liver, though the exact mechanism of destruction is not clearly understood. The small amounts of plasma hemoglobin released by intravascular destruction are normally bound to plasma haptoglobin and thus are carried to the liver. Free hemoglobin not bound to haptoglobin is oxidized in the plasma to methemoglobin, which dissociates into heme and globin. Iron is released from the heme portion, and its porphyrin ring is broken to produce biliverdin and then bilirubin. The bilirubin is conjugated by the hepatic cells into bilirubin diglucuronide, a more soluble form, which is then excreted in the bile. The life cycle of the RBC and its hemoglobin content are illustrated in Figure 20–1.

IMMUNOHEMATOLOGY

Blood Antigen Groups

At many sites on the surface of the lipoprotein membrane of the RBC, chemical structures

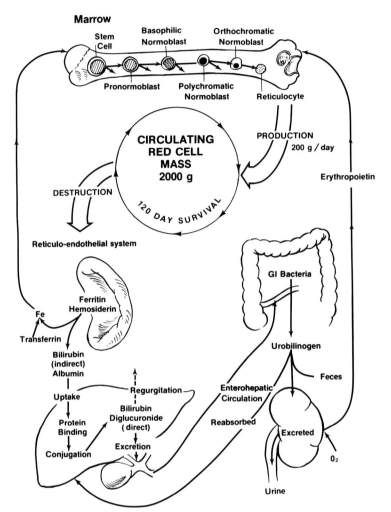

Fig 20–1.—Formation of RBCs in marrow and their destruction in reticuloendothelial system are diagrammed. Subsequent hemoglobin metabolism is also portrayed.

called "antigens" are present. These antigens are genetically determined and capable of eliciting an immune response when introduced into the tissues of another animal. Antigens are grouped according to genetic inheritance patterns. Most are proteins or protein-carbohydrate molecules. The antigens of the ABO groups chemically are short chains of identical sugar molecules on a lipid or protein backbone, with only the terminal sugar differing to dictate the A or B antigenicity. A and B antigens are found in many body tissues and are even present in certain body fluids. They are also found elsewhere in nature in animals, plants, and bacteria. This factor is believed to be the reason why people who do not have either the A or the B antigen form anti-A and anti-B antibodies early in life, these being called "natural" antibodies. Thus, people who have neither A nor B antigens (group O) form anti-A and anti-B antibodies. People who have only A antigens (group A) form anti-B antibodies, and people who have only B antigens form anti-A antibodies (Table 20–1).[30]

Less is known about the chemical structure of the hundreds of other RBC antigens that have been discovered. These antigens are demonstrated serologically after patients are found who have developed an antibody to the antigen in question. For all but the ABO system, antibody formation occurs only after sensitization of the

TABLE 20–1.—ABO BLOOD GROUPS

GROUP	RBC ANTIGENS	SERUM ANTIBODIES	FREQUENCY, % WHITE	FREQUENCY, % BLACK
O	None	Anti-A Anti-B	44	49
A	A	Anti-B	45	27
B	B	Anti-A	8	20
AB	A and B	None	3	4

host by blood that is antigenically different from his own, usually through a transfusion or transplacental hemorrhage during pregnancy. Because over 379 antigens have already been identified,[36] more than a million different combinations of these antigens are possible. For this reason, homologous blood can never be perfectly matched to the recipient and there is always the danger of antibody formation by the host after recognition of foreign antigens. This is the most important reason for the use of autologous transfusion, though both safety from hepatitis and other advantages are also secured.

Antibody Formation

Antibodies themselves are protein substances elaborated by a host in recognition of a foreign antigenic stimulus. Antibodies are produced in the reticuloendothelial system by plasma cells descended from lymphocytes. T-lymphocytes and B-lymphocytes are differentiated by the latter's villous surface on electron microscopy and by the latter's function in the production of humoral immunity. T-lymphocytes (thymus-dependent) are involved in the production of cellular immunity. Five classes of immunoglobulins are differentiated on the basis of molecular structure: IgM, IgG, IgA, IgE, and IgD. The basic immunoglobulin molecule is composed of two light chains and two heavy chains (Fig 20–2). There are two types of light chains (κ and λ) for each class of immunoglobulin. The heavy chains differ for each class of immunoglobulin and are designated γ, α, μ, δ, and ϵ. IgM molecules are usually composed of pentamers of five of the four-chain polypeptide units. The antibodies made in response to foreign RBC antigens fall into the IgM and IgG classes. The IgM molecules are the first to be produced in a primary immune response. The IgG molecules are the most important class of immunoglobulins from the standpoint of concentration. They constitute the body's secondary antibody response and are also the one immunoglobulin class that can cross the placenta.

Antibody Detection

Only with certain RBC antibodies will any visible change occur after the antigen-antibody reaction has taken place. With these, clumping or agglutination of the RBCs will be visible after they have been incubated in vitro with antibody-containing serum. In certain cases, this agglutination can be brought out by albumin in the solution. More often, the blood banker must augment the reaction by adding an antibody to human globulin (Coombs serum) to the antibody-coated RBCs to cause visible agglutination. Another technique commonly employed by the blood banker is to use enzymes to cleave off parts of the RBC membrane so that antigen sites are more vulnerable to antibody binding. The blood banker uses these techniques to iden-

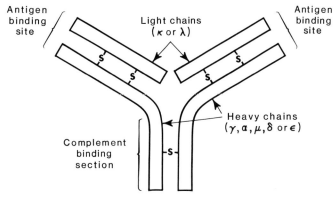

Fig 20–2.—Schematic diagram of immunoglobulin polypeptide molecule.

tify any unnatural RBC antibodies present in a recipient or a donor. In performing the antibody screen, a patient's or donor's serum is tested against RBCs known to contain all the common antigens. If a reaction is detected against a screening cell, the antibody is identified by testing the serum in question against a larger panel of antigenically typed RBCs. After the reaction pattern is demonstrated, the antibody causing it is elucidated by referring to antigens known to be present on the cells used. In the example shown in Table 20–2, when antibody screening is done with the two-cell panel, cell II reacts after incubation and the addition of Coombs serum or in papain-pretreated cells. The ten-cell panel is then set up with the serum in question. Agglutination in cells 3, 4, and 7 corresponds to the known presence of the Kell antigen on those cells alone; hence, the patient's serum antibody is identified as anti-Kell.

The time required to perform these tests is sometimes of crucial importance to the clinician faced with a hemorrhagic emergency. Usually being IgM antibodies, anti-A and anti-B react well at room temperature in saline, and the ABO grouping of a person's blood usually can be determined in as short a time as five minutes after the blood bank technologist receives the specimen. As soon as the blood type is known, "type-specific" blood (meaning that it is of the same ABO and Rh group as the patient's) can be used if the patient must be transfused on an emergency basis. While this situation is more advantageous than using O Rh-negative (universal donor) blood, it still presents substantial risks to the patient in that he might have an unknown antibody that could lead to a life-threatening hemolytic transfusion reaction. Only rarely will a patient with an antibody be able to give a history of having a known antibody or be able to identify its type, though this could be life-saving information in an emergency. Although most blood banks will release blood in an emergency situation after only "immediate" or "first-phase" testing is complete, the clinician should never forget that this blood's compatibility is still essentially only on an ABO basis. Its use before the antibody screen is complete is possible in a life-threatening situation, but such a transfusion still carries significant risk.

To rule out unnatural antibodies, the antibody screen must be performed by the blood bank. Because of the incubation times necessary to allow weaker antibodies to react, the antibody screen cannot be completed in less than 45 minutes. Before this time, the safety of any blood administered is unpredictable. If an antibody screen is positive, more time will be required to accurately identify which antibody is present. In most blood banks, the incidence of unnatural antibodies in the general patient population is 1% to 4%.[13]

At the same time that the antibody screen is being started, the crossmatch also can be

TABLE 20–2.—IDENTIFICATION OF ANTIBODIES THROUGH USE OF ANTIBODY SCREEN AND PANEL*

	SALINE			ALBUMIN			PAPAIN-PRETREATMENT	
	IMMEDIATE SPIN	30 MIN AT 20 C	30 MIN AT 4 C	IMMEDIATE SPIN	30 MIN AT 37 C	COOMBS	30 MIN AT 37 C	COOMBS
Screening cells								
I	−	−	−	−	−	−	−	−
II	−	−	−	−	−	+	+	+
Panel cells								
1	−	−	−	−	−	−	−	−
2	−	−	−	−	−	−	−	−
3	−	−	−	−	−	+	+	+
4	−	−	−	−	−	+	+	+
5	−	−	−	−	−	−	−	−
6	−	−	−	−	−	−	−	−
7	−	−	−	−	−	+	+	+
8	−	−	−	−	−	−	−	−
9	−	−	−	−	−	−	−	−
10	−	−	−	−	−	−	−	−

*See text for explanation.

started. Recipient serum is added to donor cells. As in the antibody screen, the reaction is tested with and without albumin, in cold (5 C) and warm (37 C) temperatures, and before and after incubation. Like the antibody screen, the whole crossmatching procedure takes approximately 45 minutes to complete after the blood bank receives the recipient's sample. Most blood banks no longer perform a "reverse crossmatch" (donor serum and recipient cells) because any donors with unnatural antibodies are identified by antibody screens performed on donor serum just after the blood is donated.

The delay in obtaining "safe" blood in an emergency situation can be shortened if the patient's blood has been screened for antibodies in advance of the request for crossmatch, because the sensitivity of the antibody screen is greater than that of the crossmatch. Only in extremely rare circumstances will a crossmatch detect an incompatibility when the antibody screen is negative. One situation in which this might be possible would be in a patient who had an antibody to a rare antigen present at a very low frequency in the population and not present on either RBC used for the antibody screen. The sensitivity of the antibody screen and logistic and economic reasons have led some blood banks away from the traditional type-crossmatch-hold procedure to a "type and screen" system for the ordering of blood.[13, 35, 65] Instead of grouping, screening, and crossmatching for all blood requests, only the ABO grouping and antibody screen are performed in advance. Adequate volumes of group- and Rh-specific blood are then stocked, but the crossmatch is not performed until the decision is made to transfuse. The advantages are that a large number of units of blood are not held for patients unlikely to use them, and the blood bank does not have to spend large amounts of time doing crossmatches on units that are not subsequently transfused.

HEMOLYTIC TRANSFUSION REACTIONS

Antigen-Antibody Reaction In Vivo

The antigen-antibody reaction differs in vivo in that there is no agglutination of RBCs, as in the laboratory test tube. Acute or delayed hemolysis is possible, however, with far-reaching consequences to multiple organ systems in the body.

When an antibody binds to an antigen receptor site on the surface of an RBC, a change takes place in the heavy-chain region of the antibody molecule[49, 70] (see Fig 20–2). Two events can then happen: the antibody-coated RBC can be phagocytized by macrophages in the reticuloendothelial system (extravascular hemolysis) or it can be destroyed by the interaction of the complement system (intravascular hemolysis). In most hemolytic reactions, some RBCs probably are destroyed by both mechanisms, so that categorization of reactions into intravascular and extravascular types is no longer valid. However, only certain antigen-antibody reactions bind complement. These can involve IgG or IgM molecules. One IgM molecule attached to its antigen can bind complement, but at least two IgG molecules must be bound to an RBC's surface to bind complement. Moreover, they must be 250 to 400 Å apart for C1, the first component of the complement system, to be bound.[70]

Complement

Complement is a complex system of serum proteins that work in a sequential "cascade" fashion to mediate many of the body's immune and allergic reactions. In addition to being heat-labile, the complement system differs from the antigen-antibody system in that it is not increased by immunologic stimulation. The relationship of antigen, antibodies, complement, and immune reactions has been aptly likened to an automobile's key, ignition lock, and engine.[49] A specific key (the antibody) reacts with its lock (the antigen) to start a less specific but more complex component, the engine (complement), which actually does the work.

The C1 component has three parts, C1q, C1r, and C1s, bound together by a calcium ion. After C1q recognizes and is bound to IgM or IgG, C1 is activated and cleaves multiple C4 molecules, some of which attach to the membrane of the RBC. C2 then attaches to C4 in the presence of magnesium, and the complex cleaves C3 into C3a (an anaphylotoxin) and C3b, which attaches to the RBC membrane. C3b and its attached RBC then either bind to a macrophage through the "adherence" site of C3b, or C3b acts on C5. C5 also splits into two parts. C5a is another humoral anaphylotoxin. C5b attaches to the RBC membrane and alters it so that, for the first time in this sequence of reactions, a morphologic defect can be seen with electron microscopy. C6,

C7, and C9 are then fixed, irreversibly damaging the membrane and leading to its hemolysis. All this action is referred to as the classic pathway of complement activation. In some of its nonhemolytic functions, activation of complement is possible by an alternative pathway not involving antibody.

Two theories attempt to explain the mechanism by which the complement lesion actually produces hemolysis. The "detergent mechanism" proposes that a weakened area or "leaky patch" is formed in the cell wall, owing to disorganization of the lipid bilayer. The "doughnut hypothesis" proposes that the five late-acting components of complement (C5b, C6, C7, C8, and C9) assemble themselves into a "doughnut" that extends through the RBC membrane and forms a pore through which ions easily pass. These pores are visible on electron micrographs. Through either mechanism, the membrane of the RBC is made permeable to ions that pass in until the RBC ruptures and hemolysis is complete.

Pathophysiology of the Hemolytic Transfusion Reaction

The essence of the pathophysiology of the hemolytic transfusion reaction lies in two effects of hemolysis: (1) production of hemodynamic alterations leading to renal vascular ischemia and (2) activation of the coagulation system, with subsequent production of disseminated intravascular coagulation.

Many older theories on the pathogenesis of renal failure after hemolytic transfusion reaction have been disproved. Most commonly it was held in the past that hemoglobin released from hemolyzed RBCs precipitated in the renal tubules, producing hemoglobin casts and subsequent obstruction. Some studies, however, have shown that hemoglobin casts are a late finding in hemoglobinuric renal failure, and thus probably the casts are an effect and not a cause of the renal failure.[46] Other studies have postulated a direct toxic effect of hemoglobin on the renal tubular cells, but it is now known that stroma-free hemoglobin solutions can be transfused safely, and these solutions are being investigated as a substitute for RBC transfusions.[62] Schmidt and Holland[67] also have shown that hemoglobin-free incompatible RBC stroma can produce acute renal failure in humans,[67] while compatible RBC stroma is sequestered by the reticuloendothelial system and is not toxic.[71]

The antigen-antibody reaction after an incompatible transfusion is believed to lead to renal vascular ischemia through multiple mechanisms (Fig 20–3). The antigen-antibody complex activates Hageman factor (factor XII), which in turn activates kallikreinogen to lead ultimately to the production of bradykinin,[59a] which itself is a renal vasodilator. The antigen-antibody complex also activates the complement system, which produces several vasoactive anaphylotoxins that lead to the release of histamine; histamine itself is a renal vasoconstrictor. The sympathetic nervous system, through involvement with the adrenal medulla and a direct action on the kidneys, decreases renal blood flow. The renal effects of all these vasoactive mediators is compounded by disseminated intravascular coagulation brought about by activation of the clotting system initiated by the antigen-antibody reaction. The severity of the renal vascular ischemia produced can determine the severity of the lesion produced. Most often transient ischemia will cause a functional renal failure. Acute tubular necrosis and renal cortical necrosis can be seen when the stasis and vascular thrombosis are more severe.

Clinical Presentation

Fever is the most common clinical manifestation of the hemolytic transfusion reaction. Chills, chest pain, lumbar pain, hypotension, nausea, facial flushing, and dyspnea also are commonly seen.[60] Facial flushing and a feeling of heat along the course of the vein into which the blood is running also have been described.[54] In the anesthetized patient, most symptoms will be masked and an inappropriate tachycardia and hypotension might be the only early signs. Hemoglobinuria and generalized oozing are seen later and might be the first noted signs of a hemolytic transfusion reaction in the anesthetized patient.

The hemolytic transfusion reaction is more frequent in women because of the possibility of sensitization during pregnancy and is also more frequent in older patients because of the increased likelihood of a previous transfusion. Large series report the mortality after hemolytic transfusion reactions to range between 17% and 50%.[5, 22, 60] The incidence of hemolytic transfusion reactions has decreased to one in every

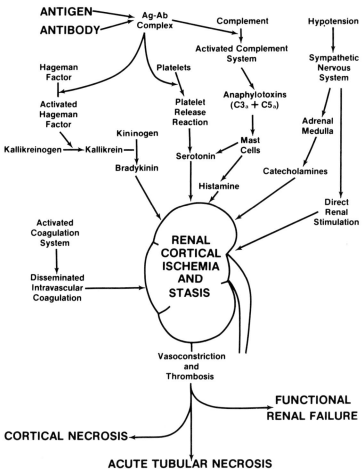

Fig 20-3.—Mechanisms of renal pathophysiology in hemolytic transfusion reactions. Schematic diagram of vasomotor alterations leading to acute renal failure after hemolytic transfusion reaction. (Data from Goldfinger.[28])

6,232 transfusions in a relatively recent series from the Mayo Clinic.[60] The hemolytic transfusion reaction remains a most dreaded clinical problem, however, because it could happen in almost any transfusion and is often preventable.

Treatment of the Hemolytic Transfusion Reaction

Therapy for the hemolytic transfusion reaction has long centered on treating the kidneys. Diuretic therapy was used early because it was believed that blockage of tubules by hemoglobin casts was the main mechanism of the renal failure.[22] Because its onset of action is so quick and the diuresis it produces is so dramatic, mannitol was a logical choice as the diuretic to be used after a hemolytic transfusion reaction had been diagnosed. The first recommendation of its use was based on only a single case, however.[7] The effect of mannitol on the kidneys is passive and purely osmotic, and evidence in the literature has shown that it does not increase renal blood flow after the hemolytic transfusion reaction[2] and it does not provide renal protection during other forms of renal ischemia.[8] Goldfinger[28] suggested that furosemide or ethacrynic acid would provide a more logical pharmacologic protection for the kidneys in a hemolytic transfusion reaction. These newer diuretics are potent and share the same mechanism of action on the kidney, although they are structurally unrelated. Their main site of action is believed to be the ascending limb of the loop of Henle, where they block the active reabsorption of chloride and increase the renal sodium, chloride, and potassium excretion, as well as the water excretion.[44] More important to this discussion, both drugs redistribute the renal blood flow to the outer cortical areas of the kidneys and increase total renal blood flow, with a decreased renal vascular resistance.[44]

The first step in the treatment for a hemolytic transfusion reaction is to stop the transfusion. The larger the amount of incompatible blood that has entered the recipient's circulation, the greater the dose of hemolyzed RBCs produced. Thus, the severity of the reaction is expected to be greater after greater volumes of incompatible blood have been administered, and the hemolytic transfusion reaction is believed to be a dose-related phenomenon.

Adequate hydration is necessary in any patient undergoing a hemolytic transfusion reaction. Hydration protects renal function and has been shown to have protective effects in other types of ischemic problems. As long as renal function is preserved and the cardiovascular system is not overloaded, crystalloid solutions can be pushed to keep the urinary flow greater than 1.5 ml/kg/hour.

Alkalinization of the urine is no longer a recommended part of the therapy in a hemolytic transfusion reaction. It was previously believed that increasing the pH of the urine prevented the formation of hemoglobin casts in the kidneys. Because the hemoglobin casts are only an effect and not a cause of the renal dysfunction seen after the hemolytic transfusion reaction, this therapy is no longer indicated. Steroids are also mentioned by some authors as part of the therapy of a hemolytic transfusion reaction.[74] There is no evidence, however, that they actually produce any beneficial effect.

Disseminated Intravascular Coagulation

Hemolytic transfusion reactions are known to activate the clotting system through several mechanisms.[28] The antigen-antibody complex activates Hageman factor (factor XII), the first factor on the intrinsic side of the clotting cascade (Fig 20-4). The antigen-antibody complex also activates platelets directly, as does the complement sequence. A phospholipid is released from the RBCs themselves, and this action also contributes to the generation of fibrin. The activation of the Hageman factor by the antigen-antibody complex is considered to be the primary means by which the coagulation system is activated, however. All of these pathways lead to disseminated intravascular coagulation in a large percentage of cases of hemolytic transfusion reaction. Thus, disseminated intravascular coagulation is the cause of the bleeding problem seen after hemolytic transfusion reactions and is also an important mechanism in the production of renal failure in these patients.

The process most commonly called "disseminated intravascular coagulation" is also referred to as "consumption coagulopathy," "defibrination syndrome," or "intravascular coagulation with fibrinolysis."[14, 51] Proponents of the last-mentioned term point out that it emphasizes the balance between coagulation and fibrinolysis, that the disease can be localized instead of disseminated, and that the coagulation process is not even always intravascular. Such disagreement about the semantics of the disease parallels the problems of understanding the etiology of the process and its laboratory diagnosis.

Seen in patients with multiple types of diseases, three processes are believed to initiate intravascular coagulation with fibrinolysis.[19] First, RBC and platelet injury can cause the release of phospholipids, which act as procoagulants and trigger the conversion of prothrombin to thrombin. Second, tissue injury can lead to intravascular coagulation with fibrinolysis through release of tissue thromboplastin (factor III), which activates the extrinsic clotting system. Third, injury to the endothelial cells of the circulatory system activates Hageman factor (factor XII) and thereby the intrinsic clotting system and other pathways, leading to increased clotting and fibrinolysis.

A long list of disease entities can lead to intravascular coagulation with fibrinolysis through one or more of these mechanisms. In addition to those instances after hemolytic transfusion reactions, the problem can be a complication of trauma, shock, septicemia, abruptio placenta, amniotic fluid embolism, cesarean section, various infections, surgery of multiple types, extracorporeal circulation, heat stroke, many types of malignancies, liver disease, and vascular aneurysms. Intravascular coagulation with fibrinolysis can be acute or chronic. Its essence is an abnormal hyperactivity of the clotting system combined with increased fibrinolysis. Excessive

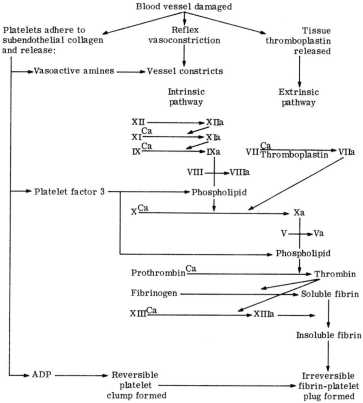

Fig 20-4.—Schematic outline of body's hemostatic mechanisms. In addition to coagulation mechanism, the importance of platelets and vasoconstriction is portrayed. (Modified from Owen et al.[59])

amounts of thrombin and plasmin are present in the circulation. Multiple organs can be affected, but the deposition of fibrin is often hard to detect. Bleeding is the most common manifestation, and renal, hepatic, and pulmonary dysfunction also are seen often.[72]

In the acute forms of intravascular coagulation with fibrinolysis, platelets and multiple clotting factors are depleted by the increased clotting activity. This condition leads to widespread clinical bleeding, which is usually the first sign of the syndrome's presence. In chronic forms of intravascular coagulation with fibrinolysis, however, increased liver and marrow production may cause clotting factor levels to be normal or even increased, complicating diagnostic problems.[58]

The diagnosis of the syndrome of intravascular coagulation with fibrinolysis is difficult because no one test is diagnostic or specific, and in some patients the diagnosis must be made by inference. The diagnosis is suspected, however, in a bleeding patient with an elevated prothrombin time, a low platelet count, and a low fibrinogen level. The increased fibrinolysis that is essential to the disease leads to the presence in the circulation of many fibrin fragments, also called "fibrin degradation products" or "fibrin split products." Although a measurement of increased levels of these fibrin split products helps to confirm a diagnosis of intravascular coagulation with fibrinolysis, other conditions correlate with elevated levels of fibrin split products, namely, peripheral venous thrombosis, pulmonary embolism, and even uncomplicated surgical procedures.[23, 58] The use of heparin during cardiopulmonary bypass can make the diagnosis of intravascular coagulation and fibrinolysis more difficult by its interference with some coagulation tests.

There are two ways of treating disseminated intravascular coagulation. The first and most important is to remove the cause itself, and the second is the use of heparin. Because the transfused incompatible blood is already circulating when disseminated intravascular coagulation is caused by a hemolytic transfusion reaction, its removal is usually impossible. Removal was achieved successfully by total exchange of blood volume in one patient when hemolytic transfusion reaction was diagnosed very early.[68] Seager et al.[68] used cardiopulmonary bypass with hypothermia and massive acute hemodilution to quickly exchange the blood volume in one patient for whom they reported a successful outcome in 1974. These authors heparinized their patient, instituted cardiopulmonary bypass, and cooled her to 30 C. They then permitted bleeding from the original stab wound, with only crystalloid replacement, until a hematocrit level of 3% was reached. The circulation was then arrested, the pump oxygenator bag was discarded, and a second oxygenator primed with O-positive RBCs was used in its place. After bypass was resumed, the patient was rewarmed and the surgery was completed.

Another method of exchange transfusion would involve the use of a continuous-flow cell-washing machine to remove circulating antibodies and cell fragments just after hemolysis has occurred. Both of these techniques to remove the cause of a hemolytic transfusion reaction usually would be impractical because of the time required to set up the equipment involved.

When the cause of intravascular coagulation and fibrinolysis cannot be removed, heparinization has been recommended to stop the coagulation process.[28] Heparin acts directly in the blood to block coagulation at many sites along the clotting cascade. Because some intravascular coagulation and fibrinolysis is present in most acute hemolytic transfusion reactions, early heparinization is recommended as an important part of the therapy of severe hemolytic transfusion reactions. The coagulation problem has reached its end stage by the time that intravascular coagulation and fibrinolysis have led to widespread hemorrhage, either from surgical wounds or from venipuncture sites that start to bleed spontaneously. At this time, heparin can do nothing to reverse the consumption of clotting factors that has already occurred. Disseminated intravascular coagulation should be treated before it reaches this stage. Thus, early heparinization with 5,000 units, repeated every four to six hours, is recommended as soon as a severe hemolytic transfusion reaction has been diagnosed. If intravascular coagulation and fibrinolysis has reached an advanced stage, the clotting factors that have been depleted by this process must be replaced. This procedure can best be done with platelet concentrates and fresh-frozen plasma.

Although ε-aminocaproic acid is a logical therapy to block the fibrinolysis seen in the intravascular coagulation with fibrinolysis syndrome, its use alone could lead to serious thrombotic problems.[52] Widespread coagulation could continue, unbalanced by increased fibrinolysis, a situation more rapidly fatal than the intravascular coagulation with fibrinolysis syndrome. The advantage of combining ε-aminocaproic acid and heparin in the treatment of intravascular coagulation and fibrinolysis is only theoretical. There is little evidence to suggest that such combined treatment is more effective than the use of heparin alone.[38]

Many physicians still consider the use of heparin in intravascular coagulation and fibrinolysis to be controversial. Although logical theoretically, the efficacy of the drug has been more difficult to prove clinically. Management of oliguria and hypotension by the usual medical means must not be overlooked while more controversial therapies are tried.

OTHER TYPES OF TRANSFUSION REACTIONS

Febrile Transfusion Reactions

Much more frequent than the hemolytic transfusion reaction is the febrile transfusion reaction. These reactions are seen in at least 1% to 2% of all transfusions. They are attributed to leukoagglutinins or antibodies of the recipient that react with the leukocytes in the transfused blood. Historically, febrile transfusion reactions were seen with increased frequency and severity because of the difficulty in eliminating pyrogens from the glass containers and reusable rubber tubing used for blood administration until recent years.[69] Since the introduction of disposable plastic blood bags and intravenous tubing, pyrogens are seldom considered to be a cause of the febrile transfusion reaction. The patient undergoing the febrile transfusion reaction shows the abrupt onset of a fever with chills, muscle aches, and sometimes nausea and a headache. The chills and fever usually begin during the blood transfusion. These are not serious reactions in that they seldom lead to permanent morbidity, but the reaction is discomforting to the patient and could prolong hospitalization. The symptoms are most worrisome to the physician, however, because fever and chills could be the first clinical signs of a hemolytic transfusion reaction. Thus, the first part of the therapy for febrile transfusion reaction is to stop the transfusion and to initiate laboratory investigation to rule out a hemolytic transfusion reaction. Once such a reaction has been ruled out, the transfusion may be continued. Symptomatic treatment can be given in the form of aspirin or acetaminophen. Just like the hemolytic transfusion reaction, the febrile transfusion reaction is usually masked by anesthesia.

Allergic Blood Reactions

Just as frequent as the febrile transfusion reaction is the allergic blood reaction. The common allergic reaction is an urticarial rash that usually consists of multiple smooth or slightly elevated patches that are either more erythematous or paler than the surrounding skin. Pruritus or itching is usually present. These allergic reactions are usually attributed to hypersensitivity to unidentified substances in the transfused plasma. The signs and symptoms of these mild allergic reactions are not part of the symptomatology of a hemolytic transfusion reaction. Thus, the transfusion need not be discontinued when a patient shows an urticarial rash. The allergic reaction is not an early sign of another more severe type of reaction.

If a patient is anesthetized or awake and has a rash but is not itching, it is unnecessary to treat him for an allergic blood reaction. The itching can be severe, however, and a patient who has this type of reaction can be given diphenhydramine. Some patients who are hypersensitive predictably develop urticaria after almost any transfusion. These patients could be pretreated with diphenhydramine, but the prophylactic use of the drug before transfusion is usually unnecessary. There is no basis either for giving diphenhydramine to patients with febrile transfusion reactions or for giving aspirin to patients with allergic transfusion reactions.

Anaphylactic Anti-IgA Reactions

More serious but fortunately very infrequent are the transfusion reactions due to antibodies to IgA proteins.[61] Certain rare patients have no IgA immunoglobulins, and in these patients an antibody occasionally develops against the whole family or a class of IgA proteins. These patients have the most severe reactions when they receive blood or any blood product. Other patients who have antibodies against a particular IgA immunoglobulin usually have a less severe reaction, but fatalities have been reported in both groups. The anti-IgA reactions are usually of the anaphylactic type. An unanesthetized patient becomes very apprehensive and often can tell you that something terrible is about to happen. There is a sudden onset of pain in the chest, abdomen, or back. The patient becomes hypotensive as anaphylactic shock develops. Flushing and rashes are seen sometimes if the reaction is progressing more slowly, and difficulty with breathing, cyanosis, and wheezing are also frequent. This reaction can be seen within minutes after a transfusion has been started and can be caused by whole blood, packed cells, plasma, plasma protein fraction, or immunoglobulins. The only blood component that can be transfused safely in such a patient is washed RBCs (fresh or frozen), because it is the only one in which all plasma IgA protein has been removed. The anti-IgA anaphylactic reaction is implicated in any case of sudden death or sudden cardiovascular collapse during a transfusion. Even in a fatal hemolytic transfusion reaction, death comes more slowly and only after renal failure or hemorrhagic diathesis has ensued.

The treatment of an anaphylactic anti-IgA reaction is the same as that for any anaphylactic reaction due to any cause. The transfusion must be stopped immediately. Epinephrine is administered in a dose of 0.5 ml of 1:1,000 diluted in saline and given slowly intravenously. Fluids are given intravenously very rapidly to counteract the generalized vasodilatation by expanding the patient's circulating blood volume. Saline, Ringer's solution, or dextran may be used, but plasma protein fraction or albumin could make the reaction worse. If the patient is wheezing and has respiratory distress, aminophylline should be given slowly intravenously. A loading dose of 5.6 mg/kg, followed by 0.5 mg/kg/hour, is recommended for adults.[80] In this type of reaction, systemic steroids may be beneficial. Careful monitoring and institution of cardiopulmonary resuscitation are essential and could be life-saving in a patient undergoing this reaction.

A more complete list of transfusion reactions is as follows:

Hemolytic
  Acute
  Delayed
Febrile
Allergic—mild
Allergic—anaphylactic
Infectious
  Hepatitis
  Sepsis from bacterially contaminated blood
  Malaria
  Syphilis
  Cytomegalovirus
  Brucellosis
  Chagas' disease
  Infectious mononucleosis
Volume overload
Hypothermia
Acidosis-alkalosis
Ammonia intoxication
Microembolization or air embolization
Transfusion hemosiderosis
Unknown effects of plasticizers
Thrombophlebitis

AUTOLOGOUS TRANSFUSION

One way of avoiding most transfusion reactions is the use of autologous blood when possible. When a patient receives his own autologous blood, as opposed to the homologous blood of a donor, there should be no possibility of a hemolytic, febrile, allergic, or infectious reaction, unless a clerical error has been made in the handling. The safety from sensitization to foreign RBC antigens and subsequent antibody formation has been referred to earlier in this chapter.

There are three main types of autologous transfusion: preoperative collection and storage, hemodilution, and intraoperative scavenging. The patient awaiting elective surgery can have 1 or more units of his own blood collected preoperatively and stored as liquid or frozen until needed during surgery. This type of autologous transfusion is especially useful for patients with rare blood types that are difficult to crossmatch because of multiple antibodies. Hemodilution is a frequently used technique in which the patient's RBCs are exchanged for crystalloids at the start of surgery, so that less hemoglobin is lost during surgical hemorrhage, and the patient's own red cells can be returned to him at the end of surgery in lieu of at least some of the homologous blood he would need. Intraoperatively, RBCs also can be scavenged from the wound, collected, washed, and retransfused by machines using centrifugation techniques (Cell Saver Autologous Blood Recovery System, Haemonetics Corporation, 8 Erie Dr., Natick, MA 01760).

BLOOD COMPONENTS

The introduction of plastic blood bags led to major changes in blood banking practice. The ease of handling and administration was only a small benefit. Much more important was the fact that plastic bags and tubing enabled blood bankers to separate whole blood into its components with relative ease by means of fairly unsophisticated equipment. These advances permit local blood banks to prepare specific components to treat patients with varying needs, often from a single donor's unit. The blood bags are manufactured with the anticoagulant contained within. Double-bag or triple or quadruple packs can be used that are hermetically sealed and enable the blood banker to separate multiple components without "entering" the blood once it has been collected from the donor. As long as the bag and closed tubing system is not entered from the exterior and all tubing connections are crimped and sealed before separation, the blood is considered to be safe from the possibility of bacterial contamination. Proper temperature must be maintained, and recommended expiration dates must not be exceeded.[75]

Blood component therapy has greatly improved the efficiency of modern blood banking. Because almost any component can be life-saving for one patient and life-threatening for another, the practicing anesthesiologist must be familiar with the components that he uses.

Whole Blood and Packed Cells

Similarities and differences exist between the two components, whole blood and RBCs (Table

20–3). Red blood cells ("packed RBCs" is no longer the preferred terminology) contain a red cell mass equal to that of whole blood, the difference being mainly in the content of plasma and some ions. To understand the differences between whole blood and RBCs, it is important to understand the effects of storage on blood. The storage lesion consists of biochemical changes in banked blood due to the anticoagulants that it contains and due to metabolism while the blood is stored outside the body (Table 20–4). The blood becomes acidic as soon as it mixes with anticoagulant. The acidity increases during storage as lactic acid builds up owing to cellular metabolism. The sodium levels are high initially because most of the citrate used as anticoagulant is in the form of trisodium citrate. The cold (4 C) temperature maintained during storage reversibly inhibits adenosine triphosphatase in the RBC membrane.[81] The weakened sodium pump allows intracellular sodium to increase. Potassium levels decrease intracellularly and increase dramatically in the plasma. Most of the ionic changes are less severe when citrate-phosphate-dextrose is used as an anticoagulant than before its development, when acid-citrate-dextrose solution was used.

In 1978, a combination of citrate-phosphate-dextrose and adenine was approved as an anticoagulant for blood storage by the FDA. The advantage of this anticoagulant is an increased storage time (up to 35 days). Although there is little change in the effects of storage, the citrate-phosphate-dextrose and adenine anticoagulant provides reduced outdating and increased flexibility

TABLE 20–3.—COMPARISON OF WHOLE BLOOD AND RBCs*

COMPONENT	WHOLE BLOOD	RBCs
Volume, ml/unit	500	300
RBC mass, ml	200	200
Hemoglobin, gm	75	75
Hematocrit, %	39	70
Leukocytes	Yes	Yes
Microaggregates	Yes	Yes
Potassium, hydrogen, ammonium	Yes	Usually
Sodium load, mEq	45	15
Citrate, ml	63	22
Plasma, ml	250	80
Albumin, gm	12.5	4
Globulin, gm	6.25	2

*Data from *Blood Component Therapy: A Physician's Handbook*.[12]

TABLE 20–4.—STORAGE LESION OF CITRATE-PHOSPHATE-DEXTROSE WHOLE BLOOD*

	DAY			
	0	7	14	21
pH	7.1	7.0	7.0	6.9
Lactate, mg/dl	41	101	145	179
Bicarbonate ion, mEq/L	18.3	15.3	11.6	10.8
Potassium, mEq/L	3.9	11.9	17.2	21.0
Sodium, mEq/L	168	166	163	156

*Data from Bailey and Bove.[4]

to the blood banker. The compositions of the anticoagulants used in acid-citrate-dextrose, citrate-phosphate-dextrose, citrate-phosphate-dextrose-adenine, and heparinized blood are shown in Table 20–5.

The changes due to storage occur whether blood is being stored as whole blood or as RBCs. The excess hydrogen, potassium, and other ions are removed only if the RBCs are separated from the plasma just before administration. If the blood is stored as "packed" cells, the metabolic changes still occur. Thus, when RBCs are chosen as a component to avoid transfusion of certain ions to critically ill patients (for example, ammonium ion to a patient in hepatic coma), the clinician may request that the RBCs be separated immediately before the transfusion and that units stored only a few days be chosen.

The major advantage of RBCs over whole blood is that the RBCs are a better component for increasing the hemoglobin level of an anemic patient. Volume overload is less likely when packed cells are used. Because the blood bank is allowed to use the plasma, platelets, and other components, the use of RBCs represents a more efficient use of non-RBC components than whole blood transfusions. Lastly, RBCs are safer for blood group switching. When certain patients with rarer types (B, AB, Rh-negative) require massive transfusion on an emergency basis, the supplying blood bank sometimes will have to switch the patient to a more common blood group. Thus, patients with type B blood are switched to type O, and patients with AB blood are switched to type A. This practice is safe as long as the recipient has no antibodies for any antigens contained in the transfused cells. With the use of RBCs instead of whole blood, a smaller load of anti-A or anti-B antibod-

TABLE 20-5.—Composition of Anticoagulants

	ACID-CITRATE-DEXTROSE	CITRATE-PHOSPHATE-DEXTROSE	CITRATE-PHOSPHATE-DEXTROSE-ADENINE	HEPARIN
Volume/unit whole blood, ml	75	63	63	30
Citric acid, mg	600	206	206	...
Trisodium citrate, gm	1.65	1.66	1.66	...
Monosodium phosphate, mg	...	140	140	46
Dextrose, gm	1.84	1.61	2.01	...
Adenine, mg	...	...	17.3	...
Heparin, units	...	...	...	2,250
Sodium phosphate, mg	...	...	...	88
Sodium chloride, mg	...	...	...	270

ies is transfused into the patient. These antibodies usually do not cause a problem with respect to the recipient's own cells, but in large amounts the antibodies can cause hemolysis in subsequent transfusions if the patient is switched back to his own type. Hence, a patient switched to type O or type A should continue to receive that type if any further transfusions are required, until two to three weeks after transfusion.

The major advantage of whole blood is that it is the best treatment for acute massive blood loss. When multiple units of blood are necessary, whole blood can be transfused more expediently than multiple components. Also, because in most blood banks the cost of RBCs is approximately that of whole blood, a large transfusion combining large volumes of RBCs and albumin-containing solutions is substantially more expensive than transfusion of an identical volume of whole blood. Although many authors have strongly recommended the use of RBCs over whole blood for a number of reasons,[18, 40, 55] the use of whole blood is still clearly justifiable in many patients.[31, 66]

Leukocyte-Poor Blood

As previously discussed, antibodies to leukocytes can cause febrile reactions to blood transfusions in some patients. Most patients with these leukoagglutinins acquire them through sensitization by a previous transfusion or pregnancy. Thus, leukocyte-poor blood is indicated for patients known to have had transfusion reactions from anti-leukocyte antibodies.

Leukocyte-poor blood was previously used also for potential organ transplant recipients. It was believed that a lower graft rejection rate could be obtained by decreasing the exposure of potential recipients to foreign-tissue antigens. These histocompatibility antigens (HLA) are located mainly on the granulocytes, lymphocytes, and platelets in whole blood. Opelz and Terasaki[57] have shown, however, that the survival rate of cadaver-donor kidney transplants was higher for patients previously transfused with multiple units of whole blood than for untransfused recipients or for those who had received frozen blood only.

Multiple filtration techniques and sedimentation techniques are available for making leukocyte-poor blood, but most blood banks make it by centrifugation, followed by removal of the plasma and buffy-coat layer of RBCs. As much as 20% of a unit's RBCs can be lost by this process also. Alternately, frozen RBCs can be used as leukocyte-poor blood, because they have a lower leukocyte count than the component prepared by centrifugation, and there is no loss of RBCs, as there is when leukocyte-poor blood is made by centrifugation.

Frozen Blood

The development of techniques of freezing blood for long-term storage brought about a great advance in clinical blood banking. Outdating has always been a problem to the blood banker because it leads to inefficiency and increased cost. With the increasing demands and the loss of certain donor sources during recent years, excessive outdating can lead to a blood banker's inability to supply blood for certain patients. A longer shelf life for a component produces fewer problems of supply for the banker. With components that become outdated in a short period, an adequate supply is difficult to maintain.

Although many techniques have been developed for freezing and thawing RBCs, most involve the use of glycerol, a trihydric alcohol with a strong affinity for water. Mixed with the blood after collection, the hypertonic glycerol prevents RBC damage by water crystals during freezing. Stored at −76 C, the blood can then be kept indefinitely. When the blood is needed, it is thawed in a water bath of 37 C, but the RBCs must then be washed to remove the glycerol. Even though the cell-washing techniques are mechanized, 30 to 45 minutes are necessary for the washing of each unit. Herein lies one of the biggest disadvantages of frozen RBCs. Thawing and washing make their availability in an emergency slower than that of cells stored at 4 C. Technician time and preparation costs are greater. More importantly, since the washing process necessitates "entering" the thawed unit, the frozen RBCs must be used within 24 hours after being thawed to avoid possible bacterial growth in the unit. Thus, there is a paradox in that the component with the longest shelf life becomes outdated the fastest after its final preparation, and units occasionally can be wasted.

Numerous advantages have been cited for the use of frozen RBCs. Their long-term storage makes them excellent for anticipation of transfusion needs in patients with extremely rare blood types due to multiple antibodies or an antibody to a high-frequency antigen. The long-term storage capability of frozen blood also makes it a useful method for predeposit autologous transfusion. As was mentioned, the freezing, thawing, and washing process removes most leukocytes from frozen blood, making it useful for patients with leukoagglutinins. Microaggregates are removed during the washing process. Plasma protein is removed with the glycerol, thus making frozen RBCs safe for patients with anti-IgA antibodies. 2,3-Diphosphoglycerate is well maintained in the frozen RBCs. The washing process removes citrate, ammonium, and potassium. The longer shelf life permits greater control of inventory to the blood banker, and subsequently less wasteful outdating. Although it was hoped that frozen RBCs would transmit less hepatitis than whole blood or packed cells, laboratory and clinical evidence has clearly shown the opposite.[1, 34, 78] Haugen noted that the large-scale use of frozen cells and washed RBCs was ineffective in reducing the incidence of posttransfusion hepatitis in humans.[34]

Platelets

In the method by which single-donor platelet concentrate is prepared, platelet-rich plasma is first separated by lightly centrifuging fresh whole blood within six hours after collection (Fig 20–5). After the platelet-rich plasma is squeezed into a satellite bag, further centrifugation separates the platelets from the rest of the plasma, all but 25 to 50 ml of which is then squeezed off. Some RBCs remain in the platelet-rich plasma after the initial centrifugation. These make the platelet-rich concentrate occasionally appear to be pink. Because of their presence, the platelet concentrates are given to ABO-compatible recipients whenever possible.

Each unit of platelet concentrate should contain a minimum of 5.5×10^{10} platelets. Optimally, this will produce an increase of between 7,000 and 10,000/cu mm in the platelet count of an adult recipient. Each unit of platelet concentrate comes from a single donor's unit of blood. Each unit of platelet concentrate, therefore, shares the same risk of posttransfusion hepatitis as there is with 1 unit of whole blood. The platelets are administered through a 170-μm filter.

At least four factors affect the viability and function of the platelets during their storage[73]: storage temperature, pH, mixing during storage, and bag composition. Platelet viability decreases sharply if the pH in stored platelet concentrates is less than 6.0. The pH decreases faster if the temperature rises above 22 C. The composition of the plastic bag in which the platelets are stored is critical to the maintenance of their pH. The greatest area of controversy over platelet storage techniques involves the optimal temperature for their storage. Most authors agree that storage at 4 C greatly reduces platelet recovery and the life span of transfused platelets, but there is disagreement as to whether platelet function is better after storage at 4 or 22 C.[79] When platelets are stored at 22 to 24 C for 72 hours, recovery should remain above 30%. The platelet life span after transfusion is 8 days. After storage at 4 C, the life span of the transfused platelets is reduced to between 2 and 3 days. A normal platelet life span is 9 to 11 days.[6]

Patients can become refractory to platelet transfusions through several antigen-antibody systems. Platelets share the ABO antigens which coat RBCs, although these antigens prob-

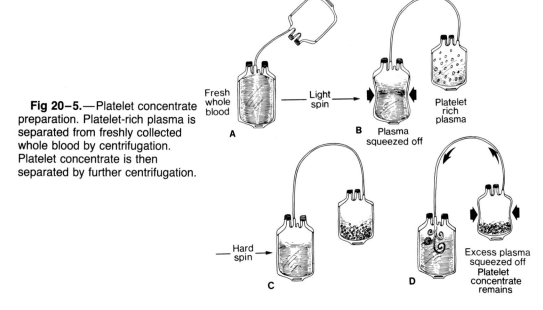

Fig 20–5.—Platelet concentrate preparation. Platelet-rich plasma is separated from freshly collected whole blood by centrifugation. Platelet concentrate is then separated by further centrifugation.

ably do not affect survival. There are also antigens that are unique to platelets. When patients become refractory to platelet transfusion, however, the usual cause of this alloimmunization is the development of antibodies to HLA antigens. For these patients, an alternative method of platelet transfusion can be used. Instead of using individual platelet concentrate units from random donors, a single donor who is HLA-compatible can undergo plateletpheresis. With this method, the equivalent of 10 or more units of platelet concentrate can be obtained from a single donor, using a machine that separates platelets from RBCs and plasma. The platelet-poor plasma and RBCs are returned to the donor, and the recipient receives all of his platelets from the single donor.

The indications for platelet transfusion are thrombocytopenia and functional defects of platelets. Thrombocytopenia is often seen on an iatrogenic basis, generally in patients receiving chemotherapeutic agents, in whom the prophylactic platelet transfusions allow the use of greater doses of the chemotherapeutic agents. Because of the absence of viable platelets in banked blood, dilutional thrombocytopenia is often seen in patients receiving massive transfusions. Spontaneous bleeding may occur after 10 to 15 units of blood have been given to an adult, unless platelet therapy is used. When there is doubt as to whether dilutional thrombocytopenia exists, a platelet count can be obtained quickly, and thus the unnecessary use of multiple units of platelet concentrate can be prevented. A minimal acceptable platelet count is difficult to define in the clinical situation. For patients who are not bleeding or who are not to undergo surgery, spontaneous hemorrhage is unlikely unless the platelet count decreases below 20,000/cu mm. Patients who are bleeding cannot generate a clot if their platelet count decreases below 50,000/cu mm.[53] However, the bleeding time (Ivy) becomes prolonged after the platelet count decreases below 100,000/cu mm.[32] Because of this factor, a level of 100,000/cu mm should probably be the minimal acceptable platelet count for patients undergoing surgical procedures.

Fresh-Frozen Plasma

Single-donor fresh-frozen plasma is made by the separation of plasma from RBCs within six hours of collection in a closed system. The plasma is then quickly frozen to −30 C. The fresh-frozen plasma can be maintained at this temperature for as long as 12 months. It is thawed in a water bath at 37 C just before use. Fresh-frozen plasma contains all of the coagulation factors except platelets and is indicated for treatment of many types of clotting factor deficiencies. Each unit contains approximately 240

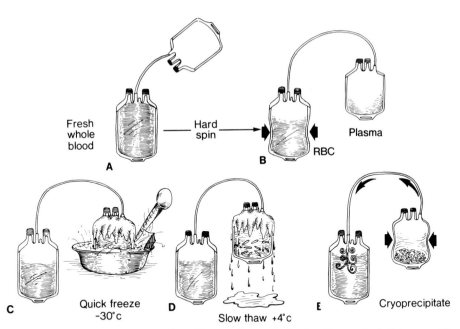

Fig 20–6.—Cryoprecipitate preparation. Plasma is separated from fresh whole blood and quickly frozen. Precipitate forms when it is thawed slowly. Concentrated by centrifugation, this precipitate is then refrozen.

ml of plasma obtained from a single donor. A unit of fresh-frozen plasma shares the same risk of transmission of hepatitis as does a unit of whole blood. Fresh-frozen plasma retains the natural ABO antibodies possessed by its donor. Thus, it is given to ABO-compatible recipients. A crossmatch is unnecessary.

Cryoprecipitate

Cryoprecipitate is a plasma fraction prepared by thawing a unit of fresh-frozen plasma at 4 C and then recovering the precipitated factor VIII protein by centrifugation. This material is then refrozen and stored at −30 C for up to 12 months. The process used for preparation of cryoprecipitate is illustrated in Figure 20–6. Each unit of cryoprecipitate comes from a single donor. Thus, it shares the same risk of hepatitis as does whole blood. Because the volume of plasma remaining with the cryoprecipitate is 25 ml or less, large amounts of factor VIII can be given to the patient without volume overload. Although there is individual variation from bag to bag, 40% to 50% of the original factor VIII activity is usually recovered from each unit of blood. Thus, each bag of concentrate should contain a minimum of 80 international units of factor VIII activity. One unit of factor VIII activity is that amount of activity present in 1 ml of normal fresh plasma. Cryoprecipitate is also a good source of fibrinogen. It is much safer for the recipient than fibrinogen concentrate prepared from pooled donor plasma because of the latter's high risk of hepatitis transmission.

Superconcentrates of lyophilized factor VIII globulin are commercially available. Although these are useful in the treatment of hemophilic patients with specific factor VIII antibodies, the concentrates carry an increased risk of hepatitis because of their pooled plasma source. Thus, they are seldom indicated. Concentrates of the vitamin K–dependent coagulation factors (II, VII, IX, and X) are also available. These preparations also carry a high risk of hepatitis transmission and are therefore less safe than fresh-frozen plasma.

Colloid Components and Blood Substitutes

The risk of hepatitis and the desirability of components that can be stored at room temperature for long periods have placed much emphasis on albumin and plasma substitutes in clinical medicine. The albumin molecule is a small pro-

to preset protocols. Difficulties are encountered in the monitoring of heparin because the effects of heparin on the coagulation system are such that most tests of coagulation are too prolonged to be accurate in the drug's presence. To obtain a clot in the presence of heparin, the coagulation system must be enhanced or the heparin must be neutralized. The quantitative protamine titration test accomplishes the latter by adding measured, increasing amounts of protamine to set volumes of patient plasma. The amount of protamine that most accurately neutralizes the heparin in the patient sample gives an indication of the amount of heparin that is present. Although the quantitative protamine titration test is very time-consuming and its methodology is too cumbersome for intraoperative use, its principle has been successfully used in a device designed to allow an automated determination of heparin levels in patients undergoing cardiopulmonary bypass (Hepcon, Hemotec, 106 Woodside Pl., 550 S. Syracuse St., Englewood, CO 80110). This instrument uses pre-manufactured protamine cassettes and optically determines in which of four blood-protamine mixtures fibrin is first forming. After initial heparinization, the Hepcon computes the amount of heparin or protamine needed for subsequent doses on the basis of an estimated blood volume. Although the machine has proved to be clinically useful, the need for an estimate of the blood volume introduces another possible inaccuracy in conclusions made from its determinations. Bull[17] pointed out that the necessity of knowing the blood volume is a drawback to any test that attempts to measure the *level* of heparin, as opposed to those tests which measure only the *effect* of heparin.

The activated coagulation time tests the effect of heparin. Hattersley[33] first described the test on whole blood and predicted its usefulness for heparin monitoring. The test is performed by drawing whole blood into a tube containing diatomaceous earth and mixing it and placing the tube in a water bath at 37 C or in a heat block. The tube is then tilted 1 minute after it is filled and at 5-second intervals thereafter. The appearance of the first unmistakable clot is the end point of the test, which normally occurs at about 1 minute 47 seconds or between 1 minute 21 seconds and 2 minutes 13 seconds.[33] As in any laboratory procedure, sources of error must be excluded, and the technique must be standardized. Waiting for a solid clot of the entire tube contents and not noting the first visible clot would falsely prolong the results. Hattersley[33] also believed that it is essential to prewarm the tube and any syringe used to collect the blood, because temperature is very critical to the activated coagulation time.[42]

The activated coagulation time of whole blood speeds the time required to generate a clot by rapidly activating factor XII, Hageman factor, with Celite. This stable, chemically inert preparation is made from fossilized diatoms. It activates the intrinsic part of the coagulation cascade through the large collective surface area of its many microscopic particles. By markedly shortening the time required for contact activation of the clotting mechanism, the activated coagulation time has none of the insensitivity of previous tests used to monitor heparin, such as the whole blood clotting time.[43] In addition to being prolonged by heparin, the activated coagulation time would be abnormal if any of the plasmatic coagulation factors other than factor VII were severely deficient. The activated coagulation time may be normal in the presence of severe thrombocytopenia, thus aiding in the differentiation between platelet problems and residual heparin at the conclusion of bypass. Hattersley[33] believed that the contributions of platelets to the clotting cascade were possibly bypassed in the activated coagulation time because of phospholipids released by hemolyzed RBCs. The linearity of the response of the activated coagulation time to increasing doses of heparin has been clearly demonstrated.[20]

Because of the variability of patient response to heparin, Bull et al.[16] recommended that a dose-response curve be constructed for each patient undergoing cardiopulmonary bypass. In this method, a baseline activated coagulation time is determined before the administration of heparin (Fig 20–9). The activated coagulation time then is measured after 2 mg/kg of heparin is administered. These points are plotted on a graph relating heparin dosage in milligrams per kilogram (ordinate) to activated coagulation time in seconds (abscissa). Having arbitrarily selected an activated coagulation time of 480 seconds as an indication of an ideal level of anticoagulation for bypass, Bull et al. then recommended extrapolating from these two points to a line at 480 seconds on the ordinate. From this extrapolation, an additional dose of heparin is predicted

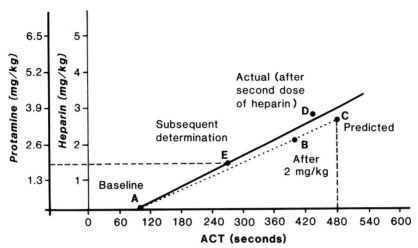

Fig 20-9.—Method of constructing dose-response curve for heparin.[16] Baseline activated coagulation time *(ACT) (A)* is plotted. Activated coagulation time is plotted after 2.0 mg/kg have been given *(B)*. Dose required to produce activated coagulation time of 480 seconds is predicted *(C)*, and actual activated coagulation time is determined *(D)* after that dose is given. Actual dose-response curve is plotted between points *B, C,* and *D*. Heparin level is later estimated by plotting subsequent activated coagulation time determinations *(E)* on graph. Amount of protamine needed for reversal is also estimated from graph, on the assumption that 1.3 mg of protamine will completely neutralize 1.0 mg of heparin.

that should increase activated coagulation time to 480 seconds. A third activated coagulation time, determined after the additional dose of heparin has been given, is a check on the accuracy of the plotted dose-response curve and the adequacy of heparinization. At later intervals in the bypass procedure, repeat values for activated coagulation time monitor the coagulation status of the patient and are used to compute subsequent doses of heparin and the dose of protamine needed for reversal of the heparin.

An automated device also is available for this type of heparin monitoring (Hemochron, International Technidyne Corporation, 138 Forest St., Metuchen, NJ 08840). The system mechanically rotates its tubes in test wells at 37 C. The timed end point is determined when a magnet in the tube is forced to rotate with the tube because of the development of fibrin. Although the device is more complicated than water baths or heat blocks used to perform the activated coagulation time, it removes subjectivity from the determination of the end point of the test and frees the anesthetist from having to tilt the tube every 5 seconds and observe it for clots.

During hypothermia (below 28 C), the activated coagulation time becomes prolonged, often being more than 1,000 seconds. The time returns to its prehypothermia range on rewarming. In spite of this problem, heparin monitoring has become accepted in cardiovascular anesthesia and is a means of increasing the safety of bypass surgery for patients. The experience of many institutions shows that heparin can be managed by empiric protocol. Because of the vagaries of patient response to this drug, however, inadequate heparinization and subsequent pump clot-off are real risks in unmonitored patients. Even if such a catastrophic complication does not result, relative underheparinization can lead to consumption of coagulation factors. Excess heparin can cause postoperative bleeding problems and require excessive doses of protamine. At the very least, heparin monitoring can allow the cardiovascular anesthesiologist to be more secure in his knowledge of the degree of heparin's effect in altering his patient's clotting system.

REFERENCES

1. Alter H.J., et al.: Transmission of hepatitis B virus infection by transfusion of frozen-deglycerolized red blood cells. *N. Engl. J. Med.* 298:637, 1978.

2. Atik M., Manale B., Pearson J.: Prevention of acute renal failure: Hemodynamic observations of transfusion reactions. J.A.M.A. 183:455, 1963.
3. Bachmann F., et al.: The hemostatic mechanism after open-heart surgery: I. Studies on plasma coagulation factors and fibrinolysis in 512 patients after extracorporeal circulation. J. Thorac. Cardiovasc. Surg. 70:76, 1975.
4. Bailey D.N., Bove J.R.: Chemical and hematological changes in stored CPD blood. Transfusion 15:244, 1975.
5. Baker R.J., Moinichen S.L., Nyhus L.M.: Transfusion reaction: A reappraisal of surgical incidence and significance. Ann. Surg. 169:684, 1969.
6. Barrer M.J., Ellison N.: Platelet function. Anesthesiology 46:202, 1977.
7. Barry K.G., Crosby W.H.: The prevention and treatment of renal failure following transfusion reactions. Transfusion 3:34, 1963.
8. Beall A.C. Jr., et al.: Mannitol-induced osmotic diuresis during renal artery occlusion. Ann. Surg. 161:46, 1965.
9. Bick R.L.: Alterations of hemostasis associated with cardiopulmonary bypass: Pathophysiology, prevention, diagnosis, and management. Semin. Thromb. Hemostas. 3:59, 1976.
10. Bick R.L., Schmalhorst W.R., Arbegast N.R.: Alterations of hemostasis associated with cardiopulmonary bypass. Thromb. Res. 8:285, 1976.
11. Bland J.H.L., Laver M.B., Lowenstein E.: Vasodilator effect of commercial 5% plasma protein fraction solutions. J.A.M.A. 224:1721, 1973.
12. Blood Component Therapy: A Physician's Handbook, ed. 2. Washington, D.C., American Association of Blood Banks, 1975.
13. Boral L.I., Henry J.B.: The type and screen: A safe alternative and supplement in selected surgical procedures. Transfusion 17:163, 1977.
14. Bowie E.J.W., Owen C.A. Jr.: Introduction: Symposium on the diagnosis and treatment of intravascular coagulation-fibrinolysis (ICF) syndrome, with special emphasis on this syndrome in patients with cancer. Mayo Clin. Proc. 49:635, 1974.
15. Bull B.S., et al.: Heparin therapy during extracorporeal circulation: I. Problems inherent in existing protocols. J. Thorac. Cardiovasc. Surg. 69:674, 1975.
16. Bull B.S., et al.: Heparin therapy during extracorporeal circulation: II. The use of a dose-response curve to individualize heparin and protamine dosage. J. Thorac. Cardiovasc. Surg. 69:685, 1975.
17. Bull M.H., Huse W.M., Bull B.S.: Evaluation of tests used to monitor heparin therapy during extracorporeal circulation. Anesthesiology 43:346, 1975.
18. Chaplin H. Jr.: Packed red blood cells. N. Engl. J. Med. 281:364, 1969.
19. Colman R.W., Robboy S.J., Minna J.D.: Disseminated intravascular coagulation (DIC): An approach. Am. J. Med. 52:679, 1972.
20. Congdon J.E., Kardinal C.G., Wallin J.D.: Monitoring heparin therapy in hemodialysis: A report on the activated whole blood coagulation time tests. J.A.M.A. 226:1529, 1973.
21. Damus P.S., Hicks M., Rosenberg R.D.: Anticoagulant action of heparin. Nature 246:355, 1973.
22. Daniels W.B., Leonard B.W., Holtzman S.: Renal insufficiency following transfusion: Report of thirteen cases. J.A.M.A. 116:1208, 1941.
23. Egan E.L., et al.: Effect of surgical operations on certain tests used to diagnose intravascular coagulation and fibrinolysis. Mayo Clin. Proc. 49:658, 1974.
24. Ellison N., Edmunds L.H. Jr., Colman R.W.: Platelet aggregation following heparin and protamine administration. Anesthesiology 48:65, 1978.
25. Ellison N., Ominsky A.J., Wollman H.: Is protamine a clinically important anticoagulant? A negative answer. Anesthesiology 35:621, 1971.
26. Estes J.W., Poulin P.F.: Pharmacokinetics of heparin: Distribution and elimination. Thromb. Diath. Haemorrh. 33:26, 1975.
27. Friedenberg W.R., et al.: Platelet dysfunction associated with cardiopulmonary bypass. Ann. Thorac. Surg. 25:298, 1978.
28. Goldfinger D.: Acute hemolytic transfusion reactions—a fresh look at pathogenesis and considerations regarding therapy. Transfusion 17:85, 1977.
29. Gollub S.: Heparin rebound in open heart surgery. Surg. Gynecol. Obstet. 124:337, 1967.
30. Greendyke R.M., Banzhaf J.C.: Introduction to Blood Banking, ed. 2. Flushing, N.Y., Medical Examination Publishing Co., 1974, p. 62.
31. Grindon A.J.: The use of packed red blood cells. J.A.M.A. 235:389, 1976.
32. Harker L.A., Slichter S.J.: The bleeding time as a screening test for evaluation of platelet function. N. Engl. J. Med. 287:155, 1972.
33. Hattersley P.G.: Activated coagulation time of whole blood. J.A.M.A. 196:436, 1966.
34. Haugen R.K.: Hepatitis after the transfusion of frozen red cells and washed red cells. N. Engl. J. Med. 301:393, 1979.

35. Henry J.B., Mintz P., Webb W.: Optimal blood ordering for elective surgery. J.A.M.A. 237:451, 1977.
36. Issitt P.D., Issitt C.H.: *Applied Blood Group Serology*, ed. 2. Oxnard, Calif., Spectra Biologicals, 1975.
37. Jeanloz R.W.: The chemistry of heparin, in Bradshaw R.A., Wessler S. (eds.): *Heparin: Structure, Function, and Clinical Implications*. New York, Plenum Press, 1975, p. 3.
38. Kazmier F.J., et al.: Treatment of intravascular coagulation and fibrinolysis (ICF) syndromes. *Mayo Clin. Proc.* 49:665, 1974.
39. Kiss J.: Chemistry of heparin: A short review on recent chemical trends. *Thromb. Diath. Haemorrh.* 33:20, 1975.
40. Kliman A.: No hepatitis after packed red cells? *N. Engl. J. Med.* 279:1290, 1968.
41. Koller F.: The physiological function of heparin. *Thromb. Diath. Haemorrh.* 33:17, 1975.
42. Kopriva C.J., et al.: Hypothermia can cause errors in activated coagulation time, abstracted. *Anesthesiology* 53:85s, 1980.
43. Lee R.I., White P.D.: A clinical study of the coagulation time of blood. *Am. J. Med. Sci.* 145:495, 1913.
44. Levin N.W.: Furosemide and ethacrynic acid in renal insufficiency. *Med. Clin. North Am.* 55:107, 1971.
45. Magnusson S.: Homologies between thrombin and other serine proteinases, abstracted. *Biochem. J.* 110:25p, 1968.
46. Mallory T.B.: Hemoglobinuric nephrosis in traumatic shock. *Am. J. Clin. Pathol.* 17:427, 1947.
47. Marcus A.J.: Platelet function. *N. Engl. J. Med.* 280:1213, 1278, and 1330, 1969.
48. Markwardt F.: Antilipemic action of heparin. *Thromb. Diath. Haemorrh.* 33:73, 1975.
49. Mayer M.M.: The complement system. *Sci. Am.* 229:54, 1973.
50. McLean J.: The thromboplastic action of cephalin. *Am. J. Physiol.* 41:250, 1916.
51. Merskey C.: Defibrination syndrome or . . . ?, editorial. *Blood* 41:599, 1973.
52. Miller R.D.: Complications of massive blood transfusions. *Anesthesiology* 39:82, 1973.
53. Miller R.D., et al.: Coagulation defects associated with massive blood transfusions. *Ann. Surg.* 174:794, 1971.
54. Mollison P.L.: *Blood Transfusion in Clinical Medicine*, ed. 5. Oxford, England, Blackwell Scientific Publications, 1972.
55. Moore F.D.: Should blood be whole or in parts?, editorial. *N. Engl. J. Med.* 280:327, 1969.
56. Moorthy S.S., Pond W., Rowland R.G.: Severe circulatory shock following protamine (an anaphylactic reaction). *Anesth. Analg.* 59:77, 1980.
57. Opelz G., Terasaki P.I.: Improvement of kidney-graft survival with increased numbers of blood transfusions. *N. Engl. J. Med.* 299:799, 1978.
58. Owen C.A. Jr., Bowie E.J.W.: Chronic intravascular coagulation syndromes: A summary. *Mayo Clin. Proc.* 49:673, 1974.
59. Owen C.A. Jr., Bowie E.J.W., Thompson J.H. Jr.: *The Diagnosis of Bleeding Disorders*, ed. 2. Boston, Little, Brown & Co., 1975; a, p. 37; b, p. 15-51; c, p. 40-41.
60. Pineda A.A., Brzica S.M. Jr., Taswell H.F.: Hemolytic transfusion reaction: Recent experience in a large blood bank. *Mayo Clin. Proc.* 53:378, 1978.
61. Pineda A.A., Taswell H.F.: Transfusion reactions associated with anti-IgA antibodies: Report of four cases and review of the literature. *Transfusion* 15:10, 1975.
62. Rabiner S.F., et al.: Evaluation of a stroma-free hemoglobin solution for use as a plasma expander. *J. Exp. Med.* 126:1127, 1967.
63. Rosenberg R.D.: Actions and interactions of antithrombin and heparin. *N. Engl. J. Med.* 292:146, 1975.
64. Rosenberg R.D.: Chemistry of the hemostatic mechanism and its relationship to the action of heparin. *Fed. Proc.* 36:10, 1977.
65. Rouault C., Gruenhagen J.: Reorganization of blood ordering practices. *Transfusion* 18:448, 1978.
66. Schmidt P.J.: Red cells for transfusion, editorial. *N. Engl. J. Med.* 299:1411, 1978.
67. Schmidt P.J., Holland P.V.: Pathogenesis of the acute renal failure associated with incompatible transfusion. *Lancet* 2:1169, 1967.
68. Seager O.A., et al.: Massive acute hemodilution for incompatible blood reaction. *J.A.M.A.* 229:790, 1974.
69. Seldon T.H.: Untoward reactions and complications during transfusions and infusions. *Anesthesiology* 22:810, 1961.
70. Sherwood G.K.: Hemolytic transfusion reactions, in *New Approaches to Transfusion Reactions*. Washington, D.C., American Association of Blood Banks, 1974, p. 1.
71. Shulman N.R., et al.: The role of the reticuloendothelial system in the pathogenesis of idiopathic thrombocytopenic purpura. *Trans. Assoc. Am. Physicians* 78:374, 1965.
72. Siegal T., et al.: Clinical and laboratory aspects of disseminated intravascular coagulation (DIC): A study of 118 cases. *Thromb. Haemost.* 39:122, 1978.

73. Slichter S.J., Harker L.A.: Preparation and storage of platelet concentrates. *Transfusion* 16:8, 1976.
74. Spellman G.G.: Corticosteroid treatment of transfusion reaction from incompatible blood of ABO type: Report of a case. *J.A.M.A.* 169:1622, 1959.
75. *Standards for Blood Banks and Transfusion Services*, ed. 9. Washington, D.C., American Association of Blood Banks, November 1978.
76. Tullis J.L.: Albumin: I. Background and use. *J.A.M.A.* 237:355, 1977.
77. Tullis J.L.: Albumin: II. Guidelines for clinical use. *J.A.M.A.* 237:460, 1977.
78. Tullis J.L., et al.: Incidence of posttransfusion hepatitis in previously frozen blood. *J.A.M.A.* 214:719, 1970.
79. Valeri C.R.: Circulation and hemostatic effectiveness of platelets stored at 4 C or 22 C: Studies in aspirin-treated normal volunteers. *Transfusion* 16:20, 1976.
80. Van Dellen R.G.: Theophylline: Practical application of new knowledge. *Mayo Clin. Proc.* 54:733, 1979.
81. Wallas C.H.: Sodium and potassium changes in blood bank stored human erythrocytes. *Transfusion* 19:210, 1979.
82. Wessler S., Gaston L.W.: Pharmacologic and clinical aspects of heparin therapy. *Anesthesiology* 27:475, 1966.
83. Wessler S., Gitel S.N.: Heparin: New concepts relevant to clinical use. *Blood* 53:525, 1979.
84. Woods J.E., et al.: The transfusion of platelet concentrates in patients undergoing heart surgery. *Mayo Clin. Proc.* 42:318, 1967.
85. Woods J.E., et al.: Effect of bypass surgery on coagulation-sensitive clotting factors. *Mayo Clin. Proc.* 42:724, 1967.

21 / Cardiac Pacemakers and Anesthesia

PAUL F. LEONARD

THE EVOLUTION of electronic cardiac pacing, as well as that of cardiac surgery, has permitted effective therapy for many patients to whom little could be offered previously. As the indications for pacing expand, the anesthesiologist encounters many patients with pacemakers who are undergoing either cardiac or noncardiac surgery. Hence, he must know the anatomy and physiology of these devices that induce myocardial contraction by the application of an electrical stimulus.

According to a 1978 report, 156,000 citizens of the United States have electronic pacemakers, or about one in 1,300 of the general population. About 60,000 pacemakers are implanted each year in the United States.[14]

INDICATIONS FOR ELECTRONIC PACING

The original indication for permanent pacing, partial or complete atrioventricular block complicated by Stokes-Adams attacks or congestive heart failure, has been extended gradually to include patients with various heart blocks or arrhythmias. For several years, permanent pacing has been widely used for symptomatic bradycardia with or without permanent atrioventricular block. Asymptomatic heart block and bradycardia are occasional indications. Surgical damage to the conduction system incident to insertion of a prosthetic valve or to repair of congenital cardiac defects produces the highest mortality of any form of heart block.[18] Temporary pacing is the initial therapy; permanent pacing is instituted if the condition persists.

Pacemakers are used as therapy for certain tachyarrhythmias. Implanted pacemakers for terminating tachycardia by applying atrial or ventricular stimuli at a rate or time specific to the patient's requirements are available. Some such pacemakers are patient-activated via a signal transmitted from an external unit.

UNIPOLAR VERSUS BIPOLAR LEADS

Cardiac pacing requires the heart muscle to be part of a complete circuit that conveys electrical signals between the pacemaker and the heart. With fixed-rate pacemakers, signals flow in one direction—from pacemaker to heart. However, to provide an appropriate response, most pacemakers sense the electrical activity of the heart; hence, signals must travel in both directions. The circuit may include a pair of wires between the pacemaker and two electrodes in or on the heart; this is termed a "bipolar system." By contrast, in the unipolar configuration, a single wire and electrode connect the pacemaker and the heart; the return circuit is completed via the conductivity of the intervening body tissue. With this arrangement, the second electrode may be a plate on the surface of the implanted pacemaker capsule or the pacemaker case itself. The two configurations are diagrammed in Figure 21-1.

Several compromises enter into the decision as to which system is most appropriate for a particular patient. Some of the differences between the systems can be anticipated by considering the effects of the spacing between the two electrodes. The closely spaced electrodes of the bipolar system supply ECG signals to the pacemaker which are less predictable and often of lower amplitude than those provided by the unipolar system. Unless the input circuit of the pacemaker has adequate amplification, low-amplitude signals will not be sensed. However, signals from bipolar electrodes are more specific to the site of implantation. Spurious signals are more likely to appear between the widely separated electrodes of the unipolar system. Sensing

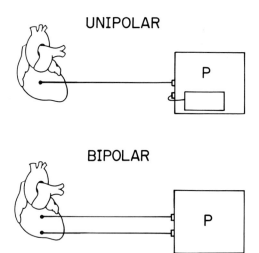

Fig 21–1.—In unipolar configuration, single lead and electrode link pacemaker *(P)* with myocardium. Circuit is completed by conductivity through body tissue to pacemaker case or to plate on its surface. Bipolar system is characterized by two leads and pair of electrodes.

circuits may be confounded by such signals, whether they arise from without the body as electromagnetic interference or within the body as skeletal muscle potentials. In one study, about half of the patients who had pacemakers with unipolar leads could inhibit their pulse generators through isometric arm exercises.[2] However, in normal activities, few patients suffer symptoms from this cause.

Conversely, the effects of stimulating signals from pacemakers are focused at the heart by the bipolar system, but these signals may be more diffuse with the unipolar system. Again the proximity of skeletal muscle may pose a problem with the unipolar system—that of muscle stimulation. Thus, a pacemaker having an attached plate electrode is implanted with this electrode on the side opposite the overlying muscle.

The brief spike artifact on the ECG that signifies the firing of the pacemaker is more prominent with the unipolar system. This characteristic is often beneficial during evaluation of pacemaker function.

The current required to trigger cardiac depolarization ("threshold current") is the same whether the unipolar or the bipolar mode is used.[19] However, the threshold for induction of ventricular fibrillation during the vulnerable period of the cardiac cycle is lower for bipolar than for unipolar electrodes with a negative cardiac electrode (which is the polarity routinely used). In all published reports but one, pacemaker-induced fibrillation has been associated with a bipolar system.[7] Fortunately, this complication is rare.

Certain electrodes made of alloys that are superior in stress resistance can be used only in the unipolar system because they corrode if used as anodes (positive electrodes).[18]

The bipolar configuration has the advantage of being relatively easy to convert into a unipolar system should one of the wires break.

PACEMAKER PLACEMENT AND RELIABILITY

Whether the system is unipolar or bipolar, most pacemaker leads are situated by transvenous placement. This technique is associated with considerably less morbidity and mortality than transthoracic placement. Leads are usually placed via the cephalic or external jugular vein, using local anesthesia and fluoroscopic guidance. Myocardial potentials and pacing threshold are measured to ensure the proper positioning of the electrodes.

A survey[9] of 313 patients who received pacemakers between 1961 and 1973 revealed that 65% survived five years. Generator reliability increased gradually during the period. A decrease in survival rate for patients who received pacemakers more recently was apparently due to the inclusion of more poor-risk patients. Death from unexpected pacing failure was extremely rare.

TYPES OF PACEMAKERS

The original pacemaker was a fixed-rate device that provided an electrical impulse to the ventricle at regular intervals regardless of cardiac activity. Subsequently, pacemakers were developed that continuously sensed the activation of the heart and tailored their output appropriately. Atrial sensing and sequential atrial and ventricular pacing are now provided by some models. Pacemakers that permit noninvasive programming of rate, stimulus duration, and sensitivity to intrinsic cardiac signals are now manufactured. The information is transmitted from an external programming device through the intervening tissue to the implanted pacemaker by magnetic or radiofrequency pulses.

Because of the many configurations available, a three-letter identification code has been established.[13] This code describes concisely the mode of operation of a pacemaker:

First letter, chamber paced
Second letter, chamber sensed
Third letter, mode of response to signal sensed
Key to symbols:
  V–ventricle
  A–atrium
  D–double chamber (atrium and ventricle)
  I–inhibited
  T–triggered
  O–not applicable

Thus, the fixed-rate ventricle-stimulating pacemaker referred to previously is designated VOO. The chamber paced is the ventricle (V), and both the chamber sensed and the mode of response to the sensed signal are designated "not applicable" (OO); this type of pacemaker has no sensing function and hence cannot respond to external signals. Because it cannot synchronize its activity with any intrinsic cardiac rhythm, it is termed "asynchronous." However, by the same token, it is virtually immune to interference, both endogenous and exogenous. Its relatively simple circuit has few components to fail. It also draws less power than some designs, which prolongs battery life. It is used chiefly in patients with chronic complete heart block.

Against these advantages must be weighed the fact that a fixed rate limits the ability of the heart to adjust its output to suit requirements. But the major concern with the fixed-rate unit is competition between spontaneous and paced depolarizations, resulting in arrhythmias.

After ventricular depolarization, there is a vulnerable period (corresponding approximately to the upstroke of the T wave) during which delivery of a stimulus may induce arrhythmias, such as ventricular premature contractions, ventricular tachycardia, and ventricular fibrillation. A significant percentage of patients with the Stokes-Adams syndrome have periods of spontaneous conducted sinus rhythm. Further, such patients also may have spontaneous ventricular activity. In either situation, the vulnerable period is random in time with respect to the asynchronous pacing stimulus. Thus, the possibility of serious arrhythmias exists whenever non-paced depolarization occurs in a patient who has this type of pacemaker.

Induction of ventricular fibrillation is less likely with the present pacemakers than it was with earlier units, which furnished a more powerful stimulus. The energy level normally required to induce ventricular fibrillation, even during the vulnerable period, is considerably greater than the level of the stimulus provided by modern pacemakers.[8] However, the threshold for depolarization may be reduced under some conditions. Fibrillation then is induced more easily.

The ventricular-synchronous pacemaker is much less likely to produce competition because its output is synchronized with intrinsic cardiac activity. As in the asynchronous unit, a single circuit links pacemaker and heart, but the circuit is bidirectional: depolarization signals (the QRS complex) flow from ventricle to pacemaker, and pacemaker stimuli flow in the opposite direction. This instrument is designated as a VVT pacemaker. When depolarization is detected, the pacemaker is immediately activated, the stimulus falling safely within the absolute refractory period of the ventricle. The pacemaker has timing circuits that establish minimal and maximal rates of stimulation. Failure to sense depolarization within a preset escape interval results in delivery of a stimulus.

The VVT pacemaker usually senses idioventricular as well as normal depolarization; competition is improbable. Although the sensing circuit of a VVT pacemaker may respond to interfering signals, the result is not pacemaker suppression but rather extra stimuli. The battery life in this type of pacemaker is relatively short; the unit delivers stimuli regardless of whether the heart requires them. The sensing circuit consumes a small amount of power. It also adds to the complexity and subtracts from the reliability of this pacemaker. Further, the pacing artifact distorts the ECG pattern when cardiac conduction is normal, which could create problems in diagnosis.

The most widely used pacemaker is the ventricular-inhibited type, and it is the instrument that usually is being referred to when the term "demand pacemaker" is applied. A more precise designation is VVI. It resembles the ventricular-synchronous unit in that the ventricle is both sensed and stimulated; it differs in being inhibited when depolarization is detected.

Thus, during periods of normal conduction, there is no pacemaker output. The QRS depolarization signal merely resets the timing circuit to zero. However, if no such signal arrives within a specific interval, the pacemaker fires, thus providing a stimulus to the ventricle and again resetting the timing circuit. Pacing of the heart at a regular rate then continues until spontaneous activity is again sensed.

The ventricular-inhibited device shares with the ventricular-synchronous unit the advantage of requiring only a single circuit between pacemaker and heart. It shares the disadvantage of greater complexity as compared to the asynchronous unit. However, because a ventricular-inhibited pacemaker provides no stimulus except when such is required, only the sensing circuit uses power when cardiac conduction is normal. Sensing requires considerably less energy than stimulating; hence, battery life tends to be prolonged.

However, if this pacemaker interprets spurious signals as indicating ventricular depolarization, it is inhibited. Thus, in the presence of interference, stimuli may not be delivered when required.

One approach to the problem of electromagnetic interference has been to design a sensing circuit that responds only to signals with the frequency characteristics of the normal QRS complex. This capability has been achieved, however, at the cost of reduced sensitivity to ventricular extrasystoles, which also may have aberrant frequency patterns. Thus, competition with an idioventricular beat is possible.

The ventricular-inhibited pacemaker does not distort the ECG when conduction in the patient is normal. However, in this circumstance, it is also impossible to examine pacemaker output or to demonstrate capture of the ventricle. ("Capture" refers to the initiation of cardiac depolarization and contraction by the pacemaker stimulus.) Therefore, most of these devices contain a magnetically activated switch. A magnet placed over the implanted generator causes it to convert to asynchronous operation, thus producing regularly recurring stimuli.

The pacing rate of a ventricular-inhibited unit converted to the asynchronous mode is significant. Manufacturers specify the relationship between the asynchronous or "magnet" rate and the battery voltage. Thus, a decline in voltage as the battery discharges can be detected, and this is the most reliable means of anticipating pacemaker battery failure.[13] Electrocardiographic patterns illustrating the timing of stimuli provided by VOO, VVT, and VVI pacemakers are shown in Figure 21–2.

The unavailability of a completely acceptable transvenous lead system for atrial placement until recently has restricted the use of pacemakers that use atrial sensing or stimulation, despite their recognized advantages in some patients. Curtis et al.[3] verified the significance of the atrial contribution in a paced heart. They used an external pacemaker that could stimulate the atria or ventricles either separately or sequentially. Patients were studied within 24 hours after cardiac surgery by means of pacing wires placed at operation. The authors found that ventricular pacing at 100 beats per minute in patients with normal sinus rhythm reduced cardiac

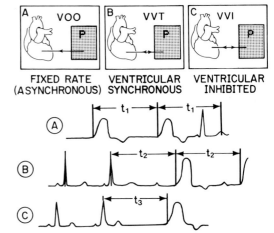

Fig 21–2.—**A,** in VOO (fixed rate or asynchronous) circuit, impulses are unidirectional, traveling only from pacemaker (P) to heart. Regularly recurring impulse occurs at interval t_1, stimulating depolarization whose ECG pattern may resemble that of ventricular premature complex. Spontaneous beat could receive pacing stimulus during its T wave. **B,** in VVT (ventricular-synchronous) circuit, impulses travel from heart to pacemaker, as well as in reverse direction. On sensing QRS complex, pacemaker fires immediately. If no complex is detected within interval t_2, stimulus discharges and triggers depolarization. **C,** impulses in VVI (ventricular-inhibited) circuit also are bidirectional, but there is no pacemaker stimulus as long as QRS complexes are sensed. Only if interval t_3 passes without detection of such a signal does pacemaker stimulate depolarization.

output by as much as 42% (average, 14%), whereas atrial and atrioventricular sequential pacing at the same rate increased cardiac output by averages of 13% and 19%, respectively.

Obel and Citron,[10] in a 1978 review of atrial-demand (AAI) and atrioventricular-sequential (DVI) pacing, noted that reliable and practical atrial lead systems "may now be available." They stated that some patients would receive pronounced clinical benefit from permanent pacing involving the atrium. However, they anticipate that most patients who are candidates for pacemakers will continue to receive ventricular-demand units and obtain satisfactory clinical results.

ELECTROMAGNETIC INTERFERENCE

Electromagnetic interference during pacemaker operation is rarely a problem when asynchronous devices are used. But with the advent of pacemakers that respond to the electrical activity of the heart, confusion of the sensing circuitry by external electrical signals became possible. The response to electromagnetic interference by a pacemaker depends on its design and on the nature and strength of the interfering signal. Generally, there is no effect on the pacemaker. However, the pacemaker may be inhibited, converted to a fixed rate in the normal range, or driven to a dangerously high rate.

Improved stability of the frequency-control circuits has virtually eliminated the problem of runaway pacemaker. Conversion to a fixed-rate operation carries with it only a slight hazard of competition-induced arrhythmia, but inhibition of a pacemaker whose stimulus is required for adequate cardiac output is life-threatening.

Pacemaker manufacturers have responded by changes in design that greatly reduce the susceptibility to interference. Improvements are primarily in two areas. Better shielding reflects or absorbs most radiated signals that are strong enough to traverse the intervening tissue and reach the unit. Better electronic filtering protects the sensing circuit from input signals whose frequency does not correspond to that of the electrical "signature" of the QRS complex.

Sources of electromagnetic interference can be categorized according to the probability that significant interference will be produced in a well-designed pacemaker.[4] Category 1 comprises devices "Unlikely to Interfere" and includes most common household appliances and small electrical shop tools. Well-shielded implanted pacemakers are not affected by microwave ovens that comply with US federal regulations. Category 2 comprises "Potentially Interfering Devices" and includes ignition systems for both large and small gasoline engines. The electrical impulse may mimic the cardiac signal and cause interference if it is near the pacemaker. Category 3 comprises "Devices Likely to Interfere" and includes equipment producing strong, pulsed signals that may not be completely rejected by filtering circuits. Electrical arc welders and high-power radio and radar transmitters are in this group. Diathermy equipment placed over a pacemaker not only may affect its output but also may damage its metal components by heat.

Because some of these interfering sources (such as radar) operate on high frequencies differing by many orders of magnitude from those in cardiac signals, it might seem that their interference should be easily rejected by the input filter. However, the filters in pacemaker circuits are preceded by diodes whose function is to protect these circuits from damage by high-power discharges from defibrillators. These diodes effectively demodulate radio-frequency signals applied to them (just as do detector circuits in radio receivers); the low frequencies of the modulation envelope remain. These low frequencies may resemble the cardiac signal sufficiently to pass through the filter and cause interference.

In the operating room, the device most likely to interfere with pacemaker operation is the electrosurgical unit. Often erroneously referred to as the "cautery," this machine can apply a modulated radio-frequency power of several hundred watts directly to the patient. For example, during prostatic resection, endocardial potentials of 8 to 16 V have been measured coincident with the use of electrosurgery.[11] Such voltages are several thousand times greater than the QRS potentials to which a pacemaker sensing circuit is designed to respond. When electrosurgery is used, the factors of power, proximity, and waveform combine to enhance the probability of pacemaker interference.

The contraindication to the use of electrosurgery in an electronically paced patient is usually relative rather than absolute. In most patients, there will be no incompatibility. In some, such as in those undergoing transurethral prostatic resection, the procedure cannot be performed without electrosurgery. When the indications are less compelling but the surgeon feels handicapped if electrosurgery is not available, the usual preparations for its use can be made but a final decision regarding its use can be deferred. The response of the pacemaker to the initial cautious application of electrosurgery should be observed closely; its use may be continued if no problem results. Assiduous monitoring of cardiac rhythm must be maintained throughout the procedure.

However, surgeon Carl Walter, commenting on electrosurgery and the patient with a pacemaker, offers the trenchant observation that "cholecystectomy can be accomplished safely without the use of electrocautery [sic; it is not electrocautery]. That technique is a nonessential convenience to the surgeon. Where increased risk is suspected, good judgment dictates omission of the questioned technique."[20]

When electrosurgery is to be used in a patient with a pacemaker, certain precautions should be observed.

1. The dispersive electrode should be situated so that the current pathway through the body between this electrode and the active electrode is as remote as possible from the pacemaker unit and the wires connecting it to the heart.

2. Both the ECG and the heart sounds should be monitored. Monitoring of the ECG is especially important in these patients because the pacing spike can be observed and pacemaker operation can be evaluated. When an isolated-input electrocardioscope is used in conjunction with an isolated-output electrosurgical unit, generally a usable tracing can be retained while electrosurgery is used. Some presently available monitor scopes are designed to exhibit reasonably clean ECG tracings regardless of the type of electrosurgical generator used. Nevertheless, stethoscope monitoring of cardiac contractions remains vital.

3. The routine admonition to use the lowest possible setting of the output control on the electrosurgical unit is especially pertinent.

4. Electrosurgery should be used in brief bursts lasting but a few seconds, with interspersed pauses sufficient to assess cardiac status.

5. If serious interference is encountered and electrosurgery is a necessity, the pacemaker generally can be converted to the fixed-rate mode by taping a magnet to the overlying skin. Conversion is verified by observing the regular pacing spikes on the ECG monitor. However, it is important to be certain of the characteristics of the pacemaker before this conversion is attempted. As was previously discussed, a few pacemakers can be programmed by pulses of radio-frequency energy. Such pacemakers are "enabled" or placed in a mode to receive these pulses by a magnetic signal. Thus, placement of a magnet over this type of pacemaker must be avoided to prevent possible random reprogramming by the electrosurgery.

ANESTHESIA FOR THE PACEMAKER PATIENT

Because cardiac pacemakers are worn by approximately 0.08% of the US population and because this group is generally of an age afflicted with a significant number of other infirmities, a number of patients with pacemakers undergo surgery.

A patient whose heart requires electronic pacing is not, by definition, placed in Physical Status I of the American Society of Anesthesiologists' classification. Nevertheless, a properly functioning pacemaker permits many patients in whom the hazard of anesthesia and operation would otherwise be almost prohibitive to withstand these stresses without incident. Obviously, continued proper function of the pacemaker is crucial, and the pacing system, as well as the patient, may be stressed during surgery. A system whose function is marginal under normal conditions may fail completely when it is most needed.

Apart from malfunction of the electronic timing circuit secondary to interference, the greatest hazard is the loss of capture. Capture may be lost as the result of increased threshold of depolarization or of inadequate stimulus. The cause of the latter may lie outside the generator as the result of electrode displacement, lead fracture, or insulation disruption, or within the generator, as with component failure or battery depletion.

Preoperative evaluation in a pacemaker clinic can be most helpful in determining whether pacing function is intact and is likely to remain so or if the system should be replaced before surgery. In addition to history and physical examination, the pacemaker clinic will generally use over-penetrated x-ray films, multiple-lead ECG, and scrutiny of the generator artifact. According to Furman,[5] evaluation of generator artifact provides the most reliable analysis of electrode disruption and surpasses roentgenography in the detection of partial lead fracture and insulation failure. In most generators, it also indicates the condition of the battery, by changes either in pacing rate or in artifact morphology. (Generators with "energy compensation" are designed to increase the duration of stimulus as battery voltage decreases. This action tends to maintain a stable output of energy but is an indication for immediate attention.)

Some assessment of pacemaker function can be made by the anesthesiologist during preoperative rounds. Return of symptoms that existed before pacemaker placement, such as light-headedness or syncope, suggests loss of capture. Palpitations may indicate loss of sensing function. As previously mentioned, with a ventricular-inhibited pacemaker operating in the inhibited mode, a weak battery is most reliably detected by magnetically converting the pacer to asynchronous operation and determining the pacing rate. This method requires the availability of the specification sheet that relates pacemaker "magnet rate" and battery voltage.

Threshold of depolarization ordinarily increases considerably during the first few weeks after implantation of the pacemaker. The threshold then tends to stabilize, although there may be a gradual upward drift thereafter. At installation, pacemaker output is set several times higher than the anticipated chronic threshold to provide a margin of safety.

Illness and operation may be accompanied by acute alterations in threshold. Sepsis produces threshold instability.[17] (Fever can alter the output voltage of the battery in an implanted pacemaker[5]; rate changes must be interpreted with caution in a febrile patient.) Lack of physical activity is often associated with an elevated threshold; pacemaker patients have reported awakening from sleep with a slow, irregular pulse and having normal pacing restored on getting out of bed and moving about.[15] (This condition warrants immediate investigation.)

Little information is available regarding the effect on threshold produced by most anesthetics and other pharmacologic agents used by the anesthesiologist. Scott[17] cautions against the use of repeated doses of succinylcholine, although such doses have been given without problems. Metocurine, with its benign cardiovascular effects[16] and the lack of associated muscle fasciculations (vigorous fasciculations are accompanied by electrical activity that a sensing circuit might confound with that of the QRS complex), appears to be an appropriate muscle relaxant for the patient with a pacemaker.

The effects of the serum potassium level on threshold are not clear-cut. One factor affecting the threshold is the ratio of intracellular to extracellular potassium. An acute elevation of extracellular potassium decreases the quotient and tends to decrease the threshold. Loss of capture associated with hypokalemia has been reported,[1] as has pacing failure induced by hyperkalemia.[12] The latter study pointed out that "the effects of potassium on the threshold for stimulation are complex and variable, depending on the absolute serum level, the intracellular-extracellular gradient, the overall electrolyte status, and the tissue involved (nodal, Purkinje, or muscle)."

Propranolol, quinidine, hypercarbia, and slight hypoxia all increase threshold. However, severe hypoxia lowers threshold. Digitalis, morphine, lidocaine, and procainamide produce little change.[6]

Although an increased threshold may produce loss of capture, a decreased threshold is also hazardous because ventricular fibrillation may then be more easily induced.[21] The most common pharmacologic agents that lower threshold are the sympathomimetic amines.

Threshold is increased by mineralocorticoids and is decreased by glucocorticoids, according to Preston and Judge.[15] They observed that these changes can be used clinically when alteration of the threshold is indicated.

Positioning under anesthesia of the patient with a pacemaker must be done with special care. Because cardiac compensatory mechanisms are compromised, sudden changes in position may produce severe hypotension. A problem unique to these patients is the possible dislodgment of the pacing electrodes or the breakage of wires secondary to position changes, if the wires are placed under tension. Blood pressure and heart sounds should be monitored especially closely when the patient is being moved.

Cessation of pacing during anesthesia may be nothing more than a normal response to a cardiac rate sufficient to suppress a pacemaker designed to be so inhibited. But loss of pacing associated with significant hemodynamic changes indicates a failure in the pacemaker system. If the cause cannot be quickly diagnosed, an isoproterenol drip should be started. Zaidan[22] recommended adding 1 mg of isoproterenol to 250 ml of 5% dextrose in water and starting the infusion at a rate of 1 to 3 µg (0.25 to 0.75 ml) per minute.

Beyond the special precautions previously discussed, the patient with a pacemaker requires anesthetic management determined by his cardiac status and by the nature of the surgical procedure. The heart block or dysrhythmia for which pacing is required is often a manifestation of an underlying cardiac disorder, such as pericarditis, coronary artery disease, calcific aortic stenosis, rheumatic heart disease, or cardiomyopathy. The anesthesiologist may choose to use a monitoring system that is rather simple or one that is quite extensive.

Decisions regarding administration of intravenous fluids are aided by monitoring urinary output and trends in the central venous pressure. A Swan-Ganz catheter can provide additional information regarding fluid balance and cardiac performance. Indirect measurement of arterial pressure is facilitated in the obese or vasoconstricted patient by use of a Doppler device. An arterial catheter can provide continuous blood pressure measurement, as well as samples for arterial blood gas and electrolyte determinations. Although some patients can be managed satisfactorily without any of these measuring techniques, continuous monitoring of the ECG and of heart sounds is important in all patients with a pacemaker.

A knowledge of the anatomy and physiology of pacemakers is useful to the anesthesiologist caring for a patient with a pacemaker. Various anesthetic techniques have been used successfully in such patients.

REFERENCES

1. Al-Abdulla H.M., Lulu D.J.: Hypokalemia and pacemaker failure. *Am. Surg.* 40:234, 1974.
2. Barold S.S.: Current problems with demand pacemakers. *Eur. J. Cardiol.* 1:339, 1974.
3. Curtis J.J., et al.: A critical look at temporary ventricular pacing following cardiac surgery. *Surgery* 82:888, 1977.
4. EMI compatibility and the pacemaker patient. *Medtronic News* 6(no. 1):6, 1976.
5. Furman S.: Cardiac pacing and pacemakers: VIII. The pacemaker follow-up clinic. *Am. Heart J.* 94:795, 1977.
6. Furman S.: Physiologic basis of cardiac pacing, in Varriale P., Naclerio E.A. (eds.): *Cardiac Pacing.* Philadelphia, Lea & Febiger, 1979, p. 59.
7. Furman S., Hurzeler P., Mehra R.: Cardiac pacing and pacemakers: IV. Threshold of cardiac stimulation. *Am. Heart J.* 94:115, 1977.
8. Green G.D.: *The Assessment and Performance of Implanted Cardiac Pacemakers.* London, Butterworth & Co., 1975, p. 31.
9. McGuire L.B., O'Brien W.M., Nolan S.P.: Patient survival and instrument performance with permanent cardiac pacing. *J.A.M.A.* 237:558, 1977.
10. Obel I., Citron P.: Atrial demand and A-V sequential pacing: Limitations and benefits. *Medtronic News* 8(no. 4):3, 1978.
11. O'Donoghue J.K.: Inhibition of a demand pacemaker by electrosurgery. *Chest* 64:664, 1973.
12. O'Reilly M.V., Murnaghan D.P., Williams M.B.: Transvenous pacemaker failure induced by hyperkalemia. *J.A.M.A.* 228:336, 1974.
13. Parsonnet V., Furman S., Smyth N.P.D.: Implantable cardiac pacemakers status report and resource guideline: Pacemaker study group. *Circulation* 50:A-21, 1974.
14. Patients write, column. *Medtronic News* 8(no. 2):5, 1978.
15. Preston T.A., Judge R.D.: Alteration of pacemaker threshold by drug and physiological factors. *Ann. N.Y. Acad. Sci.* 167:686, 1969.
16. Savarese J.J., Ali H.H., Antonio R.P.: The clinical pharmacology of metocurine: Dimethyltubocurarine revisited. *Anesthesiology* 47:277, 1977.
17. Scott D.L.: Cardiac pacemakers as an anesthetic problem. *Anaesthesia* 25:87, 1970.
18. Smyth N.P.D.: Cardiac pacing. *Ann. Thorac. Surg.* 27:270, 1979.
19. Smyth N.P.D., et al.: The significance of electrode surface area and stimulating thresholds in permanent cardiac pacing. *J. Thorac. Cardiovasc. Surg.* 71:559, 1976.
20. Walter C.W.: Cholecystectomy in patient with pacemaker. *J.A.M.A.* 218:1305, 1971.
21. Wynands J.E.: Anesthesia for patients with heart block and artificial cardiac pacemakers. *Anesth. Analg.* 55:626, 1976.
22. Zaidan J.R.: Pacemakers, in Kaplan J.A. (ed.): *Cardiac Anesthesia.* New York, Grune & Stratton, 1979.

22 / Anesthesia for Cardiovascular Diagnostic Procedures

CARL R. NOBACK
HUGO S. RAIMUNDO
SAIT TARHAN

A WIDE RANGE of patients, from the premature neonate to the debilitated elderly patient with severe coronary artery disease, may be seen for evaluation of cardiovascular physiologic and anatomical status. When noninvasive techniques are insufficient for diagnosis or when anatomical or physiologic definition is necessary before surgical intervention, these patients may require invasive cardiovascular diagnostic procedures. Among these operations are cardiac catheterization, angiography of the coronary and more peripheral arteries, and aortography.

Cardiac catheterization was described by Forssman[11] in 1929, but it was not until 1941 that Cournand and Ranges[7] used it as a diagnostic tool. Significant advances in the diagnosis and treatment of the anatomical and physiologic defects present in congenital and acquired heart disease have been made. Additional techniques are being developed, and new ones, such as the dynamic spatial reconstructor,[32] undoubtedly will be introduced. At this time, the mainstay for qualitative and quantitative determination of cardiac function remains cardiac catheterization and angiography of the heart and the great and peripheral vessels.

THE STEADY STATE AND THE ROLE OF THE ANESTHETIST

Information gathered during cardiac catheterization includes blood pressure and oxygen content of the chambers of the heart, pulmonary vasculature, aorta, and venae cavae. Abnormal communication may be evaluated with the data obtained. Because most of the blood sampling and pressure determinations at the various sites cannot be determined simultaneously, a steady cardiovascular state is required during the investigation to allow comparison of the pressures observed and oxygen saturations determined[21] to arrive at an exact diagnosis.

A steady state, with a constant heart rate, ventilation, and oxygen consumption,[14] is required for the calculation of shunt fractions and cardiac output by the Fick principle (the amount of a substance taken up by a tissue is equal to the arterial level of the substance minus the venous level times blood flow). Assessment of restrictions to flow (that is, the pressure gradient across a stenotic valve that is proportional to the square of the flow) also requires a steady state.[20] The steady state is assumed to exist when there is a minimum of anxiety in the patient, a patent airway is maintained, respirations are regular (whether spontaneous or controlled), oxygen consumption and the composition of inspired gases are unchanged, heart rate and muscular activity are stable, drugs with unknown or unpredictable effects on these factors have been avoided, and a steady state of consciousness exists.[18] These criteria are difficult to meet, but herein lies one of the major functions of an anesthetist during cardiovascular diagnostic procedures, namely, to provide as close as possible a steady state by using anesthetic techniques that produce similar physiologic changes from patient to patient, so that the final diagnosis does not need to consider changes in administered drugs. Additional roles of the anesthetist include the following: prevention, diagnosis, and treatment of complications (including resuscitation); monitoring of vital signs; comforting the patient to reduce anxiety due to unfamiliar surroundings, noise, lying on a hard table with a fluoroscopic tower overhead, and so forth; and providing the appropriate sedative, analgesic, or anesthetic technique.

ANESTHESIA FOR CARDIAC CATHETERIZATION

General Considerations

Cardiac catheterization allows the measurement of pressures in the great vessels and chambers of the heart and the determination of oxygen content at the same locations (Tables 22–1 and 22–2). Right heart catheterization is most commonly accomplished by approaches from the brachial or median cephalic vein, although the femoral or jugular veins may be used in adults and the axillary and femoral veins are optional approaches in the pediatric patient. The tip of the catheter is directed through the great veins to the right atrium, right ventricle, and pulmonary artery and finally to the pulmonary capillary wedge positions. Left heart catheterization is most commonly performed in a retrograde fashion from the femoral or brachial arteries, although left ventricular pressures can be measured by transthoracic puncture through the chest wall if passage through the aortic valve is unsuccessful.

Cardiac catheterization is not a particularly painful procedure; however, significant discomfort, nausea, or vomiting may occur during insertion or withdrawal of the catheter. The extremely young or uncooperative patient presents difficulties in management. As stated, and since accurate diagnosis is predicated on reliable data, a steady cardiorespiratory state is necessary.

Catheterization of the neonate is commonly performed on an emergency basis, either because the child is extremely ill, with deterioration imminent, or because corrective surgery is contemplated. A scheme for the classification of the severity of illness has been designed by Stanger et al.[31] (Table 22–3). Physical status may be such that sedation is unnecessary in these patients. Because of the severity of illness, cardiorespiratory arrest during the procedure is not a rarity. Most of these patients, therefore, are intubated and artificially ventilated.[23]

Respiratory Effects of Drugs

OXYGEN.—The use of supplemental oxygen in these infants is fraught with hazards. Constriction of the ductus arteriosus in infants with aortic stenosis, aortic arch interruption, or coarctation of the aorta has been blamed on increased FIO_2.[24] Infants with these lesions should receive supplemental oxygen if the PaO_2 is reduced below 35 mm Hg.[31] An increase in FIO_2 causes venous oxygen content to increase, thereby reducing the difference between venous

TABLE 22–1.—Normal Pressure Values in the Heart and Great Vessels*

PARAMETER	AVERAGE, MM HG	RANGE, MM HG
Mean right atrium	2.8	1 to 5
Right ventricle		
Systolic	25	17 to 32
End-diastolic	4	1 to 7
Pulmonary artery		
Systolic	25	17 to 32
End-diastolic	9	4 to 13
Mean	15	9 to 19
Pulmonary capillary wedge pressure	9	4.5 to 13
Mean left atrium	7.9	2 to 12
Left ventricle		
Systolic	130	90 to 140
End-diastolic	8.7	5 to 12
Systemic artery		
Systolic	130	90 to 140
Diastolic	70	60 to 90
Mean	85	70 to 105

*Modified from Yang S.Y., et al.: *From Cardiac Catheterization Data to Hemodynamic Parameters*. Philadelphia, F. A. Davis Co., 1972, p. 38.

TABLE 22–2.—Normal Oxygen Saturation in the Heart and Great Vessels*

SITE	RANGE OF OXYGEN SATURATION, %
Superior vena cava	70–75
Inferior vena cava	75–80
Coronary sinus	30–40
Right atrium	70–75
Right ventricle	70–75
Pulmonary artery	70–75
Pulmonary capillaries	98–100
Left atrium	95–98
Left ventricle	95–98
Aorta	95–97

*Modified from Wilson R.F. (ed.): *Principles and Techniques of Critical Care*. Kalamazoo, Mich., The Upjohn Company, 1976, p. 8.

TABLE 22–3.—CLASSIFICATION OF ILLNESS OF NEONATES UNDERGOING CARDIAC CATHETERIZATION*

CLASS	COMMENT
Mildly ill	Nondistressed, nonacidotic but hypoxemic babies with a PO_2 greater than 25 mm Hg, or those in controlled congestive failure
Moderately ill	(1) Intensely hypoxemic babies with a PO_2 of less than 25 mm Hg but without metabolic acidosis or (2) infants in severe congestive failure, poorly controlled with digitalis and diuretics
Critically ill	Neonates with one or more of the following: (1) requiring ventilatory assistance, (2) profound hypoxemia with acidemia, or (3) poor peripheral perfusion resulting in a shock-like pattern or pronounced acidemia (pH <7.1, base excess >-12)

*From Stanger et al.[31] Used by permission.

and arterial oxygen saturation. Small errors in calculating hemoglobin saturation for determining oxygen content could lead to large errors in cardiac output and shunt determinations.[20] Pulmonary vascular resistance and pulmonary artery pressure may be reduced by an increased FIO_2,[20] and diagnostic accuracy may be adversely affected. Between 25% and 40% oxygen can be used safely in these infants.[24]

Hypoxemia also may be a problem in these children and may manifest itself by irritability, tachypnea, intercostal or sternal retractions, increased use of the accessory muscles of breathing, increase in cyanosis, and depression of consciousness. Patients with severe pulmonic stenosis, right-to-left shunts, and inadequate aortopulmonary shunting are more likely to develop hypoxemia.[31] Partial occlusion of a stenotic pulmonary outflow tract with a catheter also may lead to hypoxemia.[16] Respiratory depression from premedicants also may result in hypoxemia, and the effect on central respiratory centers of all drugs used must be considered. Although increased FIO_2 may produce problems, oxygen can be a life-saving agent and should not be withheld if it is necessary for survival. In children with large right-to-left shunt or severe heart failure, an FIO_2 greater than 0.4 may be required.[20]

MEPERIDINE-PROMETHAZINE-CHLORPROMAZINE.—The effects of the premedicant combination, first used by Smith et al.,[29] of meperidine, chlorpromazine, and promethazine on $PaCO_2$ in infants was studied by Nicholson and Graham.[25] With a solution of 25 mg of meperidine, 6.25 mg of chlorpromazine, and 6.25 mg of promethazine per 1 ml and giving 1 ml/9 kg (20 lb) of body weight, they observed no effect on ventilation, as judged by $PaCO_2$, except in infants in congestive failure and with increased pulmonary blood flow, with or without pulmonary hypertension. These infants had either large left-to-right shunts (ventricular septal defects, patent ductus arteriosus) or left-sided lesions (aortic stenosis, hypoplastic left ventricle). Avoidance of premedicants in the acyanotic infant with congestive heart failure and respiratory difficulty should be contemplated.

DIAZEPAM.—The use of intravenously administered diazepam, 1 mg/kg, after premedication with the meperidine-promethazine-chlorpromazine mixture resulted in no alteration of $PaCO_2$.[15] Maintenance of a patent airway was similarly unaffected.

Circulatory Effects of Drugs

MEPERIDINE-PROMETHAZINE-CHLORPROMAZINE.—The anesthetist should be cognizant of the effects of the various premedicants, sedative agents, and anesthetic agents on circulatory dynamics. The introduction of the combination of meperidine, promethazine, and chlorpromazine has resulted in a decreased need for general anesthesia for cardiac catheterization.[29] Parenterally administered meperidine-promethazine-chlorpromazine decreases oxygen consumption and enhances the tendency of sick infants to develop metabolic acidosis.[1, 17] Goldberg et al.[13] showed that, in the intact unanesthetized dog, an infusion of 2 mg of meperidine, 1 mg of promethazine, and 1 mg of chlorpromazine per kilogram caused significant pulmonary vasoconstriction and systemic vasodilatation. Active pulmonary vasoconstriction was found, and promethazine and chlorpromazine were responsible. Meperidine decreases cardiac output and passively increases pulmonary vascular resistance. Meperidine also has been reported to be a coronary and systemic vasodilator and vagolytic agent. Chlorpromazine, because of its α-adrenergic blocking properties and central actions, causes vasodilatation and compensatory cardiac acceleration; however, the implications of these findings in the actual clinical setting are not clear. Promethazine may have quinidine-like properties.[22] Shackman et al.[28] observed tachycardia and decreased systemic resistance after meperidine-promethazine-chlorpromazine use in 15 adults. In 670 patients premedicated with meperidine-promethazine-chlorpromazine, Smith et al.[29] found no consistent changes in systemic or pulmonary artery pressures.

KETAMINE.—Ketamine has been proposed as a suitable anesthetic agent for cardiac catheterization because of its cardiac stability.[6] Coppel and Dundee,[5] using doses of ketamine of 10 mg/kg intramuscularly with 1 mg/kg intravenous supplementary doses in infants, found a mean maximal increase in blood pressure of 22 mm Hg systolic and 16 mm Hg diastolic four minutes after the administration of the induction dose. An increase in pressure was most dramatic (mean increase, 43 and 25 mm Hg in systolic and diastolic, respectively) in patients with coarctation of the aorta. This change was accompanied by an increase in pulmonary artery pressure and could therefore "result in erroneous data from the cardiac catheterization." Arterial pressure returned to control levels within 16 minutes, and supplementary injections did not produce a further increase in pressure. Gassner et al.[12] also observed increased pulmonary artery pressure and pulmonary blood flow in 250 infants. They postulated that such effects were secondary to effects on cardiac output because of variable effects on pulmonary vascular resistance.

Ketamine was shown to be a potent pulmonary vasoconstrictor by De Master and Fogdall,[9] even at doses as low as 0.25 mg/kg intravenously. Ketamine in doses of 2 mg/kg intravenously increases arterial pressure, heart rate, and cardiac index in normal patients and in patients with coronary artery disease.[33] The same dose in patients with valvular heart disease increases mean pulmonary artery pressure and pulmonary vascular resistance.[26] De Master and Fogdall also found that, in patients with coronary artery disease, the rate pressure product as an index of myocardial oxygen consumption increases with dosages of ketamine between 0.25 and 2 mg/kg intravenously. Edde,[10] like De Master and Fogdall, found that total pulmonary vascular resistance (mean pulmonary artery pressure divided by flow) is increased by ketamine in dosages from 1 to 4 mg/kg intravenously and that ketamine is a potent pulmonary vasoconstrictor. Ketamine, therefore, should not be used if pressure measurements are to be made within 20 minutes of administration and is probably best avoided in patients in whom accurate pulmonary artery pressures are required for diagnosis. The pressure response to ketamine is blunted by premedication with droperidol,[12] which may decrease systemic pressure,[20] mean pulmonary artery pressure, and pulmonary vascular resistance.

DIAZEPAM.—Intravenously administered diazepam, 1 mg/kg, has been used both as a primary anesthetic agent and to supplement meperidine-promethazine-chlorpromazine. Healy[15] found that this dosage minimally affected blood pressure and heart rate. While ventilation rate increased in 62% of the patients, no alteration was found in Pa_{CO_2}.

HALOTHANE.—Halothane is used commonly as an anesthetic for pediatric cardiac catheterization. In large doses, it can be a myocardial depressant and may sensitize the heart to epinephrine, with the subsequent development of arrhythmias. When used judiciously, up to 2% halothane, 30% oxygen, and 70% nitrous oxide provide an adequately anesthetized patient and allow the collection of sufficient data to arrive at an accurate diagnosis.[5, 20, 21]

ATROPINE.—Pretreatment with atropine is generally unnecessary; the drying properties are not required in the awake patient, and the potential tachycardia may be deleterious. Intensely cyanotic newborns, however, are particularly likely to experience sinus bradycardia which, because neonates have only a limited ability to increase stroke volume, may have profound circulatory effects. This group may be treated with atropine, 0.01 mg/kg, preoperatively to avoid bradycardia. This treatment decreases the cyanosis, possibly because of dilatation of a patent ductus arteriosus. Generally, hemodynamically significant bradycardias should be treated with intravenously administered atropine.

CONTRAST MEDIUM.—Choice and dose of the contrast medium also may affect outcome of the catheterization. Complications related to the use of contrast medium include arrhythmias, pulmonary edema, and cerebral and renal dysfunctions. Meglumine derivatives are safer than sodium derivatives in pediatric patients.[31] Renografin-76 has been used in doses of 4 ml/kg in children, 3 ml/kg in infants, and 1.0 to 1.5 ml/kg in premature infants. Risk of renal complications is high in neonates, and the contrast medium is diluted to a 40% concentration with saline.[31] In patients whose cardiac chambers are small or in whom the aortic arch is to be outlined, the dose of contrast medium should be 0.8 to 1.0 ml/kg.[4] The use of contrast medium should be kept to a minimum, particularly in infants, because more complications occur as a result of angiocardiography than from any other part of the catheterization procedure.[31]

Controlled Versus Spontaneous Ventilation

In the anesthetized infant undergoing cardiac catheterization, controlled ventilation may affect the data obtained. $PaCO_2$ decreases in approximately three fourths of patients for whom ventilation is controlled.[21] Similarly, mixed venous oxygen content decreases and the left-to-right shunt increases. Cardiac output may decrease with the transition from spontaneous to controlled ventilation. Two significant physiologic changes that may occur during controlled ventilation are a decrease in $PaCO_2$ and an increase in intrathoracic pressure. These findings may alter the catheterization findings, although Manners and Codman[21] found that, when coupled with the clinical findings, the differences in calculated data were not sufficient to alter the diagnosis.

Anesthesia for Pediatric Cardiac Catheterization

Premedication and Sedation

The night before the procedure, pediatric patients are given 2 mg of pentobarbital per kilogram, rectally in children less than 6 years old and orally in others. Manners[20] recommended an additional dose four hours before the procedure. Infants less than 1 year old receive nothing by mouth four hours before the procedure, whereas other children receive nothing by mouth eight hours before the procedure. Neonates undergoing emergency catheterization are neither given medications nor fasted before the procedure. Ill neonates may require nothing other than local anesthesia at the insertion site of the catheter.

Approximately 30 minutes before the procedure, children weighing more than 4.5 kg (10 lb) or older than 3 months receive an intramuscular injection of meperidine-promethazine-chlorpromazine. Each milliliter of meperidine-promethazine-chlorpromazine contains 25 mg of meperidine, 6.25 mg of promethazine, and 6.25 mg of chlorpromazine. Dosage is on a weight-related basis, 1.2 ml/9 kg (20 lb), up to 3 ml total (Table 22–4). Administration of the drug combination by this method has been satisfactory in our experience and has produced satisfactory sedation (defined as requiring no further sedation during the procedure) in more than 80% of infants.[30] If further sedation is required during the procedure, or if the patient is restless on arrival in the procedure room, an additional dose of meperidine-promethazine-chlorpromazine of one fourth to one half the original mixture can be given at intervals of one hour.[6] Infants weighing less than 4.5 kg (10 lb) and less than 3 months of age are not premedicated. They are given a small amount of brandy during the procedure, and the catheter is inserted under local anesthesia with 1% lidocaine (without epinephrine) to a maximal dose of 3 mg/kg.[6] In selected patients, we use an oral form of meperidine-promethazine-chlorpromazine (Table 22–5). The extensive sedation seen in some infants with the intramuscular injection and the pain of the injection itself are obviated, although the oral preparation is less effective. We find it unnecessary to produce heavy sedation in the pediatric group. Atropine may be used as a premedicant, in a dose of 0.01 mg/kg, for intensely cyanotic patients.

Monitoring

The ECG is monitored for all patients undergoing cardiac catheterization. Vital signs are monitored closely and, in our institution, are available from the computer operator once the catheter is in place, thus providing beat-by-beat hemodynamic data. Because neonates lose body heat more readily than other patients, temperature is monitored with a rectal thermistor, and they are placed on an insulated warming mattress. Acid-base balance is monitored, as are PaO_2 and $PaCO_2$. In neonates, a previously placed umbilical artery catheter is used to withdraw samples. Blood glucose levels are moni-

inattentiveness may occur. Because of the possibility of complications, great attention to detail is required. Pride can be taken in assisting the patient to come through an arduous procedure with a minimum of discomfort and without significant cardiorespiratory embarrassment. No single technique is correct and appropriate in every situation, and one must be aware of other techniques that may be required in specific circumstances. No method is infallible, and each technique has its shortcomings. However, it is important that, in a particular institution, a particular technique is generally followed to allow accurate assessment of the anatomical and physiologic data gathered in that institution and thereby increase diagnostic accuracy and improve patient care.

REFERENCES

1. Baum D., Brown A.C., Church S.C.: Effect of sedation on oxygen consumption of children undergoing cardiac catheterization. *Pediatrics* 39:891, 1967.
2. Benzing G. III, et al.: Simultaneous hypoglycemia and acute congestive heart failure. *Circulation* 40:209, 1969.
3. Braunwald E., Swan H.J.C.: Cooperative study on cardiac catheterization. *Circulation* 37(suppl. 3):1, 1968.
4. Cardiac Laboratory Procedure Manual, Mayo Clinic.
5. Coppel D.L., Dundee J.W.: Ketamine anaesthesia for cardiac catheterisation. *Anaesthesia* 27:25, 1972.
6. Corssen G., et al.: Ketamine as the sole anesthetic in open-heart surgery: A preliminary report. *Anesth. Analg.* 49:1025, 1970.
7. Cournand and Ranges, cited by McMichael J.: Foreword, in Verel D., Grainger R.G. (eds.): *Cardiac Catheterization and Angiography*, ed. 3. Edinburgh, Churchill Livingstone, 1978, p. v.
8. De Bakey M.E., Lawrie G.M.: Response to commentary of Hultgren et al. on 'Aortocoronary-Artery-Bypass: Assessment After 13 Years.' *J.A.M.A.* 241:2393, 1979.
9. De Master R.J., Fogdall R.P.: The effects of ketamine on the pulmonary and systemic circulations in patients with coronary artery disease. Abstracted in the Scientific Papers of the American Society of Anesthesiologists Annual Meeting, 1977, p. 721.
10. Edde R.R.: The effect of ketamine on pulmonary vascular resistance. Abstracted in the Scientific Papers of the American Society of Anesthesiologists Annual Meeting, 1977, p. 723.
11. Forssman, cited by McMichael J.: Foreword, in Verel D., Grainger R.G. (eds.): *Cardiac Catheterization and Angiography*, ed. 3. Edinburgh, Churchill Livingstone, 1978, p. v.
12. Gassner S., et al.: The effect of ketamine on pulmonary artery pressure: An experimental and clinical study. *Anaesthesia* 29:141, 1974.
13. Goldberg S.J., et al.: The effects of meperidine, promethazine, and chlorpromazine on pulmonary and systemic circulation. *Am. Heart J.* 77:214, 1969.
14. Gordon B.L., Carleton R.A., Faber L.P.: *Clinical Cardiopulmonary Physiology*, ed. 3. New York, Grune & Stratton, 1969.
15. Healy T.E.J.: Intravenous diazepam for cardiac catheterisation. *Anaesthesia* 24:537, 1969.
16. Hoffman J.I.E., et al.: Physiologic differentiation of pulmonic stenosis with and without an intact ventricular septum. *Circulation* 22:385, 1960.
17. Israel R., et al.: Evaluation of sedation during cardiac catheterization of children: Analysis of PaO_2, $PaCO_2$, pH, and base excess determinations during hemodynamic investigation. *J. Pediatr.* 70:407, 1967.
18. Korten K.: Anesthesia for diagnostic procedures. *Am. Fam. Physician* 15:103, March 1977.
19. Lown B., et al.: 'Cardioversion' of atrial fibrillation: A report on the treatment of 65 episodes in 50 patients. *N. Engl. J. Med.* 269:325, 1963.
20. Manners J.M.: Anaesthesia for diagnostic procedures in cardiac disease. *Br. J. Anaesth.* 43:276, 1971.
21. Manners J.M., Codman V.A.: General anaesthesia for cardiac catheterisation in children: The effect of spontaneous or controlled ventilation on the evaluation of congenital abnormalities. *Anaesthesia* 24:541, 1969.
22. Meyers F.H., Jawetz E., Goldfien A.: *Review of Medical Pharmacology*, ed. 5. Los Altos, Calif., Lange Medical Publications, 1976.
23. Moffitt E.A., Dawson B., O'Neill N.C.: Anesthesia for pediatric cardiac catheterization and angiocardiography. *Anesth. Analg.* 40:483, 1961.
24. Moffitt E.A., McGoon D.C., Ritter D.G.: The diagnosis and correction of congenital cardiac defects. *Anesthesiology* 33:144, 1970.
25. Nicholson J.R., Graham G.R.: Management of infants under six months of age undergoing cardiac investigation. *Br. J. Anaesth.* 41:417, 1969.
26. Savege T.M., et al.: A comparison of some car-

diorespiratory effects of althesin and ketamine when used for induction of anaesthesia in patients with cardiac disease. *Br. J. Anaesth.* 48:1071, 1976.
27. Sellick B.A.: Cricoid pressure to control regurgitation of stomach contents during induction of anaesthesia. *Lancet* 2:404, 1961.
28. Shackman R., et al.: The 'lytic cocktail': Observations on surgical patients. *Lancet* 2:617, 1954.
29. Smith C., Rowe R.D., Vlad P.: Sedation of children for cardiac catheterization with an ataractic mixture. *Can. Anaesth. Soc. J.* 5:35, 1958.
30. Standards for cardiopulmonary resuscitation (CPR) and emergency cardiac care (ECC). *J.A.M.A.* 227(suppl.):833, 1974.
31. Stanger P., et al.: Complications of cardiac catheterization of neonates, infants, and children: A three-year study. *Circulation* 50:595, 1974.
32. Swanson D.E. (ed.): The dynamic spatial reconstructor: A six-part series. *Mayo Alumnus* 15:1, 1979.
33. Tweed W.A., Minuck M., Mymin D.: Circulatory responses to ketamine anesthesia. *Anesthesiology* 37:613, 1972.
34. Verel D., Grainger R.G.: *Cardiac Catheterization and Angiocardiography*, ed. 3. Edinburgh, Churchill Livingstone, 1978, p. 139.

23 / Postoperative Management of the Cardiac Surgical Patient: General Introduction

H. MICHAEL MARSH
PETER A. SOUTHORN

SINCE the inception of cardiac surgery nearly three decades ago, the demand for it in the United States has steadily increased. In 1980, cardiac surgery for acquired heart disease was performed on approximately 130,000 adult Americans. Of the 3.1 million Americans with known coronary artery disease, about 600,000 die of the disease each year, while approximately 100,000 undergo coronary artery bypass grafting.[3, 7] Approximately 14,000 deaths occur each year from rheumatic heart disease, and 20,000 to 30,000 patients are treated with cardiac valve replacements.[2] In addition to these adults, approximately 25,000 to 30,000 babies with congenital heart defects are born each year in the United States.[2] Until the last decade, many of the infants with complex cardiac lesions were considered to be inoperable and many died. Those who survived to adulthood either had mild abnormalities or had undergone relatively simple, often only palliative, surgery. Technical advances during the past ten years have permitted physiologic correction of the heart lesions in many of these infants.

The increased demand for cardiac surgery has followed technical advances and improved survival rates. The survival of patients who have undergone cardiac surgery or general surgery in the presence of cardiac disease is largely determined by their preoperative functional state,[5, 6, 8] the standard of surgical performance, and the quality of anesthetic and postoperative supportive care. Postoperative care comprises three components: good nursing, continued accurate monitoring and support of the cardiorespiratory and other vital systems, and the prevention or treatment of complications.

Cardiac surgical patients are not a homogeneous group. Thus, in assessing the needs of the individual patient during the postoperative period, several factors should be considered. The severity of the cardiac defect varies, as do its effects on both the cardiovascular and other body systems, including the lungs and kidneys. Patients also may have concomitant noncardiac illness of varying severity, such as chronic obstructive lung disease or diabetes. Finally, the nature, duration, and complexity of the operative procedure differ among patients, even among those with similar lesions.

This chapter outlines the general principles of intensive care, specifying general procedures for the safe transfer from the operating suite to the intensive care unit and for the reception and assessment of the patient on arrival at the unit.

POSTOPERATIVE CARDIAC CARE UNIT

The postoperative cardiac care unit should be near the operating rooms. The hazards of transfer of the patient to the postoperative cardiac care unit at the end of surgery and of retransfer back to the operating room, should that be necessary, are then reduced.

Minimal standards for critical care units have been defined.[1] Each patient area in the unit should have an adjacent service area to accommodate the necessary apparatus and support systems, including underwater chest drains, mechanical ventilator, intra-aortic balloon pump, intravenous solutions and drug pumps, and monitoring equipment. One nurse can continually supervise two patients, if they are in the same room. Some patients (for example, those with infections and those who require a longer-than-normal stay in the unit) require isolation rooms and one-to-one nursing. Thus, some individual rooms also should be available. All patient areas should be visible from the central nursing station, and there must be a voice page and an additional alarm system at each bedside to allow the nurse to summon help as required. The patient should be able to be weighed daily. Adequate lighting and air conditioning are necessary.

Cardiorespiratory resuscitation equipment (a defibrillator, endotracheal intubation equipment, emergency drugs, and surgical instruments) must be available in the unit.[4] Such equipment should be checked daily for proper function and completeness. Measurements of blood gas and hematocrit levels, as well as urinalysis, are ideally performed in a small laboratory adjacent to the unit so that the results may become immediately available to the clinician. A separate conference room for discussions of patient management and for the viewing of roentgenograms is desirable. Accommodation for the medical staff in attendance is required. Finally, the patient's relatives should be provided with a pleasant waiting room nearby, with separate cubicles for those who need privacy.

STAFFING

An excellent staff, cooperating as a team, is a crucial element in providing postcardiac surgical intensive care. A physician member of the operating team should be continually available in the unit, coordinating the care for the patient. This aspect is important because several medical disciplines may be involved. The surgeon, cardiologist, and anesthesiologist should cooperate in devising a plan of management. The anesthesiologist will make a valuable contribution to the unit. His expertise in cardiopulmonary pathophysiology and respiratory support and his knowledge of resuscitative procedures are vital. Junior anesthesiologists learning these skills can gain much by working in the unit, but they should be supervised by a more experienced colleague.

Because the nursing care for these critically ill patients is both physically and psychologically stressful, the units should have an adequately trained registered nursing staff. Safety may be jeopardized if junior nurses are unsupervised, although they provide valuable help to their trained nursing colleagues and gain much knowledge and experience by working in such units. Respiratory therapists, with their knowledge of ventilators and other respiratory equipment, contribute significantly to patient care, as do trained monitoring technicians.

All medical, nursing, and paramedical staff working in the unit should be cognizant of unit policy in the management of emergencies. Ideally, all paramedical and nursing staff should be proficient in basic life support, and all medical staff should be proficient in advanced life support.[4]

TRANSFER FROM OPERATING ROOM TO POSTOPERATIVE CARDIAC UNIT

At the end of surgery, even though the patient's condition may be relatively unstable, the attention of the staff may tend to relax. During transfer, monitoring of vital signs is often temporarily reduced and facilities for treatment are diminished. On the arrival of the patient in the postoperative unit, different equipment is used for the first time. Different personnel, often unfamiliar with the patient's medical status, now become involved in his care. The surgeon and anesthesiologist responsible for the patient in the operating room should personally transfer the patient to the new attending staff, accompanying the patient to the unit to ensure that he or she is receiving appropriate care during the initial postoperative period. The unit staff have a responsibility to ensure that the equipment functions properly before the patient's arrival in the unit. They must familiarize themselves with the patient's status before dismissing their operating room colleagues.

A trolley equipped with oxygen tanks, a means for manually ventilating the patient's lungs, and a battery-powered defibrillator and two-channel oscilloscope to permit monitoring of the ECG and arterial or venous pressure is desirable. Without such a special trolley, the inability to provide adequate monitoring and support during the period from the end of surgery until arrival in the unit can be hazardous for the patient. A battery-powered intra-aortic balloon pump for assisting the patient's circulation during transfer also may be necessary. The chest tubes and draining tubes should be clamped for the shortest possible period to allow the continued accurate assessment of blood loss and to prevent clotting in the draining tubes, with the subsequent risk of tamponade.

Safe transfer to the unit is best accomplished with the patient sedated, intubated, and receiving ventilatory assistance. Only when a relatively minor and uncomplicated procedure has been performed should extubation before transfer to the unit be considered. Hemodynamic instability is frequent during the initial postoperative period, as is impaired gas exchange resulting from anesthesia, cardiac bypass, and thoracic splinting due to pain. In addition, residual effects of anesthetic agents and muscle relaxants may impair ventilatory drive and respiratory muscle function. The patient's oxygen demand also may be increased at this time, owing to shivering.

INITIAL ASSESSMENT

Immediately on arrival of the patient in the unit, monitoring and care must be begun and a rapid clinical assessment made. Immediate treatment must be available for life-threatening situations. The arterial, venous, and atrial pressure lines are reestablished and initial measurements made. Function of the intravenous infusion lines is confirmed. The ECG is analyzed. The draining tubes in the chest are checked and stripped. The initial loss of blood from the tubes is assessed and is replaced as necessary. If the patient is to be ventilated postoperatively, this is commenced. In both mechanically ventilated and spontaneously breathing patients, the adequacy of ventilation should be assessed clinically and the FIO_2 should be kept at 0.50 or above, until blood gases have been checked. The chest should be auscultated to ensure satisfactory air entry into both lungs, and the possibility of endobronchial intubation or pneumothorax should be ruled out. The patient's urinary output should be measured and fluid balance charts should be commenced. Finally, the patient's core temperature should be measured.

After this initial rapid assessment, a more detailed analysis of hemodynamic, respiratory, and other vital systems must be made. A search should be made for signs of inadequate peripheral perfusion, such as pallor, cold extremities, distention of veins, poor urinary output, and impaired consciousness. Low arterial pressure, elevated left atrial pressure, pulmonary edema, or signs of inadequate peripheral perfusion (or combinations of these) imply a low cardiac output. Low cardiac output should be confirmed by either thermodilution or dye-dilution technique. Estimations of cardiac output are extremely useful in directing therapy. A further indication of inadequate tissue perfusion and low cardiac output is a low mixed venous oxygen tension. The use of appropriate inotropic support should be commenced if needed.

With the recovery of consciousness and sympathetic tone by the patient, peripheral vasoconstriction may be noted. This condition may increase afterload on the functional left ventricle and exacerbate cardiac failure and may necessitate the use of vasodilator therapy, such as sodium nitroprusside or nitroglycerin.

The heart should be carefully auscultated for added heart sounds or murmurs, and the correct function of heart valve prostheses ensured. A full 12-lead ECG is useful. Treatment may be required for abnormal cardiac rhythms. Heart block, which requires pacemaker support, is frequent after cardiac surgery, especially when cardioplegic solutions containing high concentrations of potassium are used. Premature ventricular extrasystoles are the most common arrhythmia during the early postoperative period and are often associated with a low serum potassium level after the intraoperative use of diuretics. The effects of low serum potassium levels may be exacerbated by alkalosis. Levels of blood gases and electrolytes should be determined after surgery. Therapy is directed at correcting hypokalemia if present and at controlling the premature ventricular contractions with lidocaine. Electrocardiographic signs of potassium imbalance may be seen. Comparison with preoperative ECG findings may help in the interpretation of arrhythmias and in the diagnosis of acute myocardial infarction.

Accurate assessment of the adequacy of ventilation and of oxygenation must be made. Until proved otherwise, a patient who is "fighting the ventilator" should be assumed to be either hypoxemic or receiving an inadequate minute volume. Other causes for dyspnea, tachypnea, ventilator intolerance, or restlessness may include a low cardiac output, pain, or a full bladder. The use of intermittent mandatory ventilation may help the patient adjust to the ventilator. Arterial blood for gas analysis should be obtained within half an hour after the patient's arrival in the unit; this time is also convenient for the analysis of mixed venous blood gases and the determination of cardiac output. Appropriate adjustment of the patient's minute volume and FIO_2 can then be made. The need for positive end-expiratory pressure also should be reassessed at this time. Mixed venous oxygen tension is useful in optimizing respiratory and cardiovascular therapy and in adjusting levels of positive end-expiratory pressure.

If high inflation pressures are necessary for an adequate tidal volume, airway resistance may be increased or low lung compliance may be present. Auscultation of the chest may reveal fine crepitations, characteristic of pulmonary edema or congestion. Absent or reduced breath sounds on auscultation occur with atelectasis or pneumothorax and also with inadvertent endobronchial intubation. Pneumothorax and atelectasis may cause tracheal shifts. Bronchial breathing will be heard over a consolidated or collapsed lung.

As soon as is feasible, an anteroposterior chest roentgenogram should be obtained with a portable unit. Hilar congestion, pulmonary edema, atelectasis, accumulation of fluid or blood in the pleural space, or a pneumothorax may be detected. The roentgenogram of the chest is also important in confirming the correct placement of the distal end of the endotracheal tube in the trachea and the correct placement of the chest drains, the cardiac pacemaker wires, and the nasogastric tube.

In addition to this initial examination of the cardiovascular and respiratory systems, function of the CNS and kidneys needs to be assessed. Examination should be made to determine the level of consciousness, pupillary movement and light reflex, limb reflexes, and plantar responses. Kidney function should be closely checked, with careful hourly monitoring of urinary output. The patient may be weighed early during the postoperative period to aid in planning fluid replacement.

Blood samples should be sent early in the postoperative period for the measurement of electrolytes. Hemoglobin and hematocrit levels also need to be measured. Blood coagulation studies also may be performed at this time if indicated.

Charts should be kept both during this initial postoperative period and subsequently. These charts document the patient's cardiovascular status and therapy, the patient's respiratory support, blood and fluid loss and replacement, and other vital signs and therapy given. With the aid of such flow charts, appropriate and rational treatment may be planned.

REFERENCES

1. Committee on Guidelines of the Society of Critical Care Medicine: Guidelines for organization of critical care units, in Weil M.H., Shubin H. (eds.): *Critical Care Medicine: Current Principles and Practices.* Hagerstown, Md., Harper & Row, 1976, p. 8.
2. Fox S.M. III, Robins M.: Incidence, prevalence, and death rates of cardiovascular disease: Some practical implications, in Hurst J.W., et al. (eds.): *The Heart: Arteries and Veins,* ed. 4. New York, McGraw-Hill Book Co., 1978, p. 750.
3. McIntosh H.D., Garcia J.A.: The first decade of aortocoronary bypass grafting, 1967–1977: A review. *Circulation* 57:405, 1978.
4. Standards for Cardiopulmonary Resuscitation (CPR) and Emergency Cardiac Care (ECC). *J.A.M.A.* 227(suppl.):833, 1974.
5. Steen P.A., Tinker J.H., Tarhan S.: Myocardial reinfarction after anesthesia and surgery. *J.A.M.A.* 239:2566, 1978.
6. Tarhan S., Giuliani E.R.: General anesthesia and myocardial infarction. *Am. Heart J.* 87:137, 1974.
7. Tarhan S., White R.D., Raimundo H.S.: Anesthetic considerations for aortocoronary bypass graft surgery. *Ann. Thorac. Surg.* 27:376, 1979.
8. Vlietstra R.E., et al.: Survival predictors in coronary artery disease: Medical and surgical comparisons. *Mayo Clin. Proc.* 52:85, 1977.

24 / Postoperative Management of the Cardiac Surgical Patient: Respiratory Care

H. MICHAEL MARSH
PETER A. SOUTHORN

THE NEED for postoperative respiratory support of the cardiac surgical patient is dictated by the almost uniform occurrence of acute respiratory insufficiency during the immediate postoperative period. An essential aim of respiratory care in this postoperative period is to ensure the adequate transport of oxygen to the tissues and the optimal clearance of carbon dioxide from the tissues. This process will provide conditions that promote the rapid return to normal function of the heart and lungs, thus preventing hypoxemia, respiratory acidosis, and other pulmonary complications that might arise after cardiopulmonary bypass and surgery.

The vast majority of patients who have undergone cardiac surgery remain intubated and receive mechanical ventilatory assistance for a period immediately after the surgery. Approximately 90% of these patients can be extubated within 24 hours.[115] A smaller percentage require prolonged mechanical ventilation beyond 24 hours. In our own practice, about 10% of all patients undergoing cardiac surgery require prolonged mechanical ventilation. This last group of patients requires mechanical ventilation for an average of 3.4 days. These data can be projected into 121 bed-years per year of prolonged mechanical ventilation for cardiac surgical patients in the United States. The total cost for this prolonged mechanical ventilation, allowing $500 per bed-day, would be approximately $22 million per year. It should be noted that the total cost for surgical coronary artery grafting in the United States alone is estimated to be in excess of $1 billion per year.[56, 117, 166] Efforts at cost containment include attempts to shorten the hospital stay by hastening extubation, preventing cardiac and pulmonary complications, and dismissing the patient as soon as is safe and practical. However, rapid extubation does not necessarily hasten patient dismissal from the intensive care unit, and extubation that is too rapid may delay dismissal.[144] The basic ethical dilemma of cost-benefit justification for the surgical episode is related to the cardiac disease being treated.

PATHOPHYSIOLOGY OF PROBLEMS ENCOUNTERED

Respiratory problems contribute both to morbidity and mortality from cardiac surgery. Fortunately, advances in respiratory care have been so successful that relatively few patients now die in fulminant respiratory failure. Such was not always true.[50] The leading cause for prolonged mechanical ventilation and death during the immediate postoperative period (<30 days) is the low cardiac output syndrome.[98] This finding was confirmed by our own series of patients undergoing cardiac surgery in 1978 (Table 24-1).

Acute Pulmonary Dysfunction

The respiratory problems associated with cardiac surgery may be classified into two groups. The first produces acute dysfunction with respiratory insufficiency or failure during the immediate postoperative period. The second causes chronic pulmonary dysfunction. Acute respiratory insufficiency may be defined as an encroachment on the reserves of pulmonary func-

TABLE 24–1.—PATIENTS ADMITTED TO POSTCARDIAC SURGICAL INTENSIVE CARE UNITS (MAYO CLINIC, 1978)

	PATIENTS	
	NO.	%
Cardiopulmonary bypass patients	1,171	
Congenital heart disease		29
Coronary artery bypass grafts		30
Valve replacements		37
Ventricular aneurysms		1
Thoracic aneurysms		1
Others		2
Vascular and thoracic surgical patients	712	
Total	1,883	
Deaths	84	(4)
Intraoperative		37
Postoperative		63
Low output		(51)
Arrhythmias		(7)
Respiratory		(3)
Massive bleeding and tamponade		(2)
Mechanical ventilation		
<24 hours	1,085	
Mortality (excluding intraoperative deaths)	17	(1.5)
>24 hours	176	
Mortality	36	(20)

tion without the blood gases being abnormal and can be expressed as an increase in the ratio of respired minute volume to oxygen uptake. A normal value (mean ± 2 SD) for this ratio at rest is 25 ± 8.[87] Respiratory insufficiency commonly results from inefficient gas exchange caused by ventilation-perfusion mismatching. It may be present before operation[17] and is an almost uniform finding during the immediate postoperative period.[65, 79]

The most widely accepted definition for respiratory failure was proposed by Campbell in 1965.[30] He wrote, "Respiratory failure is present in a subject at rest breathing air at sea-level if, because of impaired respiratory function, the arterial blood Po_2 is below 60 mm Hg or the Pco_2 is above 49 mm Hg." He further pointed out that "the only condition other than respiratory failure in which blood Pco_2 is raised is nonrespiratory or metabolic alkalosis," while "the only condition other than respiratory failure causing the arterial blood Po_2 to be reduced is right-to-left cardiovascular shunting."

Campbell classified respiratory failure into two types: hypoxemia without hypercarbia (type I) and hypercarbic hypoxemic respiratory failure (type II). Hypoxemia may result from the following: (1) an increase in right-to-left shunting, in which the shunt may be intrapulmonary or cardiac; (2) an increase in lung regions with low ventilation-perfusion ratios, so-called shuntlike effect; or (3) decreased diffusion, or an increase in diffusion-perfusion mismatching.[180] Hypercarbia may result from alveolar hypoventilation associated with (1) depression of central neural drive, (2) impaired transmission of neural signals to the respiratory muscles, (3) musculoskeletal deformity and malfunction or muscular fatigue (or both), or (4) severe ventilation-perfusion mismatching. Types I and II respiratory failure are not absolutely distinct, and the patient can have type I failure early during the course of a disease—for example, pneumonia or asthma—and experience type II failure later.

One may distinguish a syndrome of severe, relentless, progressive respiratory failure, sometimes called the "adult respiratory distress syndrome."[139] It has been considered to be due to pulmonary capillary leakage, causing interstitial or frank alveolar (or both) pulmonary edema.[83] This clinical pattern may be associated with shock, trauma, or septicemia. It may also occur (1) with inflammation of the lung, that is, pneumonitis from various causes, (2) with cardiogenic pulmonary edema (as may be seen with left ventricular failure or with obstructive lesions such as mitral stenosis), (3) with pulmonary edema caused by fluid overload, or (4) with oxygen toxicity. Cardiopulmonary bypass may produce identical pulmonary lesions.

Pathogenesis

There are a number of possible causes for respiratory insufficiency and respiratory failure after cardiopulmonary bypass and cardiac surgery: "pump lung," low cardiac output syndrome, lung collapse (sputum retention) with splinting, cardiogenic pulmonary edema, and other factors (including embolus and infection).

PUMP LUNG.—Whether pump lung is a distinct entity, routinely and uniquely associated with cardiopulmonary bypass, has been controversial.[104] In 1973, Ratliff, Connell, and their associates[41, 148] reported on a series of patients undergoing cardiopulmonary bypass from whom lung biopsy specimens were obtained, both before and after operation. Biopsy specimens of the lung after bypass showed interstitial edema, perivascular hemorrhage, and miliary atelectasis. There was an intravascular accumulation of neutrophilic polymorphonuclear cells. Prolonged cardiopulmonary bypass caused intra-alveolar hemorrhage, vascular congestion, and intra-alveolar edema. Swelling of endothelial cells and type I pneumocytes with loss of granules from type II pneumocytes also has been found.[137]

Connell and others[41] examined the effects of filtering the blood and removing platelet aggregates and leukocyte breakdown products and reported that these resulted in some improvement in pulmonary function. However, pathologic changes were still present, and they increased with increasing time of cardiopulmonary bypass.

A further important cause of the pump-related pathologic changes of the lung may be overdistention and damage of the pulmonary capillaries at surgery. This condition can be caused by forward or collateral (from bronchial vessels or patent ductus) overfilling but most commonly results from back-filling of the pulmonary circulation. Back-filling results from failure of adequate decompress by venting of the left side of the heart at surgery or from attempts at increasing the filling pressure of the left ventricle to improve cardiac output while only right atrial pressure is measured, or from both of these. Large discrepancies may occur between the right and left atrial pressures during surgery. Routine monitoring of left atrial pressure has done much to mitigate this problem.[128] Likewise, the prevention of lung collapse by static inflation with pure oxygen appears to protect the lung.[137] Membrane oxygenators also produce less pulmonary damage than bubble-film oxygenators.[106] Hemodilution prime for bypass rather than the use of blood containing prime also is beneficial.[29]

Craddock and others[44] noted that complement-mediated leukostasis has a major role in acute cardiopulmonary complications after cellophane-membrane hemodialysis in renal failure. Other authors[135] noted a decrease in serum complement level after cardiopulmonary bypass. Steroids may reduce such sequestration of polymorphonuclear leukocytes in the lungs during bypass.[181]

The natural history of the pump-related changes in the lung seems to be similar to that of the adult respiratory distress syndrome. Thus, pathologic changes in pulmonary ultrastructure noted by Ratliff et al.[148] and Connell et al.[41] are similar to the findings noted by Bachofen and Weibel[14] in a series of electron micrographs of lung tissue taken from patients who had died of septicemia and are similar to changes found by Lamy and others[101] in patients with severe respiratory failure from various causes. This finding has led to widespread suspicion that the lung reacts in a nonspecific way to many different noxious stimuli. The changes seen by Bachofen and Weibel[14] included interstitial edema, leukocyte margination and degranulation, endothelial cell change, and changes in types I and II pneumocytes. These acute changes may progress either to complete repair or to replacement of normal lung cells by fibrous tissue. Disruption of lung architecture and fibrosis may be patchy, in which case the lung will function adequately at rest but will have a decreased functional reserve. More extensive damage may lead to death.

LOW CARDIAC OUTPUT.—The low cardiac output syndrome is the leading cause of death and the major reason for prolonged mechanical ventilation beyond 24 hours in the cardiac surgical patient.[98, 115] Low output is particularly frequent after surgery that requires a large ventric-

siveness in patients with cyanotic congenital heart disease (Table 24–2). Sørensen and Severinghaus showed that the increase in minute ventilation when going from an arterial oxygen tension of near 100 mm Hg to an arterial oxygen tension of 40 mm Hg was normally of the order of 10 L/minute/sq m. Markedly depressed hypoxic responsiveness was noted in persons born and living at high altitude and in patients who, late in life (average age, 18 years at time of surgery), had corrective surgery for tetralogy of Fallot. These authors postulated that this decrease in hypoxic responsiveness became fixed later in life. Blesa et al.,[22] using the increase in minute ventilation during progressive hypoxemia as a fraction of decreasing arterial oxygen saturation as their index of hypoxic responsiveness (see Table 24–2), showed that persons who had been unresponsive to a hypoxic stimulus with cyanotic disease (the cyanotic group) had an ability to recover to normal levels after correction of that cardiac lesion (the acyanotic group). They suggested that recovery took weeks and that it probably only occurred when the lesion was corrected at an early age.

The control of ventilation also may be altered during the immediate postoperative period by disorders in acid-base balance. If hypochloremic hypokalemia causes metabolic alkalosis, carbon dioxide responsiveness will be reduced. Appropriate correction of metabolic alkalosis during the postoperative period, by use of potassium salt, acetazolamide, arginine hydrochloride, or ammonium chloride (or combinations), will aid in weaning from mechanical ventilation.

TABLE 24–2.—BLUNTING OF HYPOXIC RESPONSIVENESS* WITH CHRONIC HYPOXEMIA

DETERMINATION	VALUE
Sørensen and Severinghaus[165]	$\Delta \dot{V}_{40}$ (L/min/sq m)†
Normal at sea level	9.6 ± 7.3 (n = 9)
Born at altitude	0.4 ± 1.9 (n = 9)
Tetralogy—1 year postop	0.5 ± 2.3 (n = 9)
Blesa et al.[22]	$\Delta \dot{V}/\Delta Sao_2$ (L/min/%)‡
Normal	8 ± 4 (n = 5)
Cyanotic	1 ± 3 (n = 8)
Acyanotic	7 ± 4 (n = 13)

*Mean ± SD.
†The increase in minute ventilation when going from an arterial oxygen tension of 100 to 40 mm Hg, normalized for body surface area.
‡The increase in minute ventilation during progressive hypoxemia, as a fraction of decreasing arterial oxygen saturation.

The Effects of Mechanical Ventilation

Mechanical ventilation has both advantages and disadvantages. The advantages are that it (1) decreases the work of breathing; (2) provides a constant ventilatory level, usually maintaining the blood gases constant despite changes in the patient's neural drive to ventilation; and (3) provides means for delivery of a high FIO_2 and institution of positive end-expiratory pressure if these are needed. The disadvantages of prolonged mechanical ventilation are (1) a potential increase in inefficiency of gas exchange, (2) possible trauma to the larynx and trachea, (3) possible introduction of pathogens through the endotracheal tube, bypassing normal defense mechanisms of the upper respiratory tract, (4) the potential for barotrauma and oxygen toxicity, and (5) the psychologic hazard to the patient; despite the best precautions, there is also (6) the risk of mechanical misadventure.

Possible mechanisms for the increase in inefficiency of gas exchange during mechanical ventilation are an increased mismatching of ventilation to perfusion and increased shunting of venous blood. The ideal intrapulmonary distribution of alveolar ventilation is one that matches perfectly the distribution of ventilation and perfusion, thereby resulting in a 1:1 ratio of ventilation to perfusion throughout the lung. This ideal is not, however, achieved even in healthy subjects breathing spontaneously, in whom some mismatching of ventilation to perfusion exists.[180] With mechanical ventilation, mismatching of ventilation to perfusion may increase, and lung regions with high and low ventilation-perfusion ratios may develop. Lung regions with low ventilation-perfusion ratios have a shunt-like effect and thus may interfere with oxygenation. Lung regions with high ventilation-perfusion ratios exhibit a dead-space-like effect and thus may interfere with the elimination of carbon dioxide.

Mismatching of ventilation to perfusion may be increased if either the distribution of inspired gas or the distribution of pulmonary blood flow is altered without appropriate adjustment of the other. In healthy young subjects studied while in the supine or right lateral decubitus position, intrapulmonary distribution of inspired gas, obtained using the ^{133}Xe method, becomes more uniform during anesthesia-paralysis and mechanical ventilation, compared with that during awake spontaneous breathing (Fig 24–3). By contrast, during anesthesia-paralysis and mechanical ventilation in the prone position, the distribution of inspired gas is not altered, while in sitting subjects, intrapulmonary distribution of inspired gas becomes less uniform.[150] The altered distribution of inspired gas during mechanical ventilation is presumably caused by a different pattern of expansion of the respiratory system when the muscles are paralyzed, compared with the pattern of expansion seen during active muscle contraction.[67, 149] The distribution of gas during assisted ventilation may be intermediate between that which would occur with paralysis and that which would occur with spontaneous breathing. Intrapulmonary distribution of perfusion is not significantly altered from that seen in awake subjects studied while in the supine position. In sitting subjects, intrapulmonary distribution of perfusion becomes significantly more uniform, while in subjects in the right lateral decubitus position, distribution of perfusion becomes significantly less uniform during anesthesia-paralysis and mechanical ventilation than during awake spontaneous breathing.

Subjects who are in the right lateral decubitus position have significantly increased mismatching of ventilation to perfusion during mechanical ventilation (Fig 24–4); that is, regional intrapulmonary distribution of perfusion fails to adjust to the altered regional intrapulmonary distribution of ventilation, or vice versa.[103] However, the changes in the matching of regional ventilation to perfusion occurring with anesthesia-paralysis and mechanical ventilation are not significant in subjects in the supine or sitting position. Hence, in terms of ventilation-to-perfusion relationships, the lung becomes less efficient as a gas exchanger during anesthesia-paralysis when subjects are in the lateral decubitus position.

The lung's efficiency as a gas exchanger also may decrease with anesthesia-paralysis when subjects are in the supine position, but because

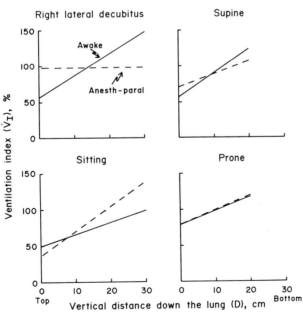

Fig 24–3.—Intrapulmonary inspired gas distribution in man in four different body positions during awake spontaneous breathing *(solid line)* and anesthesia-paralysis with mechanical ventilation *(broken line)*. Note that with mechanical ventilation, ventilation per unit lung (gas) volume ($\dot{V}_I$) became more uniform in right lateral decubitus and supine positions and less uniform in sitting position. By contrast, in prone position, anesthesia-paralysis had no effect on ventilation per unit lung (gas) volume. (From Rehder et al.[149] Used by permission.)

Gas distribution, closing capacity

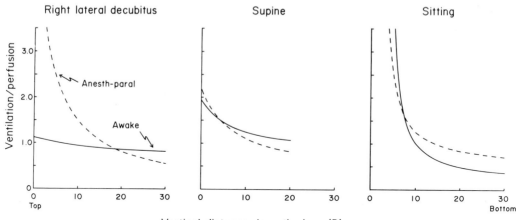

Fig 24–4.—Mean ventilation-perfusion ratios in vertically oriented lung regions from man in three different body positions during awake spontaneous breathing *(solid line)* and anesthesia-paralysis with mechanical ventilation *(broken line).* Note that with mechanical ventilation, the ventilation-perfusion distribution became less uniform in right lateral decubitus position, but was not significantly different in supine and sitting postures. (From Rehder K., Marsh H.M.: Gas exchange during anesthesia, in West J.B. [ed.]: *Pulmonary Gas Exchange.* New York, Academic Press, 1980. Used by permission.)

of the limited spatial resolution of the ^{133}Xe method, these changes are not consistently detected. Estimates of P(A-a)O_2 on the basis of studies of regional ventilation and regional perfusion showed that, for subjects in the supine position, P(A-a)O_2 increases because of increased mismatching of ventilation to perfusion. However, this P(A-a)O_2 due to ventilation-perfusion mismatching was estimated to be less than the value of P(A-a)O_2 reported in the literature for anesthetized subjects in the supine position.[114] Therefore, increased regional ventilation-perfusion mismatching alone does not totally explain the increased P(A-a)O_2 seen during anesthesia-paralysis and mechanical ventilation. With the inert gas-elimination method, which has a higher resolution than the ^{133}Xe method,[179] mismatching of ventilation to perfusion is observed to be consistently increased in both the lateral decubitus and supine positions.

Right-to-left shunting also may be determined by the inert gas-elimination method.[179] The estimates of right-to-left shunting by this method are based on increased retention of intravenously infused inert gases with low solubilities. Determination of shunts by the inert gas-elimination method does not necessitate the breathing of 100% oxygen, and it therefore excludes possible changes induced by breathing oxygen. This method indicates only the amount of shunted pulmonary arterial blood that does not perfuse ventilated alveoli, that is, direct right-to-left shunt. The estimation of shunting using this inert gas-elimination method, therefore, excludes shunted blood that originates distal to the pulmonary capillaries, that is, left-to-right shunt. The latter shunting occurs through thebesian veins or through connections between pulmonary and bronchial veins (or through both). In contrast to the inert gas-elimination method, the classic oxygen method for detecting so-called right-to-left shunt combines both types of shunts. Therefore, the amount of shunting originating distal to the pulmonary capillaries can be estimated by subtracting the shunting determined by the inert gas-elimination method from that determined by the classic oxygen method.

Increases of less than 1% in right-to-left shunt were measured by the inert gas-elimination technique in healthy young volunteers during anesthesia-paralysis and mechanical ventilation. However, in some healthy young subjects, larger increases in the shunt determined by the oxygen method may occur, suggesting that both types of shunting may be increased during mechanical ventilation in these subjects. In contrast, in heavy smokers[55] or in patients with preexisting lung disease,[157] anesthesia-paralysis and mechanical ventilation may result in large increases in shunting with the inert gas-elimination method. This alteration probably is also seen with mechanical ventilation in the absence of anesthesia and paralysis.

Respiratory Care Monitoring

The functions of the lungs include the following: gas exchange; self-protection against edema, infection, and toxicity; self-repair; filtration of venous blood; and numerous metabolic functions. These lung functions can be assessed experimentally using highly sophisticated methods.[15] Until recently, the complexity or the invasiveness (or both) of such investigations has hindered clinical application. The respiratory monitoring currently available and applicable to the postcardiac surgical patient includes blood gas analysis, measurements of ventilation and perfusion and their relationship to one another, and the recent development of clinically useful means for obtaining lung volumes and respiratory mechanics.

Blood Gas Analysis

Intermittent blood gas analysis remains an essential measurement needed for adequate management of the patient in respiratory failure. Modern blood gas analysis involves the use of a Sanz Ultramicro pH electrode,[155] a Severinghaus carbon dioxide electrode,[160] and a Clark polarographic oxygen electrode.[37] Correctly mixed heparinized samples of arterial blood must be obtained from an arterial puncture or an indwelling line. Before this sample (usually 3 to 5 ml in an adult and 1 ml in an infant) is obtained, the patient must have been in a stable state (FIO_2, positive end-expiratory pressures, and minute volume maintained constant) for 15 to 20 minutes. To make a meaningful interpretation of these results, FIO_2 should be measured, respiratory rate and tidal volume should be obtained, and airway pressures should be recorded when the sample is collected. Furthermore, the arterial puncture must be clean, and the sample should be uncontaminated with venous blood (and drawn into the syringe without bubbles) and obtained in a pain-free manner to avoid hyperventilation. The syringe, ideally made of glass, should be filled with a 1:5,000 heparin solution. The residual volume of heparin in the syringe before collection of blood should be minimal. After the blood has been collected, the syringe should be capped immediately, thoroughly mixed, and then placed in ice for transport.

Measurements are usually made at 37 C, and results should be corrected for the body temperature of the patient.[158] Spectrophotometry is often added to blood gas analysis to obtain values for oxyhemoglobin, carboxyhemoglobin, and total hemoglobin and to screen for altered hemoglobin, methemoglobin, and sulfhemoglobin.[163]

Arterial blood oxygen tension must be interpreted with knowledge of the comparable PAO_2. The latter is calculated using the alveolar air equation.[40] Inspired oxygen concentration is titrated to maintain the Pao_2 above 60 mm Hg to ensure the near-complete oxygen saturation of hemoglobin. The response of Pao_2 to increasing PAO_2 is indicative of the type of venous admixture. The Pao_2 does not respond, and the $P(A-a)O_2$ gradient widens with increasing FIO_2 when intrapulmonary shunting occurs. By contrast, the Pao_2 increases and the $P(A-a)O_2$ gradient remains relatively constant with increasing FIO_2 when ventilation-perfusion imbalance is present. Used in combination with knowledge of changes in mixed venous oxygen tension, the $P(A-a)O_2$ is also a valuable guide in achieving optimal positive end-expiratory pressure.

Mixed venous blood samples drawn from the pulmonary artery are useful in managing patients after cardiac surgery. The mixed venous oxygen tension, saturation, and content vary directly with both the arterial oxygen content (Cao_2) and the cardiac output ($\dot{Q}$) if the body's oxygen consumption remains constant. The product of the two variables ($\dot{Q} \times Cao_2$) is the oxygen delivery to the tissues. Mixed venous oxygen content ($C\bar{v}o_2$) also varies inversely with oxygen uptake ($\dot{V}o_2$) by the tissues. The combination of these factors is the Fick equation for oxygen:

$$\dot{Q} = \dot{V}o_2/C(a-\bar{V})o_2$$

Thus, mixed venous oxygen content is an effective means of assessing changes in the adequacy of tissue perfusion after cardiac surgery. It may help predict cardiovascular hemodynamic changes before circulatory collapse occurs.[172] Mixed venous oxygen content, saturation, and pressure are useful in determining optimal levels of positive end-expiratory pressure. The Fick formula for oxygen can be used to validate cardiac output determinations made by thermodilution or indicator dye-dilution techniques, especially in the low cardiac output state when the latter techniques have a greater tendency for inaccuracy. If cardiac output and the difference in arterial and mixed venous oxygen content are known, the oxygen uptake or consumption of the patient can be calculated by rearranging Fick's formula. Oxygen consumption is a useful guide for achieving optimal parenteral nutrition given to patients whose postoperative course dictates caloric support. The number of kilocalories per day required approximately equals seven times the body's oxygen consumption (milliliters per minute, standard temperature, pressure, dry).[49]

Recordings of intermittent measurements of blood gas composition on the patient chart should be performed in such a way as to permit easy analysis of trends with time and therapy.[62, 125] Computers may be useful in displays of such trends. Even with trend analysis, intermittent sampling for blood gas analysis suffers from disadvantages. First, intermittent sampling may not detect sudden changes quickly, especially when there is a time lag between ordering the sample and getting the result. Second, the information gained does not, by itself, provide a complete definition of the pathophysiologic changes in the lung.

Continuous monitoring of blood gas composition has been approached by noninvasive and invasive methods, and they are on the verge of further refinement and, thus, increasing utility. Transcutaneous noninvasive methods for Po_2 monitoring, developed by Lübbers' group,[84] are now clinically applicable to neonates. These devices rely on heating a small area of thin skin with a silver anode and creating a transcutaneous oxygen flux, which is subsequently used to permit the measurement of oxygen by polarography. A similar technique could be evolved using gas chromatography or mass spectrometry. The electrode has to be maintained at temperatures between 43 and 45 C, and burns are possible. This method is not currently considered to be of great value for critically ill adults. In both infants and adults, skin electrodes are unsatisfactory in low-flow states associated with peripheral vasoconstriction. Improvements in ear oximetry[156] allow the stable, noninvasive monitoring of blood oxygen saturation. Again, this method may be invalid in low-flow states or in patients with severe peripheral arteriolar constriction.

Invasive methods for continuous blood gas monitoring using transducers inserted into systemic arteries and the pulmonary artery also are being developed.[26, 73] Miniaturized polarographic oxygen electrodes inserted into the umbilical artery are of proved value in the care of the critically ill neonate.[42] Such electrodes also have been used to monitor Pao_2 and mixed venous oxygen content in adults.[9] Reflecting fiberoptic systems in cardiac catheters have been developed to give continuous readout of oxyhemoglobin saturation.[38] Continuous sampling techniques from an indwelling arterial or venous line to a small gas chromatograph or mass spectrometer have also been used to provide frequent measurements of Pao_2 and $Paco_2$. Indwelling electrodes for pH and $Paco_2$ are also available. Such invasive techniques are not in widespread use, and their universal clinical applicability is at present uncertain.

Expired Gas Analysis

Intermittent gas analysis using chemical methods such as Haldane or Scholander gas analyzers provides basic reference standards. These methods are, however, tedious and cannot provide continuous analyses. Continuous gas analyzers, first introduced in the early 1940s for the analysis of helium and nitrogen,[13] have now been developed for many gases. More recently, gas chromatography[178] and mass spectrometry[113] have been adapted for this purpose.

When continuous accurate measurements of respired volumes are available, expired gas analyses provide on-line estimates of oxygen consumption and carbon dioxide production, together with accurate values for $P(A-a)o_2$,

$P(a-A)CO_2$, and the physiologic and the anatomical dead space. The drawback has been the difficulty in providing continuous stable estimates of respired volume. Continuous end-expiratory estimation of carbon dioxide by itself is a useful index of adequacy of ventilation, both when the patient is being mechanically ventilated and when he is breathing spontaneously. It may be used in weaning the patient from mechanical ventilator support. A stable end-expiratory carbon dioxide percentage of less than 6% has been reported to indicate adequate spontaneous ventilation.[142]

Intermittent washout of inert gases, such as nitrogen, has been used to determine functional residual capacity,[66] estimation of the distribution of ventilation,[66] and closing capacity.[65] Helium dilution is a commonly used clinical method for measurement of functional residual capacity.[118] In 1974, Wagner et al.[179] introduced a multiple "inert" gas infusion and expired gas analysis method that is of value in determining the matching of ventilation to perfusion in the lungs and that can be adapted to the study, and perhaps monitoring, of the critically ill patient. Overland et al.[133] suggested that differential uptake of two agents, one poorly soluble in water (for example, acetylene) and one highly soluble (for example, diethyl ether), be used to estimate lung weight and pulmonary blood flow and thus monitor pulmonary extravascular water.

It remains unclear as to what improvement in cost-benefit ratio may accrue to the critically ill patient from the continuous monitoring of expired gases. Less frequent arterial blood gas analyses, more accurate estimates of caloric requirements, and better assessment of the progression of lung disease may be available from such monitoring in the future, but the current use of these techniques remains largely experimental.

Pulmonary Mechanics

Intermittent bedside measurements of vital capacity (spontaneous effort), tidal volume (spontaneous and machine-delivered), and maximal spontaneous inspiratory and expiratory pressures against airway occlusion are used in assessing the possibility of weaning the patient from mechanical ventilation.[120] Estimates of maximal inspiratory and maximal expiratory pressures in monitoring the patient with muscle weakness are particularly helpful.[21] These tests can be performed with relatively simple pieces of apparatus.

Recently, stable pneumotachography has been successfully introduced into the design of a mechanical respirator (Siemens-Elema, Servo Ventilator, Sweden) with heated Fleisch pneumotachograph screens.[161] Osborn[132] has designed a variable-orifice pneumotachograph for the same purpose, sacrificing some accuracy in flow measurement so that clogging with airway water is not a problem. By integrating gas flow with respect to time, volume change is obtained. Osborn has described techniques for providing a breath-by-breath display of change in airway pressure related to change in lung volume. The slope of this pressure-volume relationship represents the total dynamic compliance of the respiratory system. To obtain lung compliance and recoil measurements, transpulmonary pressure change must be related to changes in lung volume. Pleural pressure can be transduced using a catheter inserted into the pleural space[54] or can be estimated with an esophageal balloon.[121] Recently, a nasogastric tube with an esophageal balloon attached has been introduced for making such measurements.[105]

Because the pressure-volume relationship varies with lung volume, meaningful evaluation of compliance measurements requires that the latter be related to a given absolute lung volume, normally functional residual capacity. The latter has hitherto been difficult to measure at the patient's bedside. We have used a helium-dilution katharometer technique for this purpose and are currently exploring other tracer gas-dilution techniques using gas chromatography or mass spectrometry to measure the percentage of tracer gases. These techniques have not yet received widespread acceptance.

An index of total respiratory system compliance, the "effective" compliance, is helpful in the management of the respirator-dependent patient. As was previously mentioned, this index is found by dividing the tidal volume by the difference in airway pressure between end-inspiration and end-expiration.[57] However, its interpretation requires the realization that the index is affected not only by changes in the elastic properties of the lung or chest wall (or both) but also by changes in lung volume and possibly airway resistance. An "effective" compliance measurement, therefore, is not specific for changes in mechanical properties of the lung itself.

In the recent past, some authors suggested that optimal positive end-expiratory pressure levels can be predicted from measurements of compliance of the respiratory system.[174, 175] This technique is not now generally accepted as having much practical value. Display of breath-by-breath pressure-volume characteristics is, however, potentially of great value in the management of mechanical ventilation. The shape of the inspiratory pressure-volume curve is indicative of pulmonary compliance and resistance. Such curves have been used to calculate and subdivide the components of respiratory muscle work.[89] This subject has been recently reviewed by Wilson.[182] Acute decrease in compliance may indicate a pneumothorax or sudden atelectasis. These curves are also of value in determining the best flow rates required for lung inflation and in setting the sensitivity of ventilator inspiratory-triggering devices.[131]

Respiratory Control

Voluntary respiratory effort can be monitored continuously by means of one of a number of apnea detectors and alarms. They may detect motion of the chest wall by magnetometers,[97] change in volume of the thorax by impedance pneumography,[12] gas flow at the nose[61] or airway opening, esophageal pressure changes,[105] or a combination of these variables. The patient suffering from intermittent apnea often needs such a set of devices. Studies designed to differentiate sleep apnea syndromes serve to illustrate their usefulness. Spirometers of various types[51] have been adapted for continuous monitoring and incorporated into mechanical ventilators. An adequate ventilator alarm system is mandatory for safe care.

Pulmonary Perfusion

Pulmonary perfusion pressures and pulmonary blood flow, the balance achieved between the predicted mean capillary pressure and measured colloid oncotic pressure, and the composition of mixed venous blood may be obtained by use of balloon flotation pulmonary catheters or lines placed at surgery. The utility of ventilation-perfusion scans, pulmonary angiography, and studies of right ventricular function using echocardiography and gated blood pool scanning techniques in patients with acute respiratory failure are now being evaluated, but these techniques remain largely experimental.

Biochemical Markers

The progression from lung injury to regeneration and repair or to fibrosis, appropriately demonstrated for septicemic shock by Bachofen and Weibel,[14] cannot be easily followed in the individual patient. Repeated lung biopsy procedures on the patient who requires mechanical ventilation are difficult and dangerous, although the taking of such specimens has been recommended in protocols for extracorporeal membrane oxygenation in severe acute respiratory failure. Interruption of pulmonary ventilation and perfusion may produce biochemical and structural lung damage.[122] A search for biochemical markers and modifiers of the progression of changes in lung disease is under way.[47] A recent review[127] highlighted the biochemical and metabolic changes in lung associated with oxygen, ozone, and nitrogen dioxide toxicity. While these techniques are not currently applicable to monitoring patients in acute respiratory failure, this is the area in which rapid future advances may be expected.

Respiratory Care Management

The aims of optimal respiratory care for the patient after cardiac surgery are to (1) maximize oxygen delivery to the blood and to the tissues, using safe levels of inspired oxygen, (2) ensure adequate carbon dioxide elimination, (3) maximize the lung's reparative ability, avoiding complications such as edema, infection, barotrauma, or pulmonary fibrosis, and (4) extubate the patient at the earliest possible safe time after the surgery. It is of critical importance, particularly in managing infants and small children whose physiologic reserves are limited, to search for and identify subtle signs of deterioration before these have progressed to the point where therapy will be unsuccessful.

Mechanical Ventilation Withdrawal

One can design a decision scheme outlining a series of questions that need to be approached in managing respiratory support for postcardiac surgical patients (Fig 24–5).

The decision to commence a trial of sponta-

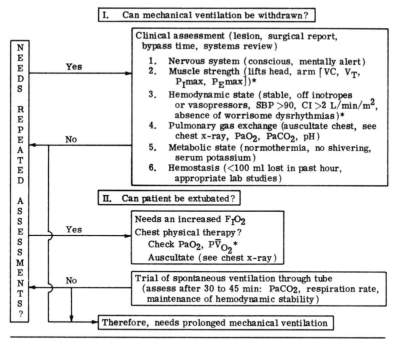

Fig. 24–5.—Scheme for managing respiratory support of cardiac patients arriving intubated from operating room.

neous breathing should be based on the following: (1) the return to an adequate level of consciousness and (2) full reversal of muscle relaxation, as judged by alertness, the ability to follow commands, and the ability to elevate the head or arm from the bed; (3) maintenance of hemodynamic stability without inotrope or vasopressor therapy, as judged by systolic blood pressure greater than 80 mm Hg, with a cardiac index above 2 L/minutes/sq m and the absence of ventricular or other serious dysrhythmia; (4) blood gas analysis showing a Pa_{O_2} of 100 mm Hg or more at an F_{IO_2} of 0.5 or less with a Pa_{CO_2} less than 45 mm Hg; (5) a normal serum potassium level; and (6) blood loss from mediastinal and intercostal chest drains of less than 100 ml/hour.

Central Nervous System

Ideally, the patient should be awake and alert. Appropriate functioning of the respiratory center and the ability to manage the airway are required for safe extubation. Coma is not necessarily a contraindication to discontinuance of mechanical ventilation, but it may suggest that continued endotracheal intubation is desirable to protect the airway and to ensure optimal pulmonary toilet in the uncooperative patient.

Transient neurologic deficits, such as confusion and delirium, commonly follow cardiac surgery. Severe cerebral damage is infrequent. Most of these syndromes reflect systemic hypotension or microembolism to the brain with air or particulate matter (or both hypotension and microembolism). Macroembolism is infrequently encountered, usually in association with valve replacement.[63] The incidence of neurologic deficits has decreased in recent years. In 1965, Gilman[69] reported a 34% incidence of impaired consciousness and disturbed behavior. Javid et al.[85] reported 53% in 1969, Tufo et al.[177] reported 44% in 1970, and Branthwaite[24] reported 19% in 1972 but only 17% in 1975.[25] These results reflect improved cardiopulmonary bypass and surgical techniques, especially the use of filters to remove aggregates from the blood returning to the patient from the extracorporeal circuit.

General principles of neurologic care that can be applied to the patient after cardiac arrest can be applied equally well to the patient having cardiopulmonary bypass and cardiac surgery.[63] Thus, monitoring of intracranial pressure and the possible, although controversial, cerebral protective effects of barbiturates should be considered when treating these patients, as should the potential value of osmotic diuretics, such as mannitol, and perhaps hyperventilation to reduce intracranial pressure. Prognosis may be indicated by signs of impaired brainstem function. At 12 to 24 hours after resuscitation, the absence of pupillary response, corneal reflex, or deep tendon reflex implies a potential cerebral death in patients who have not received opthalmoplegic agents. "Doll's eyes" or absent caloric response from the vestibular organs of the inner ear reliably predicts a vegetative state or death at this time. Decorticate or decerebrate posturing is not helpful in predicting the outcome at 12 hours, although a long persistence of either of these suggests severe disability. Some signs may indicate a favorable prognosis. Spontaneous roving horizontal eye movements at 12 to 24 hours and purposeful movements of the face, arms, or legs are signs of a good prognosis.

Cardiac Status

The patient's cardiac contractility, output, and blood pressure must be satisfactory and stable without the need for large-dose inotropic support. Inotropic drugs or intra-aortic balloon support does not contraindicate extubation and may be beneficial in maintaining cardiac output after extubation. However, the situation should have been stable and the patient should have been weaned from cardiac support before considering extubation, when the need for the muscle work of breathing and coughing will be added to the load on the heart.

Before weaning from respiratory support, dangerous cardiac arrhythmias should be absent or under control. Frequent premature ventricular contractions or short runs of ventricular ectopy are relative contraindications to the stress of a T-piece trial. Care also must be exercised when myocardial infarction is suspected.

Respiratory Status

Early extubation requires an absence of excess tracheal secretions, and the patient should be free of acute lung disease, especially that associated with a low lung compliance. Signs of pulmonary edema (including elevated left atrial pressure) should be absent. Preoperative lung dysfunction caused by diseases such as severe chronic obstructive lung disease may benefit from somewhat prolonged (12 to 24 hours) postoperative lung ventilation. A further relative contraindication to early extubation postoperatively is a bypass time greater than 2 hours, because structural changes in the lung rapidly increase when bypass times exceed this period.[10]

On blood gas analysis, the alveolar-to-arterial oxygen gradient at an FIO_2 of 1.0 should not exceed 300 mm Hg. Values less than 300 mm Hg imply that the patient will have an acceptable PaO_2 at FIO_2 of 0.5 or less. It is desirable to have satisfactory spontaneous alveolar ventilation, as indicated by the absence of carbon dioxide retention during the trial of spontaneous ventilation. Respiratory weaning is not generally successful if the physiologic ratio of dead space to tidal volume exceeds 0.6, if the vital capacity is less than 10 ml/kg body weight, and if the patient has a maximal inspiratory force of less than -20 cm H_2O. A stable respiratory status includes a hematocrit level in excess of 35% to ensure adequate oxygen transport to the tissues.

Hemostasis

The blood loss from the chest draining tubes should be less than 100 ml/hour, and the patient should have no coagulation abnormalities such that reoperation for bleeding is not contemplated.

Metabolic Status

Hyperthermia and hypothermia should be absent, as should shivering, at the time of extubation. In late extubation, it may be important to correct the metabolic alkalosis that commonly occurs during this period because of the use of potassium-losing diuretic agents, free nasogastric drainage, and the metabolism of citrate from transfused blood. Correction is required because respiratory drive may be depressed.

Weaning Trial Methods

The time-honored method for assessing the adequacy of spontaneous ventilation before extubation is to perform a trial of spontaneous breathing using an Ayre's T-piece. Blood gas analysis is performed between 30 minutes and one hour, with the patient breathing on this device. Normal values for $Paco_2$ and Pao_2 at the end of this time period imply that the patient can ventilate adequately if removed from ventilator support. If, during this period, the patient's condition deteriorates so that his respirations exceed 30/minute, his blood pressure decreases, his pulse rate increases, an arrhythmia develops, or he becomes cyanotic, somnolent, or agitated, blood is immediately drawn for blood gas determination and the patient is placed back on the ventilator. A respiratory rate in excess of 30 breaths per minute or excessive dyspnea at the end of the trial, even if arterial blood gas levels are normal, is a relative contraindication for extubation. More gentle weaning by gradually reducing rates of intermittent mandatory ventilation may occasionally be indicated, particularly in children, but is not generally necessary in adults.

The FIO_2 for the T-piece trial is set at a slightly higher percentage than that used during the preceding period of mechanical ventilation. The ECG is continually monitored, and the patient's vital signs are obtained at least every five minutes during the trial. The presence of signs of hypoxemia or hypercarbia or the development of an arrhythmia implies that the T-piece trial has not been successful.

Recently, it has been suggested that earlier extubation of patients who have undergone coronary bypass graft and who had an uncomplicated intraoperative course could be safely performed without a T-piece trial if the vital capacity were greater than 10 ml/kg body weight and the inspiratory force greater than -20 cm H_2O.[95] However, extubation achieved using such criteria[80, 141] is not associated with any decrease in length of intensive care unit stay, the duration of which is determined primarily by hemodynamic performance.[144] Further, the vital capacity and maximal inspiratory force may not reflect the patient's ability to be extubated earlier than would a successful T-piece trial performed when clinical criteria permit.[120] Thus, some patients could be extubated earlier, having completed a successful T-piece trial, yet still have an inadequate vital capacity and maximal inspiratory force according to the previous criteria.

Unless the patient is dependent on a hypoxic respiratory drive, the patient is given 100% inspired oxygen immediately before extubation. Secretions in the upper airway are thoroughly aspirated. The cuff of the endotracheal tube is deflated while positive pressure is applied, thereby forcing secretions present above the cuff into the mouth. The endotracheal tube is then removed during a forced inspiration, when the vocal cords are maximally open. The patient is instructed to immediately cough and expectorate these secretions. The patient is then given oxygen via a mask using the same inspired oxygen as was used in the T-piece trial if that was satisfactory. Initially, the patient is observed closely for laryngospasm and respiratory distress. Blood gases should be checked within an hour after extubation. Effective pulmonary toilet is begun as soon as the patient is extubated. This procedure consists of encouraging the patient to cough effectively, frequent use of an incentive spirometer, chest physiotherapy, and perhaps intermittent positive-pressure breathing.

The T-piece trial may need to be modified in certain circumstances. After prolonged intubation, a more prolonged weaning process may be needed, and for this purpose, intermittent mandatory ventilation may be useful, even in adults. Steroids may be helpful in avoiding glottic or subglottic edema. Continuous positive airway pressure may be indicated in circumstances in which decreased lung volume, airway closure, or pursed-lip breathing may occur.

Postextubation Care

An energetic program is essential to ensure secretion clearance and prevent atelectasis, infection, and respiratory failure. Good nursing is very important and includes encouraging the patient to frequently take deep breaths and cough vigorously. Supporting the patient's chest at the incision site will reduce the pain of these activities. Incentive spirometry, perhaps on an hourly basis, is effective in increasing lung volumes. Patient supervision and encouragement are required if these devices are to be used effectively.[86, 119] Percussion and vibration of the chest wall should be performed several times a day. Postural drainage and percussion aid in removal of secretions from the airway. Intermittent positive-pressure breathing as a method of clearing secretions has been criticized because lung inflation is controlled by a preset pressure. If it is used to produce a breath of given volume, intermittent positive-pressure breathing may be of benefit, especially in patients with muscle weakness and a history of chronic obstructive pulmonary disease or in those with thick, tenacious secretions and an ineffective cough.[36] To stimulate coughing and to aspirate these thick secretions, intermittent nasotracheal suction also may be needed. Flexible fiberoptic bronchoscopy should be used when these measures fail.[108] Bronchodilator drugs and heated or ultrasonic mist or nebulized water also may be useful. Careful ECG monitoring is required during the administration of β-sympathomimetic agonists, which may potentially induce tachyarrhythmias.

The patient's ability to cough effectively and cooperate in chest physical therapy depends on pain being minimized. Bromage[28] showed that postoperative pain reduces the functional residual capacity, increases transpulmonary pressures, and induces airway closure. These changes result from the restriction of diaphragmatic and chest wall movement. Correct analgesic dosage will mitigate these events. Too much opiate analgesic, however, by sedating the patient excessively, by impairing the cough reflex, and by its parasympathomimetic action that makes airway secretions more viscid, is as bad as too little. Patients vary in their analgesic requirements. The patient should receive a titrated dose rather than a set "ward-standardized" dose. To ensure proper absorption, this should be administered intravenously rather than intramuscularly. Morphine in increments of 1 to 2 mg given intravenously at 30-minute intervals is suggested for adults.

Oxygen supplementation will continue to be required after extubation. The appropriate FIO_2 will be indicated by the patient's blood gas analysis. Masks using the Venturi principle have the advantage of accurate control of the FIO_2, with no dependence of inspired oxygen tension on the patient's tidal volume. The high flow rates produced by these masks make them more comfortable for the patient than conventional low-flow masks. A disadvantage of all masks is that they have to be removed for expectoration and eating and they lack patient acceptance. For adults, nasal cannulas are an extremely useful means of administering low-flow oxygen supplementation because they can be worn without discomfort continuously below flow rates of 6 L/minute. Each liter of flow raises the FIO_2 by approximately 0.03.

Careful and continuous monitoring of the patient's respiratory condition is required in directing therapy. In addition to frequent auscultation of the chest, a roentgenogram of the chest should be obtained daily or as needed. This roentgenogram provides maximal information if it is obtained with the patient in a head-up position with a 45-degree tilt. Cardiac enlargement may cause compression of the large bronchi, especially of the bronchus to the left lower lobe.

Attention to the patient's fluid balance is important. Fluid overload will eventually result in pulmonary edema, while dehydration may make secretions more tenacious and difficult to expectorate. Uncorrected metabolic alkalosis due to continued free nasogastric tube drainage and use of potent diuretics causes impairment of respiratory drive and retention of carbon dioxide. Such conditions should be treated to make optimal the respiratory status.

CONDUCT OF PROLONGED MECHANICAL VENTILATION IN THE ADULT

If clinical assessment suggests that mechanical ventilation cannot be withdrawn, or if the weaning trial is unsatisfactory, continued mechanical ventilation will be necessary. The incidence of prolonged mechanical ventilation (>24 hours) in adults operated on in our institution is less than 10%. The incidence of prolonged mechanical ventilation is greater in children. In children aged 2 to 13 years, 20% required prolonged mechanical ventilation, while 36% of children aged less than 2 years needed this (Table 24–3). The major cause for prolonged mechanical ventilation and death in both adults and children is the low cardiac output syndrome (Tables 24–1 and 24–3 to 24–5).

The cardiac lesion for which surgery was performed also determines the time of extubation. Aortic valve replacements and coronary bypass

TABLE 24-3.—DEATHS AND MECHANICAL VENTILATION IN 430 CHILDREN LESS THAN 13 YEARS OLD UNDERGOING CARDIAC SURGERY (MAYO CLINIC, JANUARY 1976 TO JULY 1977)

MECHANICAL VENTILATION	AGE, YR		
	>2	≤2	TOTAL
Prolonged (>24 hr)			
No. of patients	61 (20)*	48 (36)*	109 (25)*
Deaths			
No.	10	12	22
%	16	25	20
Short-term (<24 hr)			
No. of patients	156	72	228
Deaths			
No.	10	18	28
%	6	25	12
None†			
No. of patients	81	12	93
Deaths	1	2	3

*Number in parentheses represents percent of whole group receiving prolonged mechanical ventilation.
†Deaths in operating room are shown here; nine late deaths are not included.

grafts in patients with good preoperative cardiac function are more likely to result in early extubation than are mitral valve replacements or repairs of congenital heart defects. The reason for this is that aortotomy and vessel grafting result in less interference with ventricular function than does ventriculotomy.

The prognosis for patients who require prolonged mechanical ventilation after cardiac surgery is better than for patients who require prolonged mechanical ventilation in the general medical and surgical intensive care units. The mortality of 20% for our patients requiring prolonged mechanical ventilation after cardiac surgery is approximately half the mortality of patients requiring prolonged mechanical ventilation in our general medical and surgical intensive care units. Patients admitted to general intensive care units after prolonged mechanical ventilation often have severe pulmonary disease in association with generalized systemic illness complicated by infection or renal failure or both. The cardiac patients, by contrast, have been well selected and prepared for the surgical episode.

The need for prolonged mechanical ventilation should be weighed against the risks of the therapy, including the risks attendant on prolonged endotracheal intubation.

Endotracheal Intubation and Airway Management

Endotracheal tubes are a frequent source of morbidity.[20] Improvement in the design of endotracheal tubes, together with better care for the intubated patient, has reduced but not eliminated these problems. Injury to the upper airway caused by endotracheal tubes is most pronounced at those points where the tube exerts maximal physical force against the sidewalls of the airway. Thus, the posterolateral surface of the larynx[107] and that length of trachea in contact with the endotracheal tube cuff[31] are areas that are most likely to be damaged. Laryngeal damage may progress through mucosal congestion to ulceration, resulting in granuloma formation, airway obstruction, and, occasionally, scarring and stenosis.[107] Acute laryngeal edema and transient laryngeal incompetence also may occur after endotracheal intubation.[78] Serious tracheal injuries resulting from intubation include stenosis, tracheomalacia, tracheoesophageal fistula, and, rarely, trachea–innominate artery fistulas.[77] The incidence of these complications appears to be related to the length of time that the tube is in place.[107] In the past, the use of low-volume, high-pressure cuffs for endotracheal tubes allowed interference with capillary blood flow in the tracheal wall.[96] This localized tracheal ischemia and the consequent pathologic changes are more likely to occur in patients in a low cardiac output state.[107] Other factors include the use of endotracheal tubes constructed from tissue-irritant materials, for example, red rubber,[78] the use of plastic tubes still containing some residual chemical such as ethylene oxide from sterilization, and inadequate sterility dur-

TABLE 24-4.—REASONS FOR PROLONGED MECHANICAL VENTILATION AFTER CARDIAC SURGERY IN 80 SURVIVORS LESS THAN 13 YEARS OLD (MAYO CLINIC, JANUARY 1976 TO JULY 1977)

REASON	NO.	%
Postoperative bleeding	5	6
Low cardiac output syndrome	23	29
Pulmonary congestion	24	30
Cardiac arrhythmia	5	6
Hypoxemia or failed weaning trial	13	16
Bronchospasm and excessive secretions	5	6
Severe respiratory distress syndrome	3	4
Metabolic acidosis or alkalosis	2	3
Total	80	100

TABLE 24–5.—CAUSES OF DEATH AFTER CARDIAC SURGERY IN CHILDREN (MAYO CLINIC, JANUARY 1976 TO JULY 1977)

CAUSE	MECHANICAL VENTILATION	
	>24 HR (N = 109)	<24 HR OR NONE (N = 321)
Low cardiac output	16	28*
Other cardiac	0	3†
Pneumonitis	3	0
Pulmonary embolus	1	0
Not reviewed	2	0
Total	22	31

*Three patients died in the operating room.
†Acute right ventricular failure, arrhythmia, myocardial infarct.

ing suctioning, with introduced infection. Finally, movement of the tube relative to the airway and the use of overly large tubes are factors that also may contribute to mechanical damage to the trachea.[107] Current use of disposable, non-tissue-toxic, plastic endotracheal tubes with large residual volume, large-diameter, low-pressure cuffs has significantly reduced the incidence of tracheal damage from the endotracheal tube.[32, 109, 116]

If nasal septal deformity does not exclude nasal intubation, the latter route is preferable to transoral intubation for both adult and child who need prolonged mechanical ventilation. Nasal intubation requires the use of a longer endotracheal tube of slightly smaller diameter than does oral intubation in the same patient, making suction more difficult but providing greater stability for fixation of the airway and improved comfort to the patient. Nasal tubes are less likely to cause nausea, retching, and coughing, which are common with oral tubes. In addition, nasal tubes are less likely to kink and cannot be bitten by the disoriented or combative patient.

Endobronchial intubation of the right mainstem bronchus is a common complication of intubation and should be checked by auscultation and roentgenography of the chest. The volume of air inserted into the cuff of the endotracheal tube should be just sufficient to produce a seal. A minimal leak can occur with inflating pressures greater than 25 cm H_2O applied to this airway.[33] The cuff pressure should be checked from time to time. When topical anesthesia is used for intubation, it should be recalled that these agents are rapidly absorbed from the mucosa and that toxic doses can be given by this route. This factor may be of particular importance for the cardiac patient, who may be receiving lidocaine for the suppression of arrhythmia. If the patient needs airway securement for mechanical ventilation or other reasons for longer than one week, tracheostomy should be considered. Lindholm[107] noted that laryngeal injury after endotracheal intubation was time-dependent, and approached 100% by the fourth day. This finding may indicate the need for tracheostomy. Since publication of that classic thesis, better construction of endotracheal tubes and the use of soft cuffs have probably reduced the rapidity with which such damage tends to occur. However, laryngeal injury is still seen. The use of tracheostomy is associated with a particular risk of mediastinal infection for the post-cardiac surgical patient who has had a median sternotomy wound. In addition, both mortality and morbidity are associated with the procedure itself. Late complications, including stenosis at the site of the tracheostomy stoma, also are relatively frequent.[107] Our experience suggests that endotracheal intubation for one week is associated with minimal risks.

Humidification, frequent careful suctioning, and attention to physical therapy of the chest, with drainage of the airway, are essential in the safe management of the patient with an artificial airway in place. Persistent collapse of a segment of lung may require fiberoptic bronchoscopy in an attempt to clear that airway in the adult patient. Fiberbronchoscopy[108] becomes necessary if adequate humidity, suctioning techniques, and chest vibration with postural drainage do not clear the bronchus within a suitable time, from six to eight hours.

Mechanical Ventilation

The ideal ventilator is volume-preset and capable of generating airway pressure in excess of 80 cm H_2O. The ventilator should be capable of controlled ventilation or assisted ventilation and, in addition, provide intermittent mandatory ventilation. Positive end-expiratory pressure is also necessary. The ventilator should be linked to an adequate humidifier[34] and have built-in alarm signals for disconnection and machine malfunction. Changes in inspired or expired (or both) gas mixture also may be monitored. Finally, ease of use and ease of cleaning and sterilization are also important considerations.

Ventilatory Support

The three essentials for adequate ventilatory support are adequate ventilation, adequate oxygenation, and adequate clearance of secretions. Unless unconscious or uncooperative, the patient should be ventilated in the ventilator-assist or intermittent mandatory ventilation mode, as opposed to the ventilator-controlled mode. This method permits the patient to control the $PaCO_2$ at near-normal levels and provides lower mean intrathoracic pressure. The patient will almost always be synchronized with the ventilator if the minute volume is adequate. For adults, the minute ventilation should be at least three times the body weight in pounds, that is, approximately three times the anatomical dead space, and the respiratory frequency should be set at levels that are suitable, that is, from 10 to 12 breaths per minute for the adult. With increasing physiologic dead space, a higher minute volume may be required than would be normal for the patient's surface area.[59, 146] Pulmonary congestion and heart failure may cause mild hyperventilation. Addition of apparatus dead space may be considered in these circumstances. The patient's synchronization with the ventilator is not affected by added dead space, which will return the $PaCO_2$ toward normal. Acute respiratory alkalosis should be avoided because of the associated changes in serum potassium concentration and serum ionized calcium levels, which will potentially interfere with cardiac function. It is rarely necessary to paralyze a patient in order to settle him on the respirator. Sedation with morphine is useful. The major risk in the use of both muscle relaxants and sedatives is hypotension.

Adequate oxygenation must be assured and can be adjusted by manipulating the FIO_2, by using positive end-expiratory pressure,[11] and by altering the patient's body position. The alteration of body position alters the gravity-dependent distribution of perfusion throughout the lung.[52] Thus, turning edematous or consolidated portions of the lung into nondependent positions may reduce the perfusion to those regions and increase perfusion toward more normal portions of lung, resulting in better gas exchange. A PaO_2 higher than 60 mm Hg is safe. When the patient first returns to the intensive care unit, the FIO_2 should be set at 0.5 unless the patient has required higher fractions in the operating room. Blood gases are obtained after a period of 30 minutes for the adequacy of the PaO_2 to be examined.

Positive end-expiratory pressure is of little benefit when hypoxemia is caused by fixed intrapulmonary or intracardiac shunt and is potentially dangerous in low cardiac output states.[140] Improvement in PaO_2 with positive end-expiratory pressure is believed to be due to an increase in functional residual capacity and possibly a decrease in airway closure, with reexpansion of areas that may have become atelectatic or edematous. The technique also may affect the distribution of ventilation and thus alter the distribution of ventilation-perfusion ratios in the lung.[1] The optimal benefit is achieved when the PaO_2 is on the steeper portion of the oxyhemoglobin dissociation curve (that is, < 60 mm Hg). A small increase in PO_2 in this situation will be associated with a large increase in arterial oxygen content and, thus, oxygen delivery to the tissues. The use of positive end-expiratory pressure in an attempt to increase PaO_2 above 60 to 70 mm Hg would then not be of great value and potentially may result in a large reduction in oxygen delivery to the tissues, because cardiac output will be decreased by the higher mean intrathoracic pressure produced. However, positive end-expiratory pressure may be useful in attempting to maintain the FIO_2 at safe levels (below 0.6) in patients in whom prolonged mechanical ventilation is required.

Several methods have been described to assess optimal positive end-expiratory pressure for a patient, including measurements of the $P(A-a)O_2$, the mixed venous oxygen tension, cardiac output,[110] and total static compliance of the respiratory system.[135, 181] The use of mixed venous oxygen tension is probably the most effective method.[110]

Reductions in cardiac output are seen with high positive end-expiratory pressure. High pressure is relatively contraindicated in patients who have undergone a Fontan procedure for tricuspid atresia or right ventricular outflow lesions or in patients in whom increases in pulmonary vascular resistance may have an adverse effect on right ventricular function.[64] The aim of treatment of these patients is to maintain pulmonary vascular resistance at a minimum. The use of positive end-expiratory pressure in such patients must be balanced with two results in mind. Increased positive end-expiratory pressure levels will, of themselves, increase pulmonary vascular resistance, but decreased lung volume and hypoxemic vasoconstriction also will increase pulmonary vascular resistance.[19] Cautious application of positive end-expiratory pressure with repeated measurements of mixed venous oxygen tension or saturation and repeated estimations of right atrial pressure and cardiac output may be needed to achieve optimal positive end-expiratory pressure levels in these circumstances. Qvist and others[145] showed that an infusion of fluids to increase blood volume during use of positive end-expiratory pressure often produces a significant increase in cardiac output and in oxygen delivery to the tissues. When high pressure levels are required, intermittent mandatory ventilation is a desirable mode of ventilation.[92]

The adequate clearance of secretions from the lung is provided by frequent suctioning and by physical therapy maneuvers of the chest. Chest physical therapy while the patient remains intubated and on prolonged mechanical ventilation is important and becomes increasingly so when the patient has a weaning problem. A comprehensive plan of care for the patient with a weaning problem includes attention to nutrition, skin care, psychologic support, and therapeutic exercise. The patient who is dependent on mechanical ventilators may become physically debilitated. Many patients may be unable to ambulate for days to weeks because of their poor hemodynamic state. Lack of mobilization and exercise causes muscle weakness, joint immobility, and decrease in cardiopulmonary endurance. There is also an increased propensity for secretion retention. These factors may add to other complications and prolong weaning.

A physical therapy program combining therapeutic exercise and other physical procedures should be initiated early during the course of management for the patient receiving prolonged mechanical ventilation.[82] These physical procedures include range-of-motion and strengthening exercises, breathing retraining exercises, chest mobilization exercises, bronchial drainage, chest clapping, vibration and shaking, and progressive ambulatory activity. Cooperation from a physical therapist in designing such programs is very valuable to the patient.

Four important complications may occur in patients who require prolonged mechanical ventilation: infections of the lung, pulmonary edema, bronchospasm, and barotrauma with pneumomediastinum and pneumothorax.[184] Necessary is attention to sterility during suctioning, to the quality and quantity of secretions from the respiratory tract, and to the free use of cultures, together with the application of appropriate antibiotics when an infection is present. Colonization of the superficial layers of mucosa in the trachea and major bronchi is frequent and can be differentiated from lung infection by the absence of significant changes on the chest roentgenogram and by the absence of high fever or of changes in the leukocyte count. Pneumothorax and pneumomediastinum are frequently seen in patients who require high levels of positive end-expiratory pressure and should be watched for with great care. Pulmonary edema may collect in distinct anatomical positions in the lungs of patients after cardiac surgery. The distribution of edema is dependent on gravitational forces, as is the distribution of perfusion. Edema fluid, therefore, tends to collect in the dependent portion of the lung. The edema may be unilateral or even lobar under certain conditions in the cardiac patient, for example, in the patient where pulmonary venous obstruction is produced during surgery. When edema collects in dependent areas, interfering primarily with gas exchange in these areas, the shunt fraction may be temporarily reduced by rotating the most edematous portion of the lung into a nondependent position. This may be achieved by prone or lateral positioning of the patient.[52] Staub[171] showed that edema does not accumulate as rapidly in the lungs of an animal that is rotated frequently from one body position to another. Therefore, rotating the edematous area to a nondependent position may result in more rapid clearance of edema fluid, thus hastening lymphatic drainage from this portion of the lung. If fluid is present in large volumes, then rotating the edematous portion of the lung may result in displacement of the fluid, and one should be careful that other portions of the lung are not drowned. Bronchospasm may dictate the need for bronchodilators.

Weaning and Extubation

After prolonged mechanical ventilation, the vital capacity, tidal volume, and maximal inspiratory and expiratory forces are valuable in indicating a suitable time for weaning. These measurements may be misleading in the immediate postoperative period,[120] and weaning at this stage can be best judged from other criteria. If the maximal inspiratory force generated from residual volume is persistently reduced far below normal range, it may be important to assess diaphragmatic function by means of fluoroscopy. Interference with one or the other phrenic nerves during cardiac surgery is not uncommon.[124] Such lesions may be reversible. Metabolic alkalosis also may prolong weaning, as may a lack of hypoxic responsiveness in patients with cyanotic congenital heart disease. Assessment of both carbon dioxide and oxygen responsiveness may be needed and can be achieved by noting minute ventilation and obtaining arterial blood gas values during periods of spontaneous breathing, as FIO_2 is reduced back toward 0.21.

Weaning from mechanical ventilatory support should be done in stages. The patient with severe difficulty in tissue oxygenation probably should be weaned through assisted ventilation to intermittent mandatory ventilation and to continuous positive airway pressure with spontaneous ventilation. Continuous positive airway pressure with spontaneous ventilation is associated with a lower mean intrathoracic pressure, in contrast to assisted ventilation with positive end-expiratory pressure. This relationship occurs because mean intrathoracic pressure is lower with continuous positive airway pressure and spontaneous ventilation than with assisted ventilation and positive end-expiratory pressure.[39] Continuous positive airway pressure with spontaneous ventilation, however, increases the work of breathing, and the patient may not tolerate this for prolonged periods. Blood gases should be assessed frequently during changes in mode of ventilation. Use of a Bird respirator attached to a walking frame (Fig 24–6) for ambulation of patients who require prolonged mechanical ventilation has been useful in increasing the rapidity with which they regain general muscle tone and strength and also in allowing them to be withdrawn from ventilatory support. In addition, attention should be given to nutrition and general care.

Summary

A general plan of care for patients after cardiac surgery and prolonged mechanical ventilation requires that the function of each of the patient's vital systems be fully reviewed at least once every 12 hours (Table 24–6). This procedure requires that a careful record be kept during the intervening period so that trends can be recognized. Treatment will be successful only

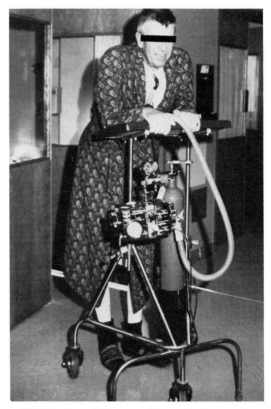

Fig 24–6.—Patient walking with frame. Note tracheostomy and Bird respirator with oxygen cylinder.

TABLE 24–6.—Checklist for Patient Needing Prolonged Mechanical Ventilation

Airway	Endotracheal tube needs suctioning? Needs tube change (oral versus nasal)? Is tube size appropriate (air leak)? Is tracheostomy required? Is patient's airway adequate? Needs positional change (supine to prone)?
Breathing	Is minute ventilation appropriate ($Paco_2$, pH)? Is oxygenation adequate (Pao_2, Fio_2)? Needs PEEP*? Secretions (nature, amount, color, culture)? Needs chest physical therapy, drugs?
Circulation	Is cardiac index (CI) adequate? Pulsus paradoxus? Is pattern of ventilation appropriate? Is any change indicated to improve CI and thus increase pulmonary flow? Any specific procedures or lesions, for example, right-to-left or left-to-right shunts (balance of systemic and pulmonary vascular resistance will affect relative flow in the two beds), or Fontan procedure (might mean changes in pulmonary vascular resistance with PEEP use could affect blood flow)?
Is feeding needed?	Greater than 3 days of starvation in noncatheterized patient suggests a definite need. Oxygen uptake? Prefer enteral route; may need parenteral route.
Is weaning problem present?	Chronic obstructive lung disease or other preexisting problem? Diaphragm paralysis? Metabolic alkalosis and hypokalemia on diuretics? Cachexia or severe congestive cardiac failure? Check vital capacity, tidal volume, maximal pressures? Screen diaphragm? Is feeding adequate? Ambulation? Intermittent mandatory ventilation may be useful? Can we change endotracheal tube to larger size to reduce resistance for spontaneous breathing trials?

*Positive end-expiratory pressure.

when every complication is immediately diagnosed and managed. The medical staff should set safe limits on the physiologic variables that are being recorded, and the nursing staff should be directed to alert a physician if these variables exceed the limits. A patient on mechanical ventilation should never be left unattended.

Attention to the respiratory system requires attention to the respirator, attention to the adequacy of ventilation and the acid-base status of the patient, attention to the adequacy of oxygenation, and checking the Fio_2, positive end-expiratory pressure, body position changes, and the adequacy of clearance of secretions. Attention to the oxygen delivery to the tissues is important, and one should remember that decreases in cardiac output may follow increases in minute ventilation or the addition of positive end-expiratory pressure.

Neurologically compromised patients may require the continuous assessment of their conscious level. Hypoxemia, carbon dioxide retention, and hypotension potentially depress the level of consciousness. Complete skin and eye care must be given to these patients, and artificial tears or chloramphenicol ointment or eyedrops are useful. In such patients, the peripheral nerves (especially the lateral popliteal), the radial nerve, and the brachial plexus are easily damaged if the limbs are improperly positioned. The facial nerve also can be damaged by pressure from the endotracheal tube, whereas pressure on the eyeball may cause retinal artery thrombosis and blindness, especially in the hypotensive patient.

To avoid urinary retention, the patient should be catheterized as required. Closed urinary drainage is useful in reducing the risk of urinary tract infection and in assessing the adequacy of renal function. Renal failure greatly increases the risk of death.[2]

The patient will not require nutritional supplements for the first 48 hours after operation. However, in this period and subsequently, adequate fluids and electrolytes must be given and any deficiencies must be corrected. Usually, fluids are restricted during the immediate postoperative period, particularly if hemodilution was used. After 48 hours, the patient will require increased caloric input over that provided by 5% glucose. An enteral route should be used; however, if that is not possible, parenteral nutrition can be used. The risk of systemic infection using parenteral nutrition is minimized by the careful attention to the site of introduction of the central venous catheter. Additional insulin may be required by these patients.

CONDUCT OF PROLONGED MECHANICAL VENTILATION IN INFANTS

Generally, in infants, the risks of continued intubation are less than the risks of cardiovascular instability with low cardiac output during at least the first postoperative night. The increased nursing skills, the use of nasotracheal intubation, the choice of a proper endotracheal tube size, a fixation-retention harness for the tube, and appropriate sedation allow emphasis to be placed on cardiovascular stability and a slow, safe progression from mechanical to spontaneous ventilation rather than on the rapidity of extubation.

The incidence of prolonged mechanical ventilation is greater for children than for adults, being highest in children less than 2 years old. The incidence of prolonged mechanical ventilation in our series of patients[115] (Table 24-3) and the changes in mortality during the last ten years for consecutive patients from various institutions[16, 23, 53, 112, 173] are shown in Tables 24-4 and 24-7.

Endotracheal Intubation and Airway Management

Major problems with endotracheal tubes in infants are related to (1) the endotracheal tube size, that is, the outside diameter and length, (2) route of insertion, and (3) blockage or obstruction of the tube.[6] For each patient, a new sterile tube should be used. The tube should be cut and inserted in the operating room, with a length adapted to each infant (Table 24-8). The type of tube used will depend on the clinical judgment of the anesthesiologist. Clear plastic, nonreactive tubes, noncuffed, up to size 5 or 6 F, are preferable. A small air leak should be present with positive-pressure ventilation (30 cm H_2O) after the tube is positioned. If necessary, the tube should be replaced in the operating room at the end of surgery to ensure that such a leak is present, or a change should be made to a nasal tube as necessary.

If the patient's condition permits, nasal tubes are preferable for patients aged up to 10 years who require mechanical ventilation for 24 hours or more. Nasal tubes cause less patient distress, are more easily fixed, and cannot be bitten or moved by the patient's tongue. Nasal tubes are particularly important when prolonged mechanical ventilation is required.[7] Fixation-retention harnesses may be useful in preventing tube movement (Fig 24-7). Metal wire adapters (Tunstall) with a special head harness provide stable fixation of the nasotracheal tube. To avoid trauma to the nose, the metal adapter tip should be positioned just outside the nose. With nasal tubes, the tube is fixed to the forehead by means of a head harness consisting of Elastoplast, foam rubber, a wire adapter, tape (clear or adhesive), and ties.

An inappropriately long tube may enter the right main-stem bronchus or, on occasion, the left main-stem bronchus. A roentgenogram of the chest should be used to verify the position of the tip of the tube in relation to the carina. Blockage or obstruction of the tube may occur with oral or nasal tubes. Damage to the nares, with nosebleeds and sinus infection, may further complicate the use of nasal tubes. Because the narrowest point in the child's airway is at the level of the cricoid cartilage, this is the maximal point for pressure with an oversized tube (inappropriately large diameter). Secretions have

TABLE 24-7.—OUTCOME AFTER CARDIAC SURGERY IN CHILDREN (SERIES PUBLISHED SINCE 1970)

AUTHOR	PATIENT NO.	AGE, MO	DEATHS NO.	%	TIME OF REVIEW, YR	TECHNIQUE
Downes et al.[53]	129*	≤24	31	24	2	Intermittent positive-pressure breathing
Stewart et al.[173]	43	≤38	10	23	3/4	Continuous positive airway pressure
Barratt-Boyes[16]	160	≤24	35	22	3 3/4	Profound hypothermia
Bonchek and Starr[23]	100	≤24	27	27	0	Standard bypass
Mayo series[115]	132†	≤24	32	24	1 1/2	Mixed
	298	<13 yr	21	7	1 1/2	
Mansfield et al.[112]	204	≤24	15	7	4	Mixed
	237	>2	4	2	4	

Required prolonged mechanical ventilation: *41%. †36%.

TABLE 24-8.—SUGGESTED SIZE AND LENGTH FOR ENDOTRACHEAL TUBES IN CHILDREN UNDERGOING CARDIAC SURGERY

SIZE*		LENGTH, CM			
OD (F)	ID, MM	ORAL	NASAL (20% LONGER)	AGE, MO	WEIGHT, KG
12	3.0	11	12	Neonate	1–3
14	3.5	11.5	12.5	Neonate	3–4
16	4.0	13–14	15.0	Neonate	3–4
18	4.5	14–15	17.5	1–6	7
20	5.0	15–16	19.2	6–18	10
22	5.5	16–17	20.5	18–36	15
24	6.0	17–18	22	48+	15

*OD indicates outer diameter; ID, inner diameter.

presented serious problems when humidification has been inadequate or excessive and when suctioning technique has not been meticulous. The suction catheter should be passed beyond the distal end of the tube into the major airways at each attempt. Kinking and mechanical obstruction of the tube also may occur with improper fixation, particularly when the tube is too long. Adequate placement and fixation, humidification, and suctioning prevent these complications. The importance of each procedure must be stressed in the care of the infant and should be frequently pointed out to the nursing staff at the bedside.

Humidification[18] and suctioning are essential for the safe care of infants. Continuous humidification of inspired gas should be provided whenever possible in the operating room and is essential after the operation. An ultrasonic nebulizer should be used with care in small infants because it can lead to fluid overload. Intratracheal instillations of saline or water are indicated to increase humidification and liquefaction of secretions, particularly in the presence of bloody or tenacious material. Saline injection should be limited to 0.5 ml each half-hour for children who weigh less than 10 kg. The amount, volume, and frequency of saline instillations should

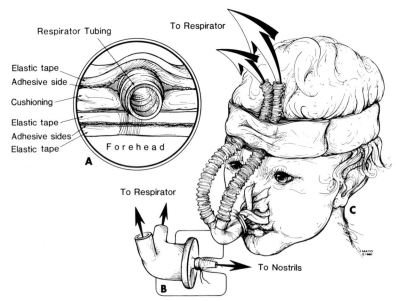

Fig 24-7.—Nasal tube, fixation-retention harness, and strapping in an infant. **A**, detail of harness as it passes over infant's forehead. **B**, endotracheal tube adapter is tied to tube. **C**, apparatus in place.

be determined by the physician. The risk of fluid overload and infection from these instillations must be considered.

Suctioning should be performed regularly and as needed. A sterile catheter should be passed, using a sterile, no-touch technique, through and beyond the end of the tube at least every 30 minutes if the presence of secretions does not demand more frequent suctioning. The suctioning procedure requires two persons. Before and after suctioning, the patient's lungs should be manually hyperinflated during approximately 30 seconds, with 100% oxygen delivered from an anesthesia bag. Suctioning for longer than 10 seconds may cause hypoxemia. The diameter of the suction catheters should be less than half the internal diameter of the endotracheal tube. Attention to sterility of all the open ends of respirator tubing is vital during these procedures.

Mechanical Ventilation

The early use of intermittent mandatory ventilation and continuous positive airway pressure with spontaneous ventilation in infants requires that the ventilator chosen for use provides these modes, in addition to the assist and control modes, at the relatively high frequencies and small tidal volumes that these infants may need. Low levels of positive end-expiratory pressure to 2.5 cm H_2O may be appropriate for most children, excluding those who have had some particular procedure, for example, the Fontan procedure, in which the technique is relatively contraindicated.

Ventilatory Support

As for adults, adequate ventilation with attention to the acid-base status of the patient, adequate oxygenation and adequate clearance of secretions, and rapid treatment of the complications of infection, pneumothorax, edema, and bronchospasm are the main aims of ventilatory support for infants. During transport from the operating room, the patient should be ventilated using a manually inflated anesthesia bag delivering 100% oxygen. In the intensive care unit, children who weigh up to 10 kg are best ventilated using intermittent mandatory ventilation or continuous positive airway pressure with spontaneous ventilation. Volume ventilators may be used when appropriate, although pressure generators are sometimes preferable. Acceptable values provide $PaCO_2$ between 30 and 45 mm Hg and PaO_2 greater than 60 mm Hg and less than 150 mm Hg at an FIO_2 of less than 0.6 and a pH from 7.3 to 7.5, with base excess or deficit in the range of ±5 mEq/L. The effective compliance should be approximately 15 ml/cm H_2O.

Weaning and Extubation

Withdrawal of ventilatory support may be started when hemodynamics are stable, minimal chest tube drainage is present, rhythm is stable, and cardiac output is adequate without significant inotropic or vasopressor support. The following sequence is useful: controlled or assisted mechanical ventilation to intermittent mandatory ventilation, to continuous positive airway pressure, to extubation, to increased oxygen concentration using a head hood or face mask, to removal of oxygen supplement. A typical procedure plan might be as follows: (1) begin intermittent mandatory ventilation at 18 breaths per minute plus spontaneous ventilation with positive end-expiratory pressure at 6 cm H_2O; (2) reduce intermittent mandatory ventilation in steps from 18 to 12 to 6 breaths per minute; and (3) decrease the continuous positive airway pressure from 6 to 3 cm H_2O when spontaneous ventilation is adequate with an FIO_2 of 0.4.

Blood gas measurements should usually be obtained with each step. After cardiopulmonary bypass procedures, the tube usually is left in place overnight for small infants. If all progresses well, by the following morning continuous positive airway pressure should be at 3 cm H_2O or less and the FIO_2 should be 0.4 to 0.5. Then the infant will be ready to be extubated shortly thereafter. Chest physical therapy should be routine whether the infant is extubated or not.

Glottic or subglottic edema after prolonged intubation in children is not uncommon.[74] Steroids may be indicated before or after extubation in this situation. Dexamethasone may be given at a dose of 2 to 4 mg intravenously 30 minutes before extubation and repeated once after two hours. Gradually decreasing this dose of steroid is not required. If stridor develops after extubation, a dilute solution of racemic epinephrine (Vaponefrin) in half doses delivered every hour for six hours may be useful. The incidence of stridor and edema is greatly lessened by ensuring an adequate air leak around the tube at the time of intubation.

The small tubes required for infants introduce a significant resistance to breathing. The infant may repeatedly fail trials of spontaneous breathing, and at this point, a trial extubation may be successful when trials of spontaneous breathing through the endotracheal tube have repeatedly failed. If extubation is to be tried, the immediate availability of intubation skills and resuscitative help is essential for at least the first two to four hours.

Summary

General care for infants after cardiac surgery requires careful attention to a systems review, as it does for adults. Nurses caring for pediatric postcardiac surgical patients should be trained both in the special techniques required for the care of infants and in those required for the care of cardiac surgical patients. Nursing coverage for all infants should be provided on a one-to-one basis, and the medical staff should be immediately available at all times while the patient is in the unit. In addition to close attention to the respiratory system, the following aspects need particular attention in the infant. Maintenance of adequate cardiac output and satisfactory hemodynamic stability is essential. Fluid balance must be accurate and blood or plasma transfusion must be provided quickly when needed to maintain an optimal blood volume. Flushing of monitoring lines and blood samples for analyses must use as small a volume as is possible, and the amount should be recorded and included in the evaluation of the fluid balance. Neonates must be maintained at a neutral thermal range. Blood sugar levels should be estimated at frequent intervals because hypoglycemia is frequent in this age group.

REFERENCES

1. Abboud N., et al.: Lung volumes and closing capacity with continuous positive airway pressure. *Anesthesiology* 42:138, 1975.
2. Abel R.M., et al.: Etiology, incidence, and prognosis of renal failure following cardiac operations: Results of a prospective analysis of 500 consecutive patients. *J. Thorac. Cardiovasc. Surg.* 71:323, 1976.
3. Agostoni E., Mead J.: Statics of the respiratory system, in Fenn W.O., Rahn H. (eds.): *Handbook of Physiology.* Section 3: *Respiration.* Washington, D.C., American Physiological Society, 1964, vol. 1, p. 387.
4. Alderson P.O., et al.: Pulmonary perfusion abnormalities and ventilation-perfusion imbalance in children after total repair of tetralogy of Fallot. *Circulation* 53:332, 1976.
5. Alexander J.I., et al.: The role of airway closure in postoperative hypoxaemia. *Br. J. Anaesth.* 45:34, 1973.
6. Allen T.H., Steven I.M.: Prolonged endotracheal intubation in infants and children. *Br. J. Anaesth.* 37:566, 1965.
7. Allen T.H., Steven I.M.: Prolonged nasotracheal intubation in infants and children. *Br. J. Anaesth.* 44:835, 1972.
8. Andersen N.B., Ghia J.: Pulmonary function, cardiac status, and postoperative course in relation to cardiopulmonary bypass. *J. Thorac. Cardiovasc. Surg.* 59:474, 1970.
9. Armstrong R.F., et al.: Continuous monitoring of mixed venous oxygen tension. *Br. Med. J.* 2:282, 1976.
10. Asada S., Yamaguchi M.: Fine structural change in the lung following cardiopulmonary bypass: Its relationship to early postoperative course. *Chest* 59:478, 1971.
11. Ashbaugh D.G., Petty T.L.: Positive end-expiratory pressure: Physiology, indications, and contraindications. *J. Thorac. Cardiovasc. Surg.* 65:165, 1973.
12. Ashutosh K., et al.: Impedance pneumograph and magnetometer methods for monitoring tidal volume. *J. Appl. Physiol.* 37:964, 1974.
13. Ayres S.M.: Use of mass spectrometry for evaluation of respiratory function in the critically ill patient, editorial. *Crit. Care Med.* 4:219, 1976.
14. Bachofen M., Weibel E.R.: Alterations of the gas exchange apparatus in adult respiratory insufficiency associated with septicemia. *Am. Rev. Respir. Dis.* 116:589, 1977.
15. Bakhle Y.S.: Epilogue, in Bakhle Y.S., Vane J.R. (eds.): *Lung Biology in Health and Disease.* Vol. 4: *Metabolic Functions of the Lung.* New York, Marcel Dekker, 1977, p. 321.
16. Barratt-Boyes B.G.: The technique of intracardiac repair in infancy using deep hypothermia with circulatory arrest and limited cardiopulmonary bypass, in Ionescu M.I., Wooler G.H. (eds.): *Current Techniques in Extracorporeal Circulation.* London, Butterworth & Co., 1976, p. 197.
17. Bates D.V., Macklem P.T., Christie R.V.: *Respiratory Function in Disease: An Introduction to the Integrated Study of the Lung,* ed. 2. Philadelphia, W.B. Saunders Co., 1971, p. 321.
18. Battersby E.F., Hatch D.J., Towey R.M.: The effects of prolonged naso-endotracheal

intubation in children: A study in infants and young children after cardiopulmonary bypass. *Anaesthesia* 32:154, 1977.
19. Benumof J.L.: Hypoxic pulmonary vasoconstriction and infusion of sodium nitroprusside, editorial views. *Anesthesiology* 50:481, 1979.
20. Bergström J., Moberg A., Orell S.R.: On the pathogenesis of laryngeal injuries following prolonged intubation. *Acta Otolaryngol.* 55:342, 1962.
21. Black L.F., Hyatt R.E.: Maximal static respiratory pressures in generalized neuromuscular disease. *Am. Rev. Respir. Dis.* 103:641, 1971.
22. Blesa M.I., et al.: Normalization of the blunted ventilatory response to acute hypoxia in congenital cyanotic heart disease. *N. Engl. J. Med.* 296:237, 1977.
23. Bonchek L.I., Starr A.: Intracardiac surgery in infants with conventional cardiopulmonary bypass, in Ionescu M.I., Wooler G.H. (eds.): *Current Techniques in Extracorporeal Circulation.* London, Butterworth & Co., 1976, p. 229.
24. Branthwaite M.A.: Neurological damage related to open-heart surgery: A clinical survey. *Thorax* 27:748, 1972.
25. Branthwaite M.A.: Prevention of neurological damage during open-heart surgery. *Thorax* 30:258, 1975.
26. Brantigan J.W.: Catheters for continuous in vivo blood and tissue gas monitoring. *Crit. Care Med.* 4:239, 1976.
27. Brigham K.L., et al.: Increased sheep lung vascular permeability caused by *Pseudomonas* bacteremia. *J. Clin. Invest.* 54:792, 1974.
28. Bromage P.R.: Extradural analgesia for pain relief. *Br. J. Anaesth.* 39:721, 1967.
29. Camishion R.C., et al.: Effect of partial and total cardiopulmonary bypass with whole blood or hemodilution priming on pulmonary surfactant activity. *J. Surg. Res.* 8:1, 1968.
30. Campbell E.J.M.: Respiratory failure. *Br. Med. J.* 1:1451, 1965.
31. Carroll R., Hedden M., Safar P.: Intratracheal cuffs: Performance characteristics. *Anesthesiology* 31:275, 1969.
32. Carroll R.G.: Evaluation of tracheal tube cuff designs. *Crit. Care Med.* 1:45, 1973.
33. Carroll R.G., McGinnis G.E., Grenvik A.: Performance characteristics of tracheal cuffs. *Int. Anesthesiol. Clin.* 12(no. 3):111, 1974.
34. Chamney A.R.: Humidification requirements and techniques: Including a review of the performance of equipment in current use. *Anaesthesia* 24:602, 1969.
35. Cheney F.W. Jr., Martin W.E.: Effects of continuous positive-pressure ventilation on gas exchange in acute pulmonary edema. *J. Appl. Physiol.* 30:378, 1971.
36. Cheney F.W. Jr., Nelson E.J., Horton W.G.: The function of intermittent positive pressure breathing related to breathing patterns. *Am. Rev. Respir. Dis.* 110(suppl.):183, 1974.
37. Clark L.C. Jr.: Monitor and control of blood and tissue oxygen tensions. *Trans. Am. Soc. Artif. Intern. Organs* 2:41, 1956.
38. Cole J.S., et al.: Clinical studies with a solid state fiberoptic oximeter. *Am. J. Cardiol.* 29:383, 1972.
39. Colgan F.J., Stewart S.: PEEP and CPAP following open-heart surgery in infants and children. *Anesthesiology* 50:336, 1979.
40. Comroe J.H. Jr., et al.: *The Lung: Clinical Physiology and Pulmonary Function Tests.* Chicago, Year Book Medical Publishers, 1955.
41. Connell R.S., et al.: The effect on pulmonary ultrastructure of Dacron-wool filtration during cardiopulmonary bypass. *Ann. Thorac. Surg.* 15:217, 1973.
42. Conway M., et al.: Continuous monitoring of arterial oxygen tension using a catheter-tip polarographic electrode in infants. *Pediatrics* 57:244, 1976.
43. Cortese D.A.: Pulmonary function in mitral stenosis. *Mayo Clin. Proc.* 53:321, 1978.
44. Craddock P.R., et al.: Complement and leukocyte-mediated pulmonary dysfunction in hemodialysis. *N. Engl. J. Med.* 296:769, 1977.
45. Craig D.B., et al.: 'Closing volume' and its relationship to gas exchange in seated and supine positions. *J. Appl. Physiol.* 31:717, 1971.
46. Crew A.D., et al.: Continuous positive airway pressure breathing in the postoperative management of the cardiac infant. *Thorax* 29:437, 1974.
47. Crystal R.G.: The biochemical basis of pulmonary function, in Lenfant C. (ed.): *Lung Biology in Health and Disease.* New York, Marcel Dekker, 1976, vol. 2.
48. Davenport H.W.: *The ABC of Acid-Base Chemistry: The Elements of Physiological Blood-Gas Chemistry for Medical Students and Physicians,* ed. 6. Chicago, University of Chicago Press, 1974.
49. Diem K. (ed.): *Documenta Geigy: Scientific Tables,* ed. 6. Ardsley, N.J., Geigy Pharmaceuticals, 1962, p. 627.
50. Dodrill F.D.: The effects of total body perfusion upon the lungs, in Allen J.G. (ed.):

Extracorporeal Circulation. Springfield, Ill., Charles C Thomas, Publisher, 1958, p. 327.

51. Donovan D.J., Johnston R.P., MacDonnell K.F.: Respiratory monitoring: Systems and devices, in MacDonnell K.F., Segal M.S. (eds.): *Current Respiratory Care.* Boston, Little, Brown & Co., 1977, p. 25.
52. Douglas W.W., et al.: Improved oxygenation in patients with acute respiratory failure: The prone position. *Am. Rev. Respir. Dis.* 115:559, 1977.
53. Downes J.J., et al.: Acute respiratory failure in infants following cardiovascular surgery. *J. Thorac. Cardiovasc. Surg.* 59:21, 1970.
54. Downs J.B.: A technique for direct measurement of intrapleural pressure. *Crit. Care Med.* 4:207, 1976.
55. Dueck R., et al.: Altered distribution of pulmonary ventilation and blood flow following induction of inhalational anesthesia. *Anesthesiology* 52:113, 1980.
56. Effler D.B.: Myocardial revascularization surgery since 1945 A.D.: Its evolution and its impact. *J. Thorac. Cardiovasc. Surg.* 72:823, 1976.
57. Egan D.F.: *Fundamentals of Respiratory Therapy,* ed. 2. St. Louis, C.V. Mosby Co., 1973, p. 92.
58. Eisenmenger V.: Die angeborenen Defecte der Kammerscheidewand des Herzens. *Z. Klin. Med.* 32(suppl.):1, 1897.
59. Engström C.-G., Herzog P.: Ventilation nomogram for practical use with the Engström respirator. *Acta Chir. Scand. Suppl.* 245:37, 1959.
60. Erdmann A.J. III, et al.: Effect of increased vascular pressure on lung fluid balance in unanesthetized sheep. *Circ. Res.* 37:271, 1975.
61. Fallat R.J., Osborn J.J.: Patient monitoring techniques, in Burton G.G., Gee G.N., Hodgkin J.E. (eds.): *Respiratory Care: A Guide to Clinical Practice.* Philadelphia, J.B. Lippincott Co., 1977, p. 950.
62. Feinstein A.R.: Quality of data in the medical record. *Comput. Biomed. Res.* 3:426, 1970.
63. Finklestein S., Caronna J.J.: Outcome of coma following cardiac arrest, abstracted. *Neurology* 27:367, 1977.
64. Fontan F., Baudet E.: Surgical repair of tricuspid atresia. *Thorax* 26:240, 1971.
65. Fordham R.M.M.: Hypoxaemia after aortic valve surgery under cardiopulmonary bypass. *Thorax* 20:505, 1965.
66. Fowler W.S., Cornish E.R. Jr., Kety S.S.: Lung function studies: VIII. Analysis of alveolar ventilation by pulmonary N_2 clearance curves. *J. Clin. Invest.* 31:40, 1952.
67. Froese A.B., Bryan A.C.: Effects of anesthesia and paralysis on diaphragmatic mechanics in man. *Anesthesiology* 41:242, 1974.
68. Geha A.S., Sessler A.D., Kirklin J.W.: Alveolar-arterial oxygen gradients after open intracardiac surgery. *J. Thorac. Cardiovasc. Surg.* 51:609, 1966.
69. Gilman S.: Cerebral disorders after open-heart operations. *N. Engl. J. Med.* 272:489, 1965.
70. Gregory G.A., et al.: Continuous positive airway pressure and pulmonary and circulatory function after cardiac surgery in infants less than three months of age. *Anesthesiology* 43:426, 1975.
71. Guenter C.A.: Chest trauma, in Guenter C.A., Welch M.H. (eds.): *Pulmonary Medicine.* Philadelphia, J.B. Lippincott Co., 1977, p. 439.
72. Guyton A.C., Lindsey A.W.: Effect of elevated left atrial pressure and decreased plasma protein concentration on the development of pulmonary edema. *Circ. Res.* 7:649, 1959.
73. Harris T.R., Nugent M.: Continuous arterial oxygen tension monitoring in the newborn infant. *J. Pediatr.* 82:929, 1973.
74. Harrison G.A., Tonkin J.P.: Laryngeal complications of prolonged endotracheal intubation. *Med. J. Aust.* 2:709, 1965.
75. Hatch D.J., et al.: Continuous positive-airway pressure after open-heart operations in infancy. *Lancet* 2:469, 1973.
76. Heath D., Edwards J.E.: Histological changes in the lung in diseases associated with pulmonary venous hypertension. *Br. J. Dis. Chest* 53:8, 1959.
77. Hedden M., Ersoz C.J., Safar P.: Tracheo-esophageal fistulas following prolonged artificial ventilation via cuffed tracheostomy tubes. *Anesthesiology* 31:281, 1969.
78. Hedden M., et al.: Laryngotracheal damage after prolonged use of orotracheal tubes in adults. *J.A.M.A.* 207:703, 1969.
79. Hewlett A.M., Branthwaite M.A.: Postoperative pulmonary function. *Br. J. Anaesth.* 47:102, 1975.
80. Hilberman M., et al.: An analysis of potential physiological predictors of respiratory adequacy following cardiac surgery. *J. Thorac. Cardiovasc. Surg.* 71:711, 1976.
81. Holley H.S., Gildea J.E.: Vocal cord paralysis after tracheal intubation. *J.A.M.A.* 215:281, 1971.
82. Holtackers T.: Personal communication.
83. Hopewell P.C., Murray J.F.: The adult respiratory distress syndrome. *Annu. Rev. Med.* 27:343, 1976.
84. Huch R., Lübbers D.W., Huch A.: Reliabil-

ity of transcutaneous monitoring of arterial Po_2 in newborn infants. *Arch. Dis. Child.* 49:213, 1974.
85. Javid H., et al.: Neurological abnormalities following open-heart surgery. *J. Thorac. Cardiovasc. Surg.* 58:502, 1969.
86. Jones N.L.: Physical therapy—present state of the art. *Am. Rev. Respir. Dis.* 110 (suppl.):132, 1974.
87. Jones N.L., et al.: *Clinical Exercise Testing.* Philadelphia, W.B. Saunders Co., 1975, p. 123.
88. Kafer E.R.: Idiopathic scoliosis: mechanical properties of the respiratory system and the ventilatory response to carbon dioxide. *J. Clin. Invest.* 55:1153, 1975.
89. Karlson K.E., et al.: Influence of thoracotomy on pulmonary mechanics: Association of increased work of breathing during anesthesia and postoperative pulmonary complications. *Ann. Surg.* 162:973, 1965.
90. Kelman G.R., et al.: The influence of cardiac output on arterial oxygenation: A theoretical study. *Br. J. Anaesth.* 39:450, 1967.
91. Kinsley R.H., et al.: Pulmonary arterial hypertension after repair of tetralogy of Fallot. *J. Thorac. Cardiovasc. Surg.* 67:110, 1974.
92. Kirby R., et al.: Continuous-flow ventilation as an alternative to assisted or controlled ventilation in infants. *Anesth. Analg.* 51:871, 1972.
93. Kirklin J.W., Rastelli G.C.: Low cardiac output after open intracardiac operations. *Prog. Cardiovasc. Dis.* 10:117, 1967.
94. Kleiber M.: Factors affecting energy exchange, in Altman P.L., Dittmer D.S. (eds.): *Metabolism.* Bethesda, Md., Federation of American Societies for Experimental Biology, 1968, p. 354.
95. Klineberg P.L., et al.: Early extubation after coronary artery bypass graft surgery. *Crit. Care Med.* 5:272, 1977.
96. Knowlson G.T.G., Bassett H.F.M.: The pressures exerted on the trachea by endotracheal inflatable cuffs. *Br. J. Anaesth.* 42:834, 1970.
97. Konno K., Mead J.: Measurement of the separate volume changes of rib cage and abdomen during breathing. *J. Appl. Physiol.* 22:407, 1967.
98. Kouchoukos N.T., Karp R.B.: Functional disturbances following extracorporeal circulatory support in cardiac surgery, in Ionescu M.I., Wooler G.H. (eds.): *Current Techniques in Extracorporeal Circulation.* London, Butterworth & Co., 1976, p. 245.
99. Lahiri S., et al.: Relative role of environmental and genetic factors in respiratory adaptation to high altitude. *Nature* 261:133, 1976.
100. Lakier J.B., et al.: Tetralogy of Fallot with absent pulmonary valve: Natural history and hemodynamic considerations. *Circulation* 50:167, 1974.
101. Lamy M., et al.: Pathologic features and mechanisms of hypoxemia in adult respiratory distress syndrome. *Am. Rev. Respir. Dis.* 114:267, 1976.
102. Landis E.M., Pappenheimer J.R.: Exchange of substances through capillary walls, in Hamilton W.F., Dow P. (eds.): *Handbook of Physiology.* Section 2: *Circulation.* Washington, D.C., American Physiological Society, 1963, vol. 2, p. 961.
103. Landmark S.J., et al.: Regional pulmonary perfusion and $\dot{V}/\dot{Q}$ in awake and anesthetized-paralyzed man *J. Appl. Physiol.* 43:993, 1977.
104. Laver M.B., Hallowell P., Goldblatt A.: Pulmonary dysfunction secondary to heart disease: Aspects relevant to anesthesia and surgery. *Anesthesiology* 33:161, 1970.
105. Leatherman N.E.: An improved balloon system for monitoring intraesophageal pressure in acutely ill patients. *Crit. Care Med.* 6:189, 1978.
106. Lee W.H. Jr., et al.: Comparison of the effects of membrane and non-membrane oxygenators on the biochemical and biophysical characteristics of blood. *Surg. Forum* 12:200, 1961.
107. Lindholm C.-E.: Prolonged endotracheal intubation. *Acta Anaesthesiol. Scand. Suppl.* 33:1, 1969.
108. Lindholm C.E., et al.: Flexible fiberoptic bronchoscopy in critical care medicine, in Shoemaker W.C. (ed.): *The Lung in the Critically Ill Patient: Pathophysiology and Therapy of Acute Respiratory Failure.* Baltimore, Williams & Wilkins Co., 1976, pp. 88–99.
109. Lomholt N.: A new tracheostomy tube: I. Cuff with controlled pressure on the tracheal mucous membrane. *Acta Anaesthesiol. Scand.* 11:311, 1967.
110. Lutch J.S., Murray J.F.: Continuous positive-pressure ventilation: Effects on systemic oxygen transport and tissue oxygenation. *Ann. Intern. Med.* 76:193, 1972.
111. Mansell A., Bryan C., Levison H.: Airway closure in children. *J. Appl. Physiol.* 33:711, 1972.
112. Mansfield P.B., et al.: Cardiac surgery under age 2 years: A review. *J. Thorac. Cardiovasc. Surg.* 77:816, 1979.
113. Marcelletti C., McGoon D.C.: Pulmonary infarction following ligation of terminally shunted pulmonary artery. *J. Thorac. Cardiovasc. Surg.* 71:746, 1976.

114. Marsh H.M., et al.: Effects of mechanical ventilation, muscle paralysis, and posture on ventilation-perfusion relationships in anesthetized man. *Anesthesiology* 38:59, 1973.
115. Mayo Clinic: Unpublished data.
116. McGinnis G.E., et al.: An engineering analysis of intratracheal tube cuffs. *Anesth. Analg.* 50:557, 1971.
117. McIntosh H.D., Garcia J.A.: The first decade of aortocoronary bypass grafting, 1967–1977: A review. *Circulation* 57:405, 1978.
118. McMichael J.: A rapid method of determining lung capacity. *Clin. Sci.* 4:167, 1939.
119. Mellins R.B.: Pulmonary physiotherapy in the pediatric age group. *Am. Rev. Respir. Dis.* 110 (suppl.):137, 1974.
120. Michel L., et al.: Measurement of ventilatory reserve as an indicator for early extubation after cardiac operation. *J. Thorac. Cardiovasc. Surg.* 78:761, 1979.
121. Milic-Emili J., et al.: Improved technique for estimating pleural pressure from esophageal balloons. *J. Appl. Physiol.* 19:207, 1964.
122. Modry D.L., Chiu C.-J., Hinchey E.J.: The roles of ventilation and perfusion in lung metabolism: Surgical implications. *J. Thorac. Cardiovasc. Surg.* 74:275, 1977.
123. Moore F.D., et al.: *Post-Traumatic Pulmonary Insufficiency: Pathophysiology of Respiratory Failure and Principles of Respiratory Care After Surgical Operations, Trauma, Hemorrhage, Burns, and Shock.* Philadelphia, W.B. Saunders Co., 1969.
124. Morriss J.H., McNamara D.G.: Residuae, sequelae, and complications of surgery for congenital heart disease. *Prog. Cardiovasc. Dis.* 18:1, 1975.
125. Muldoon S.M., et al.: Respiratory care of patients undergoing intrathoracic operations. *Surg. Clin. North Am.* 53(no. 4):843, 1973.
126. Mullan R.J., McMichan J.C., Gracey D.R.: Unpublished data.
127. Mustafa M.G., Tierney D.F.: Biochemical and metabolic changes in the lung with oxygen, ozone, and nitrogen dioxide toxicity. *Am. Rev. Respir. Dis.* 118:1061, 1978.
128. Nahas R.A., et al.: Post-perfusion lung syndrome: Role of circulatory exclusion. *Lancet* 2:251, 1965.
129. Nunn J.F.: *Applied Respiratory Physiology,* ed. 2. London, Butterworth & Co., 1977, p. 91.
130. Nunn J.F.: *Applied Respiratory Physiology,* ed. 2. London, Butterworth & Co., 1977, p. 389.
131. Osborn J.J.: Monitoring respiratory function. *Crit. Care Med.* 2:217, 1974.
132. Osborn J.J.: A flowmeter for respiratory monitoring. *Crit. Care Med.* 6:349, 1978.
133. Overland E.S., Ozanne G.M., Severinghaus J.W.: A single-breath method for determining lung weight and pulmonary blood flow from the differential uptake of two soluble gases, abstracted. *Physiologist* 18:341, 1975.
134. Pappenheimer J.R.: Capillary permeability: Deductions concerning the number and dimensions of ultramicroscopic openings in the capillary walls. *Ann. N.Y. Acad. Sci.* 55:465, 1952.
135. Parker D.J., et al.: Changes in serum complement and immunoglobulins following cardiopulmonary bypass. *Surgery* 71:824, 1972.
136. Parr G.V.S., Blackstone E.H., Kirklin J.W.: Cardiac performance and mortality early after intracardiac surgery in infants and young children. *Circulation* 51:867, 1975.
137. Pennock J.L., Pierce W.S., Waldhausen J.A.: The management of the lungs during cardiopulmonary bypass. *Surg. Gynecol. Obstet.* 145:917, 1977.
138. Peters R.M., Wellons H.A., Jr., Htwe T.M.: Total compliance and work of breathing after thoracotomy. *J. Thorac. Cardiovasc. Surg.* 57:348, 1969.
139. Petty T.L., Ashbaugh D.G.: The adult respiratory distress syndrome: Clinical features, factors influencing prognosis and principles of management. *Chest* 60:233, 1971.
140. Pontoppidan H., Geffin B., Lowenstein E.: Acute respiratory failure in the adult. *N. Engl. J. Med.* 287:690; 743; 799, 1972.
141. Pontoppidan H., et al.: Respiratory intensive care. *Anesthesiology* 47:96, 1977.
142. Prakash O., Meij S.: Use of mass spectrometry and infrared CO_2 analyzer for bedside measurement of cardiopulmonary function during anesthesia and intensive care. *Crit. Care Med.* 5:180, 1977.
143. Puyau F.A., Meckstroth G.R.: Evaluation of pulmonary perfusion patterns in children with tetralogy of Fallot. *Am. J. Roentgenol.* 122:119, 1974.
144. Quasha A.L., et al.: Early versus late extubation of patients following coronary artery bypass graft surgery. Abstracted in the Scientific Papers of the American Society of Anesthesiologists Annual Meeting, 1978, p. 211.
145. Qvist J., et al.: Hemodynamic responses to mechanical ventilation with PEEP: The effect of hypervolemia. *Anesthesiology* 42:45, 1975.
146. Radford E.P., Jr.: Ventilation standards for use in artificial respiration. *J. Appl. Physiol.* 7:451, 1955.

147. Rahn H., Fenn W.O.: *A Graphical Analysis of the Respiratory Gas Exchange: The O_2–CO_2 Diagram*. Washington, D.C., American Physiological Society, 1955.
148. Ratliff N.B., et al.: Pulmonary injury secondary to extracorporeal circulation: An ultrastructural study. *J. Thorac. Cardiovasc. Surg.* 65:425, 1973.
149. Rehder K., Knopp T.J., Sessler A.D.: Regional intrapulmonary gas distribution in awake and anesthetized-paralyzed prone man. *J. Appl. Physiol.* 45:528, 1978.
150. Rehder K., Sessler A.D., Rodarte J.R.: Regional intrapulmonary gas distribution in awake and anesthetized-paralyzed man. *J. Appl. Physiol.* 42:391, 1977.
151. Rehder K., et al.: Airway closure. *Anesthesiology* 47:40, 1977.
152. Robin E.D., Cross C.E., Zelis R.: Pulmonary edema. *N. Engl. J. Med.* 288:239; 292, 1973.
153. Rodarte J.R., et al.: New tests for the detection of obstructive pulmonary disease. *Chest* 72:762, 1977.
154. Sade R.M., et al.: Abnormalities of regional lung function associated with ventricular septal defect and pulmonary artery band. *J. Thorac. Cardiovasc. Surg.* 71:572, 1976.
155. Sanz M.C.: Ultramicro methods and standardization of equipment. *Clin. Chem.* 3:406, 1957.
156. Saunders N.A., Powles A.C.P., Rebuck A.S.: Ear oximetry: Accuracy and practicability in the assessment of arterial oxygenation. *Am. Rev. Respir. Dis.* 113:745, 1976.
157. Schuder R.J., Markello R., Olszowka A.J.: Oxygen-induced ventilation-perfusion redistribution in anesthetized patients. Abstracted in the Scientific Papers of the American Society of Anesthesiologists Annual Meeting, 1977, p. 225.
158. Severinghaus J.W.: Blood gas calculator. *J. Appl. Physiol.* 21:1108, 1966.
159. Severinghaus J.W.: Hypoxic respiratory drive and its loss during chronic hypoxia. *Clin. Physiol.* 2:57, 1972.
160. Severinghaus J.W., Bradley A.F.: Electrodes for blood pO_2 and pCO_2 determination. *J. Appl. Physiol.* 13:515, 1958.
161. Siemens-Elema Servo Ventilator 900/900 B Operating Manual. Siemens-Elema AB, S-171 95 Solna, Sweden. (Printed in Sweden.)
162. Siggaard-Andersen O.: The acid-base status of the blood. *Scand. J. Clin. Lab. Invest.* 15 (suppl. 70):1, 1963.
163. Siggaard-Andersen O., Nørgaard-Pedersen B., Rem J.: Hemoglobin pigments, spectrophotometric determination of oxy-, carboxy-, met-, and sulfhemoglobin in capillary blood. *Clin. Chim. Acta* 42:85, 1972.
164. Singer R.B., Hastings A.B.: An improved clinical method for the estimation of disturbances of the acid-base balance of human blood. *Medicine* 27:223, 1948.
165. Sørensen S.C., Severinghaus J.W.: Respiratory insensitivity to acute hypoxia persisting after correction of tetralogy of Fallot. *J. Appl. Physiol.* 25:221, 1968.
166. Special correspondence: A debate on coronary bypass. *N. Engl. J. Med.* 297:1464, 1977.
167. Stanger P., Lucas R.V., Jr., Edwards J.E.: Anatomic factors causing respiratory distress in acyanotic congenital cardiac disease: Special reference to bronchial obstruction. *Pediatrics* 43:760, 1969.
168. Staub N.C.: Steady state pulmonary transvascular water filtration in unanesthetized sheep. *Circ. Res.* 28(suppl. 1):135, 1971.
169. Staub N.C.: Pulmonary edema. *Physiol. Rev.* 54:678, 1974.
170. Staub N.C.: 'State of the Art' review: Pathogenesis of pulmonary edema. *Am. Rev. Respir. Dis.* 109:358, 1974.
171. Staub N.C.: Lung water and solute exchange, in Lenfant C. (ed.): *Lung Biology in Health and Disease*. New York, Marcel Dekker, 1978, vol. 7.
172. Stevens P.M.: Assessment of acute respiratory failure: Cardiac versus pulmonary causes, editorial. *Chest* 67:1, 1975.
173. Stewart S. III, et al.: Spontaneous breathing with continuous positive airway pressure after open intracardiac operations in infants. *J. Thorac. Cardiovasc. Surg.* 65:37, 1973.
174. Suter P.M., Fairley H.B., Isenberg M.D.: Optimum end-expiratory airway pressure in patients with acute pulmonary failure. *N. Engl. J. Med.* 292:284, 1975.
175. Suter P.M., Fairley H.B., Isenberg M.D.: Effect of tidal volume and positive end-expiratory pressure on compliance during mechanical ventilation. *Chest* 73:158, 1978.
176. Thung N., et al.: The cost of respiratory effort in postoperative cardiac patients. *Circulation* 28:552, 1963.
177. Tufo H.M., Ostfeld A.M., Shekelle R.: Central nervous system dysfunction following open-heart surgery. *J.A.M.A.* 212:1333, 1970.
178. Wagner P.D., Naumann P.F., Laravuso R.B.: Simultaneous measurement of eight foreign gases in blood by gas chromatography. *J. Appl. Physiol.* 36:600, 1974.
179. Wagner P.D., Saltzman H.A., West J.B.:

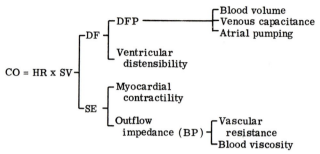

Fig 25–1.—Simplified schema outlining factors controlling cardiac pump function: cardiac output *(CO)*, heart rate *(HR)*, stroke volume *(SV)*, diastolic filling *(DF)*, diastolic filling pressure *(DFP)*, systolic emptying *(SE)*, and blood pressure *(BP)*.

pressure). The left ventricular function curve has an initial steep portion, but flattens at high ventricular filling pressures. Reduction of left ventricular filling pressure reduces stroke volume and cardiac output by only a small amount when the heart is operating on the flat part of the ventricular function curve but by a large degree when the heart is operating on the steeper part of the curve. Increases in contractility shift the curve upward and to the left, whereas decreases in contractility shift the curve downward and to the right. Increases in afterload without any concomitant change in contractile state likewise shift the curve downward and to the right. Thus, reduced stroke volume may result from (1) reduced ventricular end-diastolic volume, (2) reduced contractility, or (3) large increase in afterload. A combination of all these causes is often responsible for the low cardiac output syndrome.

Heart rate is the second determinant of cardiac output. The frequency of contraction also determines the ventricular filling period, and a rapid heart rate may limit stroke volume. However, the ability to increase the heart rate in maintaining cardiac output is important in patients whose stroke volume cannot be increased owing to compromised cardiac reserve or reduced ventricular distensibility.

With low cardiac output, the sympathetic ner-

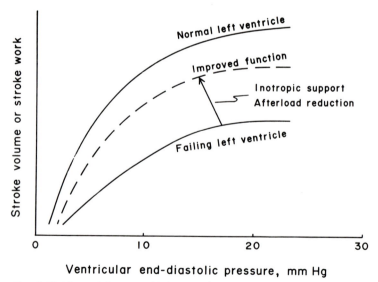

Fig 25–2.—Frank-Starling left ventricular function curves. Compared with curve of normal left ventricle, curve of failing left ventricle is displaced downward and to the right. This depressed curve may be shifted upward and to the left by the administration of inotropic drugs or vasodilator drugs.

vous system is reflexly activated to sustain both stroke volume and heart rate. At the same time, systemic vascular constriction occurs, resulting in increased impedance to outflow from the ventricle (which may further decrease cardiac output). Treatment for low cardiac output[64] proceeds through adjustment of the preload, then the afterload, and finally the contractility. α-Adrenergic vasopressors without positive inotropic effect are of limited value because they may further increase afterload without increasing myocardial contractility. By contrast, peripheral vasodilators are of great value in treating cardiogenic shock. By reducing afterload, they lower left ventricular wall tension during systole and thereby decrease myocardial oxygen requirement. At the same time, such vasodilator therapy may decrease left ventricular end-diastolic volume and thus reduce ventricular preload. The end result from the use of vasodilators on cardiac function depends on the left ventricular filling pressure.

In patients who have elevated left ventricular filling pressures, vasodilators, by decreasing systemic vascular resistance, generally increase stroke volume and cardiac output, yet the arterial blood pressure changes very little. By contrast, in patients with decreased left ventricular filling pressures, vasodilators are potentially dangerous because they can greatly reduce venous return, stroke volume, and systemic blood pressure. When cardiac output and vital organ perfusion remain inadequate despite optimal left ventricular filling pressures and optimal afterload, inotropic drugs are used to augment cardiac output.

Preventing and Treating Arrhythmias

The second aim is to maintain the heart rate within normal limits and prevent or rapidly treat arrhythmias that compromise cardiac function and oxygen demand.[66]

Arrhythmias are frequently seen during the immediate postoperative period. By producing inappropriate fast or slow ventricular rates, these arrhythmias may produce or aggravate heart failure. Furthermore, they may herald potentially lethal arrhythmias, such as ventricular fibrillation. In patients with normal or slightly elevated left ventricular end-diastolic pressure, left ventricular stroke volume can be greatly reduced by the absence of a properly timed atrial contraction.[45]

Poor myocardial oxygen delivery is particularly frequent with tachyarrhythmias. Tachycardia can lower cardiac output by reducing the time in diastole during which ventricular filling normally occurs. The decrease in diastolic time associated with increased heart rate also may reduce coronary blood flow. This combination, together with an increased myocardial oxygen demand due to an increased heart rate, may produce or aggravate myocardial ischemia.

To minimize the incidence of arrhythmias after cardiac surgery, the patient's preoperative digoxin therapy should be stopped or reduced and efforts should be made to maintain serum electrolyte values, particularly potassium, within normal limits, and to prevent acid-base disturbance or myocardial hypoxia. Removable epicardial pacemaker wires are often inserted at the end of surgery to permit rapid institution of cardiac pacing if this is required. Continuous ECG monitoring and rapid control of any arrhythmias are particularly essential during the first 48 to 72 hours after surgery.

Achieving Favorable Balance Between Myocardial Oxygen Supply and Demand

Cardiac muscle depends on aerobic metabolism. Myocardial oxygen demands result in near-maximal extraction of available oxygen from the coronary blood supply. Thus, increased myocardial oxygen demand has to be met by an increase in coronary blood flow. Postoperatively, the balance between the available myocardial oxygen supply and the myocardial demand for oxygen[9, 11, 47-50] may become critical. The importance of this balance is most readily apparent in patients with coronary artery disease, in whom the ability to increase regional coronary blood flow may be severely limited.

The two factors controlling myocardial oxygen delivery are coronary blood flow and oxygen content of coronary arterial blood. Coronary blood flow occurs primarily during diastole, particularly for the subendocardial muscle of the left ventricle. Coronary blood flow depends on (1) diastolic time, (2) coronary perfusion pressure, and (3) patency of coronary arteries. Coronary perfusion pressure, the driving force for coronary blood flow, is the difference between aortic diastolic and left ventricular diastolic pressures. The diastolic pressure time index is a useful indicator of myocardial oxygen supply;[50] it is the difference between the aortic diastolic pres-

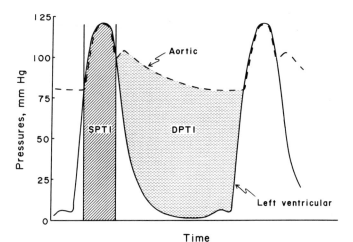

Fig 25–3.—Aortic and left ventricular pressure curves. Systolic pressure time index *(SPTI)* is the area under aortic pressure curve during systole. Diastolic pressure time index *(DPTI)* is the difference between aortic pressure and left ventricular pressure during diastole. Ratio of DPTI to SPTI is expression of the balance between myocardial oxygen supply and demand.[50]

sure and the left ventricular pressure during diastole (Fig 25–3). This index will be reduced by low aortic diastolic pressure resulting from systemic hypotension, from severe arteriosclerosis, or from severe aortic regurgitation and by increased left ventricular diastolic pressure, as may occur with heart failure. In systole, a pressure gradient is developed across the ventricular myocardial wall. Pressure is maximal in the subendocardial region and least in the epicardium. This characteristic results in the subendocardial region being almost totally dependent on diastolic perfusion for its blood flow and puts this region particularly in jeopardy with tachycardia and disease states such as coronary stenosis.

The major determinants of myocardial work and hence oxygen consumption are myocardial wall tension, contractile state of the heart, and heart rate. The myocardial wall tension is proportional to the systemic pressure developed during systole and the radius of the ventricle (law of Laplace). Thus, both systemic hypertension and dilatation of the ventricle increase myocardial oxygen requirements. The myocardial oxygen demand is increased by increasing contractility.[42] Myocardial oxygen demand is linearly and positively correlated with heart rate.

The area under the systemic pressure curve during systole (see Fig 25–3) is referred to as the tension time index[88] or systolic pressure time index[50] and is directly proportional to myocardial oxygen demand. Thus, the ratio of diastolic to systolic pressure time index is an expression of the balance between myocardial oxygen supply and demand.[50] A ratio of less than 0.5 is suggestive of subendocardial ischemia and perhaps of a poor prognosis.

In the presence of coronary artery disease, a delicate balance between myocardial oxygen supply and demand may exist because the diastolic perfusion pressure of the myocardium distal to the coronary stenosis is reduced, whereas the systolic pressure time index is nearly normal. Increase in heart rate with an increase in myocardial oxygen requirement and reduced diastolic time may produce ischemia. Increases in systemic blood pressure or in velocity of contraction likewise increase myocardial oxygen demand, and may cause myocardial ischemia. Hypotension is also potentially hazardous because it may decrease coronary blood flow distal to the stenosis.

MONITORING

Invasive monitoring is essential after cardiac surgery because clinical assessment of the patient's condition based on noninvasive measurements is often inadequate or even misleading. Furthermore, manual measurements cannot be performed frequently enough to detect the rapid hemodynamic fluctuations that can occur.

Hemodynamic Monitoring

Clinical assessment of cardiac function and its response to therapeutic interventions is best achieved by the combined measurement of cardiac output, arterial blood pressure, right atrial pressure, and left atrial pressure. Left atrial pressure in the absence of stenosis or incompetence of the mitral valve is approximately equal to left ventricular end-diastolic pressure. Other variables that should be monitored in the cardiac patient postoperatively include the ECG, drainage from the mediastinum and the precordial and pleural cavities, urinary output, and arterial and mixed venous blood gases. The mixed venous oxygen tension sampled from the pulmonary artery is a useful index of changes in cardiac output and adequacy of tissue blood flow.[93] Electrolytes must be measured, and roentgenograms of the chest should be obtained at appropriate times.

It is our routine to continuously monitor the following variables:

The heart rate and rhythm—determined by continuous ECG recording
Arterial blood pressure—measured by a pressure transducer via an indwelling arterial cannula (radial artery is frequently used)
Left atrial pressure and right atrial pressure—measured by pressure transducers through fine tissue-inert plastic catheters inserted into the two atria at surgery (As an alternative or in addition, a balloon-tipped, flow-directed pulmonary artery catheter can be used to monitor pulmonary artery and pulmonary capillary wedge pressures.)
Drainage from pericardial, mediastinal, and pleural catheters
Urinary output from urethral catheter
Fluid input
Patient weight using a weigh bed
Cardiac output[99]—determined by indicator dye-dilution or thermodilution (If the left ventricle is enlarged or cardiac output reduced, increased reliability of indicator dye-dilution measurement is achieved by injecting dye into the right atrium and sampling from a catheter inserted into the pulmonary artery at surgery, rather than by injecting dye into the left atrium and sampling from the arterial catheter.[6, 58] An alternative to dye-dilution is the thermodilution technique, which has the advantage of allowing rapid serial estimations of cardiac output.)
Temperature—monitored with rectal thermometer
Arterial and mixed venous blood gas and acid-base analysis—determined by appropriate electrodes as required
Respiratory rate, tidal volume, minute volume, peak inspiratory pressure—determined with pneumotachography and an airway pressure transducer
Roentgenogram of the chest—as required

Computer-Based Hemodynamic Monitoring

The above-listed measurements can be displayed, monitored, and analyzed using computer technology.[33, 62, 90, 91] The application of an on-line computer system to the postoperative management of cardiac surgical patients was first described by Kirklin's group in 1968.[91] An on-line digital computer permits oscilloscope display of the systolic, diastolic, and mean arterial pressures, left and right atrial pressures, heart rate, hourly chest drainage, hourly urinary output, respiration, and temperature. The computer can be used to activate audiovisual alarms if the monitored variables exceed or fall below a predetermined limit. The computer can display, for visual inspection and validation, the cardiac output dye-dilution curves and can be used to calculate the cardiac output. Such computer use also permits recall of the monitored information, both in a tabular form and in a graphic form, for various time periods. Both displays are extremely useful for trend analysis during this period of potential hemodynamic instability. Blood gas analysis and acid-base status, serum electrolytes, and other biochemical data can be manually entered and results stored for recall at any time. Likewise, nursing procedures can be entered into computer data stores. By such means, one can ensure the accuracy of the medical record and decrease the time required by nurses for charting, measuring, and recording. Systems are being developed for machine control of the intravenous administration of fluids and blood.[90] Such fluid administration may be programmed to maintain physiologic variables, such as left atrial pressure, right atrial pressure, and so forth, within predetermined limits by automatically adjusting the rate of fluid administration to the patient.

Medical logic programs are also now being developed to make therapeutic decisions on the basis of various inputs.[33] This development may be beneficial and is feasible because clinical decisions are usually based on few variables, and the number of possible therapeutic interventions in a given clinical situation is both limited and well-defined by common consensus. Depending on patient risk produced by the intervention, the computer could be programmed to suggest either that a nurse perform a certain action or give a certain drug or that the nurse recommend physician review of the situation.

We have found computer-based monitoring to be reliable and to significantly improve the quality and discipline of care offered to postcardiac surgical patients. The patient is provided with better monitoring; trend analysis improves the physician's interpretation of changes in patient status; and the nurse can devote more time to the patient's clinical condition and personal needs, free of the need for constant charting.

LOW CARDIAC OUTPUT—PATHOPHYSIOLOGY

Incidence

Persistent low cardiac output leading to shock is the most significant cause of mortality during the immediate postoperative period.[10, 29, 57, 81] The normal cardiac index in adults at rest in the supine position is 2.4 to 4.4 L/minute/sq m body surface area, with a mean of 3.5.[5] Boyd and others[10] in 1959 studied 34 patients after open-heart surgery. Fifteen of these patients had cardiac indices less than 2.0 L/minute/sq m. The cause of low output in more than half the patients in this group was unknown. This group with low output had a higher mortality and more frequent occurrence of sudden death. In 1969, Dietzman and others[29] confirmed the increased mortality in patients with low cardiac indices. The mortality associated with low cardiac output is further increased if it is associated with left ventricular failure, as evidenced by an increased left ventricular end-diastolic pressure.[60]

Clinical Diagnosis

The clinical signs of low cardiac output are those of incipient or frank shock and include restlessness, agitation, and perspiration. Pain and anxiety may cause or exacerbate such signs and should be treated appropriately. The extremities are cold and cyanotic, and the peripheral pulses are weak or absent. The blood pressure is not a reliable guide to cardiac output, but a systolic blood pressure of less than 80 mm Hg in the adult signifies a bad prognosis because it implies that the body's compensatory mechanisms are failing. Oliguria (0.5 ml/minute/kg body weight) or anuria is also of serious prognostic significance. The differential diagnosis of an oliguric state associated with low cardiac output includes postrenal and renal causes for oliguria, such as mechanical obstruction of urinary flow and acute tubular necrosis, the latter being suggested by the finding of RBCs and casts in the urine.

The widened alveolar-arterial oxygen tension gradient normally found during the initial postoperative period (see chap. 24) is further increased in the low cardiac output state. Associated with low cardiac output, there is increased oxygen extraction from blood by tissues which results in lowering of the mixed venous oxygen tension, which in turn exacerbates the effect of intrapulmonary and extrapulmonary right-to-left shunts and areas of low ventilation-perfusion in the lung.[55] In addition, left ventricular failure, resulting in left atrial pressures that exceed the colloid osmotic pressure of the plasma proteins (approximately 25 to 30 mm Hg), may produce frank pulmonary edema and, hence, also decrease PaO_2. Hypoxia will tend to rapidly increase pulmonary vascular resistance,[7] which, especially if previously elevated, will impair right heart function and further decrease cardiac output. Anaerobic metabolism by poorly perfused tissues causes acid metabolites to accumulate in the blood. The resulting metabolic

TABLE 25–1.—Hemodynamic Differentiation of the Causes of Low Cardiac Output

CAUSE	RIGHT ATRIAL PRESSURE (RAP)	LEFT ATRIAL PRESSURE (LAP)	DOES RAP EQUAL LAP?	DOES PADP* EQUAL LAP?
Hypovolemia	Low	Low	No	Yes
Cardiac tamponade	High	High	Yes	Yes
Left ventricular failure	Normal/high	High	No	Yes
Right ventricular failure	High	Normal	No	Yes or PADP>LAP (cor pulmonale)
Pulmonary embolus	High	Normal	No	No, PADP>LAP

*Pulmonary artery diastolic pressure.

acidosis will directly impair myocardial contractility[28] and may also impair cardiac output by further increasing pulmonary vascular resistance. Such metabolic acidosis may be partly compensated for by respiratory alkalosis with reduced $Paco_2$. In patients who are allowed to breathe spontaneously, rapid shallow breathing frequently occurs with low cardiac output.

Low cardiac output can be diagnosed with certainty only by measurement of cardiac output using thermodilution or dye-dilution indicator techniques or by measuring oxygen uptake and determining cardiac output utilizing the Fick equation. The capacity to perform such measurements is extremely helpful in the care of the postcardiac surgical patient. To differentiate potential causes of low cardiac output, the ability to monitor left and right atrial pressures and pulmonary artery diastolic pressure is essential. A number of hemodynamic variables are used to differentially diagnose the causes of low cardiac output (Table 25-1).

Causes

Hypovolemia

Inadequate ventricular preload due to hypovolemia is a relatively frequent cause of low cardiac output immediately after cardiac surgery. The most frequent cause is inadequate replacement of the blood lost.

Incomplete hemostasis usually results from discrete bleeding points, such as from the ventriculotomy incision and incision sites into the great vessels or atria, or from blood vessels in the chest wall. Excessive blood loss through chest drains or concealed hemorrhage may ensue. Incomplete blood volume replacement may be identified by a negative blood balance, a low cardiac output and stroke volume, and reduced left and right atrial pressures. Concealed hemorrhage is indicated when blood replacement results in an apparent positive blood balance yet the atrial pressures continue to be reduced and low cardiac output persists. Continued internal hemorrhage may lead to tamponade.

That excessive postoperative bleeding also may result from an abnormality in blood clotting is suggested by failure of the blood draining from the chest drains to clot, by generalized oozing from wounds and venipuncture sites, or by easy bruising. An abnormality is confirmed by clotting studies. An abnormal bleeding tendency may result from inadequate or excessive neutralization of heparin. Another frequent cause is a decreased platelet count either produced by a washout phenomenon associated with massive transfusion or caused by platelet adhesion to and loss in the oxygenator. Damage to platelets, RBCs, and tissues during bypass also can release thromboplastic factors and result in fibrinolytic activation.[106] Inadequate levels of clotting factors produced by the liver also may be responsible. An abnormal bleeding diathesis after cardiac surgery is frequent in patients who have had cyanotic heart disease and right-sided cardiac failure preoperatively,[41] both of which presumably depress hepatic function, including the synthesis of clotting factors.

A potential cause of postoperative hypovolemia is the use of hemodilution prime for the pump oxygenator circuit. The reduced colloid osmotic pressure resulting from the use of such fluids can promote a postoperative diuresis, which may result in a reduction of circulating blood volume. However, diuretic use is a more important cause for such hypovolemia.

The blood pressure response to hypovolemia depends on the degree of vasoconstriction present. Some reflex vasoconstriction is normally found during the first 24 to 48 hours after cardiac bypass surgery.[82] This vasoconstriction is increased by hypothermia, pain, and anxiety. The deleterious effect of hypovolemia will be exaggerated by vasodilating agents. Volatile anesthetics, morphine, and neuroleptic anesthetic agents with α-adrenergic blocking activity may induce vasodilatation, which can persist into the immediate postoperative period. Morphine given for postoperative pain relief also may produce significant vasodilatation and should be used with caution if hypovolemia is suspected.

Paradoxically, vasodilator drugs may be useful in treating the vasoconstricted and cold patient. When the patient is coming off cardiopulmonary bypass, the use of vasodilators may facilitate adequate transfusion and increase the rapidity of rewarming, particularly of the body "shell."[77] An adequate left atrial pressure must be maintained for safe use of vasodilator drugs.

Measurement of the left atrial pressure is the most reliable guide to the adequacy of blood volume replacement after cardiac surgery. The patient's clinical status, the urinary output, and the arterial blood pressure also need careful

they are anomalous in their distribution, can be directly damaged by surgery.

RESIDUAL CARDIOVASCULAR DISEASE.—Incomplete relief of cardiac lesions may lead to postoperative myocardial dysfunction. For example, residual tricuspid valve incompetence may complicate the postoperative course after mitral or aortic valve replacement.[59] Coronary artery occlusive disease may complicate aortic valve replacement.[26] Significant pulmonary artery hypertension may persist or develop after correction of an intracardiac shunt.[21, 56] Staging surgical repair of lesions such as pulmonary atresia[37] has been designed to avoid cardiac complications from pulmonary hypertension.

Cardiac function also may be impaired by inadequate repair of various congenital conditions, such as incomplete relief of right ventricular outflow obstruction in tetralogy of Fallot, incomplete closure of ventricular septal defect, and incomplete correction of valvular stenosis or incompetence.[54, 73] The prompt recognition and surgical correction of some of these defects may be life-saving.

ACID-BASE AND ELECTROLYTE ABNORMALITIES.—Severe metabolic acidosis depresses myocardial contractility and inhibits sympathomimetic action.[28] Such metabolic acidosis usually results from the low cardiac output state. Acidosis with pH below 7.25 must be corrected because it will further impair myocardial function. Sometimes inadequate perfusion during cardiopulmonary bypass is the cause. Acute renal failure is also associated with metabolic acidosis.

Rapid changes in blood pH, possibly iatrogenic in origin, may lead to rapid fluctuation in serum electrolyte concentrations. Thus, acidosis is associated with hyperkalemia, while alkalosis, if rapidly induced, may lead to hypokalemia and decreases in serum ionized calcium.

Hypokalemia predisposes to potentially dangerous arrhythmias, especially in the presence of digitalis. Hypokalemia may be produced by excessive diuretic therapy. The diuresis after a hemodilution prime also can cause hypokalemia. Hyperkalemia is frequently associated with renal failure.

The serum ionized calcium is an important determinant of myocardial contractility.[17] Ionized calcium levels less than 2 mEq/L at pH 7.40 may be associated with reduced contractility. Rapid fluctuations in serum ionized calcium may occur during the immediate postoperative period. It is important, especially when cardiac output is reduced, to give an adequate amount of calcium at this time.

Treatment

Treatment of myocardial dysfunction immediately after cardiac surgery can be exceedingly complex and difficult. Success requires meticulous attention to monitoring and to measuring the response of the patient to each therapeutic intervention. Treatment is based on several physiologic principles.

Ensuring an Optimal Filling Pressure (Preload) for the Left Ventricle

Blood is administered to increase the left atrial pressure to a value at which no further improvement in cardiac output is achieved or until the highest safe limit of left atrial pressure (approximately 20 mm Hg) is reached. Improvement in cardiac output is judged by clinical observations of urinary output and by cardiac output estimations. Because blood pressure may be maintained in the presence of a low cardiac output, the administration of blood to ensure an optimal preload is not based only on its effect on blood pressure. Concurrent use of vasodilator therapy to reduce afterload necessitates continual reassessment of left atrial pressure and adjustment of blood infusion to maintain an optimal preload.

Ensuring an Optimal Afterload by Vasodilator Therapy

Left ventricular failure is associated with a reduced stroke volume for a given left ventricular end-diastolic volume. Compensatory elevation of left ventricular end-diastolic volume to maintain stroke volume by the Frank-Starling mechanism requires further elevation of left atrial pressure to levels that can, in turn, induce pulmonary venous congestion and pulmonary edema. Decrease in left ventricular stroke volume also induces a reflex increase in peripheral vascular resistance to maintain perfusion pressure to vital organs. This increase in peripheral vascular resistance tends to further decrease left ventricular stroke volume, and a vicious circle is established. Vasodilator therapy in this situation will improve cardiac output.[22, 24, 25]

Hypotension can potentially cause ischemic heart damage and is the most serious complication associated with such therapy. Vasodilator drugs, therefore, must be administered in small doses initially, and their effect must be closely monitored. If vasodilator therapy is limited by hypotension despite optimal preload, concomitant inotropic therapy should be considered. Vasodilator therapy should not be used when hypovolemia is present.

The risk of ischemic heart damage with hypotension is mitigated by a number of factors. Reduction in arterial pressure reduces left ventricular wall stress, a major determinant of myocardial oxygen demand. Despite some reduction in blood pressure, the ratio of myocardial oxygen supply to myocardial oxygen demand is usually improved by vasodilator therapy.[71] The reduction in left ventricular end-diastolic pressure also may reduce the pressure gradient from the endocardium to the epicardium and thereby improve subendocardial blood flow.

SODIUM NITROPRUSSIDE.—Sodium nitroprusside is a nonspecific direct-acting vasodilator, acting on both the arteriolar resistance and the venous capacitance beds. By decreasing systemic vascular resistance, it may permit increases in left ventricular stroke volume. The action of the drug on the venous capacitance bed, together with any improvement in cardiac output achieved by afterload reduction, reduces pulmonary venous and right atrial pressures. In heart failure, nitroprusside usually produces only a mild to moderate decrease in arterial blood pressure, and heart rate remains unchanged. This combination of effects is useful in treating low cardiac output due to myocardial dysfunction.

Sodium nitroprusside is administered as an intravenous infusion (50 mg in 250 ml of 5% dextrose in water). Because this solution is decomposed by light, the container should be light-shielded. Once they have been prepared, solutions should not be kept for longer than four hours. The average dose of nitroprusside is 3 μg/kg/minute, with a range of 0.5 to 10 μg/kg/minute. If an inadequate reduction in blood pressure or no increase in cardiac output is seen within ten minutes at a level of 10 μg/kg/minute, the administration should be stopped. Cyanide toxicity may occur at high infusion rates or with long-term use and is implied by the development of progressive metabolic acidosis.[101]

NITROGLYCERIN.—Nitroglycerin acts primarily to dilate venous capacitance vessels.[3] As a result, left ventricular filling pressure is reduced. Unlike nitroprusside, nitroglycerin may increase or redistribute (or both) blood flow to ischemic myocardium.[75] Nitroglycerin is perhaps the vasodilator of choice in treating angina pectoris. The potential improvement in blood supply to ischemic myocardium suggests that nitroglycerin may be useful in treating postoperative myocardial ischemia. It is important to remember that hypotension and tachycardia can result from reduction in left ventricular filling pressure, and thus, paradoxically, nitroglycerin may compromise coronary perfusion pressure and worsen myocardial ischemia.

Nitroglycerin is administered sublingually (0.3 to 0.4 mg) or intravenously at an infusion rate of 0.2 to 1 μg/kg/minute (8 mg in 250 ml 5% dextrose in water).

OTHER VASODILATORS.—Hydralazine (Apresoline), tolazoline, diazoxide, α-methyldopa, ganglion-blocking drugs, and combinations of α- and β-blockers also may be used in certain instances to reduce preload and afterload. These agents may be of particular benefit in patients with long-standing hypertension of systemic or pulmonary vascular beds and have some special uses.

Inotropic Support to Improve Myocardial Contractility

SYMPATHOMIMETIC DRUGS.—Inotropic drugs, which improve myocardial contractility, are of value when cardiac output and arterial blood pressure remain inadequate despite adjustment of the left ventricular filling pressure and left ventricular afterload to optimal levels.[29, 60] The choice of an inotropic drug or a combination of such drugs depends on the desired hemodynamic effect.

Dopamine hydrochloride,[39, 84] a norepinephrine precursor, possesses predominantly β-adrenergic properties, except at high doses (above 15 μg/kg/minute), when α-adrenergic effects are more pronounced. In addition to its β-adrenergic stimulation of the myocardium, dopamine also dilates the renal vascular bed at low dosage (between 3 and 5 μg/kg/minute), a dopaminergic receptor effect. Because of its effect on the heart and renal circulation, dopamine is a useful inotropic agent in the low cardiac output state. The drug possesses less chronotropic and arrhythmogenic effects than does isoproterenol. However, tachycardia and arrhythmias can occur with its use. Furthermore, at high doses, the α-adrenergic stimulation may increase systemic vascular resistance and counteract any increase in myocardial contractility. Dopamine is administered intravenously at an initial rate of 2 to 3 μg/kg/minute (200 mg in 250 ml 5% dextrose in water). If required, this infusion can be increased to 5 to 10 μg/kg/minute, with a maximal dosage of approximately 30 μg/kg/minute.

Dobutamine possesses strong β-adrenergic stimulating action on the heart.[39, 87] At clinical dosage, the drug has a pronounced inotropic effect and causes a modest increase in heart rate.[102] Its arrhythmogenic effects appear to be less than those of isoproterenol or dopamine. Systemic and pulmonary vascular resistance decrease with dobutamine. The starting dose for infusion is 2 to 4 μg/kg/minute (250 mg in 250 ml 5% dextrose in water), and the clinical dose ranges from 2 to 20 μg/kg/minute.

Norepinephrine in low doses produces a predominantly β-adrenergic stimulatory effect on the heart, and this increases stroke volume. With larger doses, the α-adrenergic–induced increase in systemic vascular resistance may decrease cardiac output, despite the positive inotropic effect of the drug. The net effect of norepinephrine on cardiac output thus depends on the balance between the effects on contractility and the increased impedance to left ventricular ejection. Thus, with larger doses, peripheral vasoconstriction may impair vital organ tissue oxygenation and function, even though cardiac output is increased. The increase in capillary hydrostatic pressure resulting from peripheral vasoconstriction also may cause loss of intravascular fluid volume, which may exacerbate shock and make weaning from the drug difficult. Therefore, the minimal effective dose must be used and careful attention must be paid to fluid requirements during administration of the drug. The initial infusion dose of norepinephrine for a 70-kg adult is 1 to 3 μg/minute (4 mg in 250 ml 5% dextrose in water). Doses range from 0.05 to 0.2 μg/kg/minute.

Epinephrine has strong inotropic and chronotropic effects. It increases the automaticity of the heart, and arrhythmias are a potential hazard. In small doses, epinephrine stimulates predominantly the β-adrenergic receptor, causing vasodilatation. In larger doses, α-adrenergic stimulation occurs with consequent vasoconstriction. The drug is useful in augmenting cardiac output and arterial blood pressure in low cardiac output states associated with hypotension. Usual intravenous doses of epinephrine are 0.05 to 0.2 μg/kg/minute (1 mg in 250 ml 5% dextrose in water).

Isoproterenol is a selective β-adrenergic agonist with potent inotropic, chronotropic, and arrhythmogenic effects. Spontaneous ventricular rhythmicity is increased by isoproterenol, and its use is contraindicated with ventricular irritability. It may, however, be useful in heart block as an emergency measure. It significantly increases myocardial oxygen consumption. This effect, together with the potential reduction in arterial blood pressure resulting from β-adrenergic–induced systemic (and pulmonary) vasodilatation and the reduced diastolic time resulting from its chronotropic activity, can aggravate preexisting subendocardial ischemia.[18] Hence, the drug must be used cautiously in patients with myocardial ischemia or infarction. Despite these relative contraindications, isoproterenol is of value in low cardiac output associated with a decreased heart rate, increased systemic or pulmonary vascular resistance, or severe acidosis. The drug is given as an intravenous infusion (1 mg in 250 ml 5% dextrose in water) at an initial rate of 0.05 to 0.1 μg/kg/minute.

CARDIAC GLYCOSIDES.—In the absence of specific contraindications, glycosides[16] also are prescribed to patients with postoperative myocardial dysfunction. These agents improve myocardial contractility and may have a beneficial effect with supraventricular tachyarrhythmias in reducing atrioventricular conduction. Digoxin is usually the glycoside used because of its relatively short biologic half-life. The digitalizing dose is estimated at 0.9 mg/sq m of body surface area. Initially, one half of the estimated dose is administered intravenously, followed by one eighth to one fourth of the total calculated dose, given every one to two hours under careful ECG monitoring, until the desired effect is obtained or until adverse effects occur. A maintenance dose of approximately one eighth of the digitalizing dose is given daily, beginning the day after digitalization has been achieved. This dosage schedule will have to be modified and reduced if cardiac glycosides have been recently given to the patient or if the patient has renal impairment. Hypokalemia exacerbates digitalis toxicity and must be avoided.

CALCIUM.—Calcium ions have a potent but transient inotropic effect. Calcium is given as a bolus in emergency situations, particularly if the serum potassium level is elevated. The level of plasma ionic calcium is higher after the administration of calcium chloride than after the administration of either the gluconate or the gluceptate salt.[104] The usual dose of calcium chloride in an adult is 5 ml of 10% solution. The aim is to achieve a serum ionized calcium level in excess of 2 mEq/L.

Correction of Metabolic Acidosis to Promote Optimal Cardiac Contractility

Metabolic acidosis may develop secondary to low cardiac output and, if severe, will itself further depress cardiac contractility, impair sympathomimetic drug inotropic action, increase pulmonary vascular resistance, and decrease the oxygen-carrying capacity of the blood.[28, 38] To calculate the required dose of sodium bicarbonate (milliequivalents) for correction of metabolic acidosis, one multiplies the base deficit (milliequivalents/liter) by body weight (kilograms) and divides by 3. Usually, one half of this amount should be administered initially and the base deficit reestimated. Metabolic alkalosis may be detrimental and should be avoided.

Ensuring an Optimal Heart Rate to Compensate for a Low Stroke Volume

The heart rate must be kept at an adequate rate in the low cardiac output state. The heart rate can be increased using drugs or a pacemaker. Atropine increases heart rate and can be given as an intravenous bolus in doses of 0.2 to 1.0 mg. Its period of action is from 30 to 60 minutes. Isoproterenol is also a useful chronotropic drug. It is indicated either when peripheral vasoconstriction is pronounced or when its inotropic effect may be of value in a patient with bradyarrhythmia. Pacemaker stimulation to overcome a slow heart rate is especially indicated if ventricular arrhythmias, which contraindicate the use of isoproterenol, are occurring. Ventricular pacemaking will be required if there is atrioventricular dissociation. Newer pacemaker techniques, such as atrioventricular sequential pacing, may be particularly beneficial.[45]

Mechanical Assistance to the Circulation

Devices and techniques have been developed to assist the failing circulation by reducing work load and oxygen requirement of a failing heart while it recovers from cardiac surgery. They include the intra-aortic balloon pump and long-term cardiopulmonary bypass using membrane oxygenators. Intra-aortic balloon pumping is of significant benefit.[20, 27] Long-term supportive bypass may be of value after pediatric cardiac surgery when the balloon pump cannot be used.

Intra-aortic balloon diastolic augmentation[20, 80] and counterpulsation is a process whereby pressure is increased in the proximal systemic arterial tree during diastole and is reduced during systole. This action is achieved by inflating a balloon in the aorta during diastole and deflating the balloon during systole using a vacuum triggered by the R wave of the ECG just before ventricular ejection to avoid obstruction of the aorta during systole. The intra-aortic balloon is inserted into the descending aorta through the femoral artery.

Intra-aortic balloon pumping is an effective means of increasing coronary blood flow and decreasing left ventricular work, thereby improving the balance between myocardial oxygen supply and demand.[52] By increasing coronary collateral blood flow, it possibly improves the viability of ischemic zones.[76] The device is useful and can be life-saving in weaning a patient with severe myocardial dysfunction from cardiopulmonary bypass. The balloon can be left in situ for several days, with few complications. As myocardial function improves, the frequency of diastolic augmentation and counterpulsation can be reduced so that the ratio of assisted to natural beats is decreased from 1:1, through 1:2 and 1:4, to 1:8.

Reducing Body Oxygen Consumption

Postoperative acute cardiac death is frequent if the cardiac index is persistently below 2 L/minute/sq m and mixed venous oxygen tension is less than 30 mm Hg.[81] If, despite all interventions aimed at increasing cardiac output, flow is still insufficient for tissue needs, oxygen consumption must be reduced to permit vital organ survival. Reduction of tissue oxygen consumption increases mixed venous oxygen tension. Therefore, right-to-left shunting, both intrapulmonary and extrapulmonary, will have less effect on Pao_2.

Measures to reduce oxygen consumption include mechanical ventilation of the lungs, prevention of hyperpyrexia, control of anxiety, and muscle paralysis.

MECHANICAL VENTILATION OF THE LUNGS.—Normally, 1% to 3% of the body's oxygen consumption is used in respiratory work. This oxygen requirement may increase during the immediate postoperative period to 30% of the total body oxygen consumption.[100, 105] The oxygen requirement for respiratory work is particularly large when the lungs are noncompliant as a result of left ventricular failure.

In these circumstances, mechanical ventilation may be very important in reducing the oxygen requirements of the body. Mechanical ventilation, combined with the use of positive end-expiratory pressure, may also be required to improve pulmonary gas exchange in the presence of pulmonary edema.

PREVENTION OF HYPERPYREXIA.—In low cardiac output, body core temperature may increase because the poor perfusion of skin with vasoconstriction prevents normal heat loss. Fever also occurs with infection. Raised temperature increases body oxygen consumption. Hyperpyrexia should be treated with tepid sponging and cooling blankets.

CONTROL OF ANXIETY.—Agitation and restlessness increase oxygen consumption and should, if possible, be controlled by the use of a minor tranquilizer such as diazepam or haloperidol.

MUSCLE PARALYSIS.—Paralysis of skeletal muscles is occasionally used if the patient is receiving controlled mechanical ventilation. Concomitant sedation of the patient is mandatory if muscle relaxants are used. Muscle relaxation may be particularly useful when the patient is fighting the respirator or is shivering.

Removal of Excess Water and Sodium

The kidneys normally retain sodium and water after surgery. Low cardiac output may impair renal function and increase fluid retention, producing pulmonary and systemic edema. Fluids are normally restricted in the postcardiac surgical patient. If urinary output is reduced, fluid restriction must be vigorous. All fluid is given in the form of 5% dextrose in water, and fluids that contain saline usually should be avoided. If urinary output is low, diuretics such as furosemide and ethacrynic acid are given. Furosemide has an additional extrarenal effect of increasing peripheral venous capacitance.[30] Because these diuretics may be associated with loss of potassium, potassium should be replaced. With anuria, peritoneal dialysis may be used to remove excess water. Hemodialysis also is useful in renal failure, but in the low cardiac output state, low perfusion pressures may prevent conventional hemodialysis from being sucessfully used. In this situation, hemofiltration can be performed.

SYSTEMIC HYPERTENSION

Increased peripheral vascular resistance is particularly frequent after coronary artery bypass surgery.[83] In the absence of hypovolemia and myocardial dysfunction, it results in systemic hypertension. An elevated blood pressure is found in between 30% and 50% of patients immediately after coronary artery bypass surgery. Elevated blood pressure is less frequent after valve replacement surgery, but may also occur after resection of coarctation of the aorta and repair of dissecting aneurysms of the aorta.

This increased peripheral vascular resistance and systemic hypertension represent an increased afterload for the left ventricle. As a result, myocardial work and oxygen requirement are increased, which can significantly impair cardiac function and may precipitate cardiac failure. In addition, systemic hypertension immediately after operation can produce damage to and leakage from suture sites. The increased peripheral vascular resistance also will impair effective rewarming of the patient immediately after cardiopulmonary bypass, at which time the patient is often hypothermic.[77]

Increased peripheral vascular resistance after coronary artery bypass surgery has many possible causes and may be multifactorial.[83, 98] It is seen more frequently in patients who are hypertensive before surgery and in patients who have more than 50% occlusion of the left main coronary artery. Neural reflexes emanating from receptors in the coronary arteries, especially the left main coronary artery, may be involved in the genesis of this increased peripheral vascular resistance. Increased activity of the renin-angiotensin system and increased levels of circulating catecholamines are associated with the condition.[98] Other factors that may be involved include preoperative tapering of antihypertensive therapy (including propranolol), pain from the wound, a full bladder, anxiety, and hypothermia or possibly hypoxemia.

An elevated peripheral vascular resistance in the period immediately after cardiac surgery responds well to treatment with the ganglion-blocking agent trimethaphan[60] or to the nonspecific vasodilator sodium nitroprusside. The latter drug is preferable because it does not cause the tachyphylaxis often associated with trimethaphan. In addition to vasodilator therapy, pain and anxiety experienced by the patient should be treated.

ARRHYTHMIAS

Arrhythmias are frequent during the immediate postoperative period. Their successful management is based on a sound knowledge of the antiarrhythmic drug armamentarium.[32] Both tachyarrhythmias and bradyarrhythmias may be deleterious to myocardial function and can precede or cause life-threatening arrhythmia. Thus, ventricular extrasystoles or bigeminy may precede ventricular tachycardia and fibrillation. Factors that predispose to arrhythmias include the following: electrolyte imbalance, especially low serum potassium level; metabolic acidosis; myocardial ischemia or failure; digitalis excess; surgical trauma; and preexisting heart disease. Supraventricular arrhythmia also can result from atrial cannulas irritating the atrial walls. Ventricular arrhythmias are often associated with an ectopic focus of irritable myocardium. Heart block after cardiac surgery can result from surgical damage to the conduction system. Such damage is especially likely with closure of septal defects but has been minimized recently by electrophysiologic mapping of the conduction system during surgery.[68]

Arrhythmias affect cardiac function chiefly by altering the heart rate. Bradycardia will often be associated with a low cardiac output. Tachyarrhythmias also will cause the cardiac output to decrease by reducing diastolic ventricular filling time and, hence, reducing the stroke volume. By reducing diastolic filling time, coronary blood flow also may be impaired, and the resulting myocardial ischemia may further impair cardiac output. The function of some prosthetic valves may also be hampered by a rapid heart rate.

Preventive measures are routinely used to reduce the incidence of arrhythmias in the period immediately after cardiac surgery. Such measures include discontinuing or reducing the dose of digoxin before surgery, ensuring that the serum potassium level is within normal limits (both during and after surgery), and avoiding hypoxemia, hypercarbia, and anxiety during the postoperative period. Placing epicardial pacemaker wires at surgery helps ensure easy and rapid availability of means for cardiac pacing, should this be required. Continuous and careful monitoring of the ECG is essential to detect, diagnose, and treat arrhythmias.

Digitalis overdosage can produce almost any type of arrhythmia postoperatively in the cardiac surgical patient. Therefore, its administration should be carefully monitored, and if digitalis is required, the digoxin blood levels should be measured at least six hours after the last dose of the drug. Levels higher than 2.0 ng/ml are frequently associated with toxicity. Such high levels also may reduce the success rate from defibrillation by direct-current electroshock, should this be required.

Treatment of Supraventricular Tachyarrhythmias

Sinus tachycardia occurs with anxiety or pain and can occur during the administration of sympathomimetic agents, especially isoproterenol. Sinus tachycardia is often associated with low cardiac output. If no satisfactory cause is found and the tachycardia compromises cardiac performance, it can be treated with digoxin. Junctional tachycardia, a frequent arrhythmia after operation, may likewise respond to digoxin. Paradoxically, such tachycardia also may be caused by digitalis toxicity. In the latter situation, lidocaine is the drug of choice, but propranolol also can be used. Atrial flutter and fibrillation that occur for the first time during the postoperative cardiac surgical period are best treated by synchronized direct-current countershock. If this is not effective or if these arrhythmias were present before surgery, they are best treated by digitalis. Electrical pacing of the atria may convert atrial flutter to fibrillation, which is easier to control with digitalis. Electrical ventricular pacing may also be useful for the treatment of abnormally slow ventricular response to atrial fibrillation. Paroxysmal supraventricular tachycardia may be due to overdigitalization. The use of digitalis should be stopped, and potassium supplement should be given as required. Phenytoin sodium (Dilantin) is useful in treating digitalis-induced arrhythmias, including those of supraventricular origin.

Ventricular Tachyarrhythmias

Ventricular ectopic beats of recent onset, if frequent or multifocal (or both), should be treated with a bolus of lidocaine, followed by an infusion of the drug to sustain the blood level within therapeutic range. If lidocaine fails, bretylium tosylate, phenytoin, quinidine, or procainamide can be used. A treatable cause of ventricular irritability should be sought. Causes include low cardiac output, myocardial ischemia, and the use of digitalis, especially if associated with hypokalemia. Ventricular tachycardia requires urgent treatment with the intravenous administration of lidocaine, followed by synchronized direct-current countershock. β-Adrenergic blocking agents such as propranolol are useful in ventricular tachycardias that are resistant to treatment, especially those resulting from high circulating levels of catecholamines or increased sympathetic tone.

For ventricular fibrillation, the patient should receive immediate direct-current electroshock, effective cardiopulmonary resuscitation, and management as prescribed by the American Heart Association.[92]

Bradycardia

Sinus or nodal bradycardia impairing cardiac performance is first treated with atropine. If this drug is ineffective, electrical pacing is then used. Electrical pacing is also required to treat the bradycardia of heart block. Use of electrical pacing with incomplete heart block allows drugs such as digitalis to be administered that, without concomitant pacing, may convert latent heart block into complete heart block.

SPECIAL CONSIDERATIONS IN CARE OF INFANTS AND SMALL CHILDREN

Many cardiac surgical patients are infants or small children.[36, 54, 67, 73] Children currently number about 25% of our own practice. It is estimated that each year 25,000 to 30,000 American children are born with congenital cardiac defects.[34] Definitive or palliative surgery can now be performed for most conditions, but the risks remain high.[94] Because of differences in pediatric and adult physiology, the infant is more limited in its ability to compensate for or correct deviations from normal function. This factor, together with the necessary complexity of the surgery and the possible residual effects of the primary defect, results in a high incidence of myocardial dysfunction and respiratory failure during the immediate postoperative period.

The treatment of these seriously ill infants requires meticulous attention to detail by nurses and physicians trained in intensive care of infants. Particular importance is attached to identifying signs of abnormal function before deterioration has progressed to the point when therapy may be less likely to be successful. There are some special considerations involved in supporting infants through the initial postoperative period. True separation of the complications of organ dysfunction cannot be made because they are interreactive. Thus, hypoxemia and respiratory acidosis resulting from respiratory failure will compromise cardiac and renal function, and the latter organ dysfunction cannot be managed successfully until adequate oxygenation and ventilation are reestablished.

Cardiovascular Care[35, 86]

The normal cardiac index in an infant is similar to that in an adult, yet on a weight basis, a newborn has a cardiac output twice that of an adult. Normal values of left and right atrial pressures in small children are lower than those found in adults and do not reach adult values until approximately ten years of age. The normal systemic arterial pressure is lower in infants than in older children or adults. Pulmonary vascular resistance is normally elevated for six to eight weeks after birth, but thereafter decreases to values seen in older children and adults.

A major determinant of the infant's cardiac

output is its rapid heart rate. The infant heart possesses limited ability to increase stroke volume because it has a lower contractile tissue mass and is less compliant than the adult heart. Hence, the infant heart has relatively flat ventricular function curves. Manipulation of preload in the infant, therefore, must be performed with care because high preload pressures can develop rapidly and cause pulmonary and systemic congestion. Although improvement in cardiac output usually will be seen when inotropic drugs are used, output may be limited and is often largely dependent on associated chronotropic actions of these drugs. In infants after cardiac surgery, it is essential to maintain the heart at a rate that can sustain an adequate cardiac output.

Clinical monitoring of the cardiovascular system includes evaluation of the level of consciousness, urinary output, body weight, color, temperature and capillary refill of the skin, heart rate, and blood pressure. Particularly valuable clinical signs of vasoconstriction and inadequate tissue perfusion in infants and small children include the following: cold extremities; poor capillary refilling, with return of color to the skin taking longer than 3 seconds after applied pressure is relaxed; and a reduced urinary output. A reduced urinary output below an acceptable minimum of 1 ml/kg/hour, with an elevated urine osmolality in excess of 300 mOsm/L, is suggestive of hypovolemia being the cause of the vasoconstriction.

Invasive monitoring as practiced in adults is now feasible and should be used in the care of infants and small children who undergo cardiac surgery. It includes determinations of the arterial pressure, right atrial or central venous pressure, pulmonary artery pressure, pulmonary capillary wedge or left atrial pressure, and cardiac output by dye-dilution or thermodilution techniques. Miniaturization of flow-directed, balloon-tipped catheters for pediatric use has made these instruments extremely useful in monitoring pharmacologic support of the circulation and cardiac output.[72] A 5 F catheter may be used in children less than 10 years old and a 7 F catheter may be used for children 10 years old or older.

For most infants, the right atrial pressure is maintained below 10 cm H_2O, although the patient's preoperative cardiac anatomy may necessitate a different value. Thus, children with pulmonary atresia and small right ventricles may require an elevated right atrial pressure to augment right ventricular filling and sustain cardiac output.[37] By contrast, after repair of total anomalous pulmonary venous drainage, the left ventricle is initially small and the right atrial pressure should be kept as low as feasible to sustain cardiac output until the size of the left ventricle has increased.

The ECG should be monitored continuously during the immediate postoperative period. A change in heart rate may be the first indication of serious postsurgical complication, including hemorrhage, cardiac failure, or inadequate gas exchange (or combinations of these). In infants, a heart rate greater than 80 beats per minute should be maintained to sustain the cardiac output. If heart rate is slower, atropine (0.01–0.03 mg/kg/minute) or isoproterenol infusion (0.01 μg/kg/minute) should be given. Complete heart block requires electrical pacing with pacemaker wires inserted at surgery. Arrhythmias in infants and small children often compromise myocardial function, and hence, their early detection and treatment are essential and may be lifesaving.

The major causes of low cardiac output after cardiac surgery in infants and small children are myocardial injury, hypovolemia, and serious arrhythmia. Cardiac failure is also frequently seen with primary respiratory failure. In small children, sodium nitroprusside (0.1–3 μg/kg/minute) is used as an afterload-reducing agent. Isoproterenol (0.02–0.1 μg/kg/minute) and epinephrine (0.1–0.2 μg/kg/minute) with or without dopamine (2–5 μg/kg/minute) are among the most efficacious inotropic agents for the maintenance of cardiac output. A combination of dopamine and isoproterenol may be useful in augmenting cardiac output and increasing renal blood flow. Digitalis is less effective in the newborn than in the adult, but it may be of benefit to the older infant or child. In children, digoxin levels correlate poorly with therapeutic end point or toxicity. Care must be exercised in digitalis use after operation in children, who may have rapidly changing serum potassium, calcium, and magnesium levels. Hypocalcemia is relatively common in infants after cardiac surgery and must be corrected to improve cardiovascular function.

The intra-aortic balloon pump cannot easily be used for infants or children until small balloons are available, and prolonged extracorporeal membrane oxygenation and cardiopulmonary bypass in these small patients may be of particular value when all other measures have failed.

Respiratory Care

Normal infants have a reduced functional residual capacity relative to lung closing volume.[69] In heart disease, functional residual capacity may be further reduced, resulting in increased airway closure. This action may explain why an increase in functional residual capacity by use of positive end-expiratory pressure in the postoperative cardiac surgical infant can significantly improve arterial oxygen saturation.[43] High positive end-expiratory pressure, however, can collapse pulmonary capillaries and increase pulmonary vascular resistance. Use of positive end-expiratory pressure after the Fontan procedure, in which the pulmonary artery pressure is low and at best equal to the systemic venous pressure, is relatively contraindicated.

An increased pulmonary blood flow and pulmonary capillary pressure resulting from a left-to-right shunt can greatly increase an infant's airway resistance.[74] With pulmonary hypoperfusion syndromes, the occurrence of ventilation-perfusion mismatching results in an increase in the physiologic dead space, which, in turn, increases the alveolar-arterial blood oxygen tension difference. In children with unequal blood flow to the lungs secondary to shunt procedures, ventilation tends to be increased to the more compliant, less well-perfused lung, resulting in an increase in physiologic dead space and shunting.

A detailed account of the respiratory care of infants and children is presented in chapter 24.

Temperature Control

The temperature of an infant readily decreases because of the infant's large surface area, small subcutaneous fat depot, and immature thermal regulatory mechanisms. This problem is compounded by the need to nurse the infant in a seminaked state to allow monitoring access and close nursing supervision. A potentially deleterious increase in oxygen consumption, in an attempt to maintain body temperature, is minimized if the infant is kept in the neutral thermal range (skin temperature, 32 to 34 C).[31]

Infants should be nursed in a radiant heat unit. Such units are preferred because they permit much better access to the infant than does a heated incubator. Immediately after the operation has been completed, the infant is often hypothermic. The infant should be rewarmed as soon as possible at this time, and an electrical heating blanket may be of additional value for this purpose.

Hematologic Status

Oxygen delivery to tissues is relatively impaired by the physiologic anemia found during the first few postnatal months.[78] Increasing the total hemoglobin level and correcting any iron deficiency at this time may significantly improve the oxygen delivery to the tissues in infants with large left-to-right shunts. This statement also applies to infants with cyanotic heart disease in whom the physiologic anemia is blunted, although it still may occur. Occasionally infants and, more frequently, older children with cyanotic heart disease have polycythemia, which increases blood viscosity and may reduce blood flow. In this situation, improved oxygen transport to the tissues may be achieved by isovolemic reduction in the hematocrit level.

At birth, the P_{50} of the oxyhemoglobin dissociation curve is reduced because the fetal hemoglobin has low levels of 2,3-diphosphoglycerate.[79] The subsequent synthesis of adult hemoglobin moves the oxyhemoglobin dissociation curve to the right and increases the P_{50}. Cyanotic infants normally have a high P_{50} due to increased 2,3-diphosphoglycerate levels. Oxygen extraction by the tissues from arterial blood can be impaired by the rapid correction of chronic acidosis when the Bohr effect may counter the decreased synthesis of 2,3-diphosphoglycerate. Likewise, a large blood transfusion of old RBCs, low in 2,3-diphosphoglycerate, is potentially hazardous for children, especially those with cyanotic heart disease. Therefore, fresh whole blood should be used in replacing the blood lost in the chest tube drainage and the blood removed for laboratory analysis.

Fluid Balance

Fluid balance[1] is best managed by recognition of the requirement to balance fluid intake and fluid output (Table 25–2). Because of the immaturity of the infant kidney and its inability to conserve sodium,[85] this balance is especially crit-

TABLE 25-2.—BALANCE BETWEEN FLUID
INTAKE AND OUTPUT IN INFANT AFTER
CARDIAC SURGERY

FLUID INTAKE	FLUID OUTPUT
Intravenous fluids	Urine
Blood/plasma	Chest drains
Flushing fluids	Gastric drainage
Airway nebulizer	Insensible loss
Oral feeding	Blood sampling

ical in small infants. The use of potent diuretics to treat pulmonary edema and the use of free nasogastric tube drainage result in many infants being hypovolemic during the postoperative period. This process is often associated with hypokalemic, hypochloremic metabolic alkalosis. Acetazolamide (Diamox), ammonium chloride, or arginine hydrochloride may be needed to correct this hypochloremia.

Fluid Intake

Intravenous Fluids

As in adult patients, intake of water and sodium must be restricted after open-heart surgery. However, younger patients require proportionally more water than adults. The average fluid requirement of infants during the first three days after operation is shown in Table 25-3.

The degree of hydration is assessed clinically and by measuring hematocrit, plasma electrolytes, and serum and urinary osmolality. The normal serum osmolality is 285 mOsm/L. Urinary osmolality is generally slightly below plasma osmolality. The maximal urinary concentration that an infant can achieve is between 600 and 700 mOsm/L. Such an osmolality in an infant implies potentially lethal dehydration. In an older child, a urinary osmolality of 600 mOsm/L does not indicate such serious abnormality, because the kidney can concentrate the urine to 1,200 to 1,400 mOsm/L.

Sudden change in serum osmolality in infants can produce intracranial hemorrhage. To avoid this occurrence, hypertonic fluids, such as 8.4% sodium bicarbonate, are best given slowly, so that the serum osmolality does not change more than 25 mOsm/kg during a four-hour period.

Intravenous fluids required to infuse medications can easily lead to fluid overload in the infant. To avoid this, the concentration of the solution should be increased.

Blood or Plasma (or Both) Transfusion

These are given to replace blood lost from chest drains and blood removed for laboratory analysis. The hemoglobin and hematocrit levels will determine whether blood or plasma should be given. Packed cells are used when blood volume is adequate but hemoglobin level is low. Care must be taken to avoid the complications arising from administration of large amounts of banked stored blood. They include metabolic acidosis, hypocalcemia, hyperkalemia, hypothermia, the risks of jaundice, and decreased levels of 2,3-diphosphoglycerate.

Nebulizers

An ultrasonic nebulizer used in conjunction with mechanical ventilation may produce a net gain of 200 to 400 ml of body water in 24 hours. In the small infant, this process may result in water intoxication. Heated nebulizers are generally preferable.

Flushing of Monitoring Lines

Flushing volumes must be included in the fluid balance calculation. They should match the volume of blood removed for tests minus the volume of blood reinfused.

Oral Feeding

After oral feeding is commenced, the fluid volume given orally should be balanced by a comparable reduction in intravenous fluid administration.

Fluid Output

Urine

A urinary output of 1 ml/kg/hour is desirable in infants less than 1 year old. Urinary output

TABLE 25-3.—FLUID INTAKE REQUIREMENT*
IN INFANT AFTER CARDIAC SURGERY

DAYS AFTER SURGERY	FLUID REQUIREMENT, ML/SQ M/HR	COMPARABLE DAILY FLUID REQUIREMENT, ML/SQ M/DAY
1	30	720
2	40	960
3	50	1,200

*Five percent dextrose in water.

42. Graham T.P. Jr., et al.: Control of myocardial oxygen consumption: Relative influence of contractile state and tension development. *J. Clin. Invest.* 47:375, 1968.
43. Gregory G.A., et al.: Continuous positive airway pressure and pulmonary and circulatory function after cardiac surgery in infants less than three months of age. *Anesthesiology* 43:426, 1975.
44. Hancock E.W.: Cardiac tamponade. *Med. Clin. North Am.* 63(no. 1):223, 1979.
45. Hartzler G.O., et al.: Hemodynamic benefits of atrioventricular sequential pacing after cardiac surgery. *Am. J. Cardiol.* 40:232, 1977.
46. Hearse D.J., Stewart D.A., Braimbridge M.V.: Hypothermic arrest and potassium arrest: Metabolic and myocardial protection during elective cardiac arrest. *Circ. Res.* 36:481, 1975.
47. Hillis L.D., Braunwald E.: Myocardial ischemia: I. *N. Engl. J. Med.* 296:971, 1977.
48. Hillis L.D., Braunwald E.: Myocardial ischemia: II. *N. Engl. J. Med.* 296:1034, 1977.
49. Hillis L.D., Braunwald E.: Myocardial ischemia: III. *N. Engl. J. Med.* 296:1093, 1977.
50. Hoffman J.I.E., Buckberg G.D.: The myocardial supply:demand ratio—a critical review. *Am. J. Cardiol.* 41:327, 1978.
51. Horowitz M.S., et al.: Sensitivity and specificity of echocardiographic diagnosis of pericardial effusion. *Circulation* 50:239, 1974.
52. Housman L.B., et al.: Counterpulsation for intraoperative cardiogenic shock: Successful use of intra-aortic balloon. *J.A.M.A.* 224:1131, 1973.
53. Jenkins B.S., Branthwaite M.A., Bradley R.D.: Cardiac function after open heart surgery: Relation between the performance of the two sides of the heart. *Cardiovasc. Res.* 7:297, 1973.
54. Kaplan S.: Long-term results after surgical treatment of congenital heart disease. *Mod. Concepts Cardiovasc. Dis.* 46:1, 1977.
55. Kelman G.R., et al.: The influence of cardiac output on arterial oxygenation: A theoretical study. *Br. J. Anaesth.* 39:450, 1967.
56. Kinsley R.H., et al.: Pulmonary arterial hypertension after repair of tetralogy of Fallot. *J. Thorac. Cardiovasc. Surg.* 67:110, 1974.
57. Kirklin J.W., Rastelli G.C.: Low cardiac output after open intracardiac operations. *Prog. Cardiovasc. Dis.* 10:117, 1967.
58. Kirklin J.W., Theye R.A.: Cardiac performance after open intracardiac surgery. *Circulation* 28:1061, 1963.
59. Kloster F.E., Bristow J.D., Griswold H.E.: Medical problems in mitral and multiple valve replacement. *Prog. Cardiovasc. Dis.* 7:504, 1965.
60. Kouchoukos N.T., Karp R.B.: Management of the postoperative cardiovascular surgical patient. *Am. Heart J.* 92:513, 1976.
61. Kouchoukos N.T., Kirklin J.W., Oberman A.: An appraisal of coronary bypass grafting. *Circulation* 50:11, 1974.
62. Kouchoukos N.T., Sheppard L.C., Kirklin J.W.: Automated patient care following cardiac surgery. *Cardiovasc. Clin.* 3(no.3):110, 1971.
63. Kouchoukos N.T., et al.: Effect of left atrial pressure by blood infusion on stroke volume early after cardiac operations. *Surg. Forum* 22:126, 1971.
64. Lappas D.G., Powell W.M.J. Jr., Daggett W.M.: Cardiac dysfunction in the perioperative period: Pathophysiology, diagnosis, and treatment. *Anesthesiology* 47:117, 1977.
65. Linden R.J.: The heart-ventricular function. *Anaesthesia* 23:566, 1968.
66. Logue R.B., et al.: Medical management in cardiac surgery, in Hurst J.W., et al. (eds.): *The Heart, Arteries, and Veins*, ed. 4, New York, McGraw-Hill Book Co., 1978, p. 1777.
67. Mair D.D., Ritter D.G.: The physiology of cyanotic congenital heart disease. *Int. Rev. Physiol.* 9:275, 1976.
68. Maloney J.D., et al.: Identification of the conduction system in corrected transposition and common ventricle at operation. *Mayo Clin. Proc.* 50:387, 1975.
69. Mansell A., Bryan C., Levison H.: Airway closure in children. *J. Appl. Physiol.* 33:711, 1972.
70. McIntosh H.D., Garcia J.A.: The first decade of aortocoronary bypass grafting, 1967-1977: A review. *Circulation* 57:405, 1978.
71. Miller R.R., et al.: Clinical use of sodium nitroprusside in chronic ischemic heart disease: Effects on peripheral vascular resistance and venous tone and on ventricular volume, pump and mechanical performance. *Circulation* 51:328, 1975.
72. Moodie D.S., et al.: Measurement of postoperative cardiac output by thermodilution in pediatric and adult patients. *J. Thorac. Cardiovasc. Surg.* 78:796, 1979.
73. Morriss J.H., McNamara D.G.: Residuae, sequelae, and complications of surgery for congenital heart disease. *Prog. Cardiovasc. Dis.* 18:1, 1975.
74. Motoyama E.K., et al.: Application of deflation flow-volume (DFV) curve, a new non-invasive test for the assessment of respiratory failure in infants with congenital heart disease. Abstracted in the Scientific Papers of

the American Society of Anesthesiologists Annual Meeting, 1978, p. 373.
75. Myers R.W., et al.: Effects of nitroglycerin and nitroglycerin-methoxamine during acute myocardial ischemia in dogs with pre-existing multivessel coronary occlusive disease. *Circulation* 51:632, 1975.
76. Nachlas M.M., Siedband M.P.: The influence of diastolic augmentation on infarct size following coronary artery ligation. *J. Thorac. Cardiovasc. Surg.* 53:698, 1967.
77. Noback C.R., Tinker J.H.: Heat dosage vs. distribution during rewarming on C-P bypass, abstracted. *Anesthesiology* 51(suppl.): 134, 1979.
78. Oski F.A.: Designation of anemia on a functional basis. *J. Pediatr.* 83:353, 1973.
79. Oski F.A., Delivoria-Papadopoulos M.: The red cell, 2,3-diphosphoglycerate, and tissue oxygen release. *J. Pediatr.* 77:941, 1970.
80. Parker F.B. Jr., et al.: Intraaortic balloon counterpulsation and cardiac surgery. *Ann. Thorac. Surg.* 17:144, 1974.
81. Parr G.V.S., Blackstone E.H., Kirklin J.W.: Cardiac performance and mortality early after intracardiac surgery in infants and young children. *Circulation* 51:867, 1975.
82. Reid D.J., Digerness S.B., Kirklin J.W.: Changes in whole body venous tone and distribution of blood after open intracardiac surgery. *Am. J. Cardiol.* 22:621, 1968.
83. Roberts A.J., et al.: Systemic hypertension associated with coronary artery bypass surgery: Predisposing factors, hemodynamic characteristics, humoral profile, and treatment. *J. Thorac. Cardiovasc. Surg.* 74:846, 1977.
84. Rosenblum R., Frieden J.: Intravenous dopamine in the treatment of myocardial dysfunction after open-heart surgery. *Am. Heart J.* 83:743, 1972.
85. Rubin M.I., Bruck E., Rapoport M.: Maturation of renal function in childhood: Clearance studies. *J. Clin. Invest.* 28:1144, 1949.
86. Rudolf A.M.: *Congenital Diseases of the Heart: Clinical-Pathologic Considerations in Diagnosis and Management.* Chicago, Year Book Medical Publishers, 1974, p. 29.
87. Sakamoto T., Yamada T.: Hemodynamic effects of dobutamine in patients following open heart surgery. *Circulation* 55:525, 1977.
88. Sarnoff S.J., et al.: Hemodynamic determinants of oxygen consumption of the heart with special reference to the tension-time index. *Am. J. Physiol.* 192:148, 1958.
89. Sharp J.T., et al.: Hemodynamics during induced cardiac tamponade in man. *Am. J. Med.* 29:640, 1960.
90. Sheppard L.C., Kirklin J.W., Kouchoukos N.T.: Computer-controlled interventions for the acutely ill patient, in Stacy R.W., Waxman B.D. (eds.): *Computers in Biomedical Research.* New York, Academic Press, 1974, vol. 4, p. 135.
91. Sheppard L.C., et al.: Automated treatment of critically ill patients following operation. *Ann. Surg.* 168:596, 1968.
92. Standards for Cardiopulmonary Resuscitation (CPR) and Emergency Cardiac Care (ECC): I. Introduction. *J.A.M.A.* 227:837, 1974.
93. Stanley T.H., Isern-Amaral J.: Periodic analysis of mixed venous oxygen tension to monitor the adequacy of perfusion during and after cardiopulmonary bypass. *Can. Anaesth. Soc. J.* 21:454, 1974.
94. Stark J., et al.: Cardiac surgery in the first year of life: Experience with 1,049 operations. *Surgery* 69:483, 1971.
95. Starling E.H.: *The Linacre Lecture on the Law of the Heart, Given at Cambridge, 1915.* London, Longmans, Green and Co., 1918.
96. Steen P.A., Tinker J.H., Tarhan S.: Myocardial reinfarction after anesthesia and surgery. *J.A.M.A.* 239:2566, 1978.
97. Tarhan S., et al.: Myocardial infarction after general anesthesia. *J.A.M.A.* 220:1451, 1972.
98. Taylor K.M., et al.: Hypertension and the renin-angiotensin system following open-heart surgery. *J. Thorac. Cardiovasc. Surg.* 74:840, 1977.
99. Theye R.A.: Cardiac performance during anesthesia and operation. *Surg. Clin. North Am.* 45 no. 4:841, 1965.
100. Thung N., et al.: The cost of respiratory effort in postoperative cardiac patients. *Circulation* 28:552, 1963.
101. Tinker J.H., Michenfelder J.D.: Sodium nitroprusside: Pharmacology, toxicology and therapeutics. *Anesthesiology* 45:340, 1976.
102. Tinker J.H., et al.: Dobutamine for inotropic support during emergence from cardiopulmonary bypass. *Anesthesiology* 44:281, 1976.
103. Vlietstra R.E., et al.: Survival predictors in coronary artery disease: Medical and surgical comparisons. *Mayo Clin. Proc.* 52:85, 1977.
104. White R.D., et al.: Plasma ionic calcium levels following injection of chloride, gluconate, and glucepate salts of calcium. *J. Thorac. Cardiovasc. Surg.* 71:609, 1976.
105. Wilson R.S., et al.: The oxygen cost of breathing following anesthesia and cardiac surgery. *Anesthesiology* 39:387, 1973.
106. Wisch N., et al.: Hematologic complications of open heart surgery. *Am. J. Cardiol.* 31:282, 1973.

Index

A

Acid-base abnormalities: postoperative, 484
Acidosis: metabolic, correction to promote cardiac contractility, 487
Action potential configurations, 342
Adenosine triphosphate, 307
Adrenergic (*see* Beta-adrenergic blocking drugs)
Afterload, 187–189, 358
   aortic regurgitation and, 207
   mitral stenosis and, 196
   optimal
      in postoperative low cardiac output, 484–485
      vasodilators for, 484–485
   reduction
      in low heart output, 369–371
      nitrates and, 371
      nitroprusside in, 370
      prazosin in, 371
      trimethaphan in, 371
Age: at death in congenital heart disease, 73
Agenesis: of pulmonary artery, 27
Air bubbles
   cupula filling with, 322
   evacuation of, 322
   oxygenators causing, 250
Air embolism, 321–323
Airway
   management in mechanical ventilation, prolonged, 459–460
      in infant, 465–467
   obstruction
      causes of, 447
      lung dysfunction and, postoperative, 446–447
Aldosterone-renin-angiotensin system, 327–328
Allen test, 56
Allergic blood reactions, 397
Anaphylactic anti-IgA reaction, 397–398
Anastomosis
   ascending aorta-right pulmonary artery, 96–98, 99
   descending aorta to left pulmonary artery, 98–99, 100
   Potts, 98–99, 100
   subclavian-pulmonary artery, 96, 97, 98
   superior vena cava-right pulmonary artery, 101–103, 104
   Waterston, 96–98, 99
Anesthesia, 41–53
   in aneurysm
      aortic, abdominal, 265–273
      aortic, ascending, 277
      dissecting, 280–283
      thoracic, 275–287
   for angiocardiography, 429–430
   in aortic regurgitation, 222
   for arteriography, 430–431
   in arteriovenous fistula due to rupture of aneurysm, 271
   in carotid artery surgery, 289–301
      depth of, 298–299
      recommendations, 299–300
   for catheterization, cardiac, 422–429
   for children (*see* Children, anesthesia for)
   in coarctation of aorta, adult, 260–261
   contractility and, 211–212
   in coronary artery bypass, 231–241
   for diagnostic procedures, 421–433
   drug therapy effects in, 230–231
   heart rate and, 213–214
   in heart surgery, closed, 257–263
   impedance to ejection, 212–213
   induction, 48–50
      in aneurysm, aortic, abdominal, 267
      in aneurysm, aortic, abdominal, symptomatic and ruptured, 269
      in aneurysm of aortic arch, 278
      for aorta, traumatic ruptured thoracic, 286
      in children (*see* Children, anesthesia induction in)
      in coronary artery bypass, 235–236
      in high-risk cardiac patient, 50
      in valve disease, 216–217
   local, and carotid artery surgery, 292
   maintenance
      in aneurysm, aortic, abdominal, 267
      for aorta, traumatic ruptured thoracic, 286
      in coronary artery bypass, 236
      in valve disease, 216–217
   manipulations during, principles of, 210–215
   in mitral commissurotomy, closed, 258–259
   in mitral regurgitation, 218–220
   for pacemaker patient, 418–420
   in pericarditis, 259–260
   preinduction in valve disease, 216
   preload and, 210–211
   renal function and, 325–339
   in reoperation, 262–263
   rhythm and, 214–215
   in stenosis
      aortic, 220–222
      mitral, 217–218
   in valve disease, 210–223
Anesthetic(s), 41–53
   for bypass, in children, 104–105

Anesthetic(s) *(cont.)*
  cardiovascular effects of, 41–48
  inhalation, 41–44
    in carotid artery surgery, 297–298
  intravenous, 44–47
    in carotid artery surgery, 298
Anesthetist: role of, and steady state, 421–422
Aneurysm
  aortic, abdominal, 265–273
    anesthesia in, 265–273
    anesthesia induction in, 267
    anesthesia maintenance in, 267
    cardiac arrest in, 270
    disease associated with, 266
    monitoring in, 267
    postoperative care in, 272
    premedication in, 267
    preoperative assessment, 265–266
    preoperative preparation, 266–267
    ruptured, 268–269
    ruptured, mortality in, 268
    symptomatic, 268–269
    transfusion in, 270
  aortic arch
    anesthesia in, induction, 278
    cardiopulmonary bypass in, 278–279
    prosthetic replacement in, 277–280
    resection of, 277–280
  aortic, ascending, anesthesia in, 277
  dissecting, 280–285
    anesthesia in, 280–283
    classification of, surgical, 275–276
    hemorrhage in, postoperative, 285
    hypertension control in, 280
    preoperative assessment in, 280
    type I, 275
    type I, anesthesia in, 280–281
    type I, surgery of, 281
    type II, 275–276
    type II, anesthesia in, 281

  type II, resection and graft in, 282
  type III, 276
  type III, anesthesia in, 281–282
  type III, resection and graft in, 283
  pulmonary artery, 29
  thoracic
    anesthesia for, 275–287
    clinical features, 276
    pathogenesis, 275
    prognosis, 276
Angina
  aortic stenosis and, 204
  pectoris, ECG of, 228
  Prinzmetal's, 228–229
    angiography in, coronary, 229
    ECG of, 228
Angiocardiography: anesthesia for, 429–430
Angiography, 25–33
  of carotid artery, 291
  coronary, 27–33
    in angina, Prinzmetal's, 229
    in coronary artery bypass, 234–235
  of lung, 25–27
Angiotensin-aldosterone-renin system, 327–328
Anomalies
  arteriovenous *(see* Arteriovenous malformation)
  Ebstein's, 164–168
    repair, 167
  hemostatic, after bypass, in children, 114–117
  of pulmonary venous connections *(see* Pulmonary, venous connections, total anomalous)
  of pulmonary venous return, total, 26
Antiarrhythmic drugs: and preoperative assessment, 10
Antibody
  -antigen reaction, 391
  detection, 389–391
  formation, 389
Anticholinergic drugs: preoperative, 38–39
Anticoagulants
  composition of, 400

  taken before surgery, 11
Anticoagulation: and bypass, in children, 106–108
Antidiuretic hormone, 328–329
Antigen(s)
  -antibody reaction, 391
  blood, groups, 387–389
Antihypertensive drugs
  classification of, 4
  contraindications, 6–7
  side effects, 6–7
Anti-IgA reaction: anaphylactic, 397–398
Anxiety: control of, 488
Aorta
  ascending, to right pulmonary artery anastomosis, 96–98, 99
  bleeding, surgical control of, 269–270
  clamping, hemodynamic effects of, 284
  coarctation *(see* Coarctation of aorta)
  cross-clamping, 267–268
  descending, to left pulmonary artery anastomosis, 98–99, 100
  spinal cord damage after procedures on, 284–285
  thoracic, traumatic ruptured, 285–286
    anesthesia in, induction and maintenance, 286
Aortic
  aneurysm *(see* Aneurysm, aortic)
  arch aneurysms *(see* Aneurysm, aortic arch)
  incompetence, anatomical features of, 205
  intra-aortic *(see* Intra-aortic)
  pressure curves, 478
  regurgitation, 204–209
    acute, 209
    afterload and, 207
    anesthesia in, 222
    with aortic stenosis, 209
    atrial pacing in, 207
    contractility and, 207, 222
    ejection fraction in, 208
    heart rate and, 206–207, 222
    hemodynamics in, 204–206
    investigations in, 204
    nitroprusside in, 208
    oxygen balance and, myocardial, 208–209

pressure-volume loop in, 207
regurgitant flow, 206
rhythm and, 222
signs, 204
symptoms, 204
systemic vascular resistance and, 222
stenosis (see Stenosis, aortic)
valve
  disease, 200–209
  disease, preoperative assessment and, 2–3
  replacement, 221–222
Aortocaval fistula, 271
Aortography: translumbar, 430
Aortovenous fistula, 271
Arrhythmia, 341–356
  antiarrhythmic drugs, and preoperative assessment, 10
  complicating catheterization, cardiac, 428–429
  coronary artery bypass and, 241
  diagnosis, 346–354
  postoperative, 489–490
    preventing and treating, 477
  supraventricular, 347–350
  tachyarrhythmia (see Tachyarrhythmia)
  treatment, 346–354
  ventricular, 352–354
Arteries
  blood gases, 71
  brachial, perfusion of, 278
  cannula, and pressure gradients, 109
  cannulation, direct, 55
  carotid (see Carotid artery)
  catheterization of, problems of, 429
  coronary (see Coronary, artery)
  femoral (see Femoral, artery)
  great (see Transposition of great arteries)
  pressure, 55–59
  pulmonary (see Pulmonary, artery)
  radial, cannulation, wrist position for, 57
  subclavian, dissection of, 97
  supply of spinal cord, 286
  ventriculoarterial connections, 152

Arteriography
  anesthesia for, 430–431
  coronary, 430
  of neurovascular system, 430–431
  of renal system, 430–431
  of visceral system, 430–431
Arteriovenous fistula due to rupture of aneurysm, 270–272
  anesthesia in, 271
  monitoring in, 271–272
Arteriovenous malformation
  diffuse-type, 28
  pulmonary vein fistulous communication and, 27
Artifacts: in intra-aortic balloon counterpulsation, 382
Aspirin: and preoperative assessment, 12
Atelectasis, 22, 23
Atresia
  pulmonary, 139–140
  tricuspid, 147–150
    classification, 146, 147
Atrial
  contribution to preload, 185
  enlargement, and postoperative lung dysfunction, 447
  fibers, specialized, 343
  fibrillation, 348–349
    in mitral stenosis, 195–196
  flutter, 348
  function
    aortic stenosis and, 202–203
    in mitral stenosis, 195
  pacing
    in aortic regurgitation, 207
    in mitral stenosis, 195
  pressure (see Pressure, atrial)
  septal defect (see Septal defect, atrial)
  septectomy, 99–101, 102
  septostomy, balloon, 96
  tachycardia, paroxysmal, in Wolff-Parkinson-White syndrome, 350
Atrioventricular
  block, 350–352
    complete, 351–352
    first-degree, 350
    second-degree, 350–351
    third-degree, 351–352
  canal, complete, 123–125
    type A, 123–124

    type A, repair, 127
    type B, 124, 125
    type C, 125, 126
  canal defects, 120–125
    approach from right atrium, 132
  canal, partial, 120–123
    catheterization findings in, 122
    repair, 123
  connections, 152
  node reentrant tachycardia, 347
Atrium (see Atrial)
Atropine: circulatory effects of, 424
AVCO intra-aortic balloon pump console, 381–382

B

Banding: pulmonary artery, 103–104
Ball valve, 182–183
Balloon
  atrial septostomy, 96
  intra-aortic (see Intra-aortic balloon)
Basilic veins, 60
Beats: ventricular ectopic, 352–354
Bentley oxygenator (see Oxygenators, Bentley)
Beta-adrenergic blocking drugs
  coronary artery bypass and, 233–234
  taken before surgery, 10
Biochemical markers: and postoperative lung dysfunction, 454
Bird respirator, 463
Blalock-Hanlon operation, 99–101, 102
Blalock-Taussig shunt, 96, 97, 98
Bleeding
  of aneurysm, dissecting, postoperative, 285
  aorta, surgical control of, 269–270
  cumulative, in open-heart surgery, 262
  disorders, preoperative assessment and, 11–13
  sources at reoperation, 262
Block (see Atrioventricular, block)

Index

Blocking drugs
  beta-adrenergic (*see* Beta-adrenergic blocking drugs)
  neuromuscular (*see* Neuromuscular blocking drugs)
Blood, 387–412
  ABO groups, 389
  allergic reactions, 397
  antigen groups, 387–389
  cell, red (*see* Red blood cell)
  components, 398–404
    colloid, 403–404
  disorders, and open heart surgery, 14
  filter, 250
  flow
    cerebral (*see* Cerebral, blood flow)
    coronary artery, factors limiting, 227–228
    coronary, after morphine, 37
    renal, extrinsic regulation, 326
  frozen, 400–401
  gas (*see* Gas, blood)
  glucose, postoperative, in children, 494
  leukocyte-poor, 400
  pressure (*see* Pressure)
  sampling, postoperative, in children, 494
  substitutes, 403–404
  supply
    to lung, 446
    to spinal cord, 91, 285
  transfusion (*see* Transfusion)
  volume expanders, 404
  whole
    comparison with red blood cells, 398–400
    storage lesion of citrate-phosphate-dextrose, 399
BOS-5 oxygenator: primes used for, 253
BOS-10 oxygenator (*see* Oxygenator, BOS-10)
Brachial artery: perfusion of, 278
Bradycardia
  junctional, 347
  postoperative, 490
  sinus, 347
Brain: protection from ischemic and embolic phenomena, 315–324

Brock procedure, 101, 103
Bubble oxygenators, 245–246
  foreign-body particles in, 321
Bypass
  anesthesia for, in children, 104–117
  cardiopulmonary (*see* Cardiopulmonary bypass)
  in children
    emergence from, 112–113
    postbypass period, 117
  coronary artery (*see* Coronary, artery bypass)
  femoral artery to femoral vein, 240–241

C

Calcium
  coronary arteries and, 230
  in hypotension, intraoperative, 361
  postoperative, in children, 494
  for postoperative myocardial contractility, 487
  preoperative assessment and, 9
Canal (*see* Atrioventricular, canal)
Cannula: arterial, and pressure gradients, 109
Cannulation
  arterial, direct, 55
  in cardiopulmonary bypass, 254
  of femoral vein and artery, 241
  radial artery, wrist position for, 57
  technique, 56–59
Carbon dioxide elimination: and lung dysfunction, postoperative, 443–444
Cardiac (*see* Heart)
Cardiogenic shock (*see* Shock, cardiogenic)
Cardioplegia
  chemically induced, 308–311
  in children, 311
  in coronary artery surgery, 311–312
Cardioplegic solution(s)
  for bypass, in children, 111–112
  composition of, 310
  infusion of, 311
  temperature and, 313

Cardiopulmonary bypass
  in aneurysm of aortic arch, 278–279
  cannulation in, 254
  in children, 108
  embolism during (*see* Embolism, during cardiopulmonary bypass)
  emergence from, 364–368
    dobutamine in, 366
    dopamine in, 366
    epinephrine in, 365
    isoproterenol in, 365
  equipment for, 253–354
  hemodilution in, 250–252
  heparinization in, 254–255
  neurologic sequelae of, 317
  neutralization in, 254–255
  oxygenators in, 245–250
  primes for, 252–253
  techniques, 252–255
Cardiotomy
  cardiogenic shock after, 379–380
  reservoir, Q-220F, 255
Cardiovascular care, 475–497
  of children, 490–492
Cardioversion, 431
Care
  cardiovascular, 475–497
    of children, 490–492
  postextubation, 457–458
  postoperative cardiac (*see* Postoperative cardiac care unit)
  postoperative, of children, 490–494
  respiratory (*see* Respiratory, care)
Carotid artery
  angiography of, 291
  perfusion of, 278
  surgery, 289–301
    anesthesia in, 289–301
    anesthesia in, depth of, 298–299
    anesthesia in, management aims, 291
    anesthesia in, recommendations, 299–300
    inhalation anesthetic agents in, 297–298
    intravenous anesthetic agents in, 298
    monitoring in, 292–296
    monitoring in, cardiovascular, 292

monitoring in, cerebral, 292–296
muscle relaxants in, 298
preoperative assessment in, 291–292
risk factors, 290–291
surgical requirements, 290
Carotid endarterectomy (see Endarterectomy, carotid)
Catecholamines
  comparisons among, and emergence from cardiopulmonary bypass, 366–368
  for inotropic support, 364–365
Catheter
  polyethylene, placement to monitor atrial pressures, 60
  Swan-Ganz, 67, 68
  Teflon, insertion via femoral artery to thoracic aorta, 58
Catheterization
  arterial, problems of, 429
  cardiac, 422–429
    anesthesia for, 422–429
    in children, 425–427
    in children, anesthesia for, 426–427
    complications of, 428–429
    contrast medium in, 424–425
    in newborn, 423
    ventilation, controlled vs. spontaneous, 425
  in coronary artery bypass, 234–235
  findings
    in atrial septal defect, secundum, 118
    in atrioventricular canal, partial, 122
    in septal defect, atrial, 154
    in septal defect, ventricular, large, 129
    in septal defect, ventricular, small, 128
    in tetralogy of Fallot, 143
    in transposition of great arteries, complete, 154
  J-wire external jugular, technique, 63
Cell(s)
  blood, red (see Red blood cell)
  ischemia, 315

myocardial, degradation, agents protecting against, 305–306
Central nervous system: and mechanical ventilation withdrawal, 455–456
Central venous pressure, 59–66
Cephalic veins, 60
Cerebral
  blood flow
    carotid artery surgery and, 293
    "critical" human, 296–297
  function monitor, 296
  ischemia, 315–316
    global complete, in animal models, 316
    regional, in primate models, 316
  monitoring in carotid artery surgery, 292–296
  protection during bypass, in children, 113–114
Chest
  drains, in children, 494
  radiography (see Radiography, chest)
Children
  anesthesia for, 73–180
    for bypass, 104–117
    in catheterization, cardiac, 426–427
    in closed-heart surgery, 85–104
    in coarctation of aorta, 88–93
    in congenital heart disease, palliative procedures, 95–104
    dosages, intravenous, 76–77
    drugs for, 76–77
    induction (see below)
    open heart surgery, 104–173
    in patent ductus arteriosus, 85–88
    in stenosis, aortic, congenital, 137–139
    in transposition of great arteries, 162–163
    in vascular ring anomalies, 93–95
  anesthesia induction in, 78–85
    blood-gas partition coefficient, 82
    cardiac output, 82–83

child arrives asleep, 79–81
child arrives awake, 81
child arrives uncooperative, 81–82
factors affecting induction, 82
preparation, 78–82
in shunt, left-to-right, 84–85
in shunt, right-to-left, 83–84
small infants, 82
ventilation, 82
very ill infants, 82
blood sampling in, postoperative, 494
bypass for
  emergence from, 112–113
  postbypass period, 117
cardioplegia in, 311
catheterization in, cardiac, 425–427
  anesthesia for, 426–427
chest drains for, 494
electrolyte balance in, postoperative, 494
endotracheal tubes for, 78, 466
feeding of, oral, postoperative, 493
fluid balance in, postoperative, 492–493
fluid for, intravenous, postoperative, 493
fluid intake, postoperative, 493
fluid output in, postoperative, 493–494
gastric drainage in, postoperative, 494
glucose in, blood, postoperative, 494
heart surgery, outcome after, 465
hematologic status, postoperative, 492
insensible loss in, postoperative, 494
intra-aortic balloon counterpulsation in, 381
mortality
  in heart disease, congenital, 73
  after heart surgery, causes of, 460
nebulizers for, postoperative, 493
postoperative care, 490–494

Children (cont.)
  premedication of, 39, 74–78
  preoperative evaluation, 74–78
  respiratory care, 492
  temperature control, 492
  transfusion for, postoperative, 493
  urine of, postoperative, 493–494
  ventilation for, mechanical, prolonged, in infant, 464–468
Chlorpromazine
  circulatory effects of, 423–424
  procedure for use, 426, 427
  respiratory effects of, 423
Cigarette (see Smoking, cigarette)
Circulation
  arrest, total, in bypass, in children, 113
  care during coronary artery bypass, 238–241
  collateral
    in coarctation of aorta, 90
    of hand, 55–56
  compensation for valvular lesions, 190–191
  coronary, 227–230
  effects of drugs on, 423–425
  mechanical assistance to, in postoperative period, 487
  pathways in transposition of great arteries, complete, 155
  support, 357–375
    digitalis and, 372–373
    mechanical, 368
    terminology, 357
Circus movement, 349
Clamping: of aorta, hemodynamic effects of, 284
Clotting time: initial activated, 107
Coagulation
  disseminated intravascular, 394–396
  after bypass, in children, 114–116
  factors, 405
    action mechanism, 407
  hemostasis and, 404–406
  screening tests, interpretation of, 116

system
  control of, 406–409
  heparin and, 406–409
Coarctation of aorta
  adult, 260–261
    anesthesia in, 260–261
    postoperative phase, 261
  anesthesia for, in children, 88–93
  circulation in, collateral, 90
  patch graft in, 91
Collett and Edwards' classification: of truncus arteriosus, 133
Colloid components: blood, 403–404
Commissurotomy, mitral, closed, 257–259
  anesthesia in, 258–259
Complement, 391–392
Computer-based hemodynamic monitoring, 479–480
Conduction
  abnormal mechanisms, 342–346
  normal mechanisms, 341–342
Contractility, 186–187
  acidosis correction to promote, metabolic, 487
  anesthesia and, 211–212
  aortic regurgitation and, 207, 222
  mitral regurgitation and, 199, 218–219
  stenosis and
    aortic, 204, 221
    mitral, 218
Contrast medium: in cardiac catheterization, 424–425
Cor pulmonale: and emphysema, 30
Coronary
  angiography (see Angiography, coronary)
  arteriography, 430
  artery
    blood flow, factors limiting, 227–228
    bypass (see below)
    calcium and, 230
    disease, premedication in, 39
    disease, preoperative assessment and, 3
    extramural-intramural arteries, 228
    hydrogen ions and, 230

hyperventilation and, 229–230
parasympathomimetic drugs and, 229
stenosis, 31
stenosis, ostial, 32
surgery, cardioplegia in, 311–312
artery bypass
  anesthesia in, 231–241
  anesthesia in, induction, 235–236
  anesthesia in, maintenance, 236
  angiography in, coronary, 234–235
  arrhythmia and, 241
  β-adrenergic blockers and, 233–234
  catheterization in, 234–235
  circulatory care during, 238–241
  diuretics and, 233
  glycosides and, 233
  inotropes and, 239–240
  intra-aortic balloon assist and, 240
  monitoring during, 236–238
  nitroglycerin and, 235, 239
  nitroprusside and, 239
  phentolamine and, 239
  premedication in, 235
  preoperative drug intake and, 233–234
  preoperative evaluation in, 232–235
  smoking and, cigarette, 233
  temperature and, 238
blood flow after morphine, 37
circulation, 227–230
perfusion, direct, 307
vascular resistance after morphine, 37
vasospasm, with ergonovine, 229
Counterpulsation (see Intra-aortic balloon, counterpulsation)
Cross-clamping: intermittent, 306–307
Cryoprecipitate, 403
  preparation, 403
Cupula: filling with air bubbles, 322
Cyst: lung, 24–25

D

Death (*see* Mortality)
Desynchronization: complex, 346
Diabetes: and preoperative assessment, 13–15
Diazepam, 44–45
  circulatory effects of, 424
  preoperative, 36–37
  respiratory effects of, 423
Digitalis
  circulatory support and, 372–373
  preoperative assessment and, 9
Dilator: Tubbs, 258
Disk
  oxygenators, 245
  valve, 183
Diuretics, 329–330
  coronary artery bypass and, 233
  loop, 329
  osmotic, 329–330
  preoperative, 10
Dobutamine: in emergence from cardiopulmonary bypass, 366
Dopamine, 213
  in emergence from cardiopulmonary bypass, 366
Drainage: gastric, postoperative, in children, 494
Drains: chest, in children, 494
Droperidol, 45
  in carotid artery surgery, 298
Drug(s)
  anesthetic (*see* Anesthetics)
  antiarrhythmic, and preoperative assessment, 10
  anticholinergic, preoperative, 38–39
  antihypertensive (*see* Antihypertensive drugs)
  beta-adrenergic (*see* Beta-adrenergic blocking drugs)
  circulatory effects of, 423–425
  narcotic, 45–47
  neuromuscular blocking (*see* Neuromuscular blocking drugs)
  parasympathomimetic, and coronary arteries, 229
  premedicant, 35–39
  preoperative, 10–11, 35–40
  respiratory effects of, 422–423
  sympathomimetic (*see* Sympathomimetic drugs)
  therapy, effect on anesthetic management, 230–231
Dye-dilution curve, 69, 70, 71

E

Ebstein's anomaly, 164–168
  repair, 167
Ectopic beats: ventricular, 352–354
Edema
  interstitial, and mitral stenosis, 29
  pulmonary, 22
    after head injury, 25
    postoperative, 442–443
Ejection
  fraction in aortic regurgitation, 208
  impedance to ejection, 212–213
Electrocardiography
  of angina
    pectoris, 228
    Prinzmetal's, 228
  changes
    hyperkalemia causing, 9
    hypokalemia causing, 8
  monitoring, 59
    during coronary artery bypass, 237–238
Electroencephalography: intraoperative, and carotid artery surgery, 295–296
Electrolyte
  abnormalities, postoperative, 484
  balance, postoperative, in children, 494
  disturbances, preoperative assessment and, 5–10
Electromagnetic interference: with pacemaker, 417–418
Embolism
  air, 321–323
  brain protection from, 315–324
  during cardiopulmonary bypass, 317–323
  bypass devices and embolus formation, 320–321
  organ involvement by emboli, 318
  quantifying emboli, 318–320
  microembolism (*see* Microembolism)
  platelet-aggregate, 318
  pulmonary, 26
Emphysema, 21
  cor pulmonale and, 30
  pneumomediastinum and, 24
Endarterectomy, carotid
  EEG findings with various anesthetic agents in, 299
  morbidity in, 291
  mortality in, 291
Endocardial
  cushion defects, 120–125
  pacemakers, placement of, 431
Endotracheal intubation in prolonged mechanical ventilation, 459–460
  in infant, 465–467
Endotracheal tubes: for children, 78, 466
Enflurane, 43–44
  in carotid artery surgery, 297–298
Epinephrine: in emergence from cardiopulmonary bypass, 365
Equipment
  for cardiopulmonary bypass, 253–254
  for intra-aortic balloon counterpulsation, 381–382
Ergonovine: in coronary vasospasm, 229
Erythrocyte (*see* Red blood cell)
Examination: physical, 2
Exercise: and aortic stenosis, 204
Extremities: upper, superficial veins of, 61
Extubation
  postextubation care, 457–458
  in prolonged mechanical ventilation, 463
  in infant, 467–468

F

Factor(s)
  coagulation, 405
    action mechanism, 407
    inhibitors, after bypass, in children, 116–117
Febrile transfusion reaction, 396–397
Feeding: oral, postoperative, in children, 493
Femoral
  artery
    cannulation of, 241
    to femoral vein bypass, 240–241
  vein, cannulation of, 241
Fentanyl, 46–47
  in carotid artery surgery, 298
Fibrillation
  atrial, 348–349
    in mitral stenosis, 195–196
  ventricular, 354
Filter: blood, 250
Fistula
  aortocaval, 271
  aortovenous, 271
  arteriovenous (see Arteriovenous fistula)
  in pulmonary vein communication, 27
Fluid(s), in children
  balance, postoperative, 492–493
  intake, postoperative, 493
  intravenous, postoperative, 493
  management in bypass, 105
  output, postoperative, 493–494
Flutter: atrial, 348
Foam: evacuation of, 322
Fontan operation, 148
  modification of, 149
Foramen ovale: patent, 119
Force-velocity relationships: in papillary muscle (in cat), 187
Frank-Starling left ventricular function curve, 239, 476
Frozen blood, 400–401

G

Gallamine, 48
Gas(es)
  blood
    analysis, 451–452
    arterial, 71
    partition coefficient, 82
  distribution, intrapulmonary inspired, 449
  expired, analysis, 452–453
Gastric drainage: postoperative, in children, 494
Glenn shunt, 101–103, 104
Glucose: blood, postoperative, in children, 494
Glycosides
  coronary artery bypass and, 233
  for myocardial contractility, postoperative, 486–487
Graft
  in aneurysm, dissecting
    type II, 282
    type III, 283
  bypass (see Bypass)
  patch, in coarctation of aorta, 91

H

Halothane, 42–43
  in carotid artery surgery, 297
  circulatory effects of, 424
Hand: collateral circulation of, 55–56
Head injury: pulmonary edema after, 25
Heart
  afterload (see Afterload)
  arrest
    in aneurysm, aortic, abdominal, 270
    ischemic, myocardial protection during, 238
  arrhythmia (see Arrhythmia)
  catheterization (see Catheterization, cardiac)
  changes with nitrous oxide, 42
  contractility (see Contractility)
  defects (see disease below)
  diagnostic procedures, anesthesia for, 421–433
  disease, congenital
    age at death of children with, 73
    anesthesia for repair, in children, 73–180
    classification of, 73–74
    palliative procedures in, 95–104
    repair of specific defects, complete, 117–173
  disease, valvular, 181–226
    anesthesia in, 210–223
    effects of anesthetic drugs on, 41–48
    effects of neuromuscular blocking agents on, 41–48
  failure
    kidney failure and, 331–332
    vasodilators in, 370
  glycosides (see Glycosides)
  high-risk patient, anesthesia induction in, 50
  laboratory, data in preoperative assessment, 2
  open surgery
    anesthesia for, in children, 104–173
    bleeding in, cumulative, 262
    blood disorders and, 14
    von Willebrand's disease and, 15
  output, 68–70
    anesthesia induction and, in children, 82–83
    decrease in, physiologic changes with, 359–360
    low, lung dysfunction and, postoperative, 441–442
    low, postoperative, 368–373, 480–488
    low, postoperative, causes, 481–484
    low, postoperative, diagnosis, clinical, 480–481
    low, postoperative, incidence, 480
    low, postoperative, pathophysiology, 480–488
    low, postoperative, treatment, 484–488
    low, vasodilators for, 371
    oxygen saturation in, normal, 422
  perforation during catheterization, 429
  performance, determinants of, 183–190, 358–359
  postoperative care, 475–497
    unit (see Postoperative cardiac care unit)
  preload (see Preload)

pressure values, normal, 422
protection during surgery, 306–311
pumping function, optimizing, postoperative, 475–477
rate, 189–190, 359
  anesthesia and, 213–214
  aortic regurgitation and, 206–207, 222
  controlling, in low heart output, 369
  mitral regurgitation and, 199, 218
  after nitroglycerin, 38
  optimal, in postoperative period, 487
  stenosis and, aortic, 220–221
  stenosis and, mitral, 217
rhythm, and anesthesia, 214–215
suction, for bypass, in children, 108
surgery
  closed, anesthesia in, 257–263
  open (see open surgery above)
  renal dysfunction associated with, 335–336
  tamponade causing postoperative low cardiac output, 482–483
teratogens, 74
univentricular, 163–164, 165
vessels (see Vessels)
Hematologic
  disorders, and cardiovascular surgery, 13
  status, postoperative, of children, 492
Hematology: of red blood cell, 387
Hemodilution, 250–252
  historical development, 250–252
Hemodynamic monitoring, 479
  computer-based, 479–480
Hemodynamics
  in aortic regurgitation, 204–206
  in aortic stenosis, 201–202
  in mitral regurgitation, 197–198
  in mitral stenosis, 192–193
Hemoglobin-oxygen saturation curve, 106

Hemolytic transfusion reaction (see Transfusion, reaction, hemolytic)
Hemorrhage (see Bleeding)
Hemostasis
  abnormal, preoperative assessment, 75–77
  coagulation and, 404–406
  mechanical ventilation withdrawal and, 456
Hemostatic
  anomalies after bypass, in children, 114–117
  mechanisms, 395
Heparin
  coagulation system and, 406–409
  -coated vascular shunts, 283
  dose-response curve for, construction of, 409
  excess after bypass, in children, 114
  monitoring, 407–409
Heparinization: in cardiopulmonary bypass, 254–255
History, 1–2
Hormone: antidiuretic, 328–329
Hydrogen ions: and coronary arteries, 230
Hyperfibrinolysis: after bypass, in children, 114–116
Hyperkalemia
  ECG changes due to, 9
  in preoperative assessment, 8–9
Hyperpyrexia: prevention of, 488
Hypertension
  antihypertensive drugs (see Antihypertensive drugs)
  control in dissecting aneurysm, 280
  lung, 447
  in preoperative assessment, 4–5
  pulmonary artery
    shunt and, 25
    ventricular septal defect and, 28
  systemic, postoperative, 488–489
Hypertrophy
  in stenosis, subaortic, 140
  valve lesions and, 190–191
Hyperventilation: and coronary arteries, 229–230

Hypokalemia
  ECG changes due to, 8
  preoperative assessment and, 5–8
Hypoplasia: of pulmonary artery, repair, 145
Hypotension
  declamping during repair of aorta, 268
  intraoperative, 360–364
    agents used to treat, 361–364
    calcium in, 361
    sympathomimetic drugs in, 361–364
Hypothermia, 307–308
  deep, technique, 279
Hypovolemia: causing postoperative low cardiac output, 481–482
Hypoxemia: chronic, 448

I

Immunoglobulin polypeptide molecule, 389
Immunohematology, 387–391
Impedance
  to ejection, 212–213
  increase, 189
Impulse formation
  abnormal mechanisms, 342–346
  normal mechanisms, 341–342
Induction (see Anesthesia, induction)
Infant: prolonged mechanical ventilation for, 464–468
Infarction: myocardial, with normal coronary arteries, 230
Infundibular resection: closed, with pulmonary valvotomy, 101, 103
Inotropes, 213
  coronary artery bypass and, 239–240
  vs. vasodilators, 372
Inotropic
  state, 358–359
  support
    in cardiopulmonary bypass, emergence from, 365–368
    catecholamines for, 364–365
    in low heart output, 369

Inotropic *(cont.)*
  for myocardial contractility improvement, 485–487
Insensible loss: postoperative, in children, 494
Intra-aortic balloon
  assist, and coronary artery bypass, 240
  counterpulsation, 377–386
    artifacts in, 382
    in children, 381
    complications of, 385
    deflation marker adjustment, 384
    double-triggering, 383
    equipment, 381–382
    inflation marker adjustment, 383–384
    management, 382–385
    pacing spike, 383
    R wave in, 382
    technique, 380–382
    weaning from, 384–385
  placement of, 380
  pump, 368, 369
    AVCO console, 381–382
    three-segment nonocclusive, 382
  timing, 383
    landmarks, 383
Intubation, endotracheal, in prolonged mechanical ventilation, 459–460
  in infant, 465–467
Ischemia
  brain protection from, 315–324
  cellular, 315
  cerebral (*see* Cerebral, ischemia)
  myocardial changes with, 303
  myocardial preservation and, 304
Ischemic cardiac arrest: myocardial protection during, 238
Isoproterenol: in emergence from cardiopulmonary bypass, 365

J

Jugular vein
  external, 60–63
    formation and course of, 62
    J-wire catheterization technique, 63
  internal, 63–66
    puncture kit, disposable, 65
    relationships of, 64
  J-wire external jugular catheterization technique, 63

K

Ketamine, 47
  in carotid artery surgery, 298
  circulatory effects of, 424
Kidney
  arteriography of, 430–431
  autoregulation, 326
    macula densa hypothesis, 326
    metabolic mechanism in, 326
    myogenic hypothesis, 326
    prostaglandin hypothesis, 326
  blood flow, extrinsic regulation, 326
  dysfunction associated with heart surgery, 335–336
  failure, acute, 330–335
    causes of, major, 330
    classification of, 336
    heart failure and, 331–332
    prerenal failure, 331
    urinary indices of, 333
  function, 325–339
    anesthesia and, 325–339
  tubular necrosis, 332–335
  vein renin determination, 431

L

Laboratory: heart, data in preoperative assessment, 2
Leukocyte-poor blood, 400
Limb: upper, superficial veins of, 61
Lung
  (*See also* Pulmonary)
  angiography of, 25–27
  blood supply to, 446
  changes in mitral stenosis, 193–194
  collapse, 442
  cysts, 24–25
  dysfunction, postoperative
    acute, 439–445
    acute, functional changes, 443–445
    acute, pathogenesis, 441–443
    acute, pathophysiology, 439–445
    chronic, 445–448
    chronic, pathophysiology, 445–448
    chronic, restrictive defects in, 447
  dysfunction, in preoperative assessment, 3–4
  edema, postoperative, 442–443
  hypertension, 447
  infiltrates, 22
  masses, 22–23
  mechanics, 453–454
    postoperative, 444–445
  perfusion, 454
  pump, 441
  vascular disease, 445–446
  volume, postoperative, 444–445

M

Macula densa hypothesis: of renal autoregulation, 326
Magill connector, 79
Magnesium: and preoperative assessment, 9–10
Maintenance (*see* Anesthesia, maintenance)
Malformation (*see* Anomalies)
Marrow: red blood cell formation in, 388
Mayo-Gibbon pump assembly: for vertical screen oxygenator, 246
Medication (*see* Drugs)
Membrane oxygenators, 247
Meperidine, 46
  circulatory effects of, 423–424
  procedure for use, 426, 427
  respiratory effects of, 423
Metabolic disturbances: in cardiac catheterization, 429
Metocurine, 48
Microembolism
  (in dog), 319
  oxygenators causing, 250
Microembolization: during oxygenation, 320
Mitral
  commissurotomy, closed, 257–259

anesthesia for, 258–259
regurgitation, 196–200
  acute, 198
  anatomical features of, 197
  anesthesia in, 218–220
  contractility and, 199,
    218–219
  etiology, 196
  heart rate and, 199, 218
  hemodynamics in, 197–198
  investigations in, 197
  monitoring in, 218
  nitroprusside in, 219
  oxygen consumption in,
    198
  preload and, 218
  rhythm and, 218
  signs, 197
  surgery of, 220
  symptoms, 197
  vascular resistance and,
    systemic, 199
  vascular resistance and,
    systemic and pulmonary,
    219
  ventricular shape and,
    199–200
  volume infusion in, 199
stenosis (*see* Stenosis, mitral)
valve
  disease, 191–200
  disease, preoperative
    assessment and, 3
  replacement, 218,
    219–220
Models: in cerebral ischemia,
  316
Monitor: cerebral function, 296
Monitoring, 55–72
  in aneurysm, aortic,
    abdominal, 267
  in arteriovenous fistula due to
    rupture of aneurysm,
    271–272
  of atrial pressures, 60
  in carotid artery surgery (*see*
    Carotid artery, surgery,
    monitoring in)
  in catheterization, cardiac, in
    children, 425–426
  during coronary artery
    bypass, 236–238
  ECG, 59
  hemodynamic, 479
    computer-based, 479–480
  heparin, 407–409
  lines, flushing of, 493
  in mitral regurgitation, 218

myocardial, of temperature,
    312
  postoperative, 478–480
  of respiratory care, 451
  in stenosis, mitral, 217
Monoamine oxidase inhibitors:
    preoperative, 10–11
Morbidity: in carotid
    endarterectomy, 291
Morphine
  for anesthesia, 46
  coronary blood flow after, 37
  coronary vascular resistance
    after, 37
  preoperative, 36
Mortality
  in aneurysm, aortic,
    abdominal, ruptured,
    268
  in endarterectomy, carotid,
    291
  in heart disease, congenital,
    in children, 73
  after heart surgery, in
    children, causes of, 460
  hospital, in pericarditis,
    causes of, 260
Muscle
  papillary, force-velocity
    relationships in (in cat),
    187
  paralysis, postoperative, 488
  relaxants, in carotid artery
    surgery, 298
  sternocleidomastoid, 64
Myocardial
  cell degradation, agents
    protecting against,
    305–306
  changes with ischemia, 303
  contractility, improvement,
    inotropic support for,
    485–487
  dysfunction causing
    postoperative low cardiac
    output, 483–484
  infarction, with normal
    coronary arteries, 230
  monitoring, of temperature,
    312
  oxygen consumption, 308
    factors determining, 232
  oxygen supply and demand,
    balance, postoperative,
    477–478
  perfusion, factors
    determining, 232
  preservation, 303–314

  interventions affecting,
      304–306
    ischemia and, 304
    oxygen demands and,
      304–305
    oxygen supply and, 305
    substrate utilization, agents
      increasing, 305
  protection
    during bypass, in children,
      110–111
    during ischemic cardiac
      arrest, 238
Myogenic hypothesis: of renal
    autoregulation, 326

N

Narcotic agents, 45–47
Nebulizers: in postoperative
    period for children, 493
Necrosis: tubular, 332–335
Nervous system
  central, and mechanical
    ventilation withdrawal,
    455–456
  sympathetic, and valve
    lesions, 191
Neurologic
  sequelae of cardiopulmonary
    bypass, 317
  stability, and carotid artery
    surgery, 290
Neuromuscular blocking drugs
  for anesthesia, 47–48
  cardiovascular effects of,
    41–48
Neurovascular system:
    arteriography of,
    430–431
Newborn: cardiac
    catheterization of, 423
Nitrates: in afterload reduction,
    371
Nitroglycerin
  blood pressure after, 38
  coronary artery bypass and,
    235, 239
  heart rate after, 38
  in low cardiac output,
    postoperative, 485
  topical, preoperative, 37–38
  venous tone and, 211
  ventricular end-diastolic
    dimension after, 38
Nitroprusside, 213
  in afterload reduction, 370
  in aortic regurgitation, 208

Nitroprusside *(cont.)*
  coronary artery bypass and, 239
  in low cardiac output, postoperative, 485
  in mitral regurgitation, 219
  venous tone and, 211
Nitrous oxide, 41–42
  cardiovascular changes with, 42
Norepinephrine, 261

O

Open heart surgery *(see* Heart, open surgery)
Orotracheal tube, 79
  fixation of, 79
Osmotic diuretics, 329–330
Outflow resistance, 189
Oxygen
  balance, myocardial, and aortic regurgitation, 208–209
  consumption
    in mitral regurgitation, 198
    myocardial, 308
    myocardial, factors determining, 232
    reducing in postoperative period, 487–488
  demands, and myocardial preservation, 304–305
  -hemoglobin saturation curve, 106
  myocardial, supply and demand, balance, postoperative, 477–478
  respiratory effects of drugs and, 422–423
  saturation, normal, in heart and great vessels, 422
  supply, and myocardial preservation, 305
Oxygenation
  lung dysfunction and, postoperative, 443
  microembolization during, 320
Oxygenators, 245–250
  Bentley
    Spiraflo, 246
    Temptrol, 246, 247
  BOS-5, primes used for, 253
  BOS-10, 248, 249
    primes used for, 252
  Sarns pump assembly for, 254
  bubble, 245–246
    foreign-body particles in, 321
  comparisons among, 247–250
  complications of, 250
  disk, 245
  membrane, 247
  Shiley S-70, primes used for, 253
  types of, 245–247
  vertical screen, 245
    with Mayo-Gibbon pump assembly, 246

P

Pacemakers, 413–420
  anesthesia for pacemaker patient, 419–420
  electromagnetic interference with, 417–418
  endocardial, placement of, 431
  placement of, 414, 431
  reliability of, 414
  types of, 414–417
  unipolar vs. bipolar leads, 413–414
Pacing
  atrial *(see* Atrial, pacing)
  electronic, indications for, 413
Palmar arch: superficial, 56
Pancuronium, 48
Papillary muscle: force-velocity relationships in (in cat), 187
Paralysis: muscle, postoperative, 488
Parasympathomimetic drugs: and coronary arteries, 229
Patch graft: in coarctation of aorta, 91
Patent ductus arteriosus
  anesthesia for, in children, 85–88
  ligation in, 88
Patent foramen ovale, 119
Pentothal, 44
  in carotid artery surgery, 298
Perfusate: for bypass, in children, 109–110
Perfusion
  of brachial artery, 278
  of carotid artery, 278
  coronary, direct, 307
  flow, and bypass, in children, 108–109
  lung, 454
  myocardial, factors determining, 232
  reperfusion, 306–307
  -ventilation ratios, 450
Pericarditis, 259–260
  anesthesia in, 259–260
  hospital deaths in, causes of, 260
pH, 71
  hemoglobin-oxygen saturation curve and, 106
Phentolamine
  coronary artery bypass and, 239
  venous tone and, 211
Physical examination, 2
Plasma: fresh-frozen, 402–403
Platelet(s), 401–402
  abnormalities, and preoperative assessment, 12
  -aggregate emboli, 318
  concentrate preparation, 402
  dysfunction, after bypass, in children, 114
Pleural
  diseases, 23–24
  effusion, 23
Pneumomediastinum: and emphysema, 24
Po_2
  jugular bulb, and carotid artery surgery, 292
  relationship with right-to-left shunt, 87
Postcardiotomy cardiogenic shock, 379–380
Postextubation care, 457–458
Postoperative cardiac care unit, 435–438
  initial assessment in, 437–438
  staffing, 436
  transfer from operating room to, 436–437
Postoperative care: of children, 490–494
Postoperative management
  cardiovascular care, 475–497
  respiratory care, 439–474
Postoperative monitoring, 478–480
Potassium
  postoperative, in children, 494

serum, 71
Potts anastomosis, 98–99, 100
Prazosin: in afterload reduction, 371
Preinduction: in valve disease, 216
Preload, 183–186, 358
   anesthesia and, 210–211
   atrial contribution to, 185
   mitral regurgitation and, 218
   optimizing, in low heart output, 369
   stenosis and
      aortic, 221
      mitral, 217–218
   valve lesions and, 190
Premedicant drugs, 35–39
Premedication, 35–40
   in aneurysm, aortic, abdominal, 267
   in catheterization, cardiac, in children, 425
   of children, 39, 74–78
   in coronary artery bypass, 235
   in coronary artery disease, 39
   in valve disease, 216
Preoperative assessment, 1–18
   in aneurysm
      aortic, abdominal, 265–266
      dissecting, 280
   in carotid artery surgery, 291–292
   of hemostasis, abnormal, 75–77
   in valve disease, 215–216
Preoperative evaluation, 1–3
   of children, 74–78
Preoperative medication (see Premedication)
Prerenal failure, 331
Pressure
   aortic, curves, 478
   arterial, 55–59
   atrial
      left, 66–68
      monitoring, 60
   central venous, 59–66
   gradient relationships in tetralogy of Fallot, 84
   gradients, and arterial cannula, 109
   interventricular, relationships, 130
   intracardiac, normal, 67
   after nitroglycerin, 38
   pulmonary capillary wedge, 66

stump, measurement, and carotid artery surgery, 293–295
ventricular, left
   curves, 478
   end-diastolic, 238, 359
   systolic, 360
   -volume
      curve of ventricle, 186
      loop in aortic regurgitation, 207
      loop in aortic stenosis, 203
      relationships of ventricle, 188
Primes: for cardiopulmonary bypass, 252–253
Prinzmetal's angina (see Angina, Prinzmetal's)
Promethazine
   circulatory effects of, 423–424
   procedure for use, 426, 427
   respiratory effects of, 423
Propagation: slow, 346
Prostaglandin hypothesis: of renal autoregulation, 326
Prosthesis: in aortic arch aneurysm, 277–280
Pulmonary
   (See also Lung)
   artery
      agenesis, 27
      aneurysm, 29
      banding, 103–104
      hypertension (see Hypertension, pulmonary artery)
      hypoplasia, repair, 145
      left, to descending aorta anastomosis, 98–99, 100
      right, to ascending aorta anastomosis, 96–98, 99
      right, to superior vena cava anastomosis, 101–103, 104
      -subclavian anastomosis, 96, 97, 98
   atresia, 139–140
   capillary wedge pressure, 66
   cardiopulmonary (see Cardiopulmonary)
   edema (see Edema, pulmonary)
   embolism, 26
   stenosis, valvular, 140–141
   valve
      ring, repair, 145
      stenosis, 29, 140–141

valvotomy with infundibular resection, 101, 103
venous communication, fistulous, 27
venous connections, total anomalous, 168–173
   cardiac type, repair, 172
   forms of, common, 169
   infracardiac type, repair, 173
   supracardiac type, 170
   supracardiac type, repair, 171
venous return, total anomalous, 26
venous stenosis, 28
vessels, resistance
   elevation in ventricular septal defect, 129–130
   mitral regurgitation and, 219
   mitral stenosis and, 218
Pump
   assembly
      Mayo-Gibbon, 246
      Sarns, for BOS-10 oxygenator, 254
   intra-aortic balloon, 368, 369
      AVCO console, 381–382
   lung, 441
Pumping function: optimizing, postoperative, 475–477
Puncture kit: internal jugular, disposable, 65
Purkinje's fiber
   action potential, 343
   bundles, loop of, sequence of activation, 345

R

Radial artery cannulation: wrist position for, 57
Radiography, 19–33
   chest, normal, 20
   chest, preoperative, 19–25
   negative findings, 19–20
   negative findings, apparently, 21–22
   positive findings, apparently, 21
   in preoperative assessment, 2
Radiology (see Radiography)
Rashkind procedure, 96
Rastelli operation, 161
Rate (see Heart, rate)

Red blood cells
  comparison with whole blood, 398–400
  destruction in reticuloendothelial system, 388
  formation in marrow, 388
  hematology of, 387
Regurgitation
  aortic (*see* Aortic, regurgitation)
  mitral (*see* Mitral, regurgitation)
Renal (*see* Kidney)
Renin
  -angiotensin-aldosterone system, 327–328
  determination, renal vein, 431
"Reopening," 261–263
  anesthesia in, 262–263
Reoperation, 15–16
  anesthesia in, 262–263
  bleeding at, sources of, 262
  in early postoperative period, 261–263
Reperfusion, 306–307
Respirator: Bird, 463
Respiratory
  care, postoperative, 439–474
    in children, 492
    management, 454
    monitoring, 451
  control, 454
    mechanisms, defects in, 447–448
  effects of drugs, 422–423
  support, managing, 455
Reticuloendothelial system: red blood cell destruction in, 388
Rheumatic mitral stenosis: natural history of, 192
Rhythm
  anesthesia and, 214–215
  aortic regurgitation and, 222
  mitral regurgitation and, 218
  in stenosis
    aortic, 220
    mitral, 217
Ring
  anomalies, vascular, anesthesia for, in children, 93–95
  pulmonary valve, repair, 145
Roentgenography (*see* Radiography)

Ruptured thoracic aorta, 285–286
  anesthesia in, induction and maintenance, 286
R wave: in intra-aortic balloon counterpulsation, 382

S

Sarns pump assembly: for BOS-10 oxygenator, 254
Sedation: for cardiac catheterization, in children, 425
Senning repair: modified, 160
Septal defect
  atrial, secundum type, 117–120
    anatomy, pathologic, 119–120
    catheterization findings in, 118, 154
    classification, 119–120
    clinical implications, 118–119
    complications, postoperative, 120
    intraoperative management, 119–120
    patch repair, 121
    pathophysiology, 117–118
  ventricular, 125–133
    anatomical position of, 131
    anatomy, pathologic, 131–132
    classification, 125–130
    clinical implications, 130–131
    complications, postoperative, 132–133
    high, approach from right atrium, 132
    large, catheterization findings in, 129
    large, with pulmonary vascular resistance elevation, 129–130
    moderate, 125–129
    pathophysiology, 125–130
    pulmonary artery hypertension and, 28
    small, 125
    small, catheterization findings in, 128
    supracristal, repair, 132
    surgical management, 131–132

Septectomy: atrial, 99–101, 102
Septostomy: balloon atrial, 96
Shiley S-70 oxygenator: primes used for, 253
Shock, cardiogenic, 377–380
  postcardiotomy, 379–380
  self-perpetuating cycles in, 378
  supportive therapy, sequence of, 378
Shoulder: venous plexus around, 62
Shunt
  Blalock-Taussig, 96, 97, 98
  Glenn, 101–103, 104
  left-to right
    anesthesia induction in, in children, 84–85
    dye-dilution curve showing, 70
    pulmonary hypertension and, 25
  right-to-left
    anesthesia induction in, in children, 83–84
    dye-dilution curve showing, 71
    relationship with P_{O_2}, 87
  vascular
    heparin-coated, 283
    placement of, 283–284
Sinus
  bradycardia, 347
  tachycardia, 347–348
  venosus defect, 119
    repair, 121
Smoking, cigarette
  coronary artery bypass and, 233
  preoperative assessment and, 15
Sodium
  excess, removal in postoperative period, 488
  nitroprusside (*see* Nitroprusside)
  postoperative, in children, 494
  thiopental, 44
    in carotid artery surgery, 298
Spinal cord
  arterial supply of, 286
  blood supply of, 91, 285
  damage after procedures on aorta, 284–285

Staffing: postoperative cardiac
    care unit, 436
Starling curve, 184
  descending limb of, 185–186
  illustration of, 185
  valve lesions and, 190
Steady state: and role of
    anesthetist, 421–422
Stenosis
  aortic, 200–204
    anatomical features of, 202
    anesthesia in, 220–222
    angina and, 204
    with aortic regurgitation,
        209
    atrial function and,
        202–203
    congenital (see below)
    contractility and, 204, 221
    exercise and, 204
    heart rate and, 220–221
    hemodynamics in, 201–202
    investigations in, 201
    preload and, 221
    pressure-volume loop in,
        203
    rhythm and, 220
    signs, 201
    symptoms, 201
    systemic vascular resistance
        and, 221
    tachycardia and, 203–204
  aortic, congenital, 135–139
    anesthetic management in,
        137–139
    subvalvular, 136, 138
    supravalvular, 135–136
    valvular, 136, 137
  coronary artery, 31
    ostial, 32
  mitral, 191–196
    afterload and, 196
    anatomical features of, 192
    anesthesia in, 217–218
    atrial fibrillation in,
        195–196
    atrial function in, 195
    atrial pacing in, 195
    contractility and, 218
    edema and, interstitial, 29
    etiology, 191
    heart rate and, 217
    hemodynamics in, 192–193
    investigations in, 192
    monitoring in, 217
    myocardial factors in, 194
    preload and, 217–218
    pulmonary changes in,
        193–194
    rheumatic, natural history
        of, 192
    rhythm and, 217
    signs, 191
    symptoms, 191
    tachycardia in, 194–195
    vascular resistance and,
        systemic and pulmonary,
        218
    ventilation and, 218
    ventricle in, left, 194
  pulmonary
    valve, 29, 140–141
    veins, 28
  subaortic, hypertrophic
    idiopathic, 140
  tricuspid, 209
Sternocleidomastoid muscle, 64
Stomach drainage:
    postoperative, in
    children, 494
Stroke volume
  vascular resistance and,
    systemic, 189
  ventricular systolic pressure
    and, left, 360
Stump pressure measurement:
    and carotid artery
    surgery, 293–295
Subclavian
  artery, dissection of, 97
  -pulmonary artery
    anastomosis, 96, 97, 98
Succinylcholine, 47
Suction: intracardiac, for
    bypass, in children, 108
Surface cooling
  for bypass, in children,
    105–106
  technique, 279
Swan-Ganz catheter, 67, 68
Sympathetic nervous system:
    and valve lesions, 191
Sympathomimetic drugs
  in hypotension,
    intraoperative, 361–364
  for postoperative myocardial
    contractility
    improvement, 485–486

T

Tachyarrhythmia
  supraventricular, treatment
    of, 489–490
  ventricular, 490
Tachycardia
  aortic stenosis and, 203–204
  atrial, paroxysmal, in Wolff-
    Parkinson-White
    syndrome, 350
  atrioventricular nodal
    reentrant, 347
  in mitral stenosis, 194–195
  sinus, 347–348
  supraventricular, paroxysmal,
    349–350
  ventricular, 354
Tamponade: causing
    postoperative low cardiac
    output, 482–483
Teflon catheter: insertion via
    femoral artery to thoracic
    aorta, 58
Temperature, 70–71
  in bypass, in children,
    108–109
  cardioplegic solutions and,
    313
  control in children, 492
  coronary artery bypass and,
    238
  hemoglobin-oxygen saturation
    curve and, 106
Teratogens: cardiovascular, 74
Tetralogy of Fallot, 141–147
  catheterization findings in,
    143
  postoperative period in,
    145–147
  pressure gradient
    relationships in, 84
  surgical treatment of,
    143–145
Thiopental, 44
  in carotid artery surgery, 298
Thoracic
  aneurysm (see Aneurysm,
    thoracic)
  aorta, traumatic ruptured,
    285–286
    anesthesia in, induction
      and maintenance, 286
Thrombocytopenia: after
    bypass, in children, 114
Tissue valve, 183
Trachea, orotracheal tube, 79
  fixation of, 79
Tracheostomy, 463
Transfusion
  in aneurysm, aortic,
    abdominal, 270

Transfusion *(cont.)*
  autologous, 398
  postoperative, in children, 493
  reaction, febrile, 396–397
  reaction, hemolytic, 391–396
    pathophysiology of, 392
    presentation, clinical, 392–393
    treatment of, 393–394
Transposition of great arteries
  complete
    catheterization findings in, 154
    circulation pathways in, 155
    corrected, congenitally, 153
    correction of, 162
  D-Transposition of great arteries, 150–163
    anesthetic management in, 162–163
    atrial position in, 151
    operative treatment, 156–162
    position of great arteries in, 152–156
    ventricular position in, 151–152
Traumatic ruptured thoracic aorta, 285–286
  anesthesia in, induction and maintenance, 286
Tricuspid
  atresia, 147–150
    classification, 146, 147
  insufficiency, 209–210
  stenosis, 209
  valve disease, 209–210
Trimethaphan: in afterload reduction, 371
Truncus arteriosus, 133–135
  classification, anatomical
    of Collett and Edwards, 133
    of Van Praagh, 134
  pulmonary artery agenesis and, 27
  repair, 135
Tubbs dilator, 258
Tubes
  endotracheal, for children, 78, 466
  orotracheal, 79
    fixation of, 79
d-Tubocurarine, 47–48
Tubular necrosis, 332–335

U

Univentricular heart, 163–164, 165
Urinary output, 71
Urine: postoperative, in children, 493–494

V

Valve
  aortic *(see* Aortic*)*
  ball, 182–183
  disease, 181–226
    anesthesia in, 210–223
  disk, 183
  lesions, circulatory compensation for, 190–191
  mitral *(see* Mitral*)*
  pulmonary *(see* Pulmonary, valve*)*
  replacement, 181–183
  tissue, 183
  tricuspid *(see* Tricuspid*)*
  types of valves, 182
Valvotomy: pulmonary, with infundibular resection, 101, 103
Van Praagh classification
  of single ventricle, 163
  of truncus arteriosus, 134
Vasodilators, 213
  for afterload, optimal, 484–485
  in heart failure, 370
  for low heart output, 371
  vs. inotropes, 372
Vasospasm: coronary, with ergonovine, 229
Vein(s)
  arteriovenous *(see* Arteriovenous*)*
  basilic, 60
  central venous pressure, 59–66
  cephalic, 60
  femoral
    cannulation of, 241
    femoral artery to femoral vein bypass, 240–241
  jugular *(see* Jugular vein*)*
  pulmonary *(see* Pulmonary, venous*)*
  renal, renin determination, 431

tone, after nitroprusside, phentolamine and nitroglycerine, 211
  of upper limb, superficial, 61
Velocity-force relationships: in papillary muscle (in cat), 187
Vena cava: superior, to right pulmonary artery anastomosis, 101–103, 104
Venous plexus: around shoulder, 62
Ventilation
  anesthesia induction and, in children, 82
  in catheterization, cardiac, controlled vs. spontaneous, 425
  mechanical, 488
  mechanical, effects of, 448–451
  mechanical, prolonged, 458–468
    checklist for patient needing, 464
    in infant, 464–468
    weaning, in infant, 467–468
  mechanical, weaning methods, 457
  mechanical, withdrawal, 454–456
    cardiac status and, 456
    central nervous system and, 455–456
    hemostasis and, 456
    metabolic status, 456
    respiratory status and, 456
  -perfusion ratios, 450
  stenosis and, mitral, 218
Ventilatory support, 461–463
  in children, 467
Ventricle
  arrhythmia, 352–354
  atrioventricular *(see* Atrioventricular*)*
  ectopic beats, 352–354
  fibrillation, 354
  function, 184
    curves, 360
  interventricular pressure relationships, 130
  left
    end-diastolic dimension after nitroglycerin, 38
    function, 309

function curve, Frank-
Starling, 239, 476
in mitral stenosis, 194
preload, optimal, in
postoperative low cardiac
output, 484
pressure (see Pressure,
ventricular, left)
pressure-volume curve of,
186
pressure-volume
relationships, 188
septal defect (see Septal
defect, ventricular)
shape, and mitral
regurgitation, 199–200
single, Van Praagh
classification of, 163
tachyarrhythmia, 490
tachycardia, 354
univentricular heart,
163–164, 165
Ventriculoarterial connections,
152
Ventriculotomy: transverse
right, 132
Vessels
changes with nitrous oxide,
42
coronary, resistance after
morphine, 37
diagnostic procedures,
anesthesia for, 421–433
effects of anesthetic drugs on,
41–48
effects of neuromuscular
blocking agents on,
41–48

great
oxygen saturation in,
normal, 422
perforation during
catheterization, 429
pressure values for,
normal, 422
lung, disease, 445–446
neurovascular system,
arteriography of,
430–431
postoperative care of,
475–497
pulmonary (see Pulmonary,
vessels)
ring anomalies, anesthesia
for, in children, 93–95
shunt (see Shunt, vascular)
surgery of, and hematologic
disorders, 13
systemic, resistance
aortic regurgitation and,
222
mitral regurgitation and,
199, 219
stenosis and, aortic, 221
stenosis and, mitral, 218
stroke volume and, 189
teratogens, 74
Vitamin K deficiency: and
preoperative assessment,
12–13
Volume
blood, expanders, 404
infusion, in mitral
regurgitation, 199
lung, postoperative,
444–445

-pressure (see Pressure,
-volume)
stroke (see Stroke volume)
von Willebrand's disease: and
open heart surgery, 15
V wave: after nitroprusside in
mitral regurgitation, 219

W

Water
excess, removal in
postoperative period,
488
free-water clearance,
336–337
Waterston anastomosis, 96–98,
99
Weaning
from intra-aortic balloon
counterpulsation,
384–385
from mechanical ventilation,
457
prolonged, 463
prolonged, in infant,
467–468
Wenckebach's phenomenon,
350, 351
Wolff-Parkinson-White
syndrome: atrial
tachycardia in, 350
Wrist position: for radial artery
cannulation, 57